Head and Neck Oncology

Diagnosis, Treatment, and Rehabilitation

Head and Neck Oncology

Diagnosis, Treatment, and Rehabilitation

Edited by

Ernest M. Myers, M.D., F.A.C.S.

Associate Professor of Surgery, Howard University College of Medicine; Chief, Division of Otolaryngology, Head and Neck Surgery, Howard University Hospital, Washington, D.C.

Foreword by

LaSalle D. Leffall, Jr., M.D., F.A.C.S.
Professor of Surgery, Howard University College of Medicine; Chairman, Department of Surgery, Howard University Hospital, Washington, D.C.

Little, Brown and Company
Boston/Toronto/London

First Edition

Library of Congress Catalog Card No. 91-62090

ISBN 0–316–59317–6

Printed in the United States of America
MV NY

. . . He is a man who will worry, and . . . feel most keenly the burden of his responsibility . . . gentleness, compassion, tenderness do not exclude firmness . . . the bravest are the tenderest, the loving are the daring.

Rudolph Matas, *The Soul of the Surgeon*

To Joseph H. Ogura, M.D. (1915–1983)
Surgeon, Innovator, Mentor

Lindburg Professor and Chairman, Department of Otolaryngology, Head and Neck Surgery, Washington University of St. Louis School of Medicine. Past President of the Triological Society, American Laryngological Society, American Society of Head and Neck Surgery, and the Society of Academic Chairmen of Otolaryngology

Recipient of The Award of Merit from the American Academy of Ophthalmology and Otolaryngology; Bronze Medal from the University of Helsinki; Sir William Wild Gold Medal (England); Joshi Memorial Lecture Gold Medal (India); Bronze Medal from the University of Zagreb (Yugoslavia); and the Semon Medal from the University of London

One of only three in otolaryngology honored with the Casselberry Award, James Newcombe Award, and the DeRoalds Gold Medal

Author of more than three hundred articles and twenty chapters

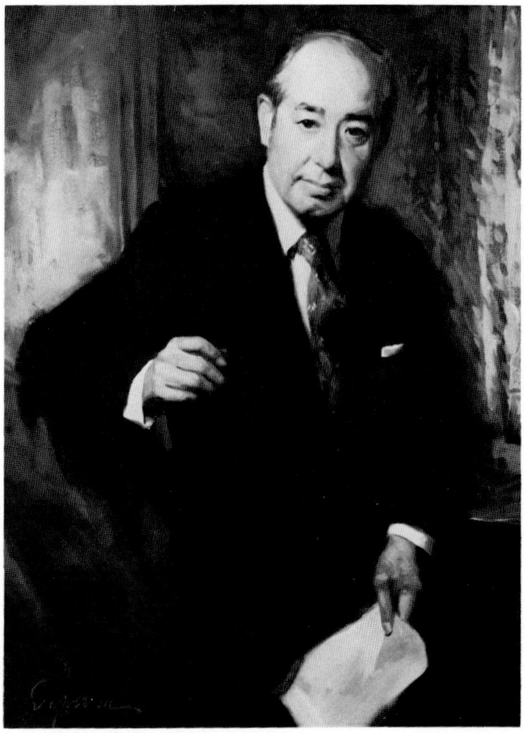

Contents

Foreword

This book addresses major problems encountered in the management of patients with cancer of the head and neck. The editor, having written several of the chapters himself, has assembled experts who have carefully detailed the essentials in their areas. Of particular importance is a glossary (Chapter 7) that is invaluable for the layman. Appropriately, the book is divided into three major topics: Diagnosis, Treatment, and Rehabilitation. The chapters in each of these groups are inclusive and informative.

Recognizing that disease prevention and health maintenance are to be encouraged, the authors emphasize the deleterious effects of tobacco and alcohol especially in head and neck cancer. Adequate attention is given to prevention and wellness as well as to diagnosis and treatment.

In endeavors of this sort, it is customary to emphasize diagnosis and therapy while placing less emphasis on the vital area of rehabilitation. The authors have made no such egregious omission, for the section on rehabilitation includes discussions on pain control, nutrition, and psychological and emotional support in addition to speech, hearing, dental, and cosmetic rehabilitation. Proper care of patients with cancer of the head and neck demands a multidisciplinary approach, which has been well-outlined in this book. The goal is minimal functional and structural impairment to the patient while appropriate therapy is instituted. One of the strengths of this book is the in-depth discussion about total rehabilitation of the patient.

Aware of the fact that it is not just that you live but how you live, the authors constantly emphasize the quality of life. This comprehensive book will be of great value for all health care personnel involved in the care of patients with cancer of the head and neck.

LaSalle D. Leffall, Jr., M.D.

Preface

. . . May I be moderate in everything except in the knowledge of this science; as far as it is concerned may I be insatiable; grant me strength and opportunity to always extend its domain. . .

The Prayer of Maimonides

Head and Neck Oncology is a concise but comprehensive multidisciplinary reference for the beginning and intermediate student of head and neck oncology. It is the culmination of over 10 years' experience with one system of patient care applied to hundreds of patients at Howard University Hospital and Cancer Center in Washington, D.C. The book is divided into three sections: Diagnosis, Treatment, and Rehabilitation. Each chapter begins with a historical perspective, followed by a concise text, augmented liberally with tables, figures, photographs, and "decision pathways." As a compact reference, it supplements the voluminous desk references. This is not a collection of dictums, but only one approach to a fascinating area of oncology.

E.M.M.

Acknowledgments

Any project begins as a dream or idea swirling about, as would a formless nebula. This dream came to fruition only with the inspiration and succor of others:

The contributors—the coauthors who wrote and endured endless revisions.

My technical support staff—Amanda Johnson (project organizer), Patricia R. Thompson, M.A., CCC-A (coauthor and reviewer), and Robert White, Jr., M.D. (coauthor and reviewer), who supported the effort tirelessly.

My immediate family—Sheila, Erica, Stacey, and Candice, who sacrificed quality time and gave me encouragement from start to finish.

My extended family—Ernest H. Myers, Ruth M. Myers, Ulysses Goodman, Horton Johnson (deceased), Ethel Johnson (deceased), Elizabeth Johnson (deceased), Wayne Myers (deceased), who always supported steadfastly any worthwhile dream.

My past professors and staff—Malcolm Stroud, M.D., Donald Sessions, M.D., Gershon Spector, M.D., Stanley Thawley, M.D., James Toomey, M.D., Barbara Bohne, Ph.D., Don Davis, and Pete Rolla, Division of Otolaryngology, Head and Neck Surgery, Washington University of St. Louis School of Medicine, who always were patient and understanding.

My past teachers—Ralph Ellison, Ph.D., and Elizabeth Trumball, M.A., Department of English, Schenley High School, Pittsburgh, who imparted a passion for clear written expression.

My technical advisors—Charles Epps, M.D., Dean, Howard University School of Medicine; Ruth Ogura, Jacqueline D. Sealey, Art Director, Printing and Reproduction, Howard University College of Medicine; Stan Griffin, Howard University Hospital Audiovisual Services; Jane Gilmore, David Klemm, Linda Culp, Peter Y. Stone, and Terese Winslow, Department of Educational Media, Georgetown University Medical Center; Laurie Anello, Susan F. Pioli and Jon Sarner, medical editors at Little, Brown and Company, who unselfishly gave their expertise.

The supportive professional staff of Howard University Hospital—William E. Matory, M.D., Chief of Ambulatory Care; C.D. Hinton, M.D., Hunter Malloy, M.D., Joseph Chapman, M.D., and Joseph Taylor, M.D., Division of Otolaryngology, Department of Head and Neck Surgery; LaSalle D. Leffall, Jr., M.D., Robert DeWitty, M.D., Warren Strudwick, M.D., Rupert Louison, M.D., and Edward L. Mosley, M.D., Department of Surgery; E. Josephine Green, M.D. (*deceased*), and Thomas E. Gaiter, M.D., Department of Family Practice and Community Medicine; Charles Curry, M.D., Juanita Archer, M.D. and Richard Adams, M.D., Department of Medicine; Wilson Jackson, D.D.S., Neal Bayley, D.D.S., Renee McCoy-Collins, D.D.S., Milton D. Bernard, D.D.S., and Thomas Pinson, D.D.S., Department of Oral and Maxillofacial Surgery; Alfred Goldson, M.D., Department of Radiotherapy; and Vincent Roux, M.D., Medical Director, who entrusted their patients to our care.

Current and past chief residents, Georgetown University Medical Center—Julio A. Ortiz McWilliams, M.D., Kirk Williams, M.D., and Nitzen Catz, M.D. (1985); Don Trotter, M.D., Scott McNamara, M.D., and Thomas Troost, M.D. (1986); Catherine P. Hudkins, M.D., Kenneth Einhorn, M.D., and Lindsey Golden, M.D. (1987); Sanjay Prasad, M.D., James Demetroulakos, M.D., Lisa Fox, M.D. (1988); Stewart Barlow, M.D., and

Nancy Juhlin, M.D. (1989); Lori Schweitzer, M.D., Betsy Vasquez, M.D., and Bruce Davidson, M.D. (1990) whose clinical assistance provided the necessary time for this project.

The patients, nurses, staff and students of Howard University Hospital—who are the ultimate inspiration for this dream. Chapter 2 is dedicated to the ongoing teachings of the late Walter L. Steihl, foremost anatomist, physician, and dedicated humanist. Other acknowledgments go to Roberto Ruiz, Camille Delgado, and Mario Fernandez (Chapter 2); Christina Davis, secretary, Radiology Department of Howard University Hospital (Chapter 4); Alvin Thomas, M.D., Pulmonary Medicine, Howard University Hospital, for his critical review of Chapter 10.

Contributing Authors

Mark V. Alexander, M.D.
Instructor in Surgery, Children's Hospital National Medical Center, George Washington University School of Medicine and Health Sciences; Attending Surgeon in Otolaryngology, Washington Hospital Center, Washington, D.C.

Ebrahim Ashayeri, M.D.
Associate Professor of Radiation Oncology, Howard University College of Medicine, Washington, D.C.

Neal Beckford, M.D.
Assistant Professor and Acting Chairman of Otolaryngology, University of Tennessee, Memphis, College of Medicine; Attending Surgeon in Otolaryngology and Maxillofacial Surgery, The University of Tennessee Medical Center, Memphis.

Mercedes J. Benitez McCrary, M.S., CCC-SLP
Speech-Language Pathologist, University Hospital, University of Medicine and Dentistry of New Jersey, Newark, New Jersey

Cheryl R. Burruss, M.D.
Instructor, Department of Anesthesiology, Howard University Hospital, Washington, D.C.

JoAnn Collier-Manning, M.D.
Instructor, Department of Radiotherapy, Howard University College of Medicine, Washington, D.C.

Gary C. Dennis, M.D., F.A.C.S.
Assistant Professor, Division of Neurosurgery, Department of Surgery, Howard University College of Medicine; Attending Surgeon and Chief, Division of Neurosurgery, Department of Surgery, Howard University Hospital, Washington, D.C.

Karen L. Beverly-Ducker, M.A., CCC-A
Director of Consumer Information, American Speech, Language and Hearing Association, Rockville, Maryland.

Roma V. Gumbs, M.D.
Assistant Professor, Department of Radiology, Howard University College of Medicine; Chief, Thoracic Radiology, Head and Neck Radiology, Howard University Hospital, Washington, D.C.

C. D. Hinton, M.D.
Clinical Professor of Otolaryngology, Howard University College of Medicine; Senior Advisory Staff, Washington Hospital Center, Washington, D.C.

James T. Jackson, D.D.S., F.A.C.D., F.I.C.D., F.A.C.P.
Professor of Prosthodontics, Howard University College of Dentistry; Director, General Practice Residency Programs, Howard University Hospital, Washington, D.C.

LaSalle D. Leffall, Jr., M.D., F.A.C.S.
Professor and Chairman, Department of Surgery, Howard University College of Medicine; Attending Surgeon, Department of Surgery, Howard University Hospital, Washington, D.C.

Robert C. Lowery, Jr., M.D.
Attending Surgeon, Cardiovascular-Thoracic Surgery, Washington Hospital Center, Washington, D.C.

Thomasine Lyles, M.S.W., L.C.S.W.
Clinical Social Worker, Social Services Department, Howard University Hospital, Washington, D.C.

Lawrence D. Mason, M.D.
Attending Anesthesiologist, Department of Anesthesiology, University of Michigan Medical Center, Ann Arbor, Michigan.

Etienne Massac, M.D.
Assistant Professor of Surgery, Howard University College of Medicine, Washington, D.C.; Chief, Division of Plastic Surgery, Howard University Hospital, Washington, D.C.

Clyde B. Mathura, Ph.D.
Associate Professor of Psychology, Coppin State University, Baltimore, Maryland.

Julio A. Ortiz McWilliams, M.D.
Attending Otolaryngologist, Fort Marelo Hospital, Humacao, Puerto Rico.

Haile Mezghebe, M.D.
Assistant Professor of Surgery, Howard University College of Medicine; Associate Director, S.I.C.U./ Trauma Howard University Hospital, Washington, D.C.

Ernest M. Myers, M.D., F.A.C.S.
Associate Professor of Surgery, Howard University College of Medicine; Chief, Division of Otolaryngology, Head and Neck Surgery, Howard University Hospital, Washington, D.C.

Sandra J. Reed, M.D.
Instructor, Department of Anesthesiology, Howard University College of Medicine, Washington, D.C.

Carolyn Sadler, B.S.N.
Clinical Nurse, Thoracic Department, Memorial Sloan-Kettering Cancer Center, New York

Calvin C. Sampson, M.D.
Professor of Pathology, Howard University College of Medicine; Attending Pathologist, and Director of Fine Needle Aspiration Biopsy Service, Howard University Hospital, Washington, D.C.

S. M. Siram, M.D., F.A.C.S.
Associate Professor of Surgery, Howard University College of Medicine; Director, S.I.C.U./Trauma, Howard University Hospital, Washington, D.C.

Tommyzee H. Suggs, M.S.W., L.C.S.W.
Clinical Social Worker, Howard University Hospital, Washington, D.C.

James S. Teal, M.D.
Professor of Radiology, Howard University College of Medicine; Chairman, Department of Radiology, Howard University Hospital, Washington, D.C.

Patricia R. Thompson, M.A., CCC-A
Associate Professor, Communication Arts and Sciences, University of the District of Columbia, Washington, D.C.

Juanita J. Watts, R.N., B.S.N.
Staff Nurse, Ambulatory Care, Howard University Hospital, Washington, D.C.

Robert M. White, Jr., M.D.
Associate Professor of Medicine, Howard University College of Medicine; Attending Physician, Howard University Cancer Center, Howard University Hospital, Washington, D.C.

Wilhelmina Wright-Harp, Ph.D.
Associate Professor and Chairperson, Communication Arts and Sciences, University of the District of Columbia, Washington, D.C.

Introduction

Echoing the African proverb—let him speak who has seen with his eyes—this book, a systematic approach to head and neck oncology, relies strongly on algorithms (see the decision tree symbols,* right), tables, photographs, and drawings. Since most readers have varied perspectives and objectives, the chapters are designated by discipline. Each chapter begins with Key Concepts, a succinct outline of the subject. This is followed by Milestones, a brief historical background. Most chapters are short, emphasizing a visual format. Others, given the nature of the topic, are more narrative. Finally, several glossaries, scattered throughout the book (Chapters 7, 18, 28), amplify and explain the more technical terms.

*Format used with permission of the editors of *MRI Decisions*, © by Physicians World Communications LP.

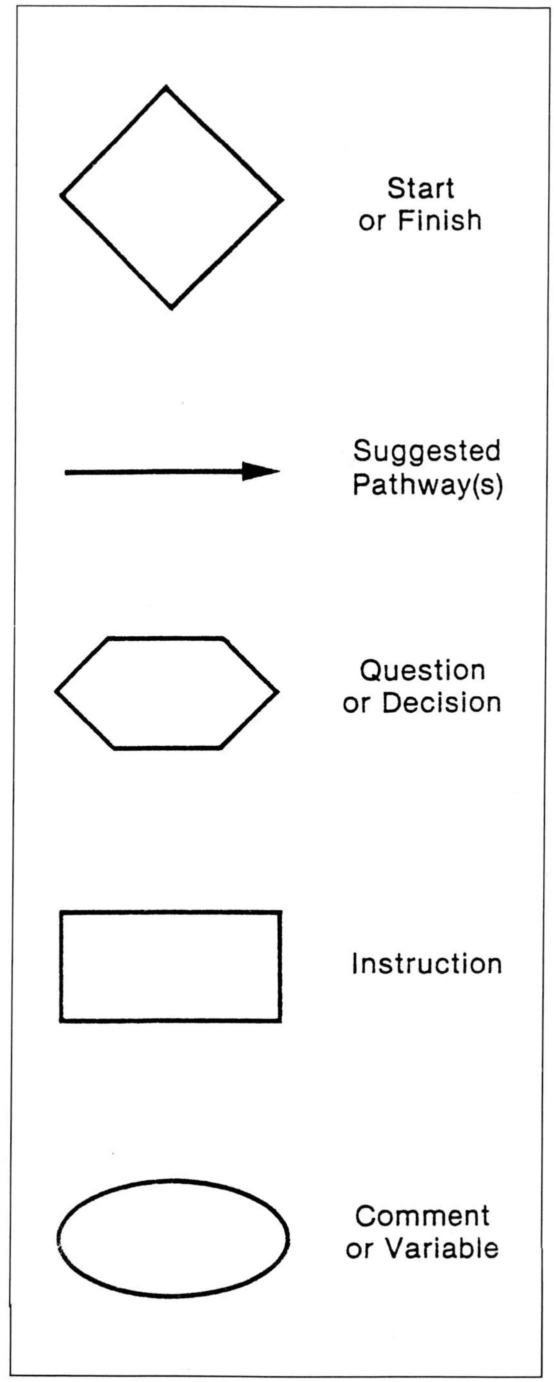

Table 1-7. Probability (p = 1.0) of head & neck cancer versus site

Site	*History*	*Symptoms/Complaints*	*Signs/Physical findings*
1. Nasopharynx	Chinese Nitrosamine exposure	Nasal obstruction Posterior epistaxis Earache Decreased hearing	Nasopharyngeal mass Extraocular dysfunction Ipsilateral serous otitis media Ipsilateral neck mass
2. Sinus/nose	Woodworker Shoe manufacturing Radiochemicals	Poor oral hygiene Midfacial numbness Nasal obstruction Anterior epistaxis	Anesthesia, infraorbital nerve Nasal mass Upper alveolar process mass Palatal mass
3. Salivary glands	Low-dose radiation History of breast malignancy	Unilateral facial or upper neck/jaw "lump"	Angle of mandible or submandibular triangle mass Facial paresis or paralysis
4. Lips	Fair-skinned white Outdoors occupation	Lower lip ulcer or sore Upper lip ulcer or sore	Ulcer—vermillion border Submental or submandibular neck mass
5. Oral cavity 6. Oropharynx	Heavy alcohol and/or tobacco usage	Earache and sore throat Halitosis Spitting up blood Sore or ulcer in oral cavity Neck lump	Exophytic or ulcerative lesion Hypoglossal paresis/paralysis Upper airway obstruction Neck mass
7. Hypopharynx	Heavy alcohol and/or tobacco usage	Earache and sore throat Dysphagia Weight loss Shortness of breath Hoarseness	Pyriform sinus or upper esophageal mass Vocal cord paralysis Lower airway obstruction
8. Larynx	Heavy tobacco usage	Hoarseness Shortness of breath "Lump" in the neck	Glottic/supraglottic mass Vocal cord paralysis Lower airway obstruction Aspiration
9. Thyroid/parathyroids	Female < 30 years Male > 40 years Low-dose radiation	Anterior/suprasternal "lump" Dysphagia Shortness of breath Hoarseness	Visceral triangle mass Vocal cord paralysis/paresis Lower airway obstruction
10. Esophagus	Black male Alcoholic Weight loss	Dysphagia Spitting up blood Chest pain	Cachexia Aspiration Hoarseness

carcinogens. As always, the ultimate burden of proof remains with the astute physician.

Physical Examination

There is no substitute for a careful general physical examination and a thorough head and neck examination (Table 1-8). The emphasis of the latter is on the ears, facies, oral cavity, oropharynx, hypopharynx/larynx, and neck. Aside from the otologic and hypopharyngeal/laryngeal examinations, no special instrumentation is required. As a basic dictum, no head and neck examination is complete without otoscopy and laryngoscopy (mirror or fiberoptic).

Diagnostic Radiology

The findings of the history and physical dictate the choice of radiologic diagnosis. The sinus and the soft-tissue neck (anteroposterior and lateral)

Table 1-8. Diagnosis of head and neck cancer

	Physical diagnosis					Basic radiology				CT scan/MRI					Pathology	
Site	*Otoscopy*	*Rhinoscopy*	*Nasopharyngoscopy*	*Laryngoscopy*	*Neck exam*	*Sinus series*	*Soft-tissue AP/Lat-neck*	*Barium swallow*	*CXR*	*Brain*	*Sinuses*	*Neck*	*Lungs*	*Mediastinum*	*Needle biopsy*	*Punch biopsy*
1. Nasopharynx	+++	+++	+++	++	+++	++	+		+++	+/-	+++	+++				+++
2. Sinus/nose	++	+++	+++	++	+++	+++			+++	+/-	+++	+/-				+++
3. Salivary glands	+	+	+	++	+++	+/-			+++		++	++			++	+/-
4. Lips				++	+++				+++							+++
5. Oral cavity				+++	+++		+/-		+++			+++				+++
6. Oropharynx	+	+	+	+++	+++				+++			+++				+++
7. Hypopharynx				+++	+++		++	++	+++			+++	+/-	+/-		
8. Larynx				+++	+++		++	+/-	+++			+++	+/-	+/-		+++
9. Thyroid/parathyroids				+++	+++		+/-	+/-	+++			++	+/-	++	+++	
10. Esophagus (cervical)				+++	+++			+++	+++			+++	+++	+++		+++

\+ Helpful.
\++ Recommended.
\+++ Preferred.
+/- Equivocal.
AP/Lat = anteroposterior/lateral; CXR = chest x-ray.

series are excellent screening examinations. However, the most accurate examinations are computed tomography and magnetic resonance imaging (see Chapter 4). These examinations have the highest yield for rapid and accurate diagnosis.

Biopsy

Sites 1 through 7, and 9 are amenable to punch or needle biopsy under local anesthesia. In the suspicious patient they are performed during the initial visit. If the diagnosis is positive, panendoscopy is performed to rule out synchronous head and neck malignancies. When the physical examination is negative, panendoscopy or other techniques (antrostomy, open biopsy) may be indicated for the high-risk patient.

The coincidental development of fiberoptic laryngoscopy, sophisticated imaging techniques, and fine-needle aspiration (biopsy) has enhanced the ability to make an early diagnosis of head and neck cancer. These exciting developments allow the head and neck diagnostician to avoid redundant and risky tests. Ultimately, they reduce the level of uncertainty and increase the level of probability. Finally, the patient benefits twofold: increased diagnostic efficiency and decreased financial costs.

TREATMENT AND PROGNOSIS

Treatment

The treatment goal is disease ablation and patient rehabilitation to the highest physiologic and psychological state. Classically, therapy consists of surgery, radiation therapy, and chemotherapy [27,28]. Early cancers are treated with either radiation or surgery. For a given lesion, if cure rates for radiation and surgery are equal, the former is chosen as the primary form of treatment [29,30]. Well-advanced or late cancers are treated by surgery and radiation. If the patient has had previous head and neck radiation, surgery may be the only curative option. As late as 1975, chemotherapy was a minor contributor and was utilized only for end-stage disease. Today, new protocols include chemotherapy as an initial and important modality (see Chapter 8) [31,32].

Prognosis

Cure rates vary markedly according to site. Characteristically, they become worse as the aerodigestive tract is transversed (see Table 1-7). Perhaps more than any other factor, the degree of cervical or distant metastasis at the time of initial presentation predicts potential survival [30,33,34].

Patterns of Failure

In addition to the presence or absence of cervical metastasis, location or site has prognostic implications. For example, locoregional control is a problem with the oral cavity (site 5), oropharynx (site 6), and larynx (site 8), whereas poor control of distant metastasis is associated with the nasopharynx (site 1).

Secondary Cancer

Life-style

Most head and neck cancers are preventable and, if detected early, curable. By far, the most important factor in the prevention of a recurrence or the development of a secondary cancer is a change in life-style. Patients who continue to smoke and drink risk developing a second head and neck malignancy.

Immune Suppression

Presently, we do not know the real impact triple modality treatment (chemotherapy, radiotherapy, and surgery) have on the immune system. It is theoretically possible that in our zeal to cure one cancer, we enhance the development of future primary malignancies.

REFERENCES

1. American Cancer Society: *1986 Cancer Facts & Figures*. New York: American Cancer Society, 1986.
2. Axtell LM, Asir AJ, Myers MH (eds): *Cancer Patient Survival*. Bethesda, MD: US Dept. of Health, Education and Welfare, 1976.
3. Lipkin A, Miller RH, Woodson GE: Squamous cell carcinoma of the oral cavity, pharnyx and larynx in young adults. *Laryngoscope* 95 : 790, 1985.
4. Shivas AA (ed): *Racial and Geographic Factors in Tumor Incidence*. Edinburgh: Edinburgh University Press, 1967.
5. Lyon JL, et al: Cancer incidence in Mormons and non-Mormons in Utah. *N Engl J Med* 244 : 129, 1976.
6. White JE, Enterline JP: Cancer in Non-White Americans. In Hickey RC (ed): *Current Problems in Cancer*. Chicago: Year Book, pp. 3–34, 1980.
7. Bang KM, Perlin E, Sampson CC: Increased cancer risks in blacks: A look at the factors. *J Natl Med Assoc* 89(4) : 383, 1987.
8. Phillips CW, Lacey LFP: Cancer profiles from several high-risk Chicago communities. *J Natl Med Assoc* 79(7) : 701, 1987.
9. Neighbors HW, Jackson JS: Barriers to medical care among adult blacks: What happens to the uninsured? *J Natl Med Assoc* 79(5) : 489, 1987.
10. Lindue G: The influence of social class in the survival of cancer patients. *Am J Public Health* 59 : 267, 1964.
11. Lipworth L: Socioeconomic factors in the progress of cancer patients. *J Chronic Dis* 23 : 105, 1970.
12. Baquet CR, et al: *Cancer Among Blacks and Other Minorities*. National Cancer Institute, DHRS Publication No. (NIH) 86-27185. Washington, DC: Government Printing Office, 1986.
13. Wynder EL: The epidemiology for cancers of the upper alimentary and upper respiratory tracts. *Laryngoscope* 88 : 50, 1978.
14. Wynder EL, Hoffman B: Tobacco and tobacco smoke. *Semin Oncol* 3 : 5, 1976.
15. Stockwell HG, Lyman GH: Impact of smoking and smokeless tobacco on the risk of cancer of the head and neck. *Head Neck Surg* 9 : 104, 1986.
16. Rao RS, Desai PB: The challenge of head and neck cancer in India (Editorial). *Head Neck Surg* 11 : 487, 1989.
17. Cooper GM, et al: Transforming activity of DNA of chemically transformed and normal cells. *Nature* 284 : 418, 1980.
18. Friend SH, Drya TP, Weinberg RA: Oncogenes and tumor-suppressing genes. *N Engl J Med* 10 : 618, 1988.
19. Busch H. Oncogenes and other new targets for cancer chemotherapy. *J Res Clin Oncol* 107 : 1, 1984.
20. Nowell P. The clonal evolution of tumor cell populations. *Science* 194 : 23, 1976.
21. Johns ME. The clonal assay of head and neck tumor cells: Results and clinical correlations. *Laryngoscope* 92 (Suppl 28) : 1, 1982.
22. Batsakis JG: *Tumor of the Head and Neck: Clinical and Pathological Considerations*. Baltimore: Williams and Wilkins, 1979.
23. El Badawi SA, et al: Squamous cell carcinoma of the pyriform sinus. *Head Neck Surg* 5 : 508, 1983.
24. Close LG, et al: Microvascular invasion in cancer of oral cavity and oropharynx. *Arch Otolaryngol Head Neck Surg*. 113 : 1191, 1987.

25. Kassirer JP: Sounding board: Our quest for diagnostic certainty. *N Engl J Med* 320(22) : 1489, 1989.
26. Sox HC, et al: *Medical Decision Making*. Boston: Butterworth, 1988.
27. Marks JE, et al: Floor of mouth cancer: Patient selection and treatment results. *Laryngoscope* 93 : 475, 1983.
28. Marks JE, et al: Carcinoma of the oral tongue: A study of patient selection and treatment results. *Laryngoscope* 91 : 1548, 1981.
29. Kaplan MJ, et al: Stage II glottic carcinoma: Prognostic factors and management. *Laryngoscope* 93 : 725, 1983.
30. Mizono GS, et al: Carcinoma of the tonsillar region. *Laryngoscope* 96 : 240, 1986.
31. Adjuvant chemotherapy for advanced head and neck squamous carcinoma: Final report of the head and neck contracts program. *Cancer* 60(3) : 301, 1987.
32. Chang TM: Induction chemotherapy for advanced head and neck cancers: A literature review. *Head Neck Surg* 10 : 150, 1988.
33. St. Pierre S, Bake SR: Squamous cell carcinoma of the maxillary sinus: Analysis of 66 cases. *Head Neck Surg* 5 : 508, 1983.
34. Wolf GT, et al: Definite vs adjuvant radiotherapy. *Arch Otolaryngol* 111 : 716, 1985.

2

History and Physical Examination

JULIO A. ORTIZ McWILLIAMS

KEY CONCEPTS

Clinical Presentations; Functional Anatomy; History; Physical; Site Analysis

MILESTONES

1829	Glottiscope	Babington
1855	Indirect Laryngoscopy	Garcia
1857	Mirror Laryngoscopy	Czermak
1968	Fiberoptic Laryngoscopy	Sawashinice and Hirose
1981	Video Laryngoscopy	Yanagisawa

The three goals of the history and physical examination are preliminary diagnosis, disease assessment, and the establishment of a doctor-patient relationship. To fulfill these goals, this chapter outlines basic data collection, describes the head and neck examination, and highlights fundamental diagnostic concepts.

GENERAL CONSIDERATIONS

Early Diagnosis

Head and neck tumors are ascribed to five major anatomic regions. Reflecting distinctive symptomatology, each region contains several major sites and subsites. Tumors arising from within each region present locally, regionally, or both. In general, the clinical presentations correlate with early, advanced, or late pathogenesis. More important than regional classification and assignment, subtle complaints indicative of malignancy must be differentiated from benign conditions. In short, the physician must be suspicious of persistent innocent complaints that indicate early malignancy.

Subtle Presentation

Since many early head and neck malignancies mimic common benign diseases (i.e., sinusitis, pharyngitis), early diagnosis requires diligent follow-up and a high index of suspicion. It is imperative to pursue chronic "benign" symptoms. Such complaints as a persistent sore throat, earache, or vague "lump" must be investigated carefully.

Silent Presentation

What is even more discouraging is that many patients, even with advanced disease, are asymptomatic. *The silent head and neck areas are the nasopharynx, paranasal sinuses, base of the tongue, supraglottic larynx, and pyriform sinus (Figure 2-1).* Classically, disease in these areas presents as unilateral hearing loss, nasal obstruction, or neck mass [1–3].

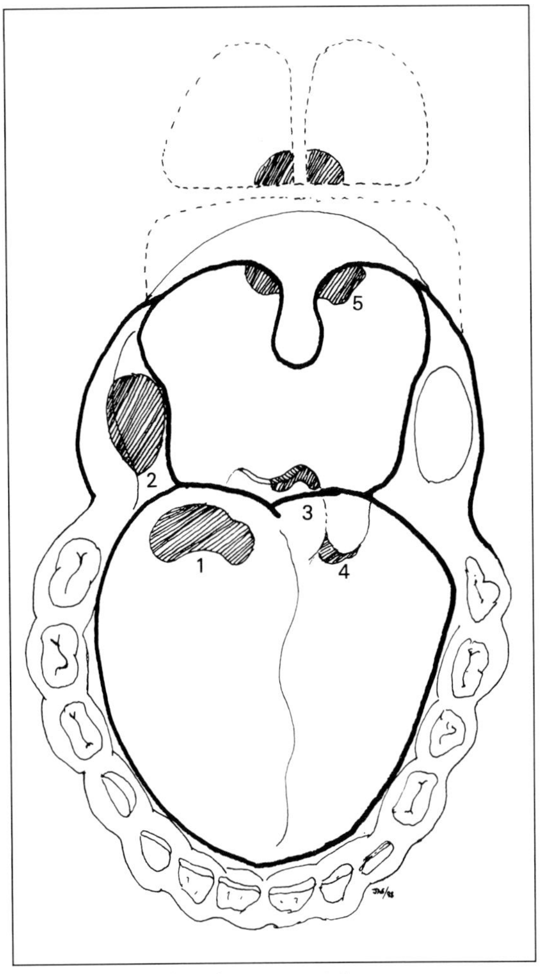

Figure 2-1. The silent areas. These areas include subsites where tumors are asymptomatic in the early stages. *1*-Base of tongue; *2*-tonsils; *3*-supraglottis; *4*-hypopharynx; and *5*-nasopharynx. Not included in this figure are the paranasal sinuses.

Regions

As outlined in Chapter 1, the 10 head and neck sites have 50 subsites that are divided into five major anatomic regions (Figure 2-2). After the patient interview, the principal complaints are assigned to one of the following regions.

Regions I and II: Face/Sinonasal Tract

Facial lesions (region I) present as erythematous, granulomatous skin eruptions or nonhealing ulcers [4]. The primary sinonasal tract (region II) manifestations are rhinorrhea, epistaxis, and nasal obstruction. Secondary manifestations are neck mass or unilateral hearing loss [5]. Unfortunately in region II, the late or secondary manifestations are the most common initial presentations.

Regions III and IV: Oro- and Aerodigestive Tracts

Regions III and IV are associated with the following common complaints: sore throat, dysphagia, otalgia, hoarseness, and neck mass. The predominant primary region III manifestations are sore throat and dysphagia [6]. Secondary manifestations for both, but especially region IV, are neck mass, otalgia, and dyspnea. In region IV, the aerodigestive tract, the upper portion (supraglottis) is part of the digestive tract as well as the airway, so complaints may be difficult to ascribe regionally. If the lesion is in the upper aerodigestive tract (supraglottis), sore throat and dysphagia are the primary (local) manifestations. With lower airway lesions, hoarseness and airway obstruction predominate [7].

Region V: Neck

The neck mass is discussed extensively in Chapter 3. The origins are cervical viscera (thyroid, parathyroid, and neurovascular structures), adjacent structures (salivary glands), distant organs (breast, lung, gastrointestinal, genitourinary), or one of the head and neck regions [8].

HISTORY

Data Base

An accurate history gleaned from directed questioning and attentive listening is indispensable for defining disease progression. The data base is the beginning of the formal history (Table 2-1). The essentials are name, sex, birthdate, age, residence, telephone number, marital status, race or nationality, occupation, and closest relative or friend.

Chief Complaint

The chief complaint is the catalyst that prompts the patient to seek medical advice. Head and

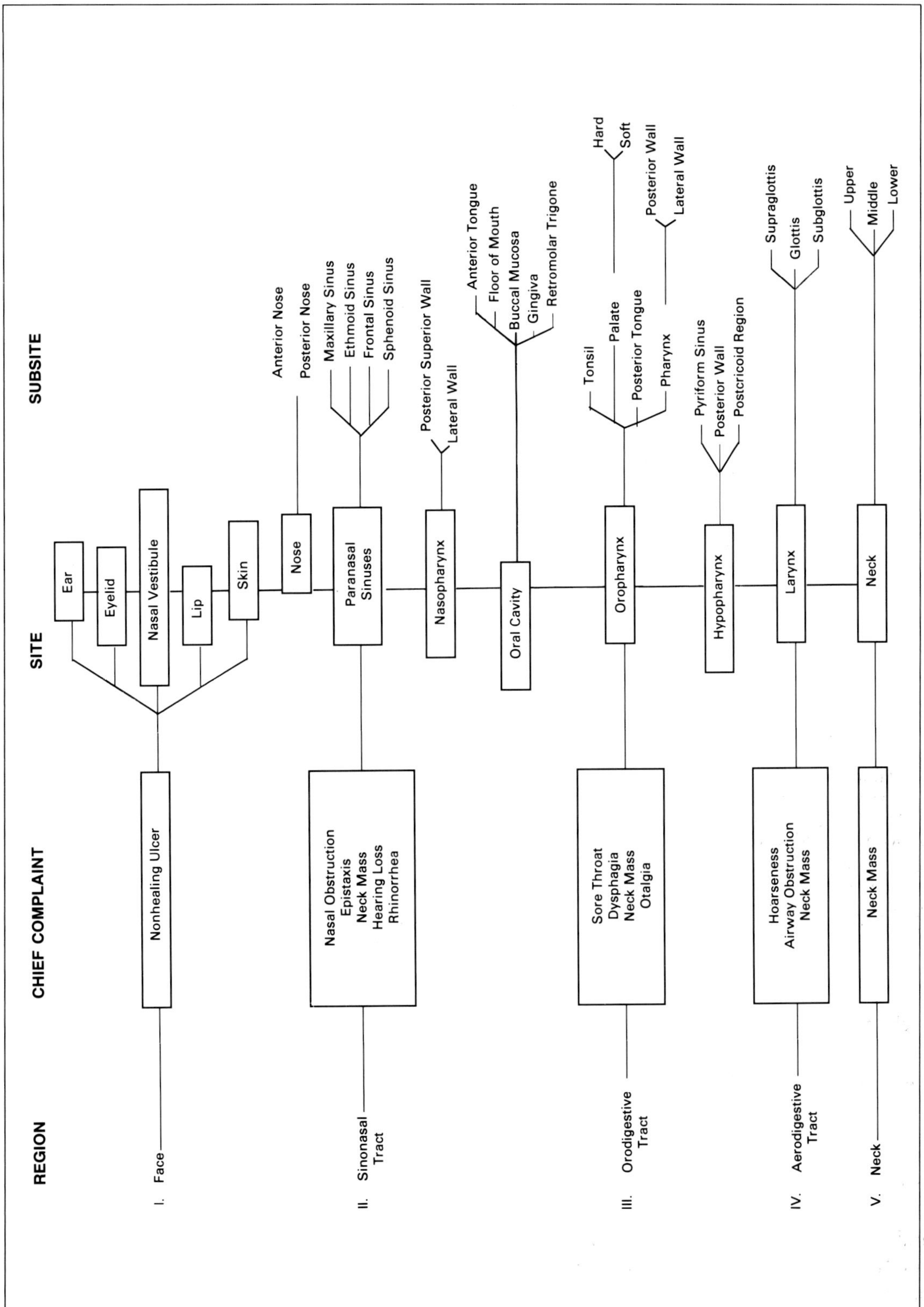

Figure 2-2. Correlation of chief complaints to regions and sites.

Table 2-1. History: data collection

Verify
1. Name
2. Address
3. Telephone
4. Age
5. Sex
6. Birthdate
7. Occupation
8. Nationality/ethnic group/race
9. Close relatives

Chief complaint (CC): Correlate with the five major head and neck regions:
- I. Face
- II. Sinonasal tract
- III. Orodigestive tract
- IV. Aerodigestive tract
- V. Neck

History of present illness (HPI):
1. Onset
2. Primary symptoms
3. Secondary symptoms
4. Progression
5. Duration
6. Extent
7. Associated problems
8. Site and subsite

Past medical history (PMH):
1. Medical illnesses
2. Medications
3. Allergies
4. Hospitalizations
5. Operations
6. Habits
7. Carcinogen exposure
8. Previous carcinoma
9. AIDS risk factors
10. Occupation
11. Radiation exposure
12. Family history of cancer

neck chief complaints are assigned to one or more anatomic regions. The most common, but not necessarily the only chief complaints for each region are as follows:

Region I (face): skin lesion (nonhealing ulcer or swelling).
Region II (sinonasal tract): rhinitis, sinusitis, nasal obstruction, rhinorrhea, or epistaxis.
Region III (orodigestive tract): sore throat, dysphagia.
Region IV (aerodigestive tract): upper—sore throat and dysphagia; lower—hoarseness and airway obstruction.
Region V (neck): neck mass or masses.

History of the Present Illness

Patient Narrative

The history of the present illness, a succinct narrative of the disease process, includes the time of onset, location, progression, severity and frequency of complaints, associated problems (e.g., weight loss, dyspnea, headache, visual changes), and pertinent negatives. In addition, the patient's general appearance, demeanor, expression, and emotions are recorded.

Goal

The history of the present illness fulfills three goals: (1) identification of the major region (site or subsite), (2) determination of the preliminary disease stage, and (3) assessment of the patient's reaction and tolerance to the malady.

Past Medical History

The past medical history should include the following:

1. Medical illnesses: all significant illnesses, including heart diseases, hypertension, diabetes, pulmonary disease, psychiatric, and cerebrovascular problems.
2. Medications: dosage and frequency.
3. Allergies: reactions to medications, food, and contrast media.
4. Hospitalizations: all major hospitalizations.
5. Operations: all major procedures.
6. Habits: tobacco consumption (pipe, cigar, chewing, and cigarette on a per day per year or pack years basis), alcohol consumption (amount/day/year), drug and chemical dependency.
7. Carcinogens: radiation, chemicals [9–11].
8. Previous malignancy.
9. AIDS risks factors: homosexuality/bisexuality, blood transfusion prior to 1983, intravenous drug abuse, multiple sexual partners, hemophilia [9].
10. Occupation: nickel refining, woodwork-

ing, leather working, asbestos, military service, exposure to radioactive materials [10].
11. Carcinogens: irradiation (6–40 years previously) to the thyroid, salivary glands, and larynx.
12. Family history of cancer.

Review of Systems

For the head and neck, the emphasis is as follows:

1. Eyes: visual assessment (blindness, acuity, fields).
2. Ears: prior disease or hearing loss.
3. Respiratory: pulmonary disease (presence and severity).
4. Cardiac disease: a history of myocardial infarction (low risk versus high risk), hypertension, stroke [12].
5. Gastrointestinal: symptoms suggestive of gastrointestinal malignancy.
6. Neurologic: any evidence of cerebrovascular disease.
7. Psychiatric: the ability to handle stress (e.g., depression) [13].

PHYSICAL EXAMINATION

The head and neck examination is divided into an external and internal examination whose methodology encompasses direct/indirect visualization and palpation (Table 2-2) [11, 14]. The external examination includes lips, facial skin, eyes, ears, and sinuses. The internal examination requires illumination and instrumentation.

External Examination

The physical examination begins with inspection. A wealth of information is obtained by careful observation of demeanor, level of discomfort, speech, airway, and evidence of alcoholism or heavy tobacco usage. The external examination, an assessment of facial symmetry, speech patterns, and airway, includes the following:

Symmetry

Observe for asymmetry of the eyes (ptosis, proptosis), face (facial palsy, edema), and neck (mass).

Table 2-2. Physical examination of the head and neck regions

Region	*Inspection*	*Palpation*	*Auscultation*	*Special techniques*
Face				
Skin	+	+		Oto, In
Eyes	+	+		Oto, Fund, In★
Ears	+	+		Oto, In★, In
Lips	+	+		In
Sinonasal				
Nasopharynx	+			Oto, Fund, In, In★
Sinuses	+	+		Oto, Fund, In, In★
Nose	+			Oto, Fund, In, In★
Orodigestive				
Oral cavity	+	+		Oto, In
Otopharynx	+	+		Oto, In
Aerodigestive				
Larynx		+	+	In
Hypopharynx		+		In
Neck	+	+	+	In

+ = Emphasis. In★ = Indirect nasopharyngoscopy.
Oto = Otoscopy.
Fund = Fundoscopy.
In = Indirect laryngopharyngoscopy.

Speech

Characteristic speech is associated with nasopharyngeal, oropharyngeal, and hypopharyngeal lesions. The hyponasal voice is produced by nasopharyngeal, posterior nasal, and palatal lesions (region II). The muffled voice is associated with lesions of the base of the tongue, epiglottis, and posterior pharyngeal wall (region III). Tongue-tied speech implicates the oral cavity, especially the anterior tongue and floor of the mouth.

Airway

Suprasternal retractions, accessory muscle usage, cyanosis, high-pitched stridor, tachycardia, and tachypnea are signs of severe airway obstruction. Airway obstruction in head and neck cancer patients often develops slowly and insidiously, producing a low-pitched stridor, dysphagia, and mild dyspnea on exertion. High-pitched stridor or aphonia implicates a glottic lesion. Despite severe airway compromise, many patients are asymptomatic at rest due to gradual metabolic compensation. Obviously, early intervention of airway problems even in compensated patients results in decreased mortality and morbidity.

Skin

Examination of the skin consists of visual inspection and palpation.

Ears

Standard otoscopy is performed (Figure 2-3). Remember that otalgia and serous otitis are subtle complaints of head and neck cancer.

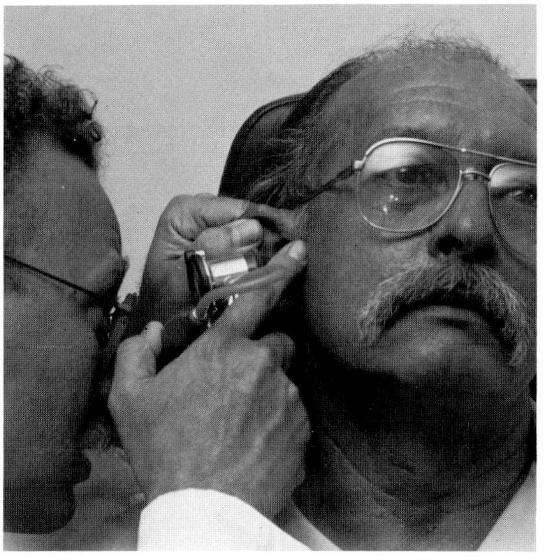

Figure 2-3. Otoscopy with the battery-powered, self-contained, closed or open-headed otoscope. Many skilled clinicians use an ear speculum and headlight (or head mirror only) for this examination.

Eye

Proptosis, exophthalmos, ptosis, and strabismus implicate sinonasal or orbital disease. Head and neck malignancies may extend into the skull or parapharyngeal space and affect extraocular movements and visual acuity.

Nose and Sinuses

Examination of the nose and sinuses consists of both an external and internal examination. The external examination includes inspection and palpation. Inspect the upper and middle face for asymmetry and tenderness. Palpate the nasal dorsum and bony pyramids. Test, with touch and pinprick, for infraorbital hypothesia; its presence suggests a sinonasal tract lesion.

Lower Face, Mandible, and Parotids

The lower face, mandible, and parotids are inspected and palpated. The examination includes bimanual palpation, especially for lesions of the mandible, floor of the mouth, and tongue. Mental nerve sensation is assessed routinely; anesthesia implies nerve invasion (Figure 2-4).

Neck Examination

A complete description of a neck mass includes tenderness, size, firmness, consistency, mobility, and auscultation. The neck is palpated in the submental, submandibular, carotid, and parotid regions, usually from behind the patient. Instruct the patient to swallow as the suprasternal area is palpated. Palpate the hyoid and thyroid cartilage. Mobilize the larynx and feel the grating sensation, the absence of which suggests a cricoid lesion. The thyroid gland is

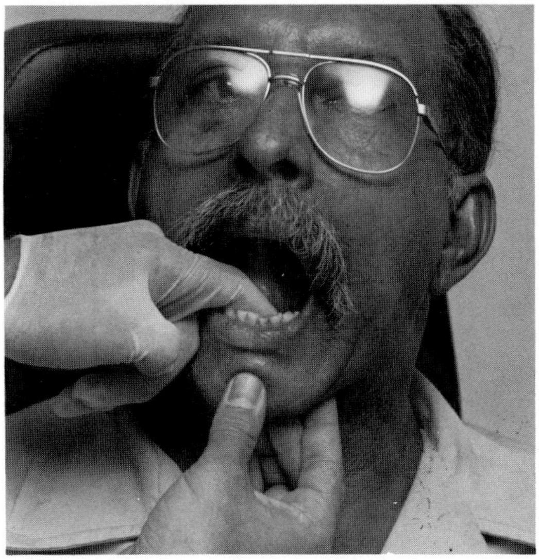

Figure 2-4. Bimanual palpation of the oral cavity and oropharynx. A finger cot or glove is mandatory for the internal examination.

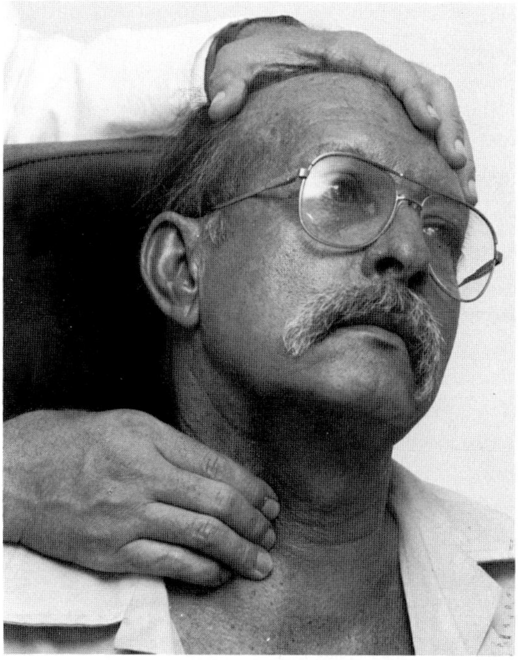

Figure 2-5. Palpation and auscultation (*not shown*) of the neck. Usually, the physician stands behind the patient and palpates both sides simultaneously.

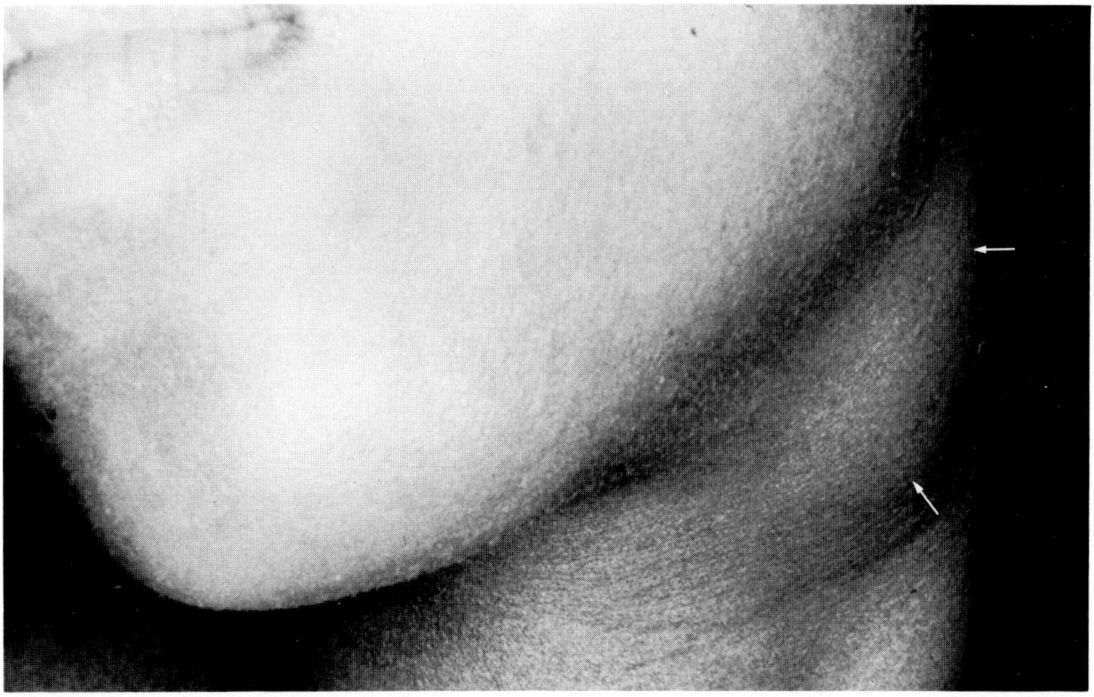

Figure 2-6. Second branchial cyst. A long-standing asymptomatic mass in a 27-year-old woman was confused initially with a parotid neoplasm.

grasped between the thumb, index, and middle fingers. Displace the sternocleidomastoid by a gentle bidigital grasp; palpate the deep cervical fat pad and carotid sheath. Flex and rotate the head to decrease muscle tension and facilitate palpation (Figures 2-5 through 2-11).

Internal Examination

The basic requirements for the internal examination are illumination (headlight or head mirror), laryngeal mirrors (sizes 3–6), nasopharyngeal mirrors (sizes 0–2), and topical anesthesia (Figure 2-12). Other more sophisticated instruments are the Hopkins (rod) and Machida (fiberoptic) laryngoscopes (Figure 2-13). They provide excellent aerodigestive

Figure 2-7. Large second branchial cyst, presenting in the posterior cervical triangle.

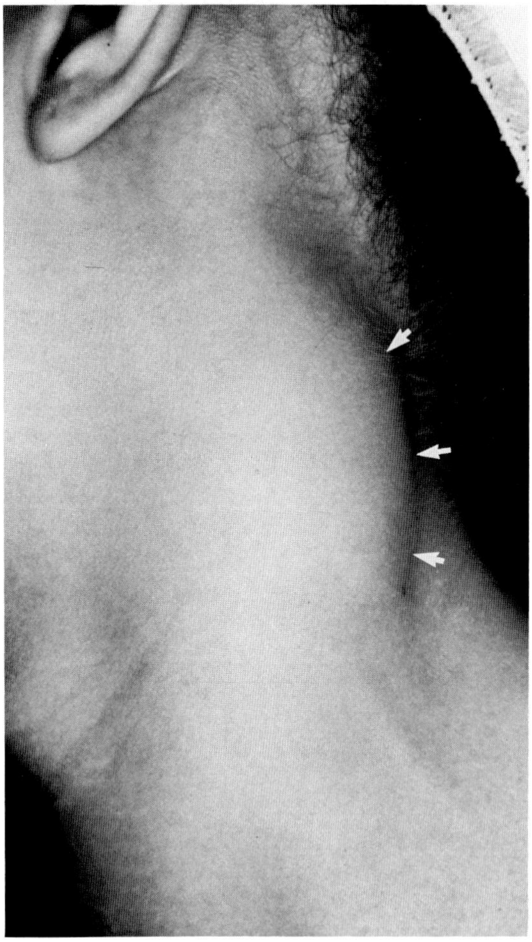

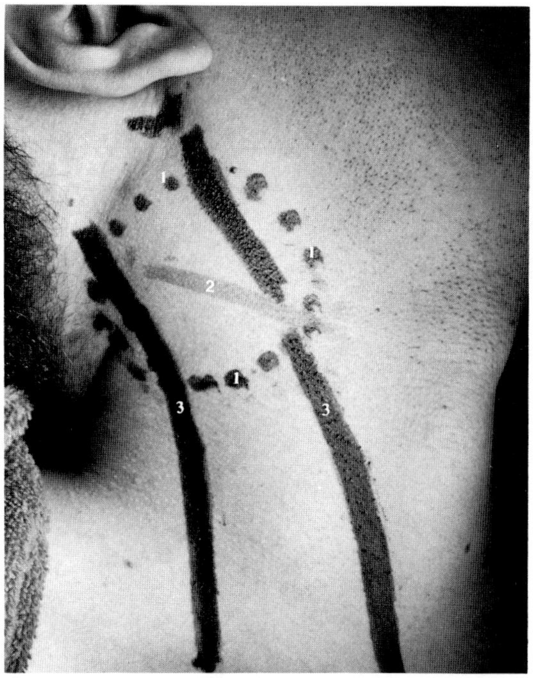

A

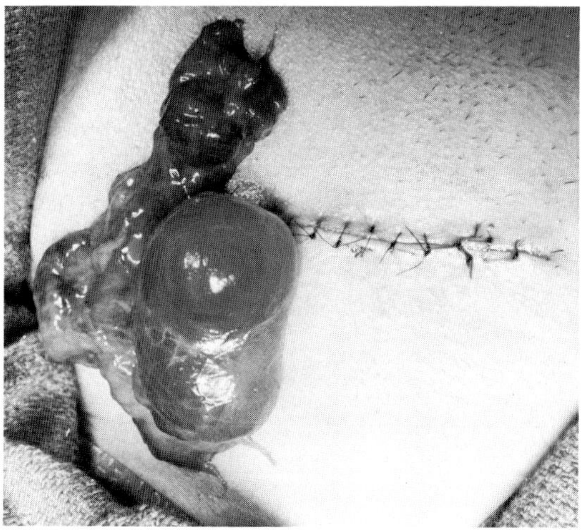

B

Figure 2-8. Deep cervical lymphangioma. A. Preoperative view. *1* = mass; *2* = proposed incision; *3* = anterior and posterior margins of the sternocleidomastoid muscle. B. The cystic specimen with attached lymph nodes.

Figure 2-9. Submandibular gland mixed tumor. A–D. Preoperative views in a 40-year-old man who had a slowly enlarging left submandibular mass spanning 20 years. The full beard camouflages the mass.

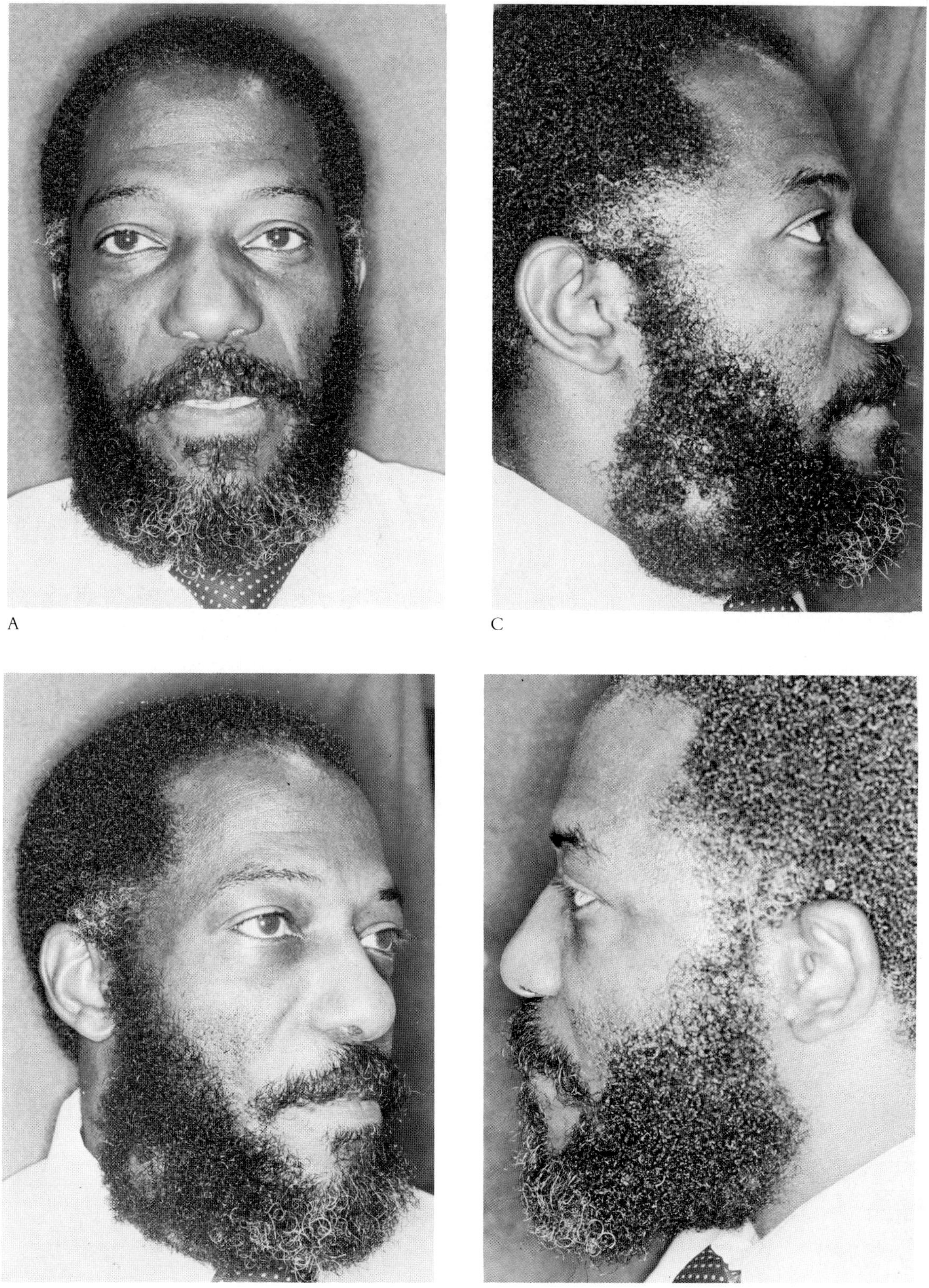

A C

B D

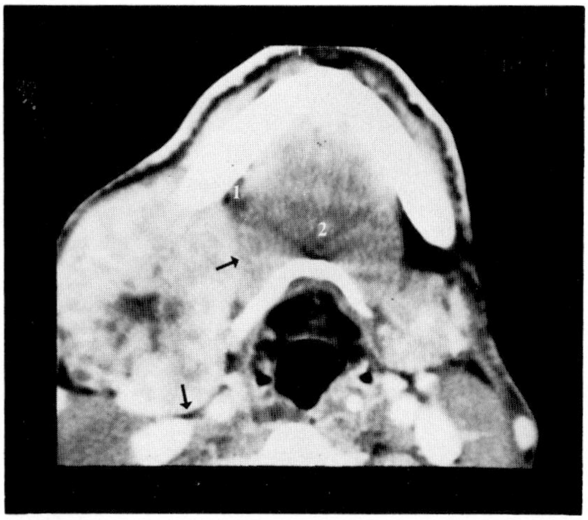

E

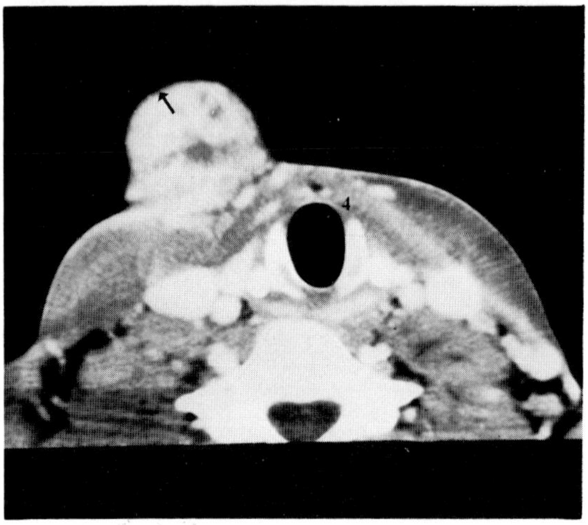

F

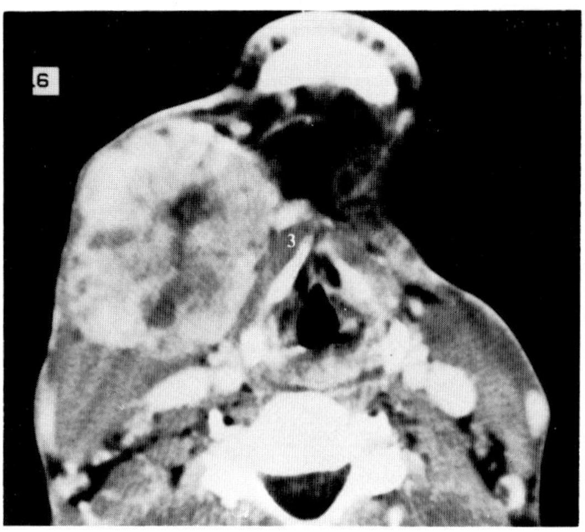

G

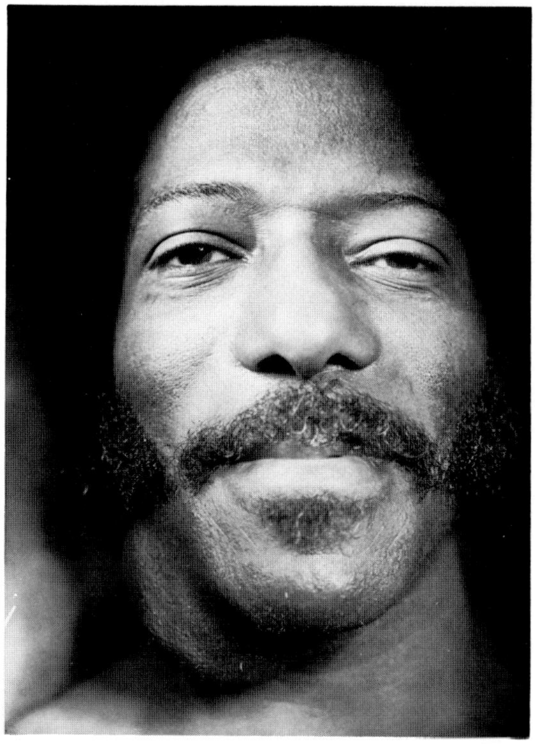

H

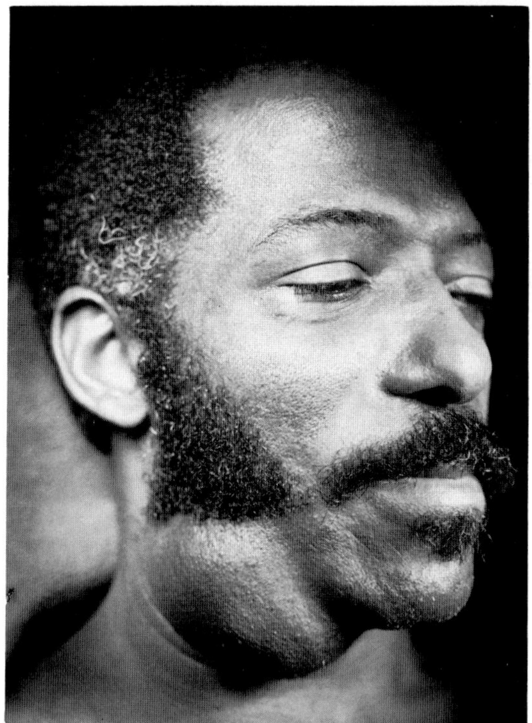

I

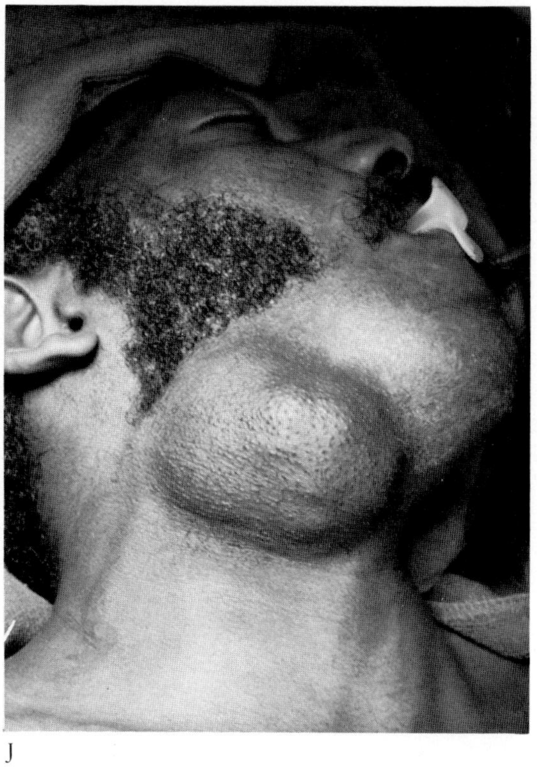

J

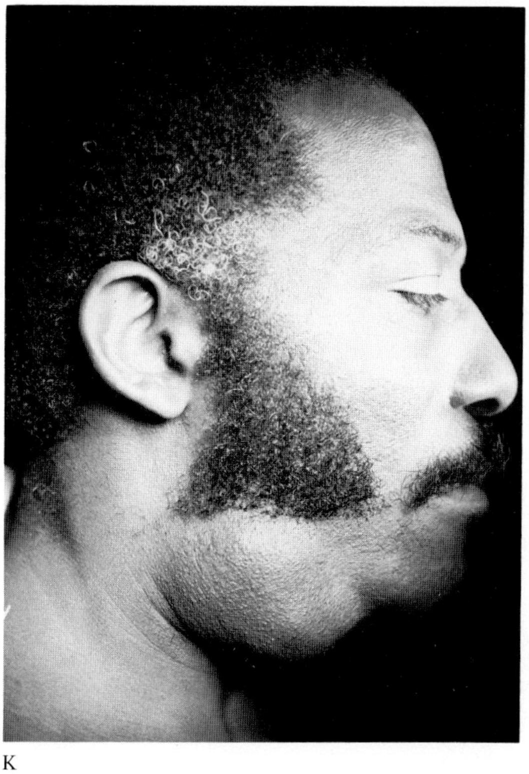

K

Figure 2-9 (continued). E–G. CT scans demonstrate the full extent of the mass from the angle of the mandible to the midtrachea. *1* = mandible; *2* = tongue; *3* = thyroid cartilage; *4* = cricoid cartilage. H–K. Intraoperative views without the beard demonstrate the magnitude of the problem. A fine-needle aspiration showed findings consistent with benign mixed tumor.

Figure 2-9 (continued). L–M. The multilobulated mass incorporates the submandibular gland. Its removal reveals the submandibular triangle, posterior belly of the digastric muscle (*pbd*), hypoglossal nerve (*hy*), and hyoglossal muscle (*hg*).

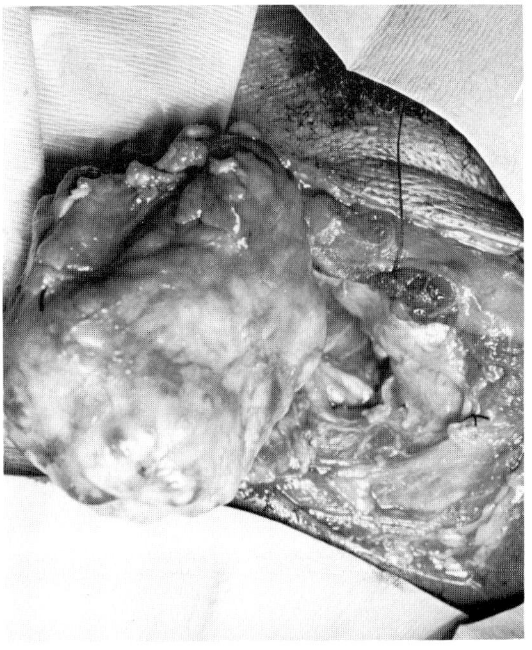

L

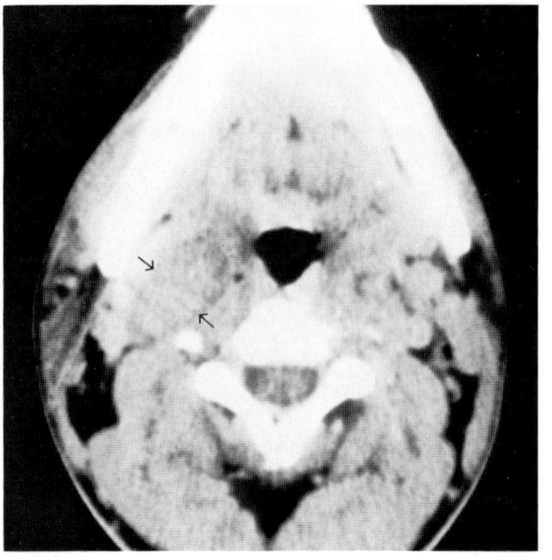

Figure 2-10. Sympathetic neuroma. This is a deep carotid sheath mass in a muscular 25-year-old man whose complaint was dull, unrelenting, right-sided neck pain. CT scan with contrast demonstrated a homogeneous mass within the carotid sheath from the skull base to the larynx. A sympathetic neuroma was removed. The patient has a postoperative Horner's syndrome.

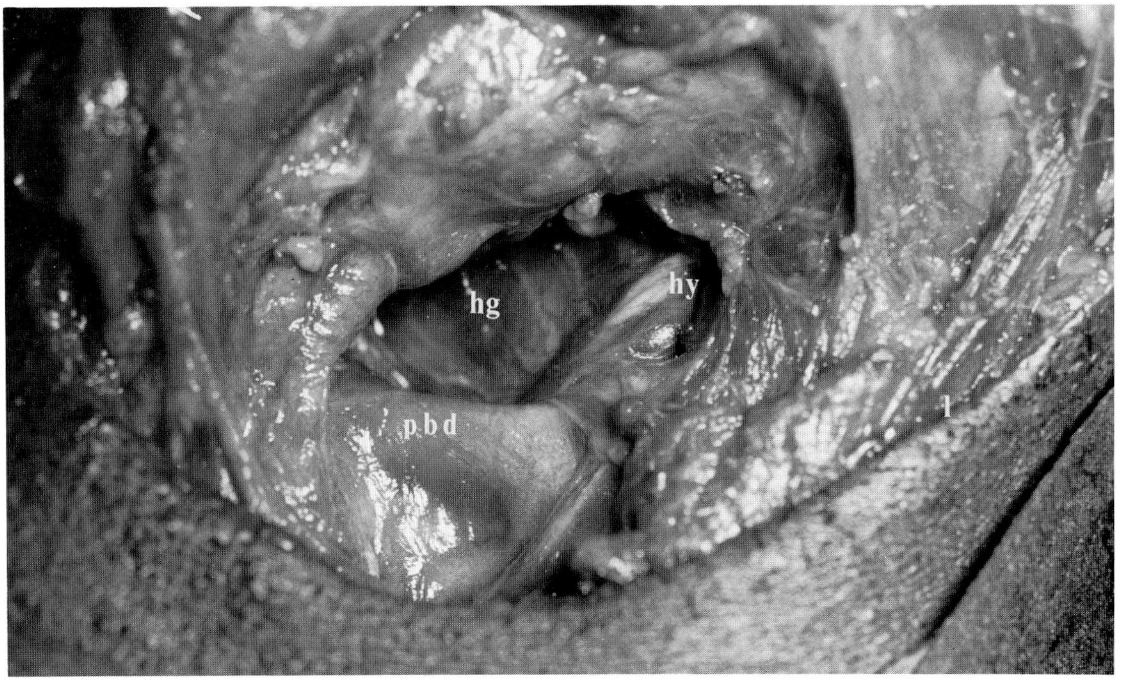

M

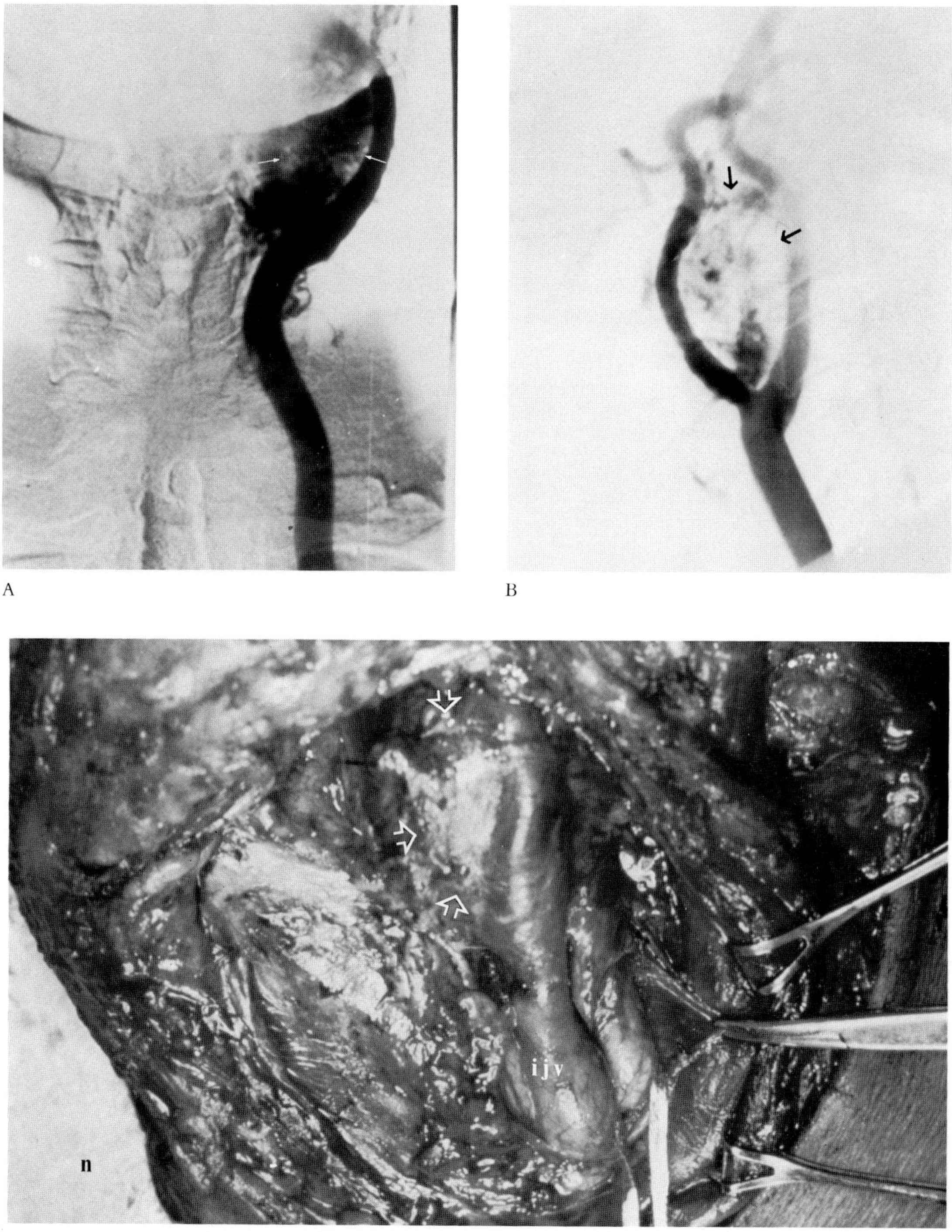

A B C

Figure 2-11. Carotid body tumor. A slowly enlarging, tender, compressible left neck mass was found on physical examination in a 72-year-old woman. Angiography confirmed a highly vascular lesion between the external and internal carotid arteries. Exposure of the carotid sheath (*c*) revealed the mass deep to the posteriorly displaced internal jugular view (*ijv*). A. Lateral view. B. Frontal view. C. Deep lateral.

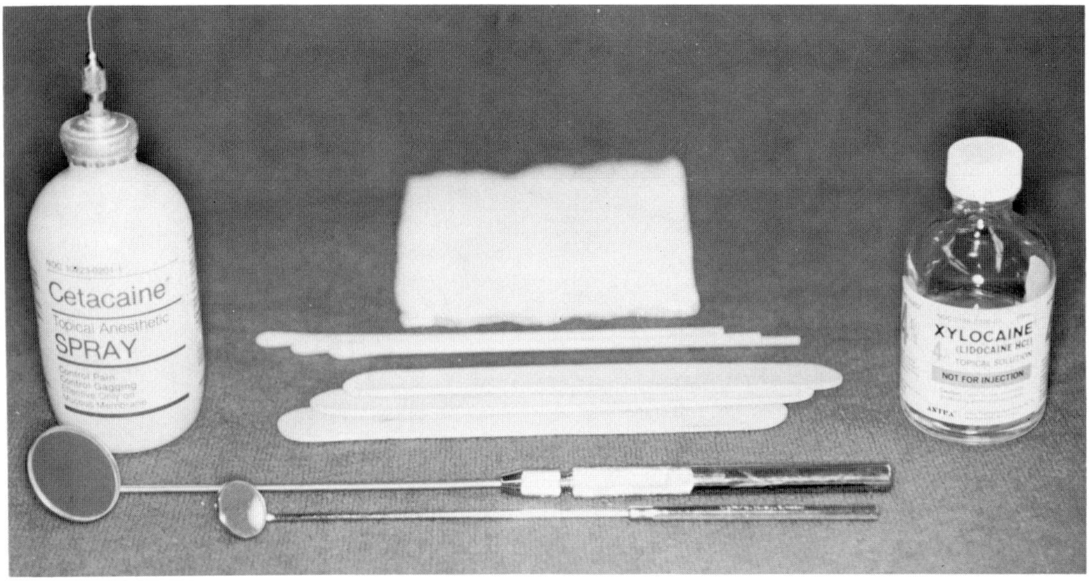

Figure 2-12. The basic equipment for indirect mirror laryngoscopy and nasopharyngoscopy: topical anesthesia, gauze sponges, tongue blades, and mirrors.

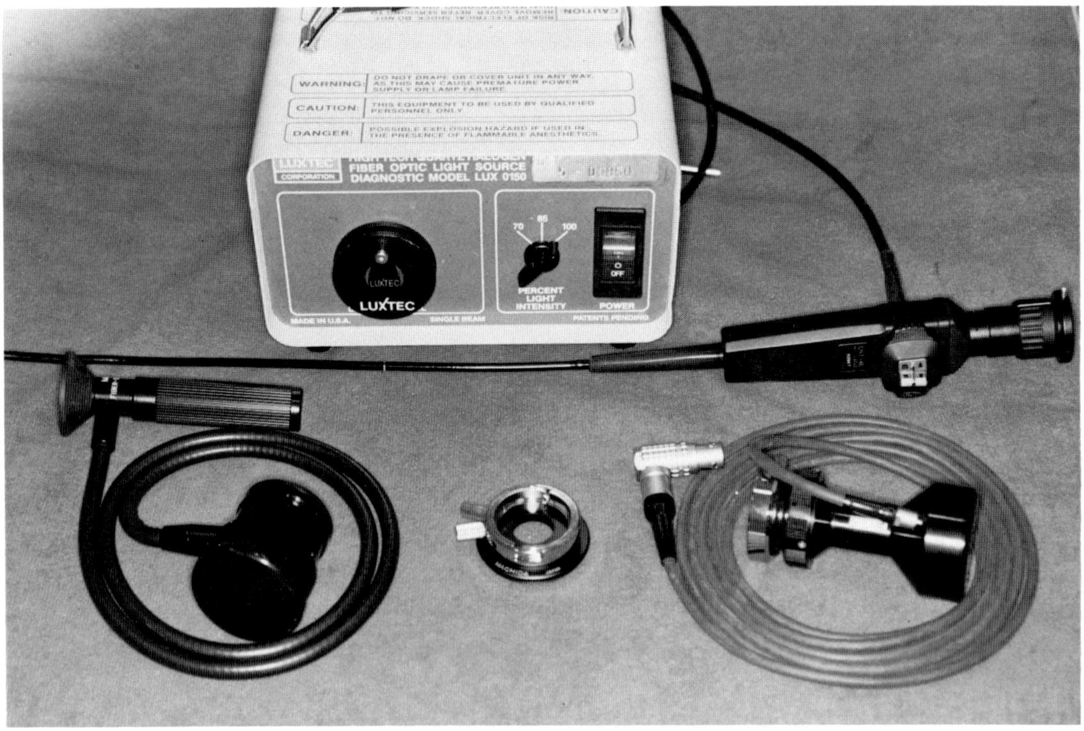

A

Figure 2-13. Fiberoptic nasopharyngoscopy and laryngoscopy. A. The basic equipment (beginning clockwise, centrally): 45-mm adapter for 35-mm SLR camera, observer attachment, light source, flexible fiberoptic laryngoscope, and television camera. (continued)

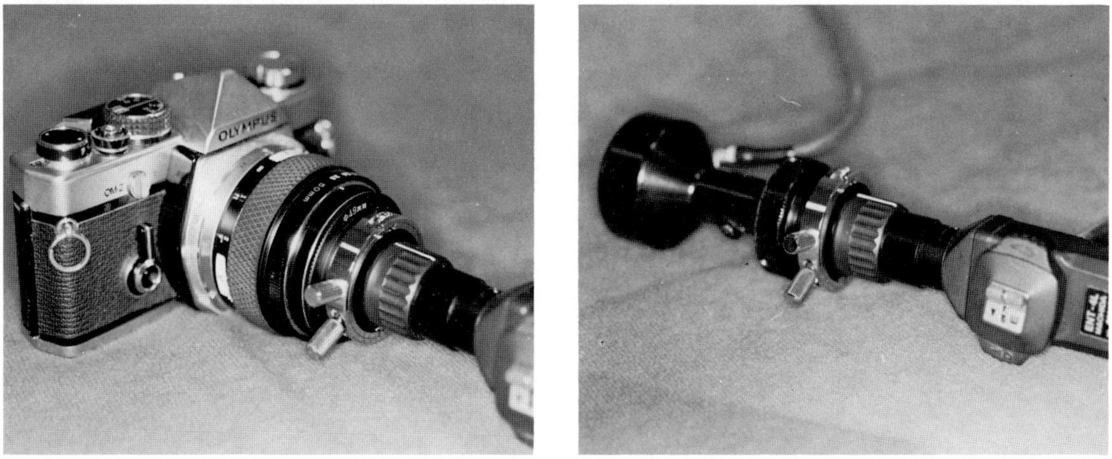

B C

Figure 2-13 (continued). B. Fiberoptic laryngoscope attached to 35-mm SLR camera via 45-mm adapter. C. Television camera attached to fiberoptic laryngoscope.

Figure 2-14. Mirror examination with the headlight or head mirror is the standard examination. Gentle tongue immobilization and avoidance of the tongue base (gag reflex) facilitate the procedure. For problem patients, topical anesthesia is necessary to attenuate the gag reflex.

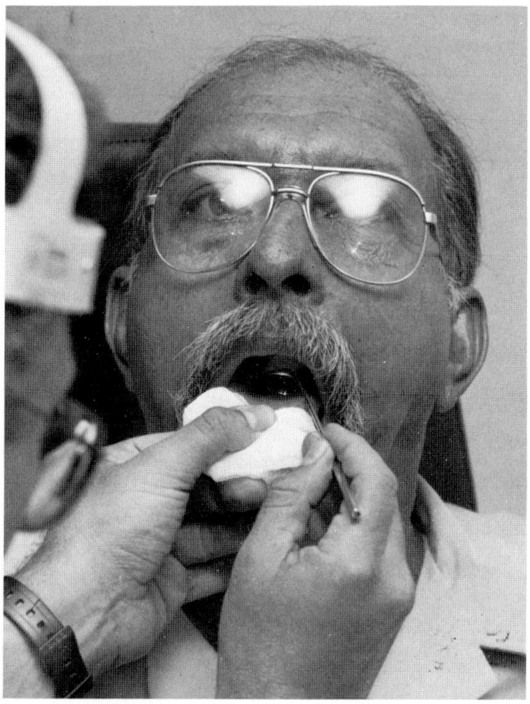

tract examinations with minimal patient discomfort. After anesthetizing the nose with 2% pontocaine or 4% xylocaine spray, the scope is passed through the nose, over the soft palate to the nasopharynx, oropharynx, hypopharynx, and larynx.

The internal examination includes the nose, nasopharynx, oral cavity, oropharynx, hypopharynx, and larynx.

Nose

Aided by a mirror and nasal speculum, the nasal fossae are inspected for inferior turbinate or septal displacement, masses with associated secondary nasal obstruction, mucosal ulceration, and necrosis.

Oral Cavity

With excellent illumination, inspect the floor of the mouth, teeth, gingivae, tongue, tonsils, retromolar trigone, palate, buccal mucosa, and dentition. Some key findings are trismus, impaired tongue mobility or fixation, hypoglossal palsy, tonsillar asymmetry, palatal palsy, and any erythematous or ulcerative lesion. Follow with bimanual palpation.

Nasopharynx

The nasopharynx is visualized either indirectly (by mirror) or directly (by laryngoscope). Indirect largygoscopy is performed by depressing the tongue and inserting the laryngeal mirror past the soft palate. After rotating the mirror superiorly 90 degrees, the choanae, eustachian tubes (especially Rosenmüller's fossae), and posterior pharyngeal wall are inspected. Significant findings are edema, irregularity, nasal vault asymmetry, ulceration, and bleeding.

Hypopharynx and Larynx

The patient sits and faces the examiner (Figure 2-14). The tongue is grasped firmly, pulled anteriorly and inferiorly. The patient is instructed to breathe rhythmically as a warm laryngeal mirror is placed in the oropharynx. With the mirror directed 90 degrees inferiorly, the base of the tongue, epiglottis, lateral pharyngeal walls, pyriform sinuses, and endolarynx are visualized well (Figure 2-15). Ulceration, swelling, pooling of saliva, and vocal cord dysfunction are the significant findings.

REGIONAL ANALYSIS

This section analyzes four of the five major anatomic head and neck regions. The emphasis is on the correlation of complaints with pathogenesis. The fifth region, the neck, is discussed in Chapter 3.

Region I: Face

Chief Complaint

A nonhealing ulcer or enlarging skin eruption is often the chief complaint (Figure 2-16). Facial

Figure 2-15. Schematic view of the larynx and hypopharynx with indirect or direct laryngoscopy. *1* = epiglottis, *2* = valleculae, *3* = false cords, *4* = true vocal cord, *5* = pyriform sinus (left).

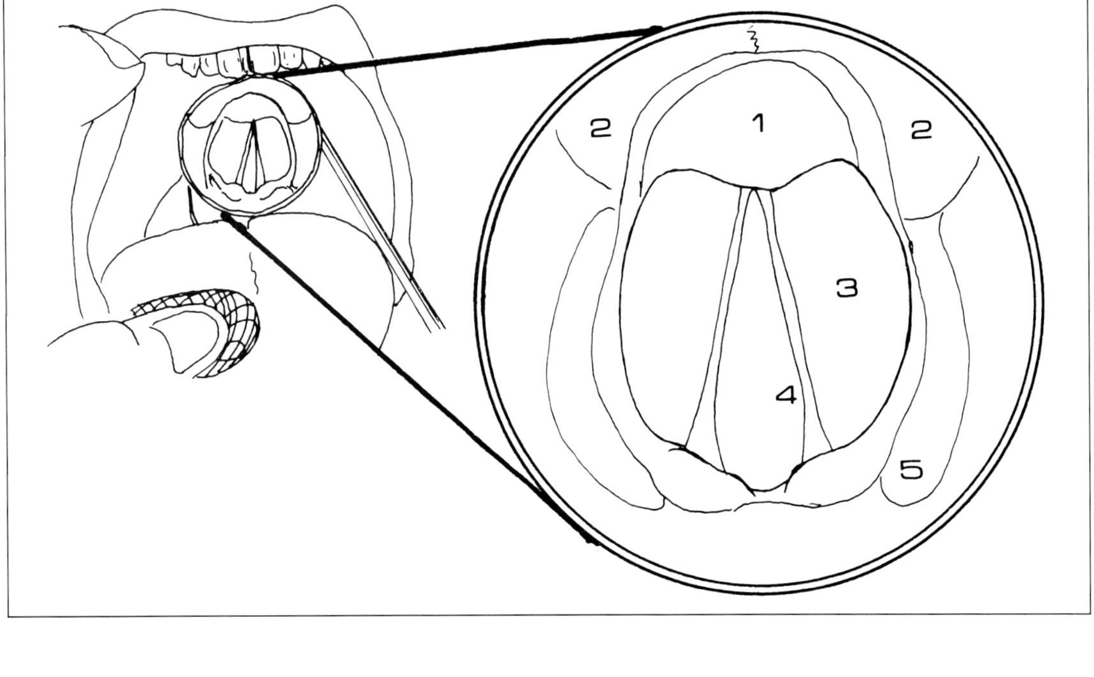

Table 2-3. Clinicopathologic correlation of nasopharyngeal tumor extension

Presentation	*Signs and symptoms*	*Anatomic site*	*Pathologic correlation*
Early	Postnasal irritations (S)	Nasopharynx	Impaired cillia
	Halitosis (S)	Nasopharynx	Accumulated secretions
	Blood streak (0)	Nasopharynx	Mucosal ulceration
Advanced	Cervical node (0)	Posttriangle	Metastasis/retropharynx
	Ear symptoms (S)	Eustachian tube	Obstruction/infiltration
	Nasal obstruction (S)	Nasopharynx, choanae	Large obstructive tumor
	Bleeding (0)	Nasopharynx	Ulceration
Late	Headache (S)	Trigeminal nerve or mininges	Intracranial or perineural invasion
	Diplopia (0)	Orbit, cavern-ous sinus	Involvement of cranial nerve VI
	Ophthalmoplegia (0)	Orbit, cavern-ous sinus	Involvement of cranial nerves III, IV, VI
	Loss of corneal reflex (0)	Orbit, cavern-ous sinus	Involvement of cranial nerve VI
	Decreased lacrimation (0)	Pterygoid canal	Involvement of greater petrosal nerve V
	Ptosis (0)	Carotid artery	Involvement of sympathetic fibers
	Hoarseness (0)	Parapharyngeal space	Involvement of cranial nerve X
	Dysphagia (0)	Parapharyngeal space	Involvement of cranial nerves IX, X
	Trismus (0)	Parapharyngeal space	Involvement of pterygoid muscles
	Drooping shoulders (0)	Parapharyngeal space	Involvement of cranial nerve XI

Sign = objective (0); symptom = subjective (S).

lesions are classed as either primary or secondary. A primary lesion exclusively involves the skin, while a secondary lesion reflects advanced underlying disease or metastasis.

The most common primary skin pathology is basal and squamous cell carcinoma [15]. The exposed areas, forehead, nose, lips, and cheeks, are the usual sites.

Secondary facial involvement suggests advanced upper and midfacial tumors from the orbit, nose, and paranasal sinuses. Lower facial involvement originates from advanced mandibular and parotid gland tumors. Large oropharyngeal tumors, affecting the buccal region, invade submucosally, causing edema and erythema. The breast, lung, and gastrointestinal and genitourinary tracts are the most common sites of distant metastases.

Signs

Lesions greater than 2 to 3 cm imply progressive disease and a poor prognosis [15]. Unfavorable lesions grow rapidly, fix to underlying structures, and involve the ear, periorbita, nose, and deep neck.

Pathogenesis

The early signs are a nonhealing ulcer and skin paresthesias (perineural spread) [15].

The intermediate findings are subcutaneous fixation and invasion of adjacent sites, that is,

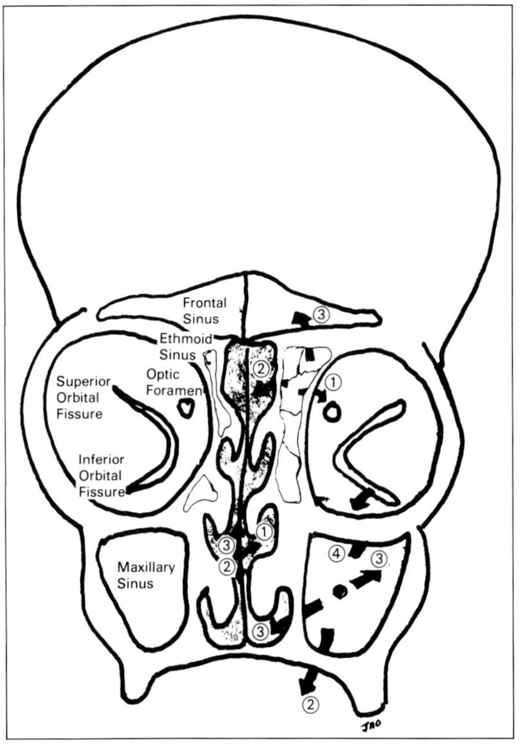

Figure 2-17. Region II: Patterns of tumor spread—nasal and paranasal sites.

Symptoms

Symptoms include headache, visual complaints, nasal obstruction, and loose teeth.

Pathogenesis

The maxillary sinus is the most commonly involved subsite.

Maxillary Sinus

Early maxillary sinus carcinoma mimics sinusitis. Advanced and late symptomatology reflects five routes of potential spread (Table 2-5) [10, 21–23].

Ethmoid Sinuses

Ethmoid tumors spread along four potential routes: laterally, into the orbit; superiorly, into the anterior cranial fossa; posteriorly, into the sphenoid sinus; and inferiorly, into the nose. Early orbital symptoms are pain and retro-orbital headache; advanced signs are diplopia, proptosis, and blindness. Invasion of the anterior cranial fossa may cause unexplained personality changes and anosmia.

Table 2-5. Maxillary sinus pathogenesis

	Symptoms and signs	
Route	***Early***	***Late***
Anterior (soft tissue)	Bulging cheek Loss of nasolabial fold Facial asymmetry Infraorbital nerve involvement	Skin induration Fixation Ulceration
Posterior (pterygomaxillary space)		Infratemporal space Skull base: Trigeminal hypesthesia Trismus Eustachian tube involvement
Medial (nasal vault)	"Sinusitis" "Rhinitis"	"Polyposis" Nasal Obstruction
Superior (orbit)	Infraorbital nerve involvement	Ophthalmoplegia Lower lid swelling Diplopia Blindness
Inferior (alveolar process palate)	Submucosal swelling Loose teeth Poorly fitting dentures	Exuberant granulation Oral-antral fistula

Table 2-6. Orodigestive tract

		Symptoms		*Signs*			
Site	***Subsite***	***Early***	***Late***	***Early***	***Late***	***Pathogenesis***	***Salient features***
Oral cavity	Floor of mouth Anterior tongue	Sore throat "Lump in throat"	Speech complaints	Bleeding Erythematous lesion	Tongue paralysis Neck mass Mandibular invasion Tongue fixation	Erythematous lesion Loose teeth Impaired tongue mobility Soft tissue involvement Mandibular involvement Neck mass	Early: Sore throat Bleeding Odynophagia Late Dysphagia Neck mass Loose teeth Speech complaints Earache Localized pain
	Alveolar process	Sore throat "Lump in throat"	Paresthesias Odynophagia	Mandibular invasion Gingival lesion	Anesthesia V_3 Loose teeth Neck mass		
	Retromolar trigone	Silent	Odynophagia Sore throat	Bleeding lesion	Trismus Anesthesia, V_3 Neck mass		
	Buccal mucosa	Silent	Sore throat	Bleeding lesion	Parotid obstruction Facial paralysis Neck mass		
Oropharynx	Palate	Silent	Sore throat Halitosis Odynophagia Nasal regurgitation	Bleeding lesion	Serous otitis Neck mass	Early nasopharyngeal and pterygoid involvement Neck mass	Early Bleeding Neck mass Earache Sore throat Late Decreased hearing Odynophagia Dysphagia Airway obstruction Localized pain
	Base of tongue	Silent	Sore throat Earache Dysphagia Halitosis	Neck mass Lesion (hidden)	Bleeding		
	Tonsil	Silent	Sore throat Earache Odynophagia Dysphagia Shortness of breath	Neck mass Lesion	Serous otitis media Bleeding		

Sphenoid Sinus
Malignancies in the sphenoid sinus are characterized by headache, diplopia, or cranioneuropathies [24].

Salient Features
Most sinus carcinomas present initially with late symptoms and signs: proptosis, diplopia, ptosis; Horner's syndrome; cavernous sinus invasion; and parapharyngeal space involvement.

Region III: Orodigestive Tract (Sites 5 and 6)

Twenty five percent of all head and neck tumors originate from the orodigestive tract (oral cavity and oropharynx) [25]. The early symptoms are nonspecific: sore throat or a "lump" in the throat (Table 2-6). Pain usually signifies advanced disease. A persistent sore throat or the feeling of a lump in the throat must be investigated aggressively.

Region IV: Aerodigestive Tract—Hypopharynx (Site 7)

Chief Complaint
Despite the various anatomic subsites, the common presenting symptom is sore throat. Unlike an infected sore throat, malignant pain usually is specific and chronic (Table 2-7).

Symptoms
Symptoms include sore throat, earache, and dysphagia.

Pathogenesis
The patterns of spread define symptomatology. Lateral pharyngeal tumors spread laterally and posteriorly: posterior pharyngeal wall tumors spread superiorly or inferiorly [26]. Pyriform sinus tumors, relatively asymptomatic, grow submucosally, and involve the paraglottic space or the posterior cricoid area. Pyriform lesions present with hoarseness, dysphagia, aspiration, and early neck metastasis. Otalgia indicates progressive disease caused by superior laryngeal nerve invasion. Early dysphagia is associated with problems handling liquids, late dysphagia affects both liquids and solids. In addition to dysphagia, odynophagia, dyspnea, hoarseness, weight loss, drooling, persistent cough, excessive secretions, and hematemesis occur singly or in combination. Dyspnea suggests tracheal wall invasion, vocal cord paralysis, or airway obstruction.

Salient Features
The subtle early complaints accurately reflect pathogenesis.

Region IV: Aerodigestive Tract—Larynx (Site 8)

Chief Complaint
The larynx is composed of three subsites: the supraglottis, glottis, and subglottis. The aerodigestive complaints reflect the origin of the lesion such as hoarseness (glottis and subglottis) versus problems with deglutition (supraglottis) (see Chapter 14).

Symptoms
The supraglottis shares deglutition with the hypopharynx; thus early complaints may be ascribed to either subsite (Figure 2-18). Glottic and subglottic lesions are characterized by vocal and airway symptoms. Airway compromise presents early with glottic and subglottic lesions. It is only in the later stages that supraglottic tumors compromise the airway.

Pathogenesis
Both supraglottic and glottic lesions produce gradual, insidious airway obstruction.

Salient Features
Laryngeal lesions are characterized by very early and obvious airway complaints. Airway obstruction and aspiration indicate late disease; neck metastasis occurs early with supraglottic but late with glottic malignancies [3].

Table 2-7. Aerodigestive tract

Site	Subsite	Symptoms: Early	Symptoms: Late	Signs: Early	Signs: Late	Pathogenesis	Salient features
Larynx	Supraglottis	"Lump in throat" Sore throat Earache	Hoarseness Hot potato voice Dysphagia Odynophagia Shortness of breath	Exophytic or ulcerative lesion Neck mass	Vocal cord paralysis Hemoptysis Stridor Airway obstruction	Preepiglottic space Base of tongue Vocal cord paralysis Early unilateral or bilateral cervical metastasis	Early: Sore throat or vague complaints Intermediate: Voice change Late: Airway complaints Frequent early cervical metastasis
	Glottis	Hoarseness	Shortness of breath	Vocal cord lesion	Vocal cord paralysis	Paraglottic space	Early: Hoarseness
	Subglottis	Shortness of breath Hoarseness	Sore throat	Subglottic lesion without cord paralysis	Subglottic lesion with cord paralysis	Preepiglottic space Thyrohyoid membrane Cricoid membrane	Late: Airway complaints Neck mass
Hypopharynx	Lateral pharynx	Sore throat Odynophagia	Decreased hearing		Trismus	Airway involvement	Early: Hoarseness Airway complaints Late: Cervical metastasis
	Posterior pharynx	Sore throat		Exophytic lesion		Paratracheal involvement	
	Pyriform sinus	Sore throat Earache	Hoarseness Shortness of breath		Hoarseness Aspiration Airway obstruction	Cricothyroid membrane Paraglottic space	
	Posterior pharynx Posterior cricoid	Sore throat Odynophagia	Dysphagia		Aspiration	Base of tongue Early unilateral and bilateral cervical metastasis	Early: Cervical metastasis Sore throat Earache Late: Airway obstruction Aspiration

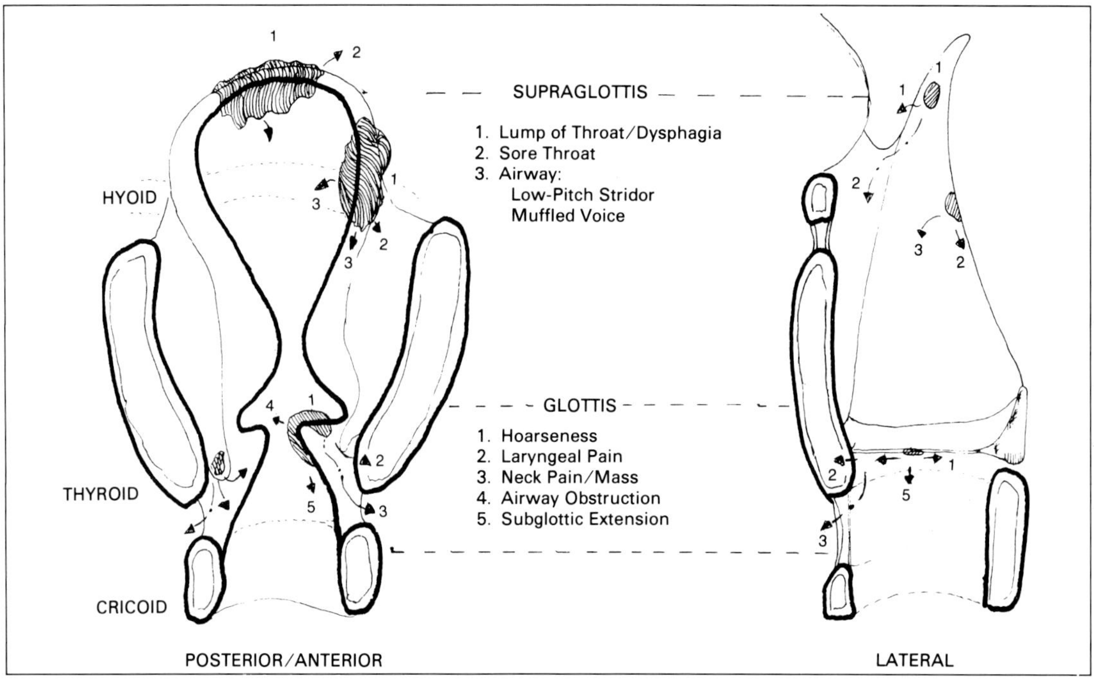

Figure 2-18. Aerodigestive tract complaints.

REFERENCES

1. Becker S. Atijan RA: Nasal and paranasal malignancies. Otolaryngol Clin North Am 18(3) : 491, 1985.
2. Millon R, Cassisi NJ: Oropharynx. In: *Management of Head and Neck Cancer*. Philadelphia: Lippincott, 1984.
3. Spector JG: *Diagnosis and Treatment of Cancer of the Larynx: Self-Instructional Package*. Rochester, MN: American Academy of Otolaryngology, 1978. Pp 28–30.
4. McGregor I, McGregor FM: Lips. In: *Cancer of the Face and Mouth: Pathology and Management for Surgeons*. New York: Churchill Livingstone, 1986.
5. Batsakis J: *Tumors of the Head and Neck: Clinicopathological Considerations*. Baltimore: Williams & Wilkins, 1974. P 195.
6. Batsakis SR: Malignant Neoplasms of the Oral Cavity. In Cummings C, et al (eds): *Otolaryngology: Head and Neck Surgery*. St. Louis: Mosby, 1986.
7. Millon R, Cassisi NJ: Larynx. In: *Management of Head and Neck Cancer*. Philadelphia: Lippincott, 1984.
8. Batsakis J, McBoney T: Metastatic neoplasms to the head and neck. *Surg Gynecol Obstet* 133 : 673, 1971.
9. Castro K, et al: Acquired immunodeficiency syndrome: Epidemiology and risk factors for transmission. *Med Clin North Am* 76(3) : 635, 1986.
10. Rice DH: Benign and malignant tumors of the ethmoid sinuses. *Otolaryngol Clin North Am* 18(1) : 117, 1985.
11. Vaughn C, et al: Work-up and treatment planning for head and neck cancer. *Otolaryngol Clin North Am* 18(3) : 403, 1985.
12. Weitz H, Goldman L: Non-cardiac surgery in the patient with heart disease. *Med Clin North Am* 71(3) : 478, 1987.
13. Jesse RH: General Considerations. In Suen J, Myers EN (eds): *Cancer of the Head and Neck*. New York: Churchill Livingstone, 1981.
14. Lee KJ, Vris J: Otolaryngology: Head and Neck Physical Diagnosis—Ambulatory Surgery and Office Procedures. In Kee K, Stewart C (eds): *Head and Neck Surgery*. Orlando, FL: Grune & Stratton, 1986.
15. Goepert H, et al: Perineural invasion in squamous cell skin carcinoma of the head and neck. *Am J Surg* 148 : 542, 1984.
16. Neel BH: Nasopharyngeal carcinoma. *Otolaryngol Clin North Am* 18 : 481, 1985.
17. Snow J: Carcinoma of the nasopharynx in children. *Ann Otol Rhinol Laryngol* 84 : 820, 1975.
18. Som P, Biller H, et al: Tumors of the para-

pharyngeal space preoperative evaluation: Diagnosis and surgical approaches. *Ann Otol Rhinol Laryngol* 122 : 5, 1981.
19. Stell PM, et al: Surgical approaches to tumors of the parapharyngeal space. *Am J Otolaryngol* 2 : 93, 1985.
20. Heeneman H, et al: *The Parapharyngeal Space: Anatomy and Pathologic Conditions with Emphasis on Neurogenous Tumors. Self-Instructional Package,* (2nd ed). Rochester, MN: American Academy of Otolaryngology, Pp 24–26.
21. Bennett M: Paranasal sinus malignancies. *Laryngoscope* 80 : 933, 1970.
22. Robinson P: Cancer of the head. *JAMA* 219 : 336, 1971.
23. St. Pierre S, Baker S: Squamous cell carcinoma of the maxillary sinus: Analysis of 66 cases. *Head Neck Surg* 5 : 509, 1983.
24. Moore G, et al: Abducens nerve paralysis: A potential presentation of sphenoid sinus cancer. *Otolaryngol Head Neck Surg* 94 : 249, 1985.
25. Beerkhold RE: Carcinoma of oral cavity: Symposium on squamous cell cancer of the head and neck. *Otolaryngl Clin* 18 : 445, 1985.
26. Schuller, D: *Management of Epidermoid Cancer of the Oral Cavity: Self-instructional package (Sipac).* Rochester, MN: American Academy of Otolaryngology, 1980. Pp 28–29.

3

Neck Mass

ERNEST M. MYERS

KEY CONCEPTS

Simpson's Dictums; Basic Workup; Differential Diagnosis; Special Neck Masses

MILESTONES

1902	Head and Neck Lymphatics	Polya
1938	Thyroid Lymphatics	Rouviere
1942	Treatise on the Lymphatic System	Drinker
1944	Head and Neck Cancer and Cervical Metastasis	Martin
1955	Microscopic Cervical Metastases	Frazell and Foote
1973	Fine-Needle Aspiration	Crile and Hawk

In 12 percent of all head and neck cancer patients, a neck mass is the only presenting sign [1]. This medical and surgical challenge requires careful consideration and systematic investigation. A comprehensive understanding of physiology and anatomy is paramount to avoid glaring and possibly deadly errors (Table 3-1). Haphazard and confused workups waste time, money, and life. Efficient diagnosis and logical management dramatically affect prognosis. Finally, the proper workup of the occult neck mass is an esthetic and intellectually rewarding endeavor.

BASIC WORKUP

History

Duration

Until recently, Skandelakis's "rule of sevens" was invaluable: a mass present for 7 days is inflammatory; 7 months, neoplastic; 7 years, congenital (Table 3-2) [2]. Today, acquired immunodeficiency disease (AIDS) alters this aphorism drastically [3–6]. Therefore, it is imperative that the physician obtain an accurate social and personal habits history.

Age

In the pediatric population, most neck masses are congenital or inflammatory, whereas in the adult, neoplasm is the primary consideration.

Sex

In women, there is a higher association of occult neck metastasis from the genitourinary systems, breast, and thyroid (Table 3-3). Overall, head and neck malignancies predominate in men by a 4 : 1 ratio.

Race

In general, there is a higher association of head and neck malignancies, especially of the oropharynx, oral cavity, larynx, and esophagus, in blacks as compared to whites.

Habits

As stated in Chapter 1, a strong history of tobacco or alcohol usage or radiation exposure implicates malignancy in the adult.

Table 3-1. Systems found in the neck

System	*Structure*
Integument	Scalp Neck skin Beard
Cardiovascular	Carotid artery Thyrocervical trunk Subclavian artery Innominate artery Internal jugular vein External jugular vein
Nervous	Sympathetics Nodose ganglia Sympathetic trunk Parasympathetics Carotid body Lingual nerve Facial nerve Glossopharyngeal nerve Spinal accessory nerve Hypoglossal nerve Superior laryngeal nerve Recurrent laryngeal nerve Peripheral nerves Phrenic nerve Brachial plexus
Endocrine	Thyroid gland Parathyroids
Gastrointestinal	Salivary glands Tongue Pharynx Esophagus
Hematopoietic	Thymus Lymph nodes Thoracic duct
Musculoskeletal	Cervical spine Mandible Scapula Clavicle Cervical musculature
Respiratory	Larynx Trachea Lungs (apices)

Physical Examination

The foundation of the diagnostic inquiry is the physical examination (see Chapter 2). Precise location of the primary site as well as the cervical metastasis is the beginning of an efficient workup. The physical examination is exhaustive. In addition to a thorough head and neck examination, the following systems are emphasized: the integumental, neurologic, gastrointestinal, respiratory, lymphatic, musculoskeletal, endocrine, and genitourinary systems (Table 3-4).

Table 3-2. Simpson's dictums

1. Adult neck masses are considered neoplastic, until proven otherwise.
2. Most neck masses originate from the head and neck.
3. Location is most important.
4. Histology determines treatment.
5. Some primaries remain occult.
6. Avoid incisional biopsy.

Source: Adapted from Simpson GT: The evaluation and management of neck masses of unknown etiology. *Otolaryngol Clin North Am* 13(3) : 489, 1980.

Table 3-3. Occult metastasis: site predilections

Site	*Rank*
1. Nasopharynx	1
2. Sinuses/nose	7
3. Salivary glands	6
4. Lips	10
5. Oral cavity	5
6. Oropharynx	2
7. Hypopharynx	3
8. Larynx	9
9. Thyroid/parathyroids	4
10. Cervical esophagus	8

Location

More than any other factor, location is the most helpful (Tables 3-5 and 3-6). For example, a left-sided supraclavicular neck mass has a strong association with an intra-abdominal malignancy. The more proximal the location (level I, II, or III), the more likely the primary lesion is in the head and neck (Figure 3-1). Conversely, the more distal the location (level IV or V), the more likely the origin is below the clavicle. Bilaterality most frequently is associated with metastasis from the nasopharynx, supraglottis, base of the tongue, and midline oral cavity.

Pain

Most malignant neck masses are asymptomatic. However, pain associated with fixation is almost pathognomonic for malignancy.

Table 3-4. Occult neck mass: system versus pathology

System	*Neoplasm*
Integument	Melanoma
Musculoskeletal	Osteogenic sarcoma Rhabdomyosarcoma
Nervous	Neuroblastoma Retinoblastoma
Vascular	Hemangioma Glomus jugulare, vagale Carotid body tumor Angiofibroma
Respiratory	Bronchogenic cancer Undifferentiated cancer Adenocarcinoma
Gastrointestinal	Esophageal cancer Stomach cancer Biliary tract cancer Pancreatic cancer Colon cancer
Genitourinary	
Male	Testicular cancer
Female	Cervical cancer Uterine cancer Ovarian cancer
Both	Renal cell cancer Bladder cancer
Endocrine	Breast cancer
Hematopoietic	Hodgkin's disease Lymphoma

Consistency

Malignancies are rubbery or rock-hard. Fluctuant or cystic masses are inflammatory, hematologic, or congenital in origin.

Fixation

As previously noted, fixation implies malignancy and signifies a poor prognosis.

Diagnostic Radiology

The routine films are the chest, neck (soft tissue), and sinus series (see Chapter 4). If there are signs of an oral cavity or oropharyngeal origin, a panorex or bone scan is ordered.

Laboratory

Basic laboratory screening includes complete blood count (CBC) and differential, multichannel hematologic screening, urinalysis, and possibly HIV titers. Based on the history, intermediate PPD, a viral panel or HIV titer is requested.

Panendoscopy and Biopsy

Endoscopy remains the diagnostic cornerstone and is included in most comprehensive workups (Tables 3-7 and 3-8). However, time and cost-effectiveness dictate selectivity. This depends

Table 3-5. Neck mass: site versus level

		Level				
Site	*Preauricular*	*I*	*II*	*III*	*IV*	*V*
1. Nasopharynx	+	−	+ + +	+ +	+ +	+ +
2. Sinus/nose	+ + +	+/−	+ + +	−	−	−
3. Salivary glands	+ + +	+ +	+ + +	+ +	−	−
4. Lips	−	+ + +	+ +	−	−	−
5. Oral cavity	−	+ + +	+ + +	+ +	+	−
6. Oropharynx	−	+ +	+ + +	+ +	+	−
7. Hypopharynx	−	−	+/−	+ + +	+ + +	+ +
8. Larynx	−	−	+ +	+ + +	+ + +	+ +
9. Thyroid/parathyroids	−	−	−	+ +	+ + +	+ +
10. Cervical esophagus	−	−	−	−	+ + +	+ + +

+ + + Likely.
+ + Probable.
+ Possible.
− Unlikely.
+/− Equivocal.

Table 3-6. Cervical metastasis: site versus location

Site	*Submental/ Submandibular*	*Jugulodigastric*	*Midjugular*	*Distal Jugular*	*Posterior Cervical*
1. Nasopharynx[c]		+	+	+	
2. Sinus/nose[a]		+			
3. Salivary glands	+	+			
4. Lips[b]	+				
5. Oral cavity[c]	+	+			
6. Oropharynx[c]	+	+	+		
7. Hypopharynx[c]			+		
8. Larynx[b]			+		
9. Thyroid/ parathyroids			+	+	
10. Esophagus[a]				+	+

+Primary presentation.
[a]Late cervical metastasis.
[b]Rare cervical metastasis; supraglottic larynx is exception in the larynx.
[c]Early cervical metastasis (particularly retromolar trigone, buccal mucosa and base of tongue).

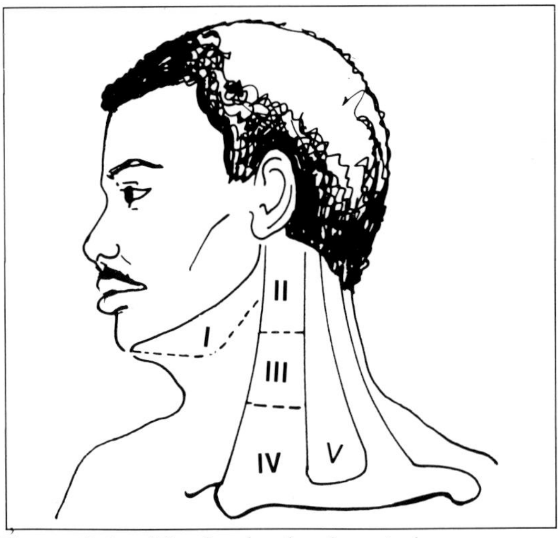

Figure 3-1. The five levels of cervical metastasis. Level I includes the submental and submandibular triangles. Levels II, III, and IV include the deep cervical fat pad or anterior cervical triangle. Level V is the posterior cervical triangle.

on the initial suspicion of the system that is involved. If after a thorough head and neck examination and a general physical examination no obvious lesions are found, panendoscopy and biopsy are performed for level I through III neck masses. During panendoscopy, if no obvious lesion is found endoscopically, blind biopsy of the nasopharynx tonsil, tongue, and

Table 3-7. Basic workup

Physical examination
- Scalp and skin
- Head and neck
- Thorax and lungs
- Breasts and axillae
- Abdomen
- Pelvis and genitalia
- Rectum

Laboratory
- CBC
- Multiphasic Screening
- Urinalysis
- HIV*
- PPD*

Diagnostic radiology
- Chest anteroposterior and lateral
- Soft tissue anteroposterior and lateral neck*
- Sinus series*
- Panorex*
- CT scan*

Endoscopy
- Indirect nasopharyngoscopy
- Indirect laryngoscopy
- Flexible endoscopy*

Empirical trial of antibiotics*

*When so indicated by chief complaint, history, or physical examination.

Table 3-8. Special diagnostic workups

System	Laboratory	Diagnostic radiology	Endoscopy	Fine-needle aspiration	Special studies	Other considerations
Respiratory	Arterial blood gases Tubercular skin tests HIV	CT—lung CT—mediastinum	Bronchoscopy Esophagoscopy	Possibility	Mediastinoscopy	Pulmonary function studies Flow loop studies
Gastrointestinal						
Salivary glands	Rheumatoid factor HIV	CT—neck Sialogram	No	Possibility	Salivary gland scan	No
Upper/lower GI tract	SMA-12 Stool guaiac	Upper/lower GI series CT—abdomen	Fiberoptic panendoscopy	No	Liver-spleen scan Gallbladder series	Laparoscopy
Vascular	No	CT—neck CT—sinuses CT—brain	No	No!!	Angiography	Visual fields/acuity Audiometry
Endocrine						
Breast	SMA-12	Mammography CT—lung CT—mediastinum	No	Yes	Assay for estrogen receptors	Bone scan
Thyroid	Serum calcium Serum phosphorus Triiodothyronine (T_3) Thyroxine (T_4) Thyroid-stimulating hormone Calcitonin	Technetium scan Iodine scan CT—neck CT—mediastinum	Laryngoscopy	Yes!!	Sonography	Barium swallow
Genitourinary	Urinanalysis Acid phosphatase SMA-12	CT—abdomen CT—pelvis Bone scan Intravenous pyelogram	Uroscopy	Possible under CT or sonographic control	Laparoscopy	Urine for creatinine clearance, protein, gonadotropins
Hematopoietic	CBC HIV Bone marrow	CT—neck CT—mediastinum CT—abdomen	Nasopharyngoscopy Laryngoscopy	Yes	Liver-spleen scan Lymphangiogram	Anergy panel

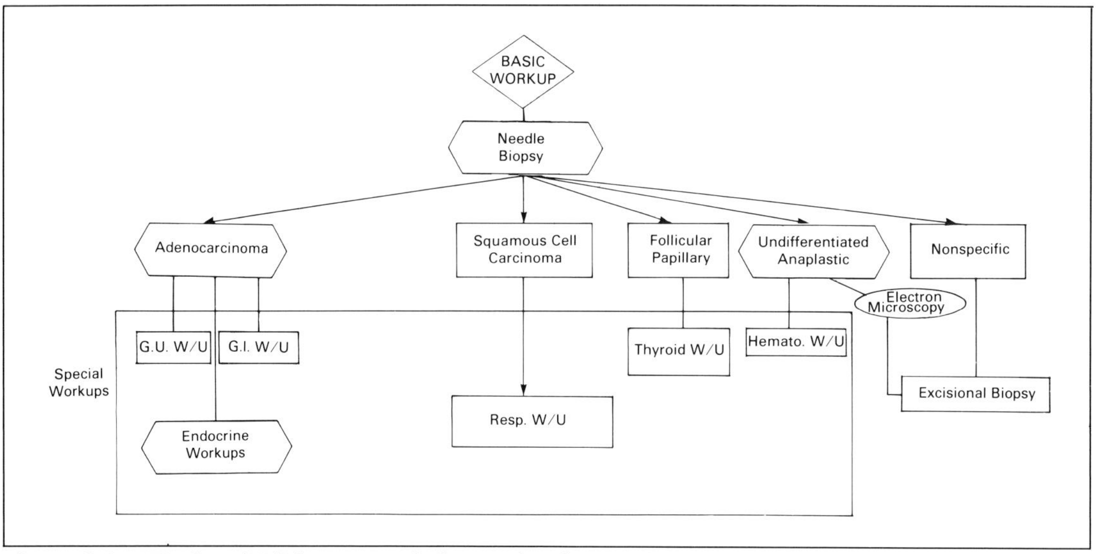

Figure 3-2. Workup (*W/U*) versus pathology. The ultimate decision as to subsequent workup(s) is predicated upon histopathology. For small masses, needle biopsy should be performed under sonographic control. *G.U.* = genitourinary; *G.I.* = gastrointestinal; *Resp.* = respiratory; *Hemato.* = hematologic.

hypopharynx ipsilateral to the lesion is performed; realistically, the yield is poor.

Needle Biopsy

For selected neck masses, fine-needle aspiration in lieu of panendoscopy streamlines the workup [8,14–18]. Fine-needle aspiration is indicated for level IV or V masses, whereas masses involving other levels require panendoscopy (Figure 3-2). To ensure safety and accuracy, fine-needle aspiration under sonographic control is recommended (Figure 3-3).

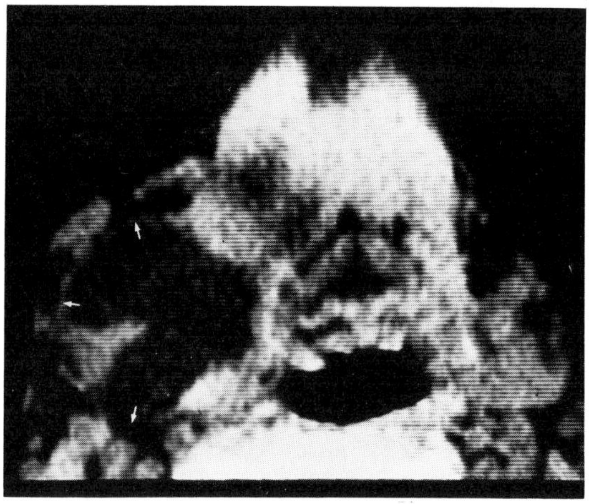

Figure 3-3. Fine-needle aspiration of this large, fluid-filled mass in a 23-year-old man unveiled chronic inflammation and many lymphocytes. The mass involved the submandibular and anterior cervical triangles. Neck exploration revealed a cystic hygroma.

DIFFERENTIAL DIAGNOSIS

Infection

Regardless of location, if the neck mass is tender or associated with overlying erythema, "infection" is included in the differential diagnosis. This is a very strong consideration if the patient is young (age 20–40 years) or denies the common neoplastic risk factors. Three infectious diseases are confused with malignancy: AIDS, tuberculosis, and syphilis. As a general dictum, for cost-effectiveness and safety, infection is ruled out before other diagnoses are pursued.

AIDS

Yearly, the number of AIDS cases escalates exponentially. In some geographic areas it approaches epidemic proportions (i.e., subequatorial Africa and large North American and

European urban areas). First the sexual proclivities of the patient are determined, since homosexuality and bisexuality are associated strongly with this condition. Has the patient had a sexual liaison with a known drug addict, prostitute, or bisexual? Second, race and ethnicity are important, since AIDS is more common in blacks, Haitians, and Hispanics. Third, the location and description of the mass is considered; AIDS manifests as multiple, bilateral rubbery nodes. Fourth, AIDS lymphadenopathy is associated with generalized adenopathy in the groin and axillae. Fifth, has the patient indulged in past or present intravenous drug abuse? Finally, some clinicians have found a synchronous association with other malignancies [6]. If the diagnosis is suspected, a human immune viral (HIV) assay is obtained.

Tuberculosis

Despite stringent public health measures, the incidence of tuberculosis remains surprisingly high. Many physicians do not realize that tuberculosis is associated with unilateral or bilateral cervical lymphadenopathy (scrofula) (Figure 3-4). If tuberculosis is suspected, the patient is queried as to life-style and contact with known tuberculosis patients. Classically, tuberculosis occurs in populations living in crowded and transient conditions. A patient's living arrangements are extremely important in determining the likelihood of contracting the disease. When tuberculosis is suspected, a chest x-ray and PPD are obtained.

Figure 3-4. A 47-year-old renal dialysis patient slowly developed a large anterior cervical triangle mass. Incisional biopsy after panendoscopy revealed granulomas consistent with atypical tuberculosis. Computed tomography (CT) scan shows a cystic mass occupying the left carotid sheath.

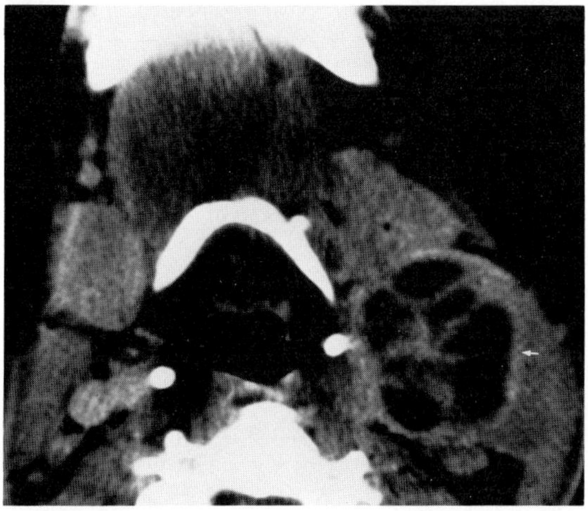

Syphilis

As with the previous infections, syphilis or lues is related to life-style. Cunnilingus and fellatio, particularly with bisexuals or homosexuals, is associated with syphilis. Oral syphilis presents initially as an ulcer on the lips, tongue, or buccal mucosa that rapidly heals. This is followed by regional lymphadenopathy (ipsilateral or contralateral), either submental or submandibular. When suspected, a VDRL or, more specifically, fluorescent treponemal antibody absorption (FTA-ABS) test is obtained.

Lymphomas

Lymphomas are a heterogenous group of malignant neoplasms of the lymphoreticular system characterized by local or generalized lymphadenopathy (see Chapter 4). Head and neck lymphomas are rare but are easily diagnosed when the physician is vigilant. If a patient is between 15 and 40 or between 60 and 80, this diagnosis is a definite possibility. In the first age group (15–40), this is a strong consideration if infections or carcinogens are nonexistent. However, in the older age group (60–80), carcinoma is a strong possibility.

Hodgkin's Disease

Hodgkin's disease presents in the neck (60–80%) within a single lymph node chain and spreads secondarily to other regional groups. Hodgkin's disease is associated with constitutional symptoms such as fever, night sweats, and weight loss. The neck nodes are rubbery, nontender, and may be accompanied by hepatosplenomegaly. The diagnosis is determined by the histologic relationship of lymphocytes and histiocytes. Reed-Sternberg cells are almost pathognomonic. Depending on the stage (Table 3-9), the treatment is either chemotherapy or radiation therapy.

Table 3-9. Classification of lymphomas

Stage I	One node chain
Stage II	Two or more lymph node chains, ipsilateral to the diaphragm
Stage III	Lymph node involvement of two or more chains, above and below the diaphragm
Stage IV	Generalized disease

Non-Hodgkin's Lymphoma

Non-Hodgkin's lymphoma is characterized by cervical lymphadenopathy and Waldeyer's ring involvement, without associated constitutional symptoms. Note the similarities to AIDS. The general overall physical findings are indistinguishable from lymphomas disease. Pathologic analysis (excisional biopsy) is characterized by well-differentiated lymphocytes, histiocytes, or poorly differentiated lymphocytes. The last finding may be confused with anaplastic carcinoma. If the diagnosis is equivocal, electron microscopy is very helpful. Depending on the stage, the treatment is either chemotherapy or radiotherapy.

Diagnosis

Classically, lymphomas are located in the posterior cervical triangle, either ipsilateral or bilateral. A thorough general physical examination is performed, emphasizing the axillae, groin, and abdomen (liver, spleen). The CBC and differential may show a high white count or lymphocytosis, but more often it is normal. Excisional biopsy is preferable to fine-needle aspiration, since small samples are difficult to analyze. The following workup is suggested for diagnosis and accurate staging: chest and abdominal computed tomography (CT) scans, bone marrow aspirate, and possibly lymphangiogram.

Extracervical Malignancy

Breast Cancer

Breast cancer is a definite consideration if the mass is in the supraclavicular (level V) area. Of course, when suspected, a careful breast and axillary examination is extremely important. Although rare in men, this diagnosis is still possible. After a thorough physical examination, chest x-ray and fine-needle aspiration are suggested. Early needle aspiration is both cost-effective and efficient.

Lung Cancer

Although not common, bronchogenic adenocarcinoma metastasizes to the neck, especially to levels IV and V. A screening chest x-ray usually confirms the diagnosis. For the suspicious chest lesion, the following workup is suggested: (1) mediastinal and lung CT scan, (2) flexible bronchoscopy with cytology or brush biopsy, (3) mediastinoscopy, and (4) percutaneous (fluoroscopy or CT guided) transthoracic needle biopsy.

Gastrointestinal Malignancy

The classic head and neck physical finding with gastrointestinal malignancy is a left supraclavicular or Virchow's node. Masses in this area are highly suspicious for gastrointestinal malignancies. The order of suspicion is esophagus, stomach, and pancreas. Again, fine-needle aspiration is invaluable for tissue diagnosis. The workup is as follows: (1) upper and lower gastrointestinal series, (2) abdominal CT scan, and (3) fiberoptic panendoscopy or colonoscopy.

Genitourinary Malignancy

Genitourinary malignancies, especially renal cell carcinomas, metastasize to the neck (level V). In the female patient, ovarian or cervical cancer is a possible source for neck metastasis. Rectal and pelvic examinations are followed by (1) abdominal and pelvic CT scan, (2) intravenous pyelogram, (3) barium enema, (4) retrograde urography, and (5) laparoscopy. Appropriate consultation is most helpful in determining the magnitude and scope of the workup.

SPECIAL NECK MASSES

Special neck masses are masses that arise from areas other than the classic cervical triangles.

Parotid Space

The parotid space is a rhomboid-shaped space bounded by the zygomatic arch and skull base (superior), superficial cervical fascia (lateral),

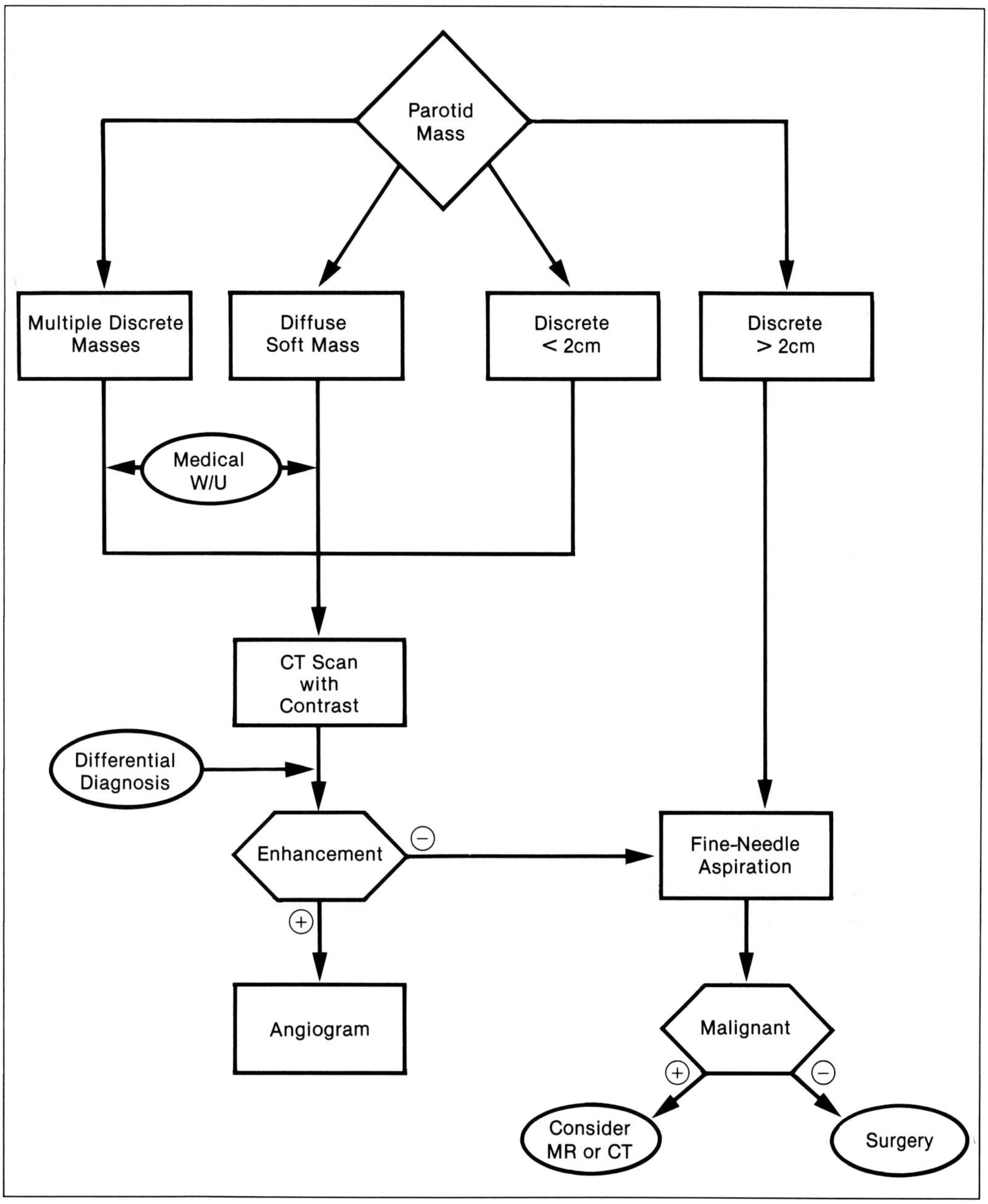

Figure 3-5. The parotid mass. The initial diagnostic decision is predicated on whether the mass is diffuse or discrete. MRI or CT scan is the definitive diagnostic modality. Medical workup includes chest x-ray, intermediate PPD, and HIV titers when indicated.

buccinator (anterior), ascending ramus and parapharyngeal space (medial), and the styloid process (posterior).

Contents
The contents within the parotid space are (1) superficial and deep parotid lobes, (2) facial nerve, (3) ascending ramus, and (4) deep facial and parotid lymphatics (see also Chapter 2).

Lymphatics
The lymphatics consist of afferents (orbit, paranasal sinuses, scalp external auditory canal) and efferents (submandibular nodes, superior deep cervical lymph nodes) (see also Chapter 16).

Neoplasms
The parotid space may be involved by metastases from the parapharyngeal space and paranasal sinuses; primary malignant and benign parotid neoplasms; cavernous hemangiomas; benign, malignant neoplasms of the mandible; and lymphomas (Table 3-10; Figures 3-5 through 3-8).

Parapharyngeal Space

The parapharyngeal is a potential, inverted, cone-shaped space, roughly bounded by the skull base (superior), ascending ramus (lateral), pterygoids (medial), parotid gland (posterolateral), superior constrictor (medial), carotid sheath (posterior), buccinator muscle fascia (anterior), and hyoid bone (inferior or apex) (see Figure 3-9).

Contents
The contents of the parapharyngeal space may be divided into three components. The prestyloid compartment includes the internal max-

Figure 3-6. Moderate size tail of parotid mass in a 45-year-old man. Superficial parotidectomy revealed a Warthin's tumor.

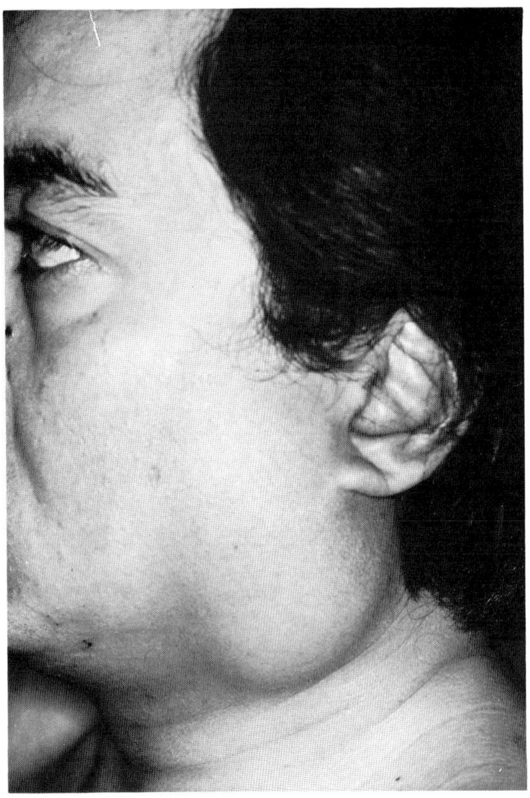

A

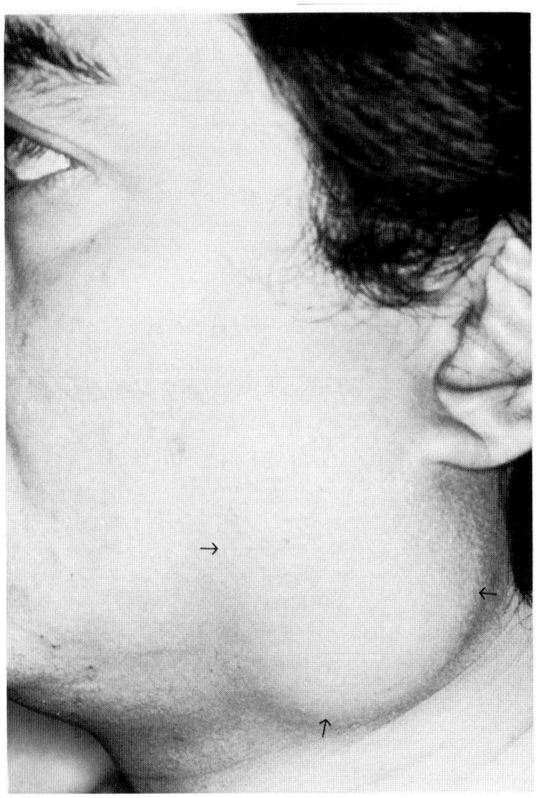

B

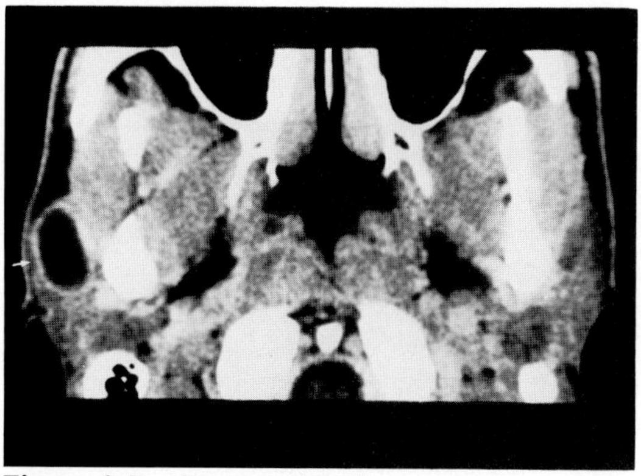

Figure 3-7. Despite several courses of antibiotics over 6 months, this cystic preauricular mass persisted. Fine-needle aspirate was consistent with pleomorphic adenoma. Superficial parotidectomy confirmed the pathologic diagnosis.

Table 3-10. Parotid space mass

Medical Workup
HIV
Rheumatoid factor
Mumps titer
Heterophile
PPD
Differential diagnosis
Parotid neoplasm
Masseter hypertrophy
Mandibular neoplasm
Parapharyngeal space neoplasm
Arteriovenous malformation
Facial neuroma

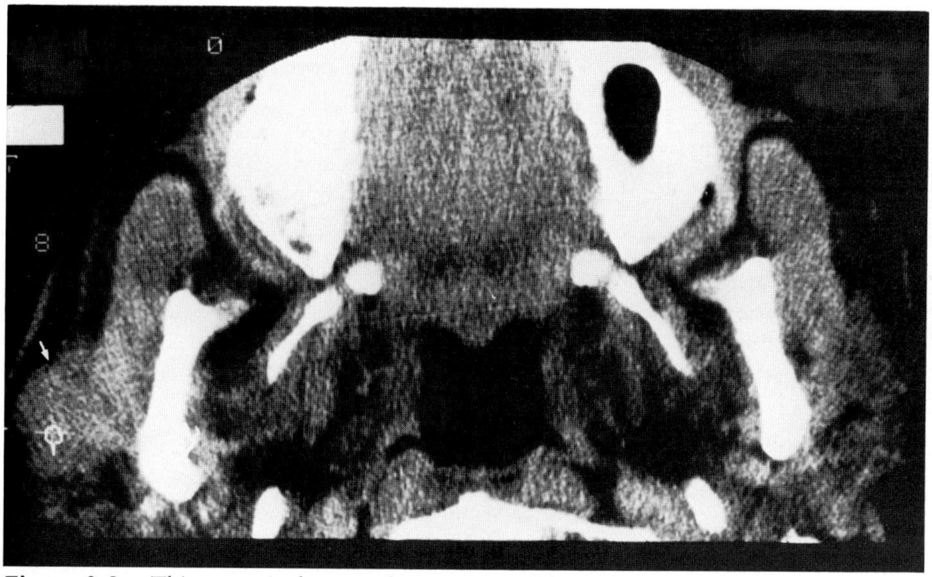

Figure 3-8. This preauricular mass has a more solid consistency; however, the diagnosis is again pleomorphic adenoid.

illary artery; and inferior alveolar, lingual, and auriculotemporal nerves.

The poststyloid compartment encompasses the internal carotid artery; internal jugular vein; cranial nerves IX, X, and XII; sympathetic chain; and lymph nodes.

The third component is the retropharyngeal space and medial extension of parapharyngeal space.

Lymphatics and vessels

Parapharyngeal space lymphatics are afferents from the nasopharynx (node of Rouviere, anterior and posterior pharyngeal wall, and submandibular nodes) and efferents to the superior deep cervical lymph nodes, spinal accessory chain, and transverse cervical chain. The vessels include the carotid artery and internal jugular vein (Figure 3-10).

Neoplasms

Lymphoma, carcinoma of the nasopharynx, deep parotid lobe neoplasms, glomus jugulare and vagale are neoplasms found in the parapharyngeal space.

DIAGNOSTIC ORCHESTRATION

After the first visit, a rapid workup is initiated. If the head and neck examination is negative, several systems are investigated simultaneously. This pursuit along several pathways is guided by both history and neck mass location. Depending on the patient and the vagaries of each institution, a workup is completed within 7 to 10 days.

Rapid Diagnosis

An example of a rapid diagnostic workup is as follows (Table 3-11):

Day 1: History and physical examination.
Indirect and/or direct endoscopy.
Initiation of basic workup.
Scheduling of special procedures.
Trial of antibiotics.
Tentative scheduling of panendoscopy or fine-needle aspiration (for day 6).

Days 2–4: Special procedures.

Day 5: Review of special procedure results with the patient.

Day 6: Panendoscopy with frozen section. If the frozen section is equivocal, a sample is sent for electron microscopy.

Day 7: Final pathologic interpretation and discussion with the patient.

If the biopsy is nonspecific or anaplastic, a delay of 1 to 2 weeks is required for electron microscopic interpretation. It is urged strongly that a sample of the original biopsy (panendoscopy or fine-needle aspiration) be reserved for this contingency. In general, speed and accuracy are of utmost importance. After all, who is to say how long the tumor has been present? Furthermore, delays usually are preceded and compounded by patient or physician procrastination (see Chapter 19).

Frozen Section

At the time of panendoscopy or needle biopsy, a frozen section is obtained (see Chapter 4). This has several advantages: First, it determines if a second sample must be obtained; second, it dictates whether a fresh sample for electron microscopy should be sent; and third, it enables

Table 3-11. Neck masses: common diagnostic pitfalls

Low index of suspicion for a head and neck malignancy

Prolonged observation of either a symptomatic or asymptomatic neck mass or masses

Premature open neck biopsy without an adequate workup:
- History
- Complete physical examination, including indirect nasopharyngoscopy and laryngoscopy
- Diagnostic radiology

Inadequate incisional or excisional biopsy (sampling error)

Incomplete review of pathologic specimens (needle, punch, or incisional biopsy)

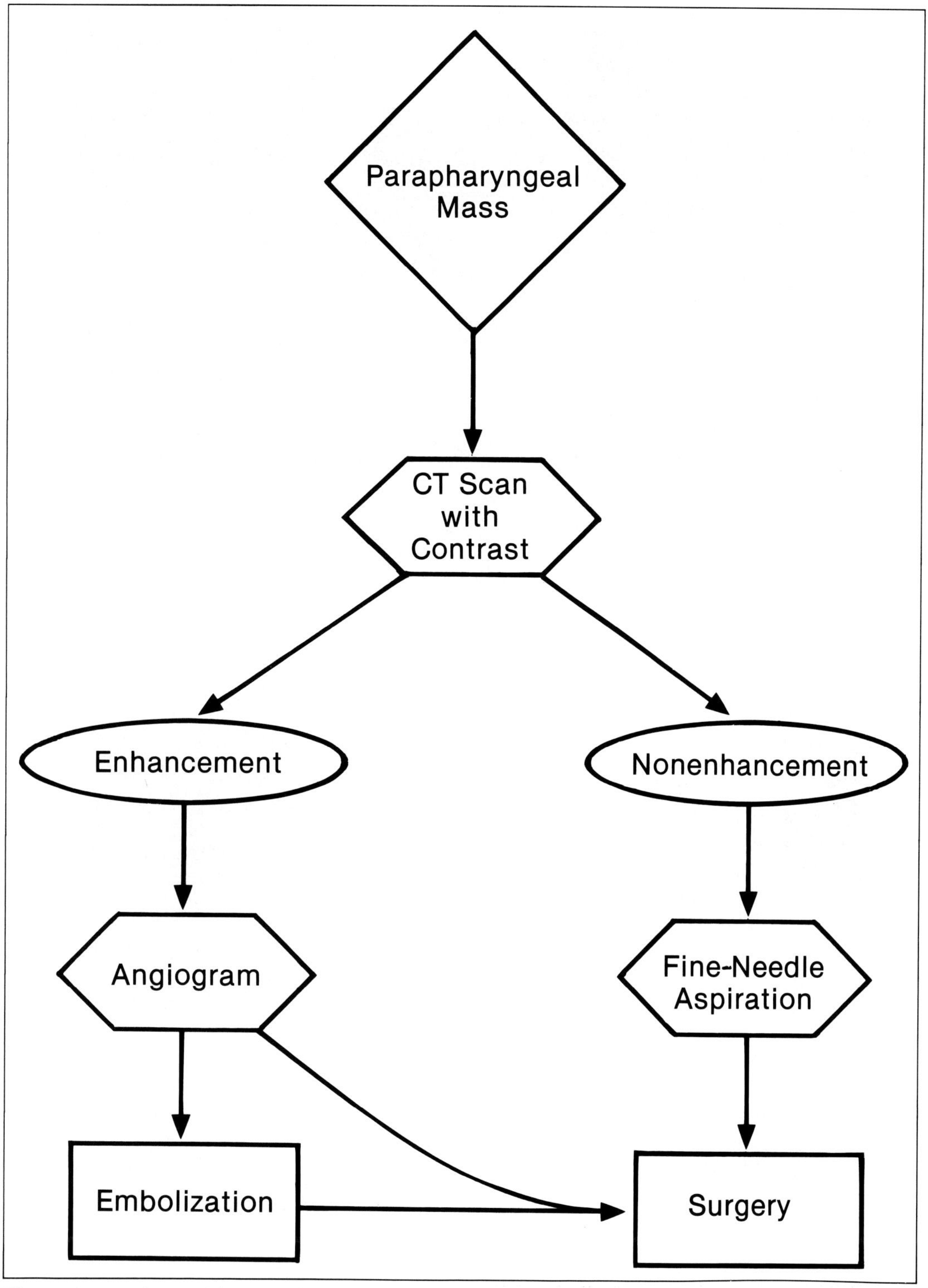

Figure 3-9. The parapharyngeal mass. Enhanced lesions require angiography. Fine-needle aspiration is indicated for unenhanced lesions.

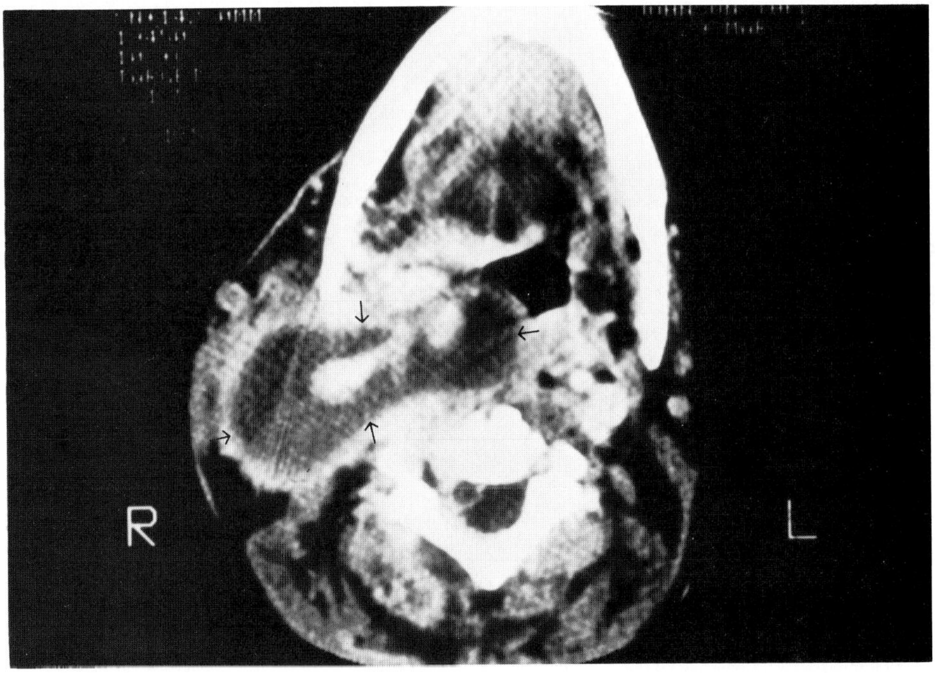

A

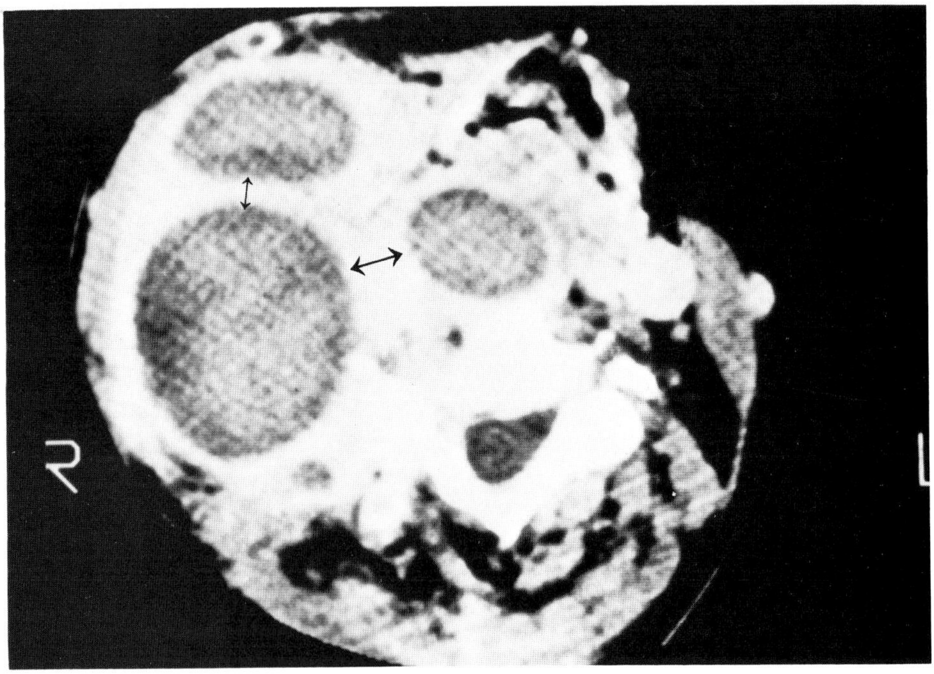

B

Figure 3-10. CT scan, neck. A huge vascular mass in a 54-year-old woman that slowly began 10 years ago after removal of a supraclavicular lymph complicated by a brisk hemorrhage. It spans the entire neck. A. Angle of the mandible. B. Middle. (continued)

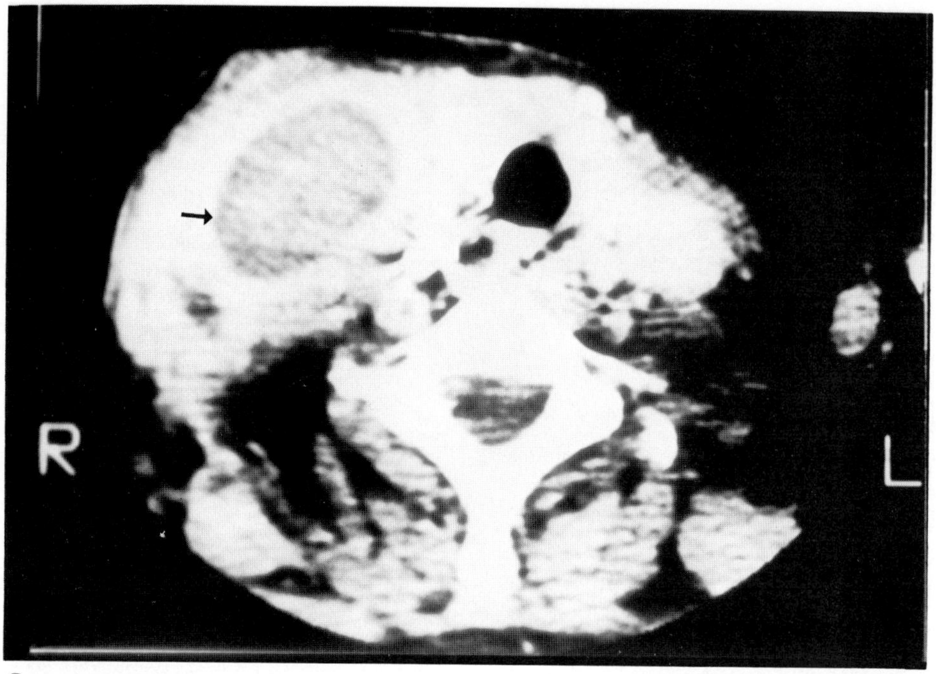

C

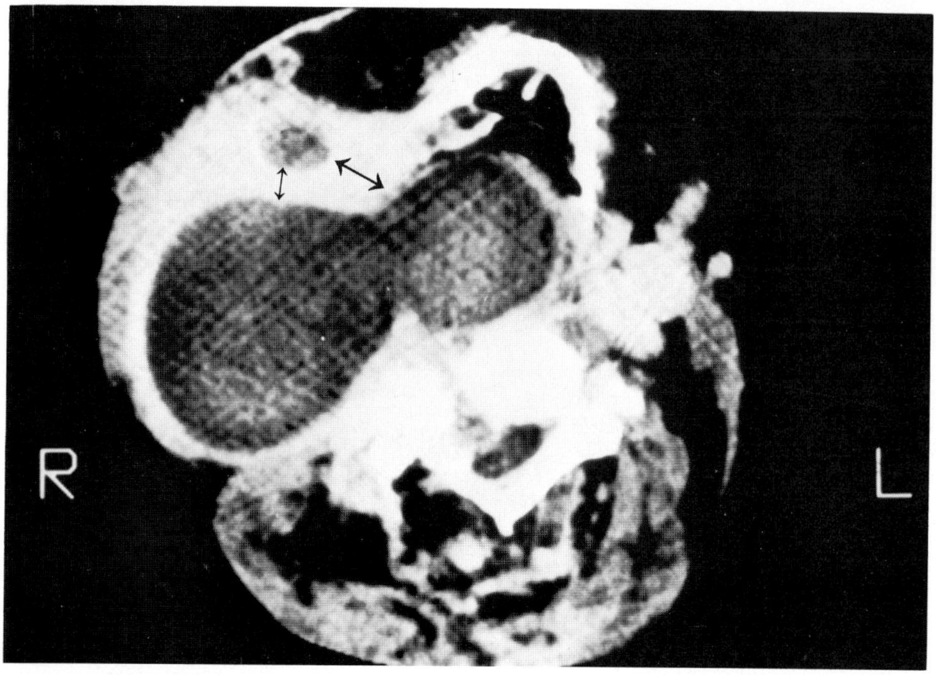

D

Figure 3-10 (continued). C. Thoracic inlet. D. Contiguous with the retropharyngeal and parapharyngeal spaces, its removal required a multidisciplinary team (neurosurgeon, cardiovascular surgeon, and otolaryngologist). Under hypotensive anesthesia, a post-traumatic arteriovenous malformation was removed.

the senior oncologist to initiate a treatment plan. The goal by day 7 is a diagnosis and a preliminary treatment plan (see Chapters 5 and 7).

MANAGEMENT OF OCCULT METASTASIS

Despite an exhaustive workup, 20 percent of the malignant neck masses remain occult [19–21]. In such cases the entire head and neck is radiated from the skull base to the thoracic inlet (see Chapter 9).

N_1 (Stage II) Neck

While undergoing radiotherapy the patient is observed carefully for a primary lesion [10]. If one emerges, it is treated in conjunction with the neck metastasis. However, if there is partial or no response, full-course radiotherapy is followed by neck dissection [10] (see Chapter 16).

$N_{2/3}$ (Stage III, IV) Neck

A patient in this category is started on induction chemotherapy and followed by surgery and radical radiotherapy (see Chapter 8).

REFERENCES

1. Simpson GT: The evaluation and management of neck masses of unknown etiology. Otolaryngol Clin North Am 13(3) : 489, 1980.
2. Skandelakis JE, et al: Tumors of the neck. *Surgery* 48 : 375, 1960.
3. Heyward WL, Curran JW: The epidemiology of AIDS in the U.S. Sci Am 259(4) : 72, 1988.
4. Man JM, et al: The international epidemiology of AIDS. *Sci Am* 259(4) : 82, 1988.
5. Rosenberg RA, Schneider KL, Cohen NL: The head and neck presentation of acquired immuno deficiency syndrome. *Laryngoscope* 94 : 642, 1984.
6. Knowles DM, et al: Lymphoid neoplasia associated with the acquired immuno deficiency syndrome (AIDS). *Ann Intern Med* 168 : 744, 1988.
7. Martin H, Morfitt HM: Cervical lymph node metastasis as the first symptom of cancer. *Surg Gynecol Obstet* 78 : 133, 1944.
8. Lindberg R: Distribution of cervical lymph node metastatic tracts. *Cancer* 29 : 1446, 1972.
9. Johnson JT, et al: Cervical lymph node metastasis. *Arch Otolaryngol* 111 : 534, 1985.
10. Jesse RH, Neff LD: Metastatic carcinoma in cervical nodes with an unknown primary. *Ann Otol Rhinol Laryngol* 84 : 152, 1975.
11. Comess MS, Beahrs OH, Dockey MB: Cervical metastasis from occult carcinoma. *Surg Gynecol Obstet* 133 : 607, 1957.
12. Millon RR, Cassisi NJ: The Natural History of Squamous Cell Carcinoma. In: *Management of Head and Neck Cancer*. Philadelphia: Lippincott, 1984.
13. Rush BF: Diagnostic and therapeutic approach to an isolated metastatic lymph node in the lower one-third of the neck. *Surg Rounds*, Dec 1984. Pp 32–38.
14. Sheikh FA, et al: Final diagnosis by fine-needle aspiration biopsy for definitive operations in breast cancer. Am J Surg 154(5) : 470, 1987.
15. Som PM, et al: Tumors of the parapharyngeal space and upper neck: MRI imaging characteristics. *Radiology* 164 : 823, 1987.
16. Cohen JP, Cho HT: The role of needle aspiration biopsy in the selection of patients for thyroidectomy. *Laryngoscope* 98 : 35, 1988.
17. Rodriguez AP, et al: Fine-needle aspiration of parotid tumors. *Am J Surg* 158 : 342, 1989.
18. Hessan H, Stiansis M, Sharkey FE: Genital tract carcinoma metastasis. *Arch Otolaryngol* 111 : 534, 1985.
19. Cece JA, et al: Complications in the management of large glomus jugulare tumors. *Laryngoscope* 97 : 152, 1987.
20. Fried MP, et al: Cervical metastasis from an unknown primary. *Ann Otolaryngol* 84 : 152, 1975.
21. Richard JM, et al: Prognostic factors in cervical lymph node metastasis in upper respiratory and digestive tract carcinomas: Study of 1,713 cases during a 15 year period. *Laryngoscope* 97 : 97, 1987.

4

Radiology

ROMA V. GUMBS AND JAMES S. TEAL

KEY CONCEPTS

Anatomy; Imaging; Pathology

MILESTONES

1895	X-rays	Roentgen
1896	Plain Radiography	MacIntyre
1897	Barium Esophagography	Cannon
1939	Laryngeal Tomography	Howes
1957	Laryngography	Powers et al.
1973	Computed Tomography (CT)	Hounsfield, Ambrose
1977	Magnetic Resonance Imaging (MRI)	Hinshaw
1978	Head and Neck CT	Archer et al. and Mancuso et al.
1984	Head and Neck MRI	Stark et al.; Dillon et al.
1988	Contrast Head and Neck MRI	Vogl et al.

In 1895 Roentgen accidentally discovered x-rays. Within a year, MacIntyre [1] produced x-ray images of the neck in both patients and cadavers. Later, mucosal abnormalities were accentuated by the use of topical iodized oil [2,3,4]. Conventional tomography was the first available technique to delineate the deeper structures of the larynx and hypopharynx [5,6]. Today, computed tomography (CT) permits better evaluation of these areas as well as the oral cavity, oropharynx, and other structures in the neck (Table 4-1). Such detailed information facilitates the staging of both primary tumors and metastatic lymphadenopathy [7–12].

Recently, nuclear magnetic resonance has been employed for medical imaging [13]. It is devoid of ionizing radiation and poses no known biologic risks at field strengths currently utilized for imaging. Without altering the patient's position, images can be generated in axial, sagittal, coronal, and oblique planes. Contrast resolution of magnetic resonance imaging (MRI) exceeds that of CT, but spatial resolution at the present time is less. MRI is the preferred modality for evaluating the posterior fossa and the white matter of the central nervous system [14,15]. The introduction of paramagnetic contrast agents, such as gadolinium diethylenetriamine penta-acetic acid (Gd-DTPA), has enhanced intra-axial and extra-axial tumor identification [16,17]. The multiplanar capability of MRI is exploited for critical assessment of the skull base, tongue base, laryngeal ventricles, and anterior commissure [18,19]. MRI is contraindicated, however, in patients with cardiac pacemakers, cochlear implants, ferromagnetic intracranial aneurysm clips, and suspected metallic objects in the eye. Patients with claustrophobia, even when sedated, may not tolerate the confines of the magnet.

Table 4-1. Sites versus imaging modalities

Head and Neck Site	*Plain Films*	*Computed Tomography*[a]	*Magnetic Resonance Imaging*[a]	*Barium Swallow*	*Other*[b]
Base of skull	+	+ + +	+ + +		Angiography
Nasopharynx	+	+ +	+ + +		Angiography
Paranasal	+	+ + +	+ + +		Angiography
Salivary glands	+	+ + +	+ +		Salivary gland scan
Lips		+			
Oral cavity		+ + +	+ +		
Oropharynx	+	+ + +	+ +		
Hypopharynx	+	+ + +	+ +	+	
Larynx	+	+ + +	+ +	+	
Thyroid/parathyroid		+ + +		+	Thyroid scans/ sonography
Cervical esophagus		+ + +	+	+ + +	

+ = Helpful; + + = Recommended; + + + = Preferred.
[a]CT and MRI are frequently complementary.
[b]Angiography, if a vascular lesion is suspected.

SKULL BASE

Anatomy

The cranium is divided into the calvarium superiorly and the skull base inferiorly. The frontal, temporal, and occipital bones contribute to both the calvarium and the skull base. The skull base is primarily cartilaginous bone, while the calvarium is membranous bone. The skull base forms the floor of the anterior, middle, and posterior cranial fossae (Table 4-2 and Figure 4-1) [20].

Imaging

Plain Films

The submentovertex (base) view is adequate for preliminary skull base evaluation. Most of the foramina (Table 4-2) are visualized on this view. There is good definition of the clivus and the greater wings of the sphenoid bone forming the anterior wall of the middle cranial fossa. For better delineation of the floor of the sella and the foramina rotundum, this view is supplemented by the Caldwell and Waters views.

Complex Motion Tomography

This technique was once used extensively to evaluate the skull base and the petrous portion of the temporal bone. It has been replaced by high-resolution, thin-section CT.

Angiography

Normal vascular structures can be confused with skull base tumors due to dilatation or aberrant location. Tortuosity and aneurysms of the internal carotid artery can simulate pituitary adenomas and craniopharyngiomas. Glomus tumors must be differentiated from aberrant internal carotid arteries or abnormal jugular bulbs associated with dehiscence of the anterior wall of the jugular fossa. Angiography is essential not only for defining the nature of the mass but also for preoperative embolization in selected tumors.

Computed Tomography

Skull base CT usually is performed in the axial projection with the scanning angle parallel to Reid's baseline as contiguous 1.5- or 2-mm sections are obtained. Coronal scans are useful for completely evaluating the sella turcica, the petrous portions of the temporal bones, and the middle and posterior fossa foramina. Most scanners when equipped with high-resolution algorithms give excellent bony detail.

Magnetic Resonance Imaging

MRI's multiplanar capability is a tremendous asset in evaluating skull base lesions, especially those of the sellar, juxtasellar, and cerebellopontine angle areas. Gd-DTPA, recently approved as a paramagnetic contrast agent, shortens T1 and T2 relaxation times. It does not cross an intact blood-brain barrier but is incorporated by the normal pituitary gland and stalk, which lack a blood-brain barrier. It also is incorporated by intracranial neoplasms, inflammatory and gliotic tissue, and subacute infarcts when the blood-brain barrier has been disrupted [16,17].

Pathology

The common skull base tumors are neural tumors, meningiomas, pituitary adenomas, and craniopharyngiomas.

Neural Tumors

Schwannomas and Neurofibromas

Nerve sheath tumors are classified as schwannomas or neurofibromas, with schwannomas being encapsulated and neurofibromas unencapsulated. On plain films, nerve sheath tumors enlarge their respective foramina, and the borders remain sclerotic. They tend to be hypo- or isodense or a mixture of the two on noncontrast CT and show variable enhancement following intravenous contrast infusion (Figure 4-2). Neuromas commonly are avascular or hypovascular on angiography. With MRI, these lesions are hypointense on T1-weighted images and hyperintense on T2-weighted sequences (Figure 4-3). Neuromas demonstrate strong enhancement on T1-weighted images following Gd-DTPA injection.

Glomus Tumors (Chemodectomas)

Glomus tumors arise from nonchromaffin paraganglionic cells. The two most common sites in the skull base are the jugular bulb (glomus jugulare) and the middle ear (glomus tympanicum). The patients typically present with tin-

Table 4-2. Major foramina of the skull base

Foramen	*Structure(s)*
Anterior cranial fossa	
Foramen cecum	Nasal veins
Cribiform plate	Olfactory nerve
Middle cranial fossa	
Superior orbital fissure	Cranial nerves III, IV, V_1, VI Superior ophthalmic vein
Optic canal	Cranial nerve II Ophthalmic artery
Foramen rotundum	Cranial nerve V_2
Foramen ovale	Cranial nerve V_3 Emissary vein or sinus Accessory meningeal branch of internal maxillary artery (variable)
Foramen spinosum	Middle meningeal artery
Foramen lacerum	Meningeal branches of ascending pharyngeal artery Fibrocartilage
Greater palatine foramen	Greater (descending) palatine artery Greater (anterior) palatine branch of the sphenopalatine nerve
Lesser palatine foramen	Lesser palatine nerve Branches of greater palatine artery
Posterior cranial fossa	
Carotid canal	Internal carotid artery Sympathetic nerve fibers
Jugular foramen	Internal jugular vein Cranial nerves IX, X, XI Meningeal branches of ascending pharyngeal artery
Hypoglossal canal	Cranial nerve XII
Stylomastoid foramen	Cranial nerve VII
Foramen magnum	Medulla oblongata Spinal portion of cranial nerve XI Vertebral arteries and veins Anterior and posterior spinal arteries

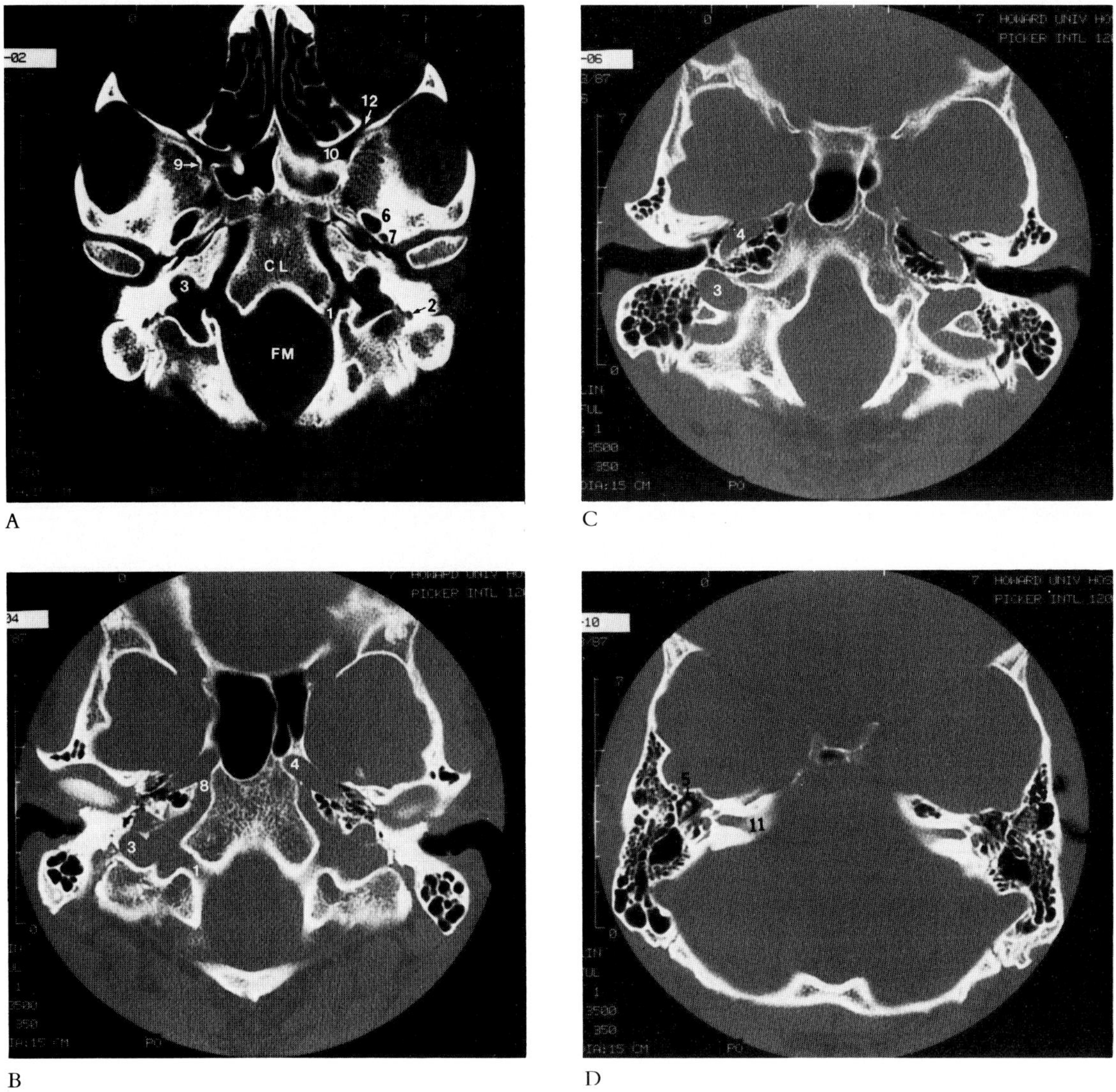

Figure 4-1. 2-mm high-resolution axial CT scans of the skull base. *1* = hypoglossal canal (XII); *2* = stylomastoid foramen (VII); *3* = jugular fossa (IX, X, XI); *4* = carotid canal; *5* = middle ear; *6* = foramen ovale (V_3); *7* = foramen spinosum (middle meningeal artery); *8* = foramen lacerum; *9* = foramen rotundum (V_2); *10* = pterygopalatine fossa; *11* = internal auditory canal; *12* = inferior orbital fissure; *FM* = foramen magnum; *CL* = clivus.

nitus and hearing loss. Otoscopy may show a pulsatile middle ear mass. Radiographic findings include irregular, erosive expansion of the jugular foramen, erosion of the petrous tip, and clouding or sclerosis of the mastoid air cells [21]. On contrast CT, these tumors frequently are well circumscribed and highly vascular. Arteriography should be performed to confirm vascularity and to identify synchronous tumors. Preoperative embolization may decrease intraoperative bleeding (see Chapter 13).

Chordomas

Chordomas, derived from notochord remnants, commonly are located in the clivus, dorsum sellae, and sacrum. On plain films, they

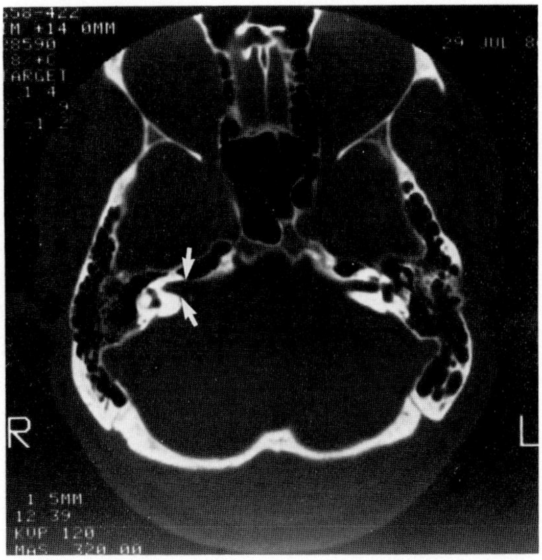

A

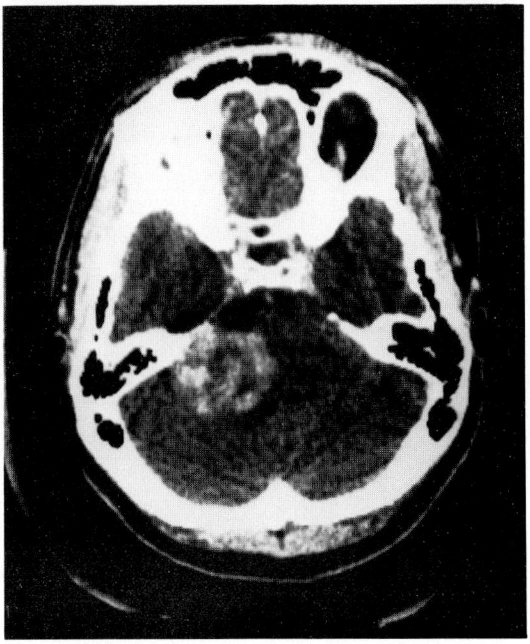

B

Figure 4-2. Acoustic neuroma. A. A 1.5-mm section of skull base shows enlargement and truncation of the right internal auditory canal (*arrows*). B. CT scan with contrast reveals heterogeneous enhancement of a large right cerebellopontine angle mass.

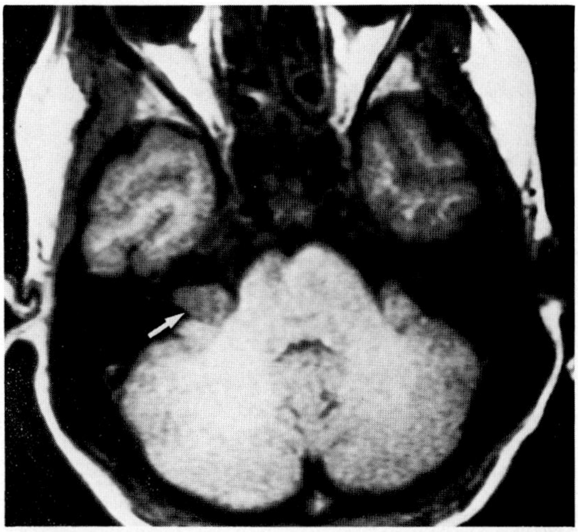

A

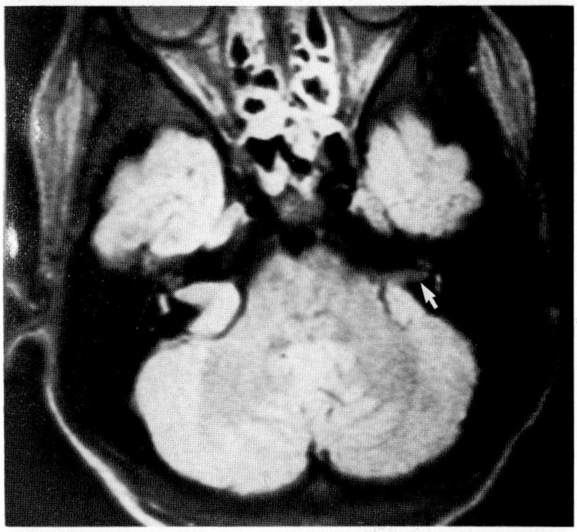

B

Figure 4-3. Acoustic neuroma in a 14-year-old girl with neurofibromatosis. A. T1-weighted (600/20) image shows a slightly hypointense right cerebellopontine angle mass (*arrow*). B. The mass becomes hyperintense on the T2-weighted (2500/40) sequence. *Arrow*-normal left eighth cranial nerve.

frequently contain calcification and demonstrate bony destruction. Similar findings are appreciated on CT with heterogeneous enhancement following contrast infusion. On MRI these masses are of variable intensity, frequently being dark on T1-weighted images and bright on T2-weighted images. MRI is superior to CT in detecting brainstem involvement. Nasopharyngeal extension is appreciated equally by both modalities [22].

Sellar and Juxtasellar Lesions

The most common lesions of the sellar and juxtasellar areas are pituitary adenomas and craniopharyngiomas. A partial listing of other entities includes optic chiasm and hypothalamic gliomas, meningiomas, and internal carotid artery aneurysms.

Pituitary Adenomas

Pituitary adenomas are grouped into microadenomas and macroadenomas. Microadenomas, less than 10 mm in size, are confined to the sella (Figure 4-4). They may secrete prolactin (the majority), growth hormone, or adrenocorticotrophic hormone (ACTH). Microadenomas, presenting as intraglandular focal lesions, sometimes erode the sellar floor and/or anterior wall. Macroadenomas, greater than 1 cm in size, are frequently nonsecretory [23] and are associated with remodeling of the sellar floor, suprasellar extension, and cavernous sinus invasion (Figure 4-5).

Nonhemorrhagic microadenomas and macroadenomas are hypointense or isointense on T1-weighted images (see Figure 4-4) [24]. Immediately following contrast administration, microadenomas are usually hypointense on T1-weighted MR images in reference to contrast enhancing normal pitituitary tissue. Microadenomas usually demonstrate contrast enhancement with both modalities. Macroadenomas, enhancing strongly on postcontrast CT images, are difficult to separate from the cavernous sinuses and internal carotid arteries, but on MRI the arteries appear as signal voids and can be delineated from the macroadenomas.

MRI also shows hemorrhage, cystic change, and extension into the clivus and sphenoid sinus. Sagittal images depict the relationship to the optic chiasm, suprasellar cisterns, hypothalamus, and brainstem. Cavernous sinus involvement is demonstrated better on coronal image [24]. This information aids the surgeon in deciding between a subfrontal or transsphenoidal approach (see Chapter 13). MRI with intravenous Gd-DTPA infusion is probably the preferred modality for imaging sellar lesions.

Craniopharyngiomas

Craniopharyngiomas are predominantly childhood tumors but are found in all ages. They develop from the squamous epithelial rests of

Figure 4-4. Pituitary microadenoma. T1-weighted (500/30) coronal image shows a hypointense mass (*arrow*) in the left side of the pituitary gland with bulging of the superior surface.

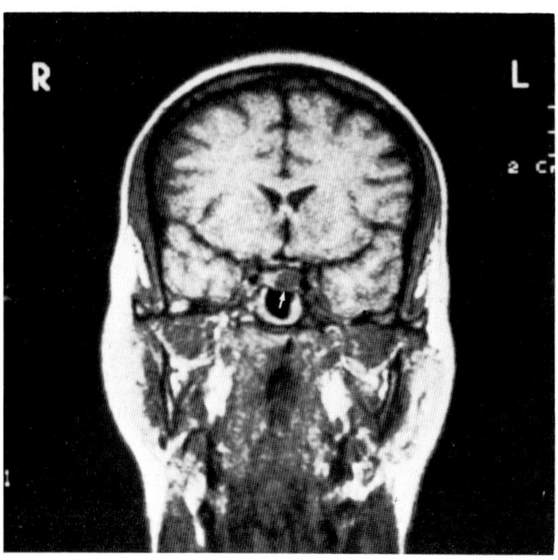

Figure 4-5. Pituitary macroadenoma. Contrast-enhanced coronal CT image shows an enhancing mass arising from the sella and extending into the suprasellar cisterns. There is focal calcification (*arrow*) at the border of the mass. *S* = sphenoid sinus.

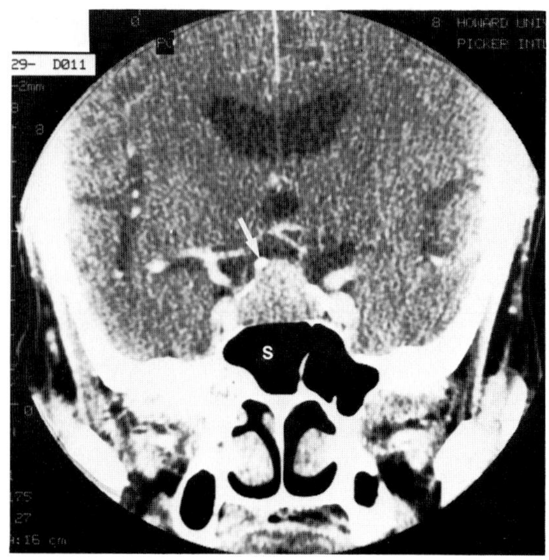

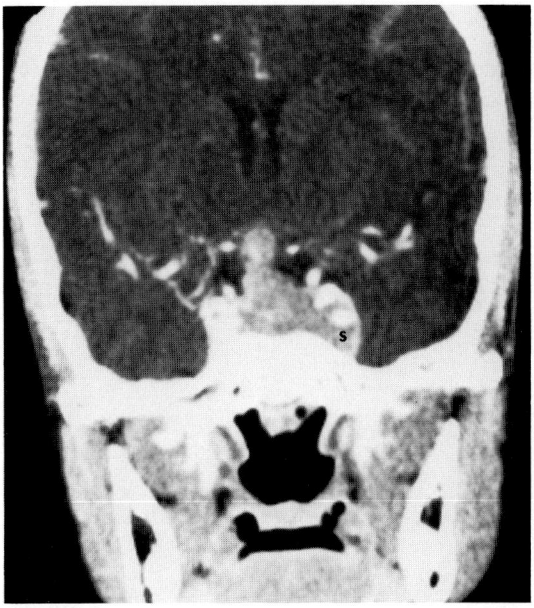

A

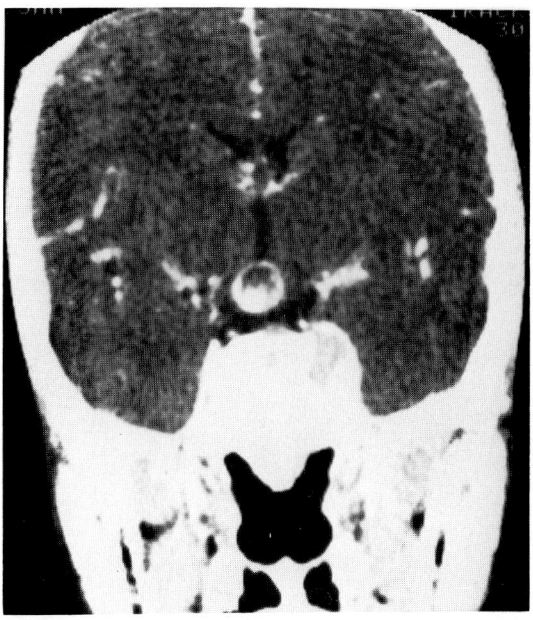

B

Figure 4-6. Coronal CT images of a craniopharyngioma in a 6-year-old girl. A. An enhancing mass extends out of the sella into the suprasellar area and into the left cavernous sinus (*s*). B. Image 4.5 mm posterior to A clearly shows the cystic component.

Rathke's pouch and occur mainly in the suprasellar area. Plain film findings include sellar enlargement, "amputation" of the dorsum sella, and calcification, features that also are identified easily on CT scan (Figure 4-6). With MRI, the noncalcified components of these tumors are bright on T2-weighted images but show variable intensity on the T1-weighted sequences [25]. Craniopharyngiomas are differentiated from pituitary adenomas by the more frequent occurrence of calcification and cystic changes. Radiographic calcification is present in only 1 to 6 percent of pituitary adenomas, whereas it is detected in 75 to 90 percent of children and 40 to 50 percent of adults with craniopharyngiomas.

Meningiomas

Forty percent of meningiomas occur along the sphenoidal wing, parasellar area, and olfactory groove, with an additional 10 percent occurring in the posterior fossa. The involved bone is usually sclerotic. On CT scan, meningiomas usually appear as dural-based, well-circumscribed, densely enhancing lesions associated with variable amounts of edema (Figure 4-7A, D, and E). The typical angiographic appearance is a well-circumscribed mass, often having a spokewheel appearance and showing a dense vascular stain extending into the venous phase (Figure 4-7B and C). They frequently are isointense (low field) or hypointense (high field) on T1-weighted images and iso- or hyperintense on T2-weighted images (Figure 4-7F). MRI is extremely useful in evaluating vascular encasement, invasion, and displacement [26]. These lesions typically demonstrate marked T1 hyperintensity following Gd-DTPA infusion.

Primary Bone Lesions

Chondromas and Chondrosarcomas

Since the skull base develops partly or wholly from cartilage, the most common primary bone lesions are chondromas and chondrosarcomas, occurring frequently at the spheno-occipital synchondrosis. Bone erosion is well-defined in chondromas and poorly marginated in chondrosarcomas. On angiography, the lesions usually are avascular, although chondrosarcomas

Figure 4-7. Meningiomas. A. CT scan without contrast shows a hyperostotic mass of the left sphenoidal wing with a small amount of surrounding edema (*arrows*). B. Anteroposterior view of left internal carotid artery injection of a left sphenoidal wing meningioma (different patient from A). Middle cerebral artery (*long arrow*) is elevated, and both the anterior cerebral artery (*short arrows*) and supraclinoid internal carotid artery (*arrowheads*) are shifted to the right by a vascular mass (*open arrows*) arising from the left sphenoidal wing. C. Venous phase of B (lateral view). The vascular stain (*arrows*) in the well-circumscribed mass is still apparent. D and E. CT images of a left middle fossa meningioma (*M*) extending through Meckel's cave into the posterior fossa with marked edema (*E*) in the left frontal and parietal lobes. F. Right cerebellopontine angle meningioma. T2-weighted (2000/50) image shows a hyperintense mass causing elevation of the proximal right posterior cerebral artery (*arrowhead*) and slight right-to-left displacement of the midportion of the basilar artery (*short arrows*).

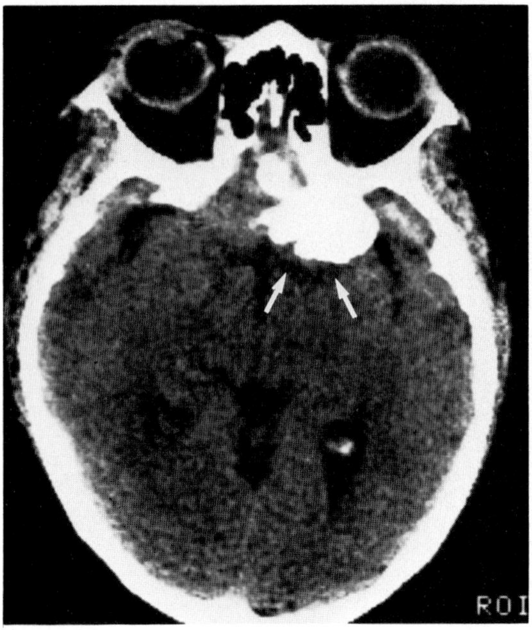

A

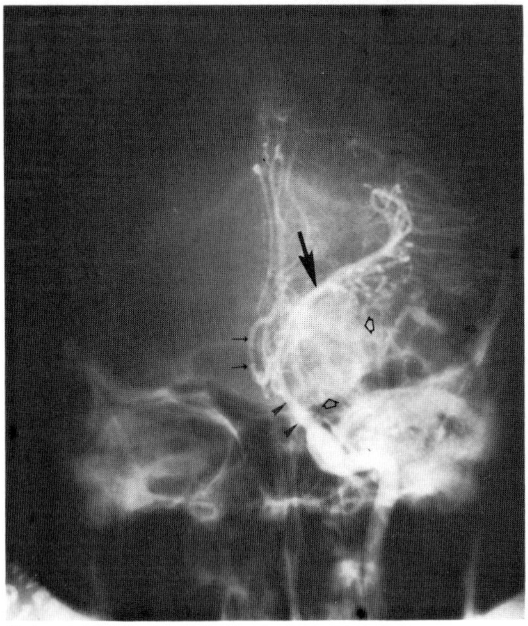

B

may be hypervascular. Both chondromas and chondrosarcomas enhance on postcontrast CT images. Chondrosarcomas, like most tumors, have been found to be relatively dark on T1-weighted images, becoming bright on the T2-weighted sequences [22].

Cholesteatomas (Epidermoids)

Skull base cholesteatomas are termed primary or secondary. Primary cholesteatomas develop from embryonic epithelial rests behind an intact tympanic membrane. The majority of cholesteatomas are secondary or postinflammatory in origin. They develop from epithelial cells sequestered in the middle ear after tympanic membrane perforations. The accumulation of the breakdown products (keratin) of the epithelial cells causes pressure erosion of the surrounding structures. The lesions radiographically appear lucent with smooth, well-circumscribed, sometimes sclerotic margins. On CT the lesions have low attenuation due to their keratin content. Enhancement is variable, depending on the amount of surrounding inflammation. Cholesteatomas are bright on T1-weighted sequences and dark on T2-weighted images.

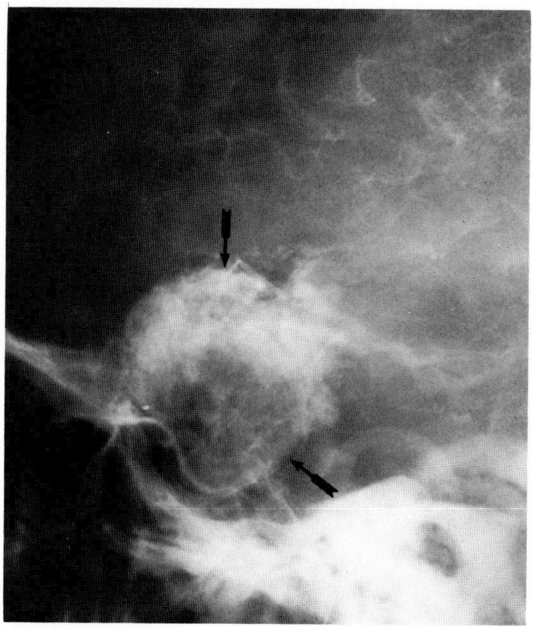
C

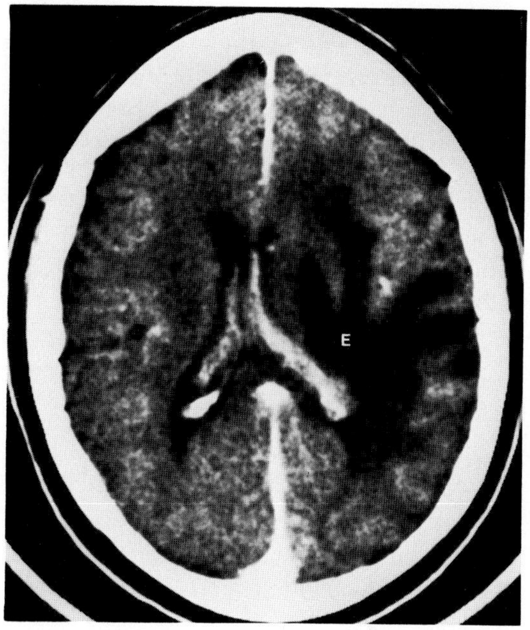

E

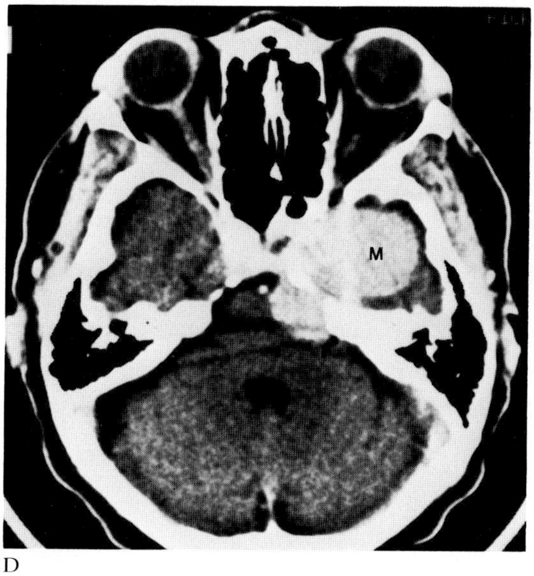

D

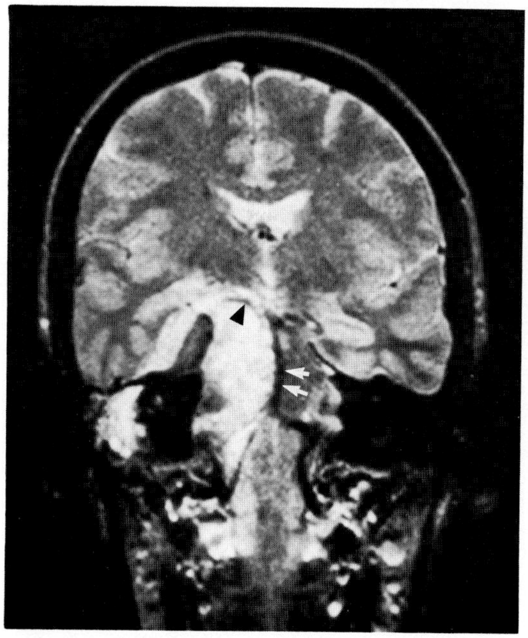
F

Secondary Bone Lesions

Metastatic disease to the skull base is unusual, with the most common sites of origin being the prostate, lung, and breast. Whereas plain radiographs will often show the bony changes (although not usually as well as CT), CT and MRI better demonstrate the soft-tissue component. Direct extension to the skull base from nasopharyngeal and paranasal sinus malignancies is possible (see Nasopharynx and Paranasal Sinuses/Nose).

NASOPHARYNX (Site 1)

Anatomy

The nasopharynx, lying posterior to the nasal cavity, is bounded by the sphenoid sinus and the clivus superiorly, the soft palate inferiorly, and the prevertebral muscles at C1 and C2, laterally and posteriorly. The superior pharyngeal constrictor muscle and the pharyngobasilar fascia form the walls of the nasopharynx. The tensor and levator veli palatini muscles contribute to the lateral walls. These muscles originate in part from the eustachian tube and affect its function. The eustachian tube orifice is anterior to the torus tubarius and Rosenmüller's fossa (lateral pharyngeal recess) (Figure 4-8). In children, the adenoids contribute significantly to posterior wall thickness [27].

The foramen lacerum, in the roof of the nasopharynx, is an important potential pathway for tumor access to the cavernous sinus. The internal carotid artery runs just above this foramen as it enters the posterior cavernous sinus (see Figure 4-1).

The parapharyngeal space, lateral to the nasopharynx, contains the internal carotid artery, the internal jugular vein, cranial nerves IX through XII, and the cervical sympathetic chain (see Chapter 3).

Figure 4-8. CT images of upper nasopharynx. *1* = eustachian tube orifice; *2* = torus tubarius; *3* = lateral pharyngeal recess (Rosenmüller's fossa); *PM* = pterygoid muscle.

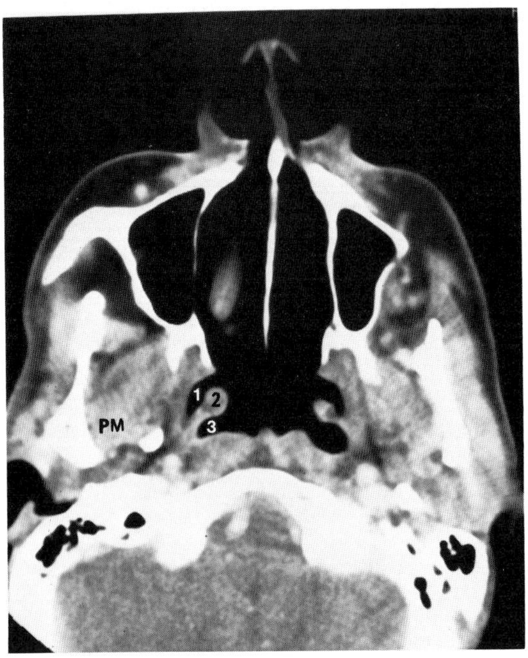

Imaging

Plain Films

On lateral skull films, nasopharyngeal tumors may be seen as soft-tissue masses beneath the sphenoid sinus and clivus, distorting the nasopharyngeal air column. Submentovertex views may show a mass, skull base destruction, and foraminal enlargement.

Computed Tomography

Current-generation CT scanners provide excellent display of the nasopharynx and surrounding structures [27]. Axial scanning is performed during intravenous contrast infusion parallel to Reid's baseline. Five-millimeter contiguous scans are obtained from the skull base to the mandibular alveolar ridge. If skull base involvement is suspected, direct coronal scans are obtained.

Magnetic Resonance Imaging

MRI with a head coil effectively images the nasopharynx. Its soft-tissue detail exceeds that of CT, making early detection or invasion of soft-tissue planes possible [28]. With MRI, the pharyngobasilar fascia and lymphoid tissue are separated from contiguous muscles, thus better defining the tumor margins.

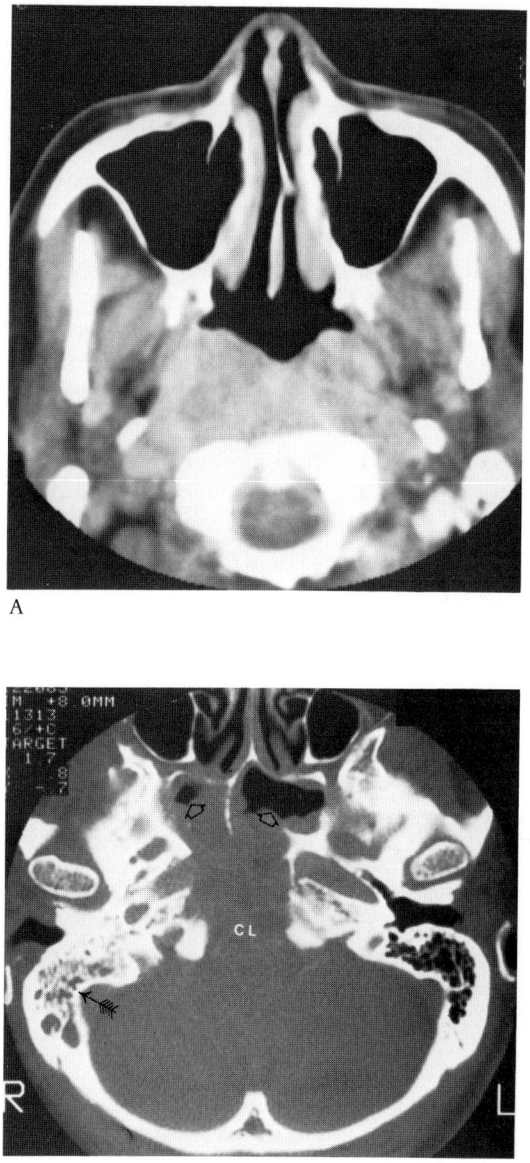

A

B

Figure 4-9. Nasopharyngeal carcinoma. A. There is marked thickening of the posterior wall of the nasopharynx. B. CT image of the skull base. The clivus (*CL*) is eroded, and tumor extends into the sphenoid sinuses (*open arrows*). There is loss of aeration of the right mastoid air cells (*feathered arrow*).

Pathology

Malignant Tumors

Squamous cell carcinomas, keratinizing and nonkeratinizing, account for approximately 80 percent of all nasopharyngeal carcinomas. Adenoid cystic carcinomas, adenocarcinomas, and lymphomas also occur in this area [29]. Rhabdomyosarcoma is the most common childhood malignancy at this site.

Most nasopharyngeal carcinomas are exophytic and arise from the lateral or posterior walls [30]. Early infiltration around the levator veli palatini muscle can lead to levator and eustachian tube dysfunction with secondary serous otitis media and mastoiditis (Figure 4-9). The carcinoma may grow superiorly toward the skull base or inferiorly toward the soft palate and oropharynx. If the tumor invades the parapharyngeal space, dysfunction of cranial nerves IX through XII as well as the cervical sympathetics may occur [28,30]. Tumor migrating along the internal carotid artery into the cavernous sinus can affect cranial nerves III through VI. Anterior extension into the nasal cavity (Figure 4-10), posterior ethmoidal air cells, maxillary sinus, and orbits frequently occurs.

Figure 4-10. Nasopharyngeal non-Hodgkin's lymphoma. Soft-tissue mass thickens the posterior nasopharyngeal wall with direct extension into the right nasal cavity.

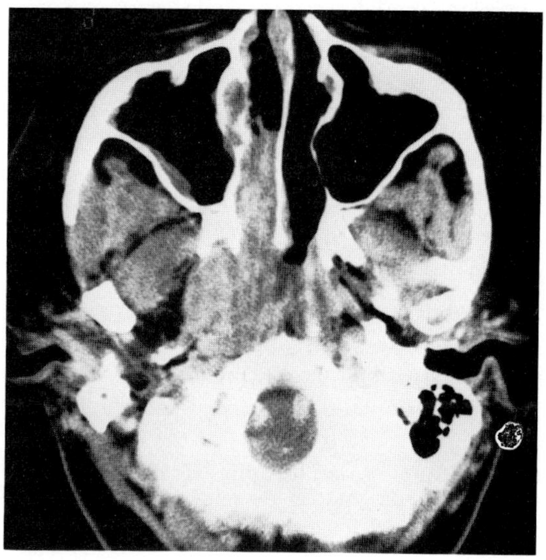

Nasopharyngeal carcinomas appear intermediate in intensity on T1-weighted sequences obtained at low MR field strengths. Subtle spread along the eustachian tube and gross extension into the nasal cavity, pterygopalatine fossa, and middle cranial fossa can be detected [28].

The lymphatics from the posterior and lateral nasopharyngeal walls drain to the retropharyngeal and jugulodigastric nodes. In a high percentage, the adenopathy is bilateral [29].

Benign Tumors

The juvenile angiofibroma, originating in the nasopharynx and posterior nares, is the most common benign tumor of the nasopharynx. It is locally invasive, unencapsulated, and highly vascular. It is typically found in young males who present with nasal stuffiness, epistaxis, and facial deformity. Characteristically, it grows through and expands into the pterygomaxillary fossa, displacing the posterior maxillary wall anteriorly. Orbital extension is through the inferior and superior orbital fissures. Anterior extension into the nasal cavity accounts for stuffiness and bleeding. Contrast CT is currently the imaging modality of choice. The role of MRI has not been determined presently. If surgery is contemplated, angiography defines the feeding vessels for possible preoperative embolization. The arterial supply usually originates from the ipsilateral internal maxillary artery and occasionally the ipsilateral internal carotid artery and the contralateral external carotid artery.

PARANASAL SINUSES/NOSE (Site 2)

Anatomy

Nose

The mobile, anterior nose consists of cartilage and skin. The maxillae, inferiorly, and the nasal bones, superiorly, constitute the lateral bony elements. The nasal floor (hard palate) is composed of the palatal process of the maxilla and the horizontal palatine bone. The nasal bone, nasal process of the frontal bone, and the cribriform plate (ethmoid) constitute the roof of the nose. Cribriform plate perforations allow for the passage of the olfactory nerve rootlets.

Internally, the nasal cavity is divided equally by the midline nasal septum (composed of cartilage anteriorly), the vomer, and the perpendicular plate of the ethmoid posteriorly. The conchae or turbinates are three bony projections from the lateral nasal wall. The superior and middle conchae are protuberances of the ethmoid bone, while the inferior concha is a separate bone. The respective meatus from the paranasal sinuses lie inferior and lateral to the conchae. The lacrimal gland drains through the nasolacrimal duct into the inferior meatus. In addition, the sphenopalatine foramen, connecting the nasal cavity to the pterygomaxillary fossa, is behind the middle concha [31].

Paranasal Sinuses

The paranasal sinuses develop as evaginations of the nasal mucosa. Rudimentary maxillary, ethmoid, and sphenoid sinuses are present at birth, while the frontal sinuses develop postnatally [32].

Maxillary Sinus

The maxillary sinuses are fairly symmetric in size. They are related to the orbit superiorly, the nasal cavity medially, and the maxillary alveolar process inferiorly. Drainage is through the maxillary ostia into the middle meatus of the nasal cavity.

Frontal Sinus

The frontal sinuses, variable in size and frequently absent, originate from the ethmoid sinuses and drain into the middle meatus. These sinuses extend within the diploë of the frontal bone, frequently into the supraorbit between the roof of the orbit and the floor of the anterior cranial fossa. Septae usually are found within the frontal sinuses.

Ethmoid Sinus

The ethmoid sinuses lie between the orbits and the upper nasal cavity. Each sinus contains between 3 and 18 septated air cells that are divided into anterior, middle, and posterior groups. The anterior and middle groups drain into the middle meatus, while the posterior group drains into the superior meatus. The ethmoidal air cells may encroach into adjacent paranasal sinuses and be indistinguishable from supraorbital extension of the frontal sinus.

Sphenoid Sinus

Although the anlagen of the sphenoid sinuses are present at birth, most of their development occurs after age 3. Lying superior to the nasopharynx, these paired sinuses are usually asymmetric in size and shape. The sella and anterior cranial fossa lie immediately above the sphenoid sinuses, with the cavernous sinuses and internal carotid arteries laterally located. They drain through the sphenoethmoidal recesses located above and behind the superior nasal conchae.

Imaging

Plain Films

In routine radiography, the four standard views are the Caldwell, Waters, lateral, and submentovertex (Table 4-3) projections.

Computed Tomography

CT should be performed in both the axial and coronal projections with 5-mm contiguous sections. Intravenous contrast helps to distinguish inflammatory from malignant masses.

Magnetic Resonance Imaging

T2-weighted images have been most useful in separating carcinoma from associated inflammation. Most tumors are of low to intermediate intensity, while inflammation is bright [33]. Further work in this area, however, is needed.

Pathology

Nose

Primary tumors of the nasal cavity are rare; involvement usually is secondary to spread from a maxillary malignancy. However, there are two lesions peculiar to the nose: esthesioneuroblastoma and inverting papilloma.

Esthesioneuroblastomas (Olfactory Neuroblastomas)

Esthesioneuroblastomas arise from the neurosensory receptor cells of the olfactory mucosa high in the nasal fossa. They are slow growing with local invasion into the ethmoid and sphenoid sinuses and intracranially [31,32]. They enhance on postcontrast CT images. Metastases to the cervical nodes and the lungs occur in about 20 percent.

Inverting Papilloma

The inverting papilloma, a benign lesion, presents as a unilateral, expansile nasal mass that

Table 4-3. Paranasal sinus series

Sinus	Caldwell View	Waters View	Submentovertex View	Lateral View
Frontal	Superior and lateral walls	Superior and lateral walls	Anterior and posterior walls	Anterior and posterior walls
Ethmoid	Lamina papyracea	Separates anterior cells from posterior, lacrimal bone	Anterior and posterior cells	Roof
Maxillary	Medial wall and roof	All walls except anterior	Posterolateral	Floor and posterior roof
Sphenoid	—	—	Lateral and anterior walls	Roof and posterior walls
Nose	Nasal septum and turbinates	Nasal septum and turbinates	—	Nasal bone and hard palate

displaces without destroying the nasal septum. It frequently spreads into the ipsilateral ethmoid and maxillary sinuses, nasopharynx, and skull base. Thinning and frank destruction of the lateral nasal wall are common. Postsurgical recurrence occurs in 25 to 50 percent of cases. A small percentage demonstrates cellular atypia or foci of invasive squamous cell carcinoma [32].

Paranasal Sinuses

Primary Malignancies

The overwhelming majority of paranasal sinus malignancies (80–90%) are squamous cell carcinomas of the maxillary antra (80%) [34]. Sixty percent of the patients have bony destruction and local extension upon initial presentation (Figure 4-11).

Adenocarcinomas constitute less than 10 percent of the malignancies in this area. They have a predilection for the ethmoid sinuses. There is an increased incidence in hardwood (furniture industry) workers.

Adenoid cystic carcinomas (cylindromas) arise in the minor salivary glands lining the paranasal sinuses. The highest incidence is in the maxillary antra. Perineural spread is a common pathologic feature.

Nodal metastases are unusual in carcinomas of the paranasal sinuses, with adenocarcinomas having the highest frequency and squamous cell the lowest. The lateral retropharyngeal and jugulodigastric nodal chains are the usual sites.

Non-Hodgkin's lymphomas account for most of the nonepithelial malignancies in the paranasal sinuses and nose [35]. Sinus involvement may reflect regional head and neck or systemic disease (see Chapter 3).

All of these malignancies present as masses that may completely fill the sinuses. Squamous cell carcinomas show bony destruction with extrasinus spread identified as loss of the fat planes surrounding the bony walls (Figure 4-11) [32]. Adenocarcinomas, adenoid cystic carcinomas, and lymphomas have a higher pro-

Figure 4-11. Maxillary sinus carcinoma. A. Soft-tissue mass fills the left maxillary antrum, eroding the medial wall and extending into the nasal cavity. The lateral wall is also destroyed with extension into the infratemporal fossa (*arrow*). (Figure Continued.)

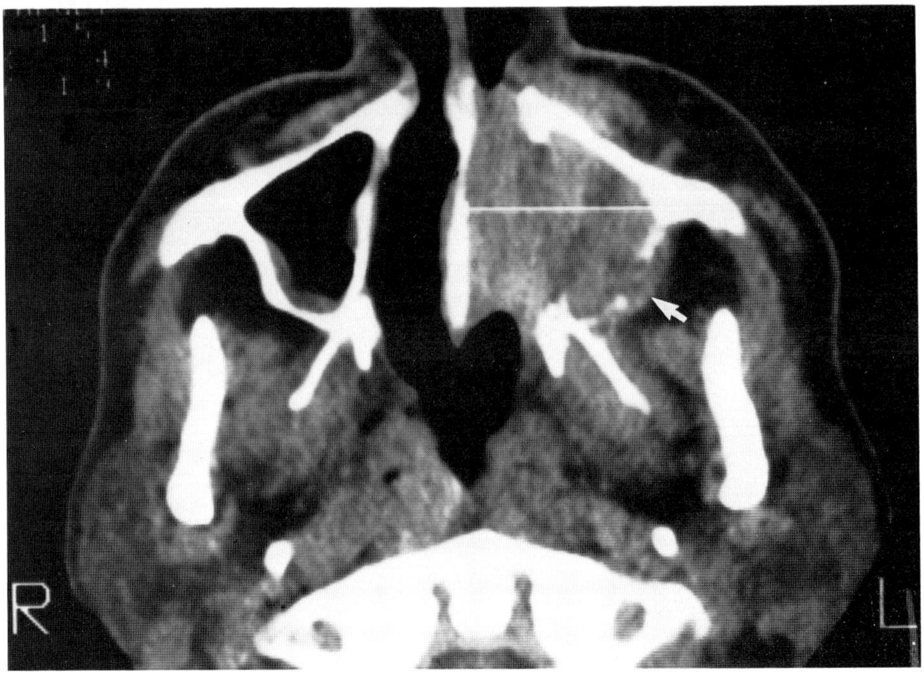

A

pensity for expansion rather than invasion [32]. A similar expansile pattern is consistently seen with mucoceles that may coexist with neoplasms. Both MRI and contrast-enhanced CT scans can separate the malignancy from a secondary mucocele [33].

Secondary Malignancies
Metastatic disease, distinctly uncommon, presents as destructive bony lesions that must be differentiated from primary malignancies. The most common sources for distant metastasis are kidney, lung, and breast.

MAJOR SALIVARY GLANDS (Site 3)

Anatomy

There are three major paired salivary glands: parotid, submandibular, and sublingual. There are an estimated 600 to 1000 minor salivary glands in the upper aerodigestive tract, with the greatest concentration in the palate.

Parotid Gland

The parotid gland, the largest of the salivary glands, is found in the preauricular area, posterior to the masseter muscle and overlying the ramus of the mandible. This gland contains

Figure 4-11. (continued) B. The floor of the maxillary antrum and the hard palate are destroyed by the soft-tissue mass (*M*).

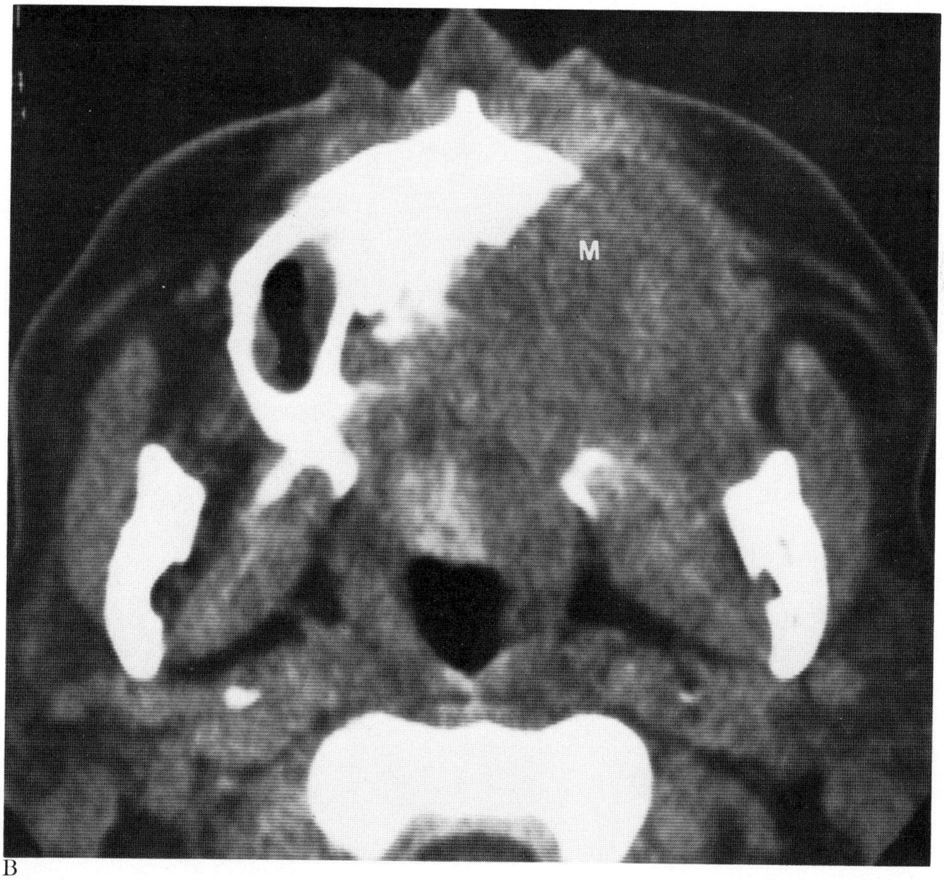

B

more fat than the other salivary glands, a fact that makes its identification easy on CT and MRI.

The parotid (Stensen's) duct leaves the anterior aspect of the gland superficial to the masseter muscle and passes through the buccinator muscle into the oral cavity opposite the second upper molar tooth.

The facial nerve, exiting at the stylomastoid foramen and running through the parotid gland, creates a surgical plane and divides the gland into the so-called superficial and deep lobes. There are numerous lymph nodes superficial to and within the gland. These nodes drain the scalp, external ear, orbit, and face (see Chapters 3 and 16).

Submandibular Gland

The submandibular gland, the second largest of the major salivary glands, lies both superficial and deep to the mylohyoid muscle. The submandibular (Wharton's) duct leaves the deep portion of the gland, runs forward in the floor of the mouth between the mylohyoid and hyoglossus muscles, and empties lateral to the frenulum [36].

The submandibular lymph nodes drain the gland itself, the lips, anterior two-thirds of the tongue, and the nose (see Chapter 3).

Sublingual Gland

The sublingual glands, lying on the mylohyoid muscle, have numerous efferent ducts that empty directly into the floor of the mouth. Occasionally, an accessory duct may join the submandibular duct [36].

Imaging

The goals of imaging are separation of intrinsic from extrinsic lesions, tumor definition, and identification of associated adenopathy. In the parotid gland, lesion location relative to the facial nerve is very helpful.

Computed Tomography

CT usually is performed in the axial projection with 5-mm contiguous sections. Intravenous bolus injection of contrast medium combined with drip infusion separates muscle, adenopathy, and juxtaglandular masses from the glands. Coronal images, performed as needed, delineate the skull base and parapharyngeal space [37].

Magnetic Resonance Imaging

MRI for imaging the salivary glands is currently under investigation. Preliminary studies suggest CT and MRI are equivalent [38,39]. MRI is much less affected by dental amalgam and may depict the facial nerve.

Pathology

Salivary gland tumors account for less than 3 percent of all head and neck malignancies. The majority of tumors (80%) occur in the parotid gland, with most (80%) of these being benign.

Benign Neoplasms

The two most common benign tumors are the pleomorphic adenoma and Warthin's tumor. The pleomorphic adenoma occurs most commonly in the superficial lobe of the parotid gland. It is composed of epithelial and myoepithelial cells. Warthin's tumor consists of oncocytic cells in a lymphoid stroma [40]. These tumors can be bilateral. Recurrences even after 20 years are frequent.

On CT, the benign lesions, regardless of etiology, are well-circumscribed with variable

Figure 4-12. Pleomorphic adenoma. There is a well-circumscribed lesion (*P*) in the superficial lobe of the right parotid gland.

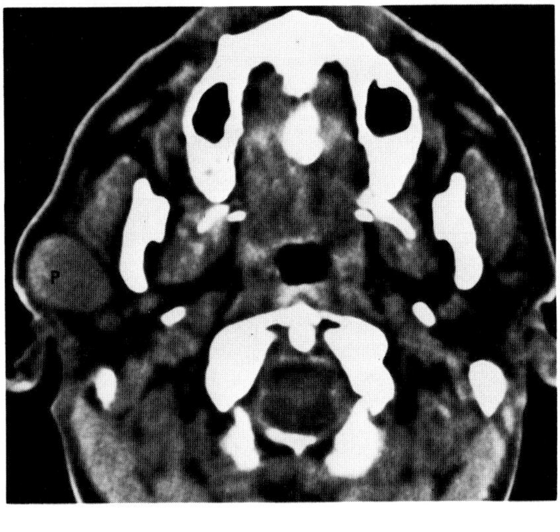

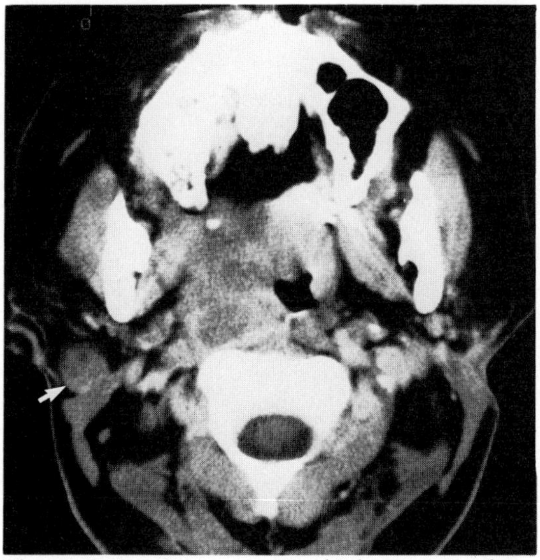

Figure 4-13. Recurrent Warthin's tumor in the right parotid gland. A Warthin's tumor had been resected from the right gland 17 years earlier. A well-circumscribed mass (*arrow*) in the posterior portion of the parotid gland abuts the sterno-cleidomastoid muscle. Also noted is lymphoma of the nasopharynx.

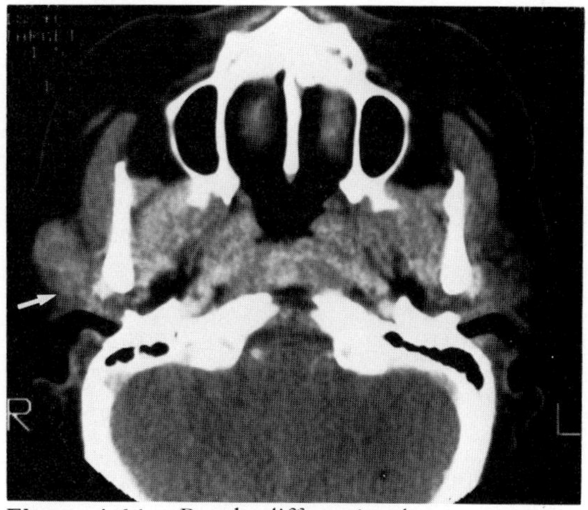

Figure 4-14. Poorly differentiated squamous cell carcinoma. The posterior border (*arrow*) of the mass is ill-defined and merges with the rest of the right parotid gland.

enhancement after contrast infusion (Figures 4-12 and 4-13) [37]. On MRI, these lesions are well-defined, homogeneous, and usually of low to intermediate signal intensity on T1-weighted images [39,41].

Malignant Neoplasms

Mucoepidermoid carcinomas, arising from ductal epithelium, account for less than 10 percent of all salivary gland tumors, but 90 percent occur in the parotid gland. Low-grade tumors are encapsulated, whereas high-grade tumors are infiltrative [40]. The adenoid cystic carcinoma is the most common malignant tumor of the submandibular and sublingual glands. Slow growing, it arises from the intercalated duct and tends to invade nerves.

Both CT and MRI are nonspecific; malignant and benign lesions may be well-demarcated or poorly defined (Figure 4-14). Malignancy is suggested only by infiltration and invasion of adjacent structures [37,39].

Due to abundant lymphatics, parotid metastases are common, usually from melanomas and skin carcinomas. Both CT and MRI can separate adjacent lymph nodes from the salivary glands; however, intraparotid nodes may be confused with primary tumors.

ORAL CAVITY AND OROPHARYNX (Sites 5 and 6)

Anatomy

The oral cavity includes the oral tongue, floor of the mouth, buccal mucosa, hard palate, and retromolar trigone. The oropharynx is separated from the oral cavity by the tonsillar pillars, soft palate, and base of the tongue. The soft palate forms the superior border of the oropharynx and separates it from the nasopharynx. The posterior and lateral pharyngeal walls compose the remainder of the oropharynx [11].

Imaging

CT and MRI, complementing the physical examination, are the primary imaging modalities. Local spread with deep extension especially in the base of the tongue, is appreciated much better than on physical examination (see Chapter 2).

MRI surpasses CT in delineating the normal fascial planes and theoretically demonstrates tumor infiltration earlier than CT [19,42]. MRI is affected much less by dental amalgams that cause marked artifacts on CT. In general, T1-

weighted images separate tumor from fat, and T2-weighted images differentiate tumor from muscle. Gd-DPTA shows promise in delineating tumor from surrounding edema [43].

Pathology

Squamous cell carcinomas constitute the majority of malignancies in the oral cavity and oropharynx, with tumors of the former being better differentiated and less aggressive than those of the latter. Adenocarcinomas, minor salivary gland tumors, and lymphomas compose the remainder.

Excluding the lips, the oral tongue and floor of the mouth are most affected. Tongue lesions occur mainly on the lateral surface (Figure 4-15), extending into the remainder of the tongue as well as into the base. Floor of the mouth lesions are commonly found within 2 cm of the anterior midline (Figure 4-16). They usually spread along the mandibular periosteum into the sublingual and submandibular trian-

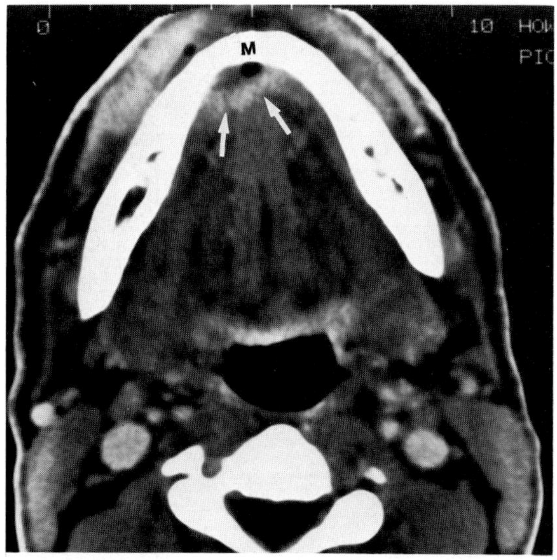

Figure 4-16. Squamous cell carcinoma of the floor of mouth. There is an enhancing lesion of the anterior floor of mouth (*arrows*) with cavitation just behind the mandible (*M*).

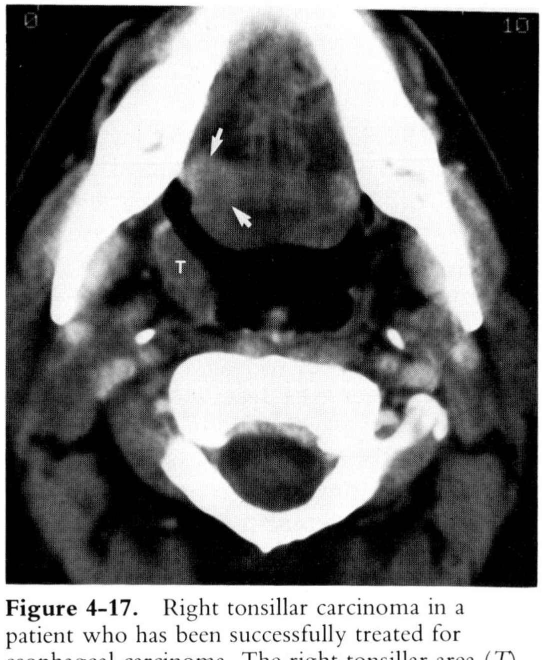

Figure 4-17. Right tonsillar carcinoma in a patient who has been successfully treated for esophageal carcinoma. The right tonsillar area (*T*) is enlarged. Tumor has spread to the tongue base (*arrows*).

Figure 4-15. Squamous cell carcinoma of the oral tongue. Contrast-enhanced CT image shows an enhancing lesion of the right posterolateral tongue (*open arrows*).

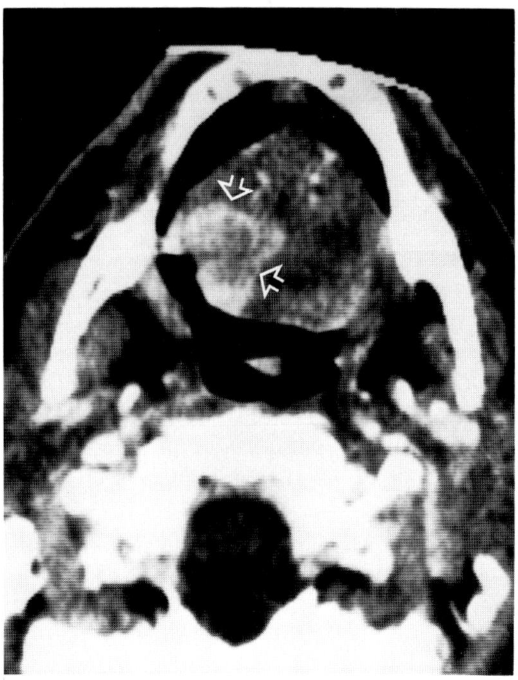

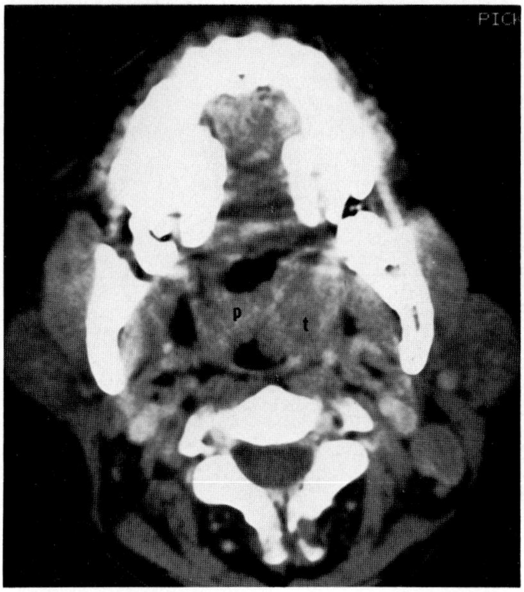

A

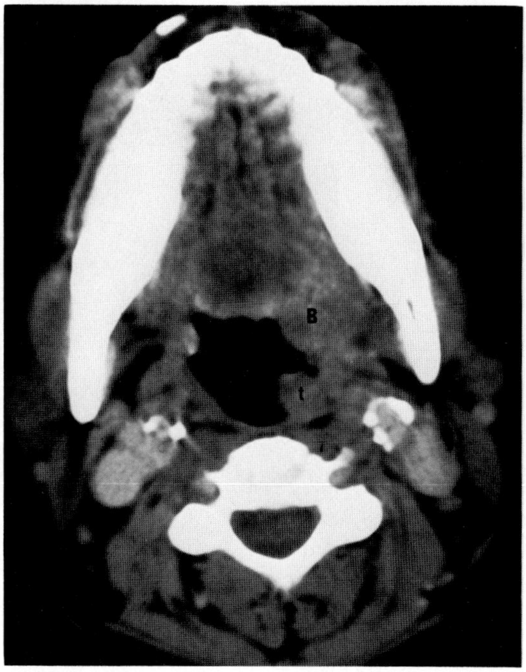

B

Figure 4-18. Left tonsillar carcinoma. A. Mass involves the left tonsillar area (*t*), soft palate (*p*), and right tonsil. Ring-enhancing left posterior triangle node is present. B. Inferiorly the mass infiltrates the tongue base (*B*). The left tonsil (*t*) is still enlarged.

gles. Retromolar trigone carcinomas can easily extend to the tonsillar areas, thus behaving as tonsillar carcinomas. Lateral extension into the buccal mucosa, mandible, and masticator space also is frequent. Nodal metastasis in oral cavity lesions is to the jugulodigastric and submandibular nodes (see Chapter 16).

The most frequent subsite of oropharyngeal carcinoma is the tonsils. Tonsillar lesions spread to the base of the tongue, oral tongue, hypopharynx, soft palate, and nasopharynx (Figures 4-17 and 4-18). Retromolar trigone involvement may appear as mandibular or cheek swelling. Soft palate tumors, found mostly on the oral surface near the tonsillar pillars (Figure 4-19), spread to the tonsils or nasopharynx. Base of the tongue lesions are infiltrative and clinically underestimated. Lymphatic drainage from oropharyngeal lesions is to the jugulodigastric, retropharyngeal, and spinal accessory chains.

On contrast-enhanced CT scans, primary lesions show varying degrees of enhancement (see Figures 4-18 and 4-19). Involved nodes may be homogeneous or display ring enhancement (see Figure 4-19A and C) suggestive of necrosis. On the T1-weighted MR images, tumor appears isointense or slightly hypointense to muscle. The T2-weighted sequences are critical in separating the "bright" tumor from the "dark" adjacent muscles [19,42].

LARYNX AND HYPOPHARYNX (Sites 7 and 8)

Anatomy

The anatomy of the larynx and hypopharynx is reviewed extensively in Chapters 2 and 14.

Larynx

The supporting structures of the larynx are the thyroid and cricoid cartilages and the hyoid bone. The thyroid cartilage is the most prominent external feature of the larynx, forming the Adam's apple in the male. It articulates with the cricoid cartilage inferiorly and the hyoid bone superiorly. The arytenoid cartilages, two small pyramid-shaped structures, articulate with the cricoid cartilage. The true vocal cords attach

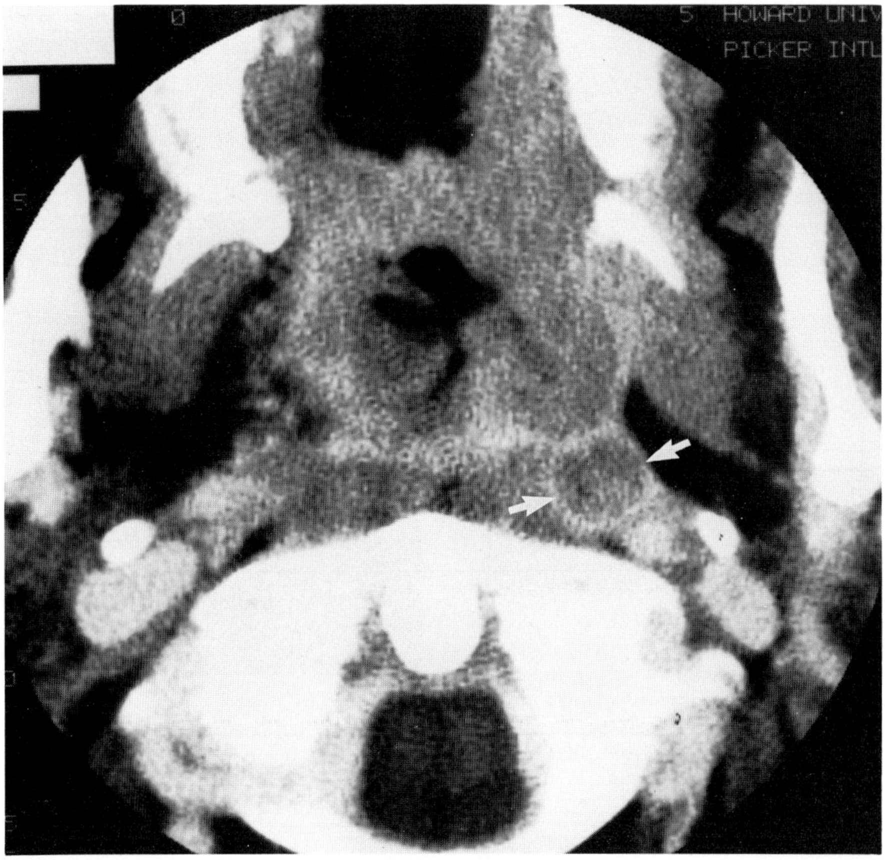

A

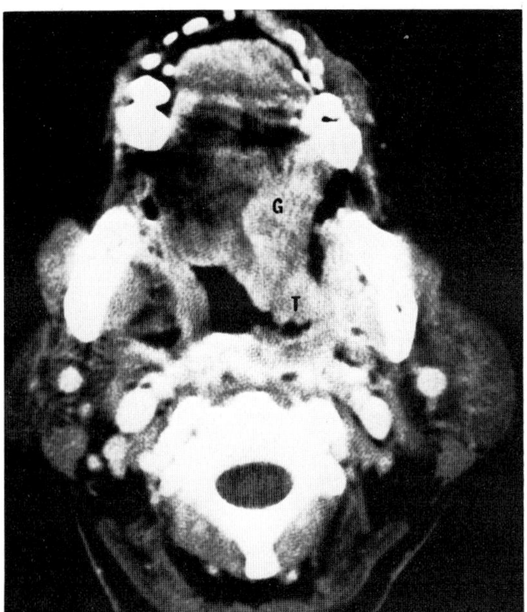

B

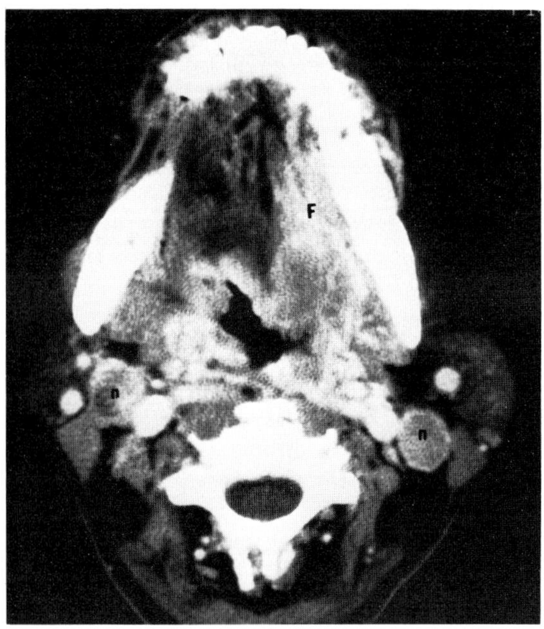

C

Figure 4-19. Soft palate carcinoma. A. There is central ulceration of the soft palate. A ring-enhancing, left lateral retropharyngeal node (*arrows*) is present. B. There is inferior extension to the left tonsil (*T*) and oral tongue (*G*). Tumor also involves the right tonsil and the posterior pharyngeal wall. C. Tumor surrounds the oropharynx and is also seen in the left floor of the mouth (*F*). Necrotic nodes (*n*) are present in both internal jugular chains.

anteriorly to the vocal processes of the arytenoids.

The endolarynx is composed mainly of the epiglottis, the true and false vocal cords, and the aryepiglottic folds. Axial CT sections of the superior portion of the arytenoids define the level of the false cords. The airway is usually pear-shaped, and a small amount of soft tissue can be seen in the anterior midline. On T1-weighted MR images, fat and mucous glands in the false cords give a bright signal. The true vocal cords, inferior to the false cords, are separated from the latter by the laryngeal ventricle. On axial CT sections, the soft-tissue density of the vocalis muscles at the level of the cricoarytenoid articulation delineates the true cord level. The airway also assumes a more triangular configuration. The normal CT appearance of the larynx is shown in Figure 4-20.

Hypopharynx

The hypopharynx usually is considered part of the alimentary tract, being continuous with the oropharynx above and the cervical esophagus below. It encompasses the pyriform sinuses, the posterior pharyngeal wall, and the postcricoid space.

Imaging

Soft-Tissue Radiography

Cervical soft-tissue radiography is an economical screening examination. Ulcerations and masses of the larynx and hypopharynx show as abnormalities of the air-mucosa interface.

Barium Swallow

The barium swallow frequently is ordered for patients who present with dysphagia or odynophagia. It can demonstrate lesions of the pyriform sinuses, posterior pharyngeal wall, and the base of the tongue. After laryngeal or pharyngeal surgery, the barium swallow documents swallowing abnormalities (see Chapter 25).

Computed Tomography

CT represents a significant advance over the prior imaging modalities of laryngography and conventional tomography [8,9]. It is invaluable in tumor staging by identifying spread to the preepiglottic and paraglottic spaces, the anterior and posterior commissures, and the postcricoid area [10]. Scanning is usually performed in the supine position in the plane parallel to the vocal cords. Five-millimeter contiguous sections are obtained from the tip of the epiglottis to the inferior border of the cricoid cartilage. Intravenously administered iodinated contrast facilitates the separation of adenopathy from the numerous vascular structures of the neck [44]. However, CT has serious limitations in evaluating superficial glottic lesions, distinguishing edema from tumor, and detecting microscopic cartilaginous invasion [10,45].

Magnetic Resonance Imaging

The quality of images generated with surface coils are almost comparable to those of CT [46,47]. The multiplanar (axial, sagittal, etc.) capability of MRI allows optimization of imaging plane according to tumor location. Spread of tumor in the craniocaudad direction is sometimes overestimated on axial images. The axial views are therefore supplemented by sagittal projections for evaluating the anterior commissure, the preepiglottic space, and the tongue base. Coronal views can be added for further clarification of tumor spread across the laryngeal ventricle and hence the feasibility of conservation surgery (see Chapter 14). Reformatted sagittal and coronal CT images suffer from image degradation and therefore do not provide the same information as direct sagittal and coronal MR images.

MRI may detect early cartilaginous invasion more precisely than CT scan [48]. If further studies substantiate this initial impression, MRI may have a profound impact on management

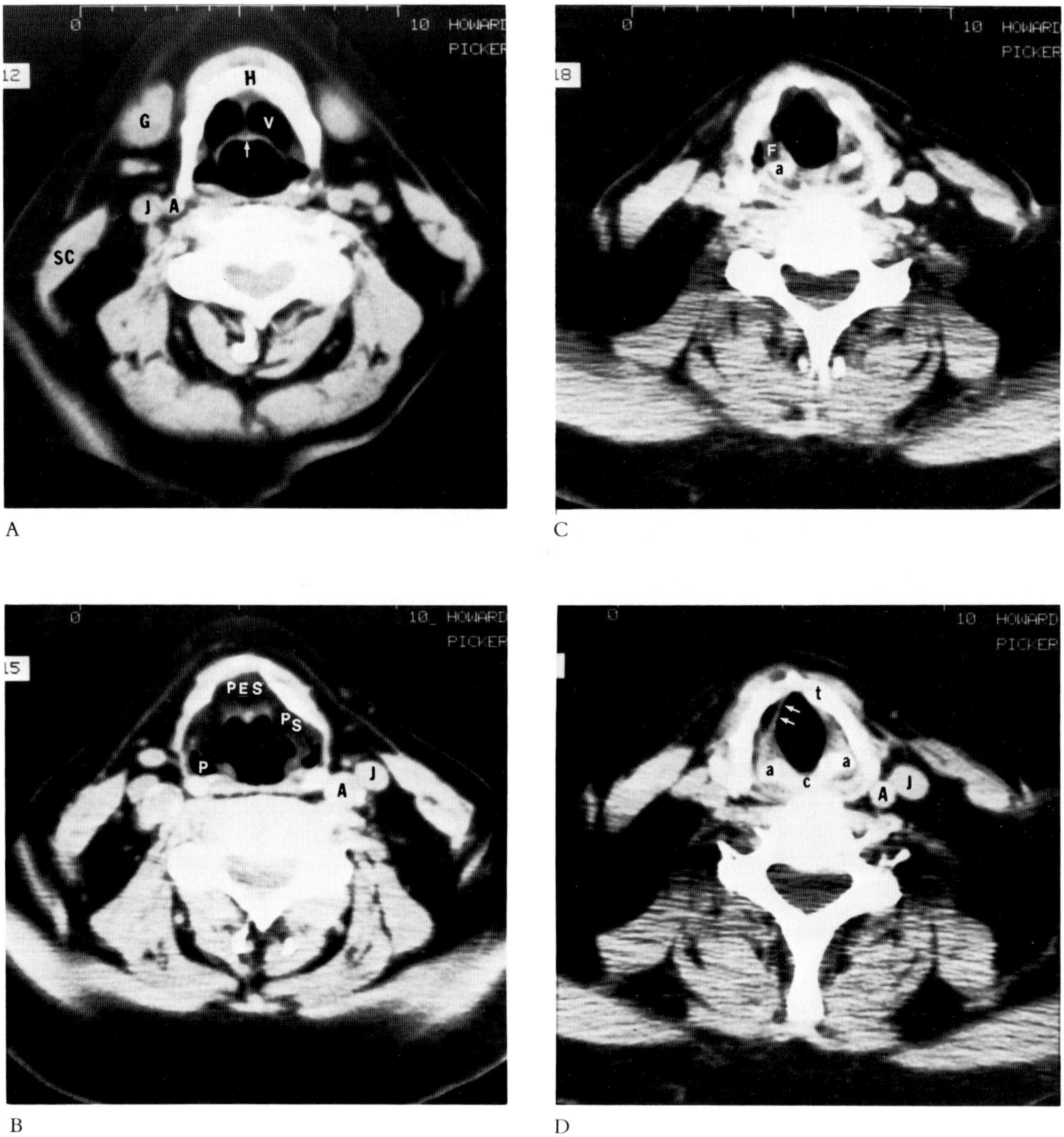

Figure 4-20. Normal axial CT images of the larynx at levels of (A) free tip of the epiglottis; (B) preepiglottic space; (C) false vocal cord; (D) true vocal cord; and (E) subglottic space. *A* = carotid artery; *a* = arytenoid cartilage; *c* = cricoid cartilage; *F* = aryepiglottic fold; *G* = submandibular gland; *H* = hyoid bone; *J* = internal jugular vein; *P* = pyriform sinus; *PES* = preepiglottic space; *PS* = paralaryngeal space; *SC* = sternocleidomastoid muscle; *t* = thyroid cartilage; *TG* = thyroid gland; *V* = vallecula; *arrow* = epiglottis; *double arrows* = true vocal cord.

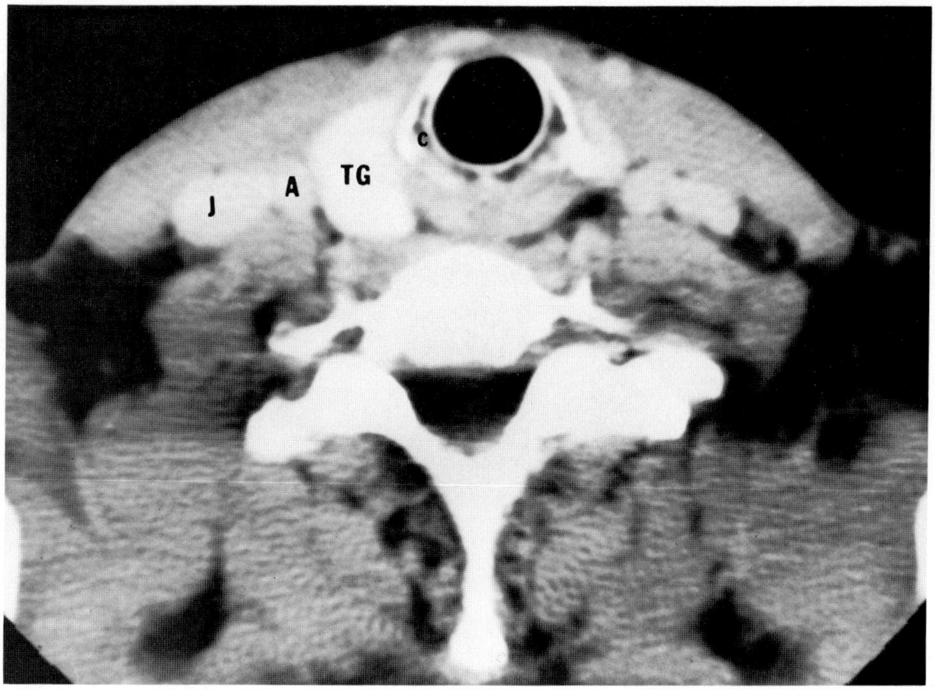

E

decisions, as cartilage invasion precludes most conservation laryngeal surgery.

Pathology

Larynx

Laryngeal neoplasms, the majority being squamous cell carcinomas, are located in three subsites. Most, 60 to 70 percent, arise from the glottis or true vocal cords. Supraglottic tumors, 25 to 30 percent, involve the structures superior to the true vocal cords, while subglottic tumors occur below the true cords. Primary tumors of the subglottis are rare.

Glottis

Neoplasms of the glottis usually occur on the anterior two-thirds of the true vocal cords (Figure 4-21A). Local spread is to the anterior and posterior commissures, the contralateral true cord, and the subglottis (Figure 4-21B). Nodal spread is uncommon.

Supraglottis

Tumors in the supraglottis arise from the false cords, laryngeal ventricle, epiglottis, and aryepiglottic folds. The most common area is the epiglottis. Supraglottic lesions are less well-differentiated than those of glottic origin and have a higher incidence of metastatic lymphadenopathy. Epiglottic tumors frequently bulge into the laryngeal vestibule, invade the preepiglottic space, and extend inferiorly to the false cords and aryepiglottic folds (Figure 4-22). Aryepiglottic fold tumors present as fold asymmetry. Large supraglottic tumors may invade the arytenoid (posteriorly) and the paraglottic and preepiglottic (anteriorly) spaces (Figure 4-23).

Hypopharyngeal Neoplasms

Less well-differentiated than those of the larynx, hypopharyngeal tumors metastasize early and may present silently as neck masses (see Chapters 2, 3, and 6). Most of these tumors arise in the pyriform sinuses (Figure 4-24). They may infiltrate the aryepiglottic folds and arytenoid, cricoid, and thyroid cartilages and extend into the cervical soft tissues [44]. Since the apices of the pyriform sinuses are at the level of the true cords and cricoid cartilage, lesions involving the

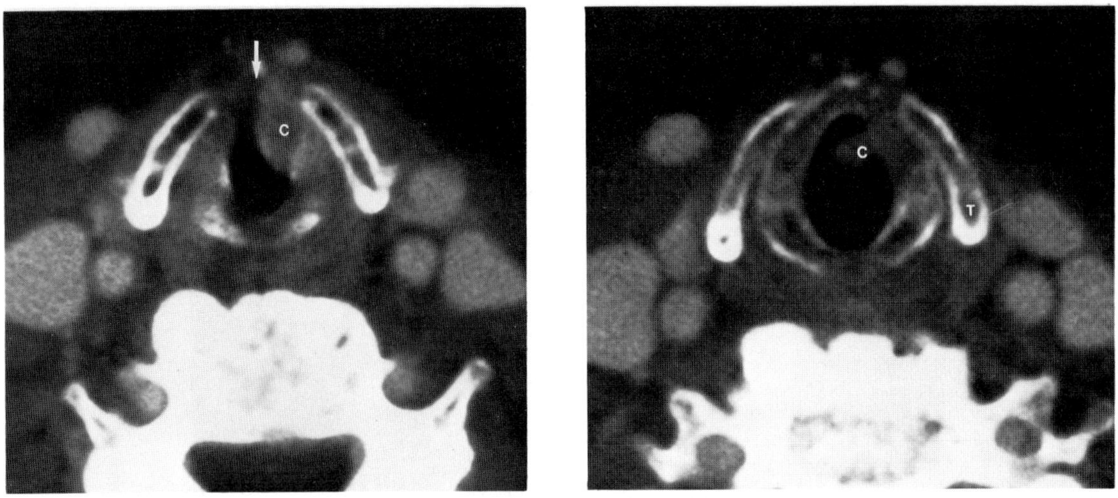

A B

Figure 4-21. Glottic carcinoma. A. CT image shows a soft-tissue mass (*C*) of the anterior left true vocal cord extending to the anterior commissure (*arrow*). B. CT image through the cricoid cartilage. Carcinoma (*C*) extends into the subglottic space with erosion of the cricoid cartilage. *T* = thyroid cartilage.

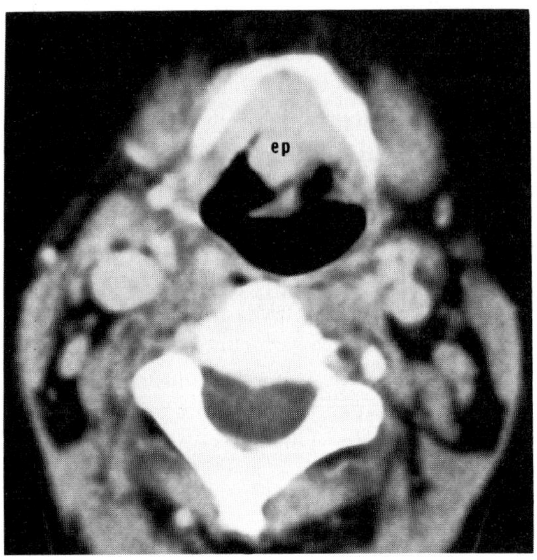

Figure 4-22. Epiglottic carcinoma. Lobulated mass involves the epiglottis (*ep*) and obliterates the normal fat in the preepiglottic and paralaryngeal spaces.

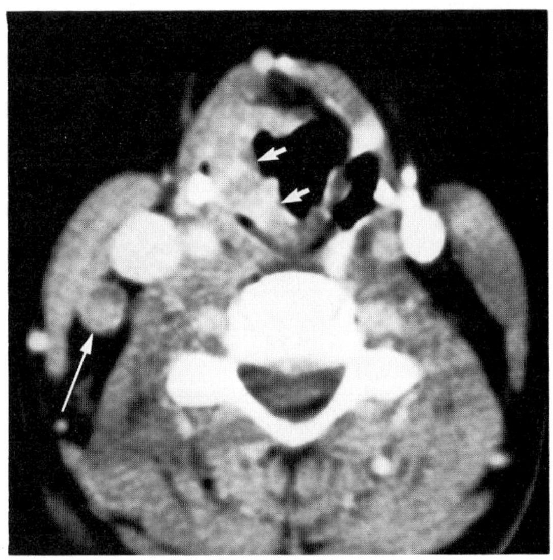

Figure 4-23. Squamous cell carcinoma of the right aryepiglottic fold. The right fold is enlarged (*short arrows*), and tumor extends into the right paraglottic space. Note enlarged necrotic right posterior triangle node (*long arrow*).

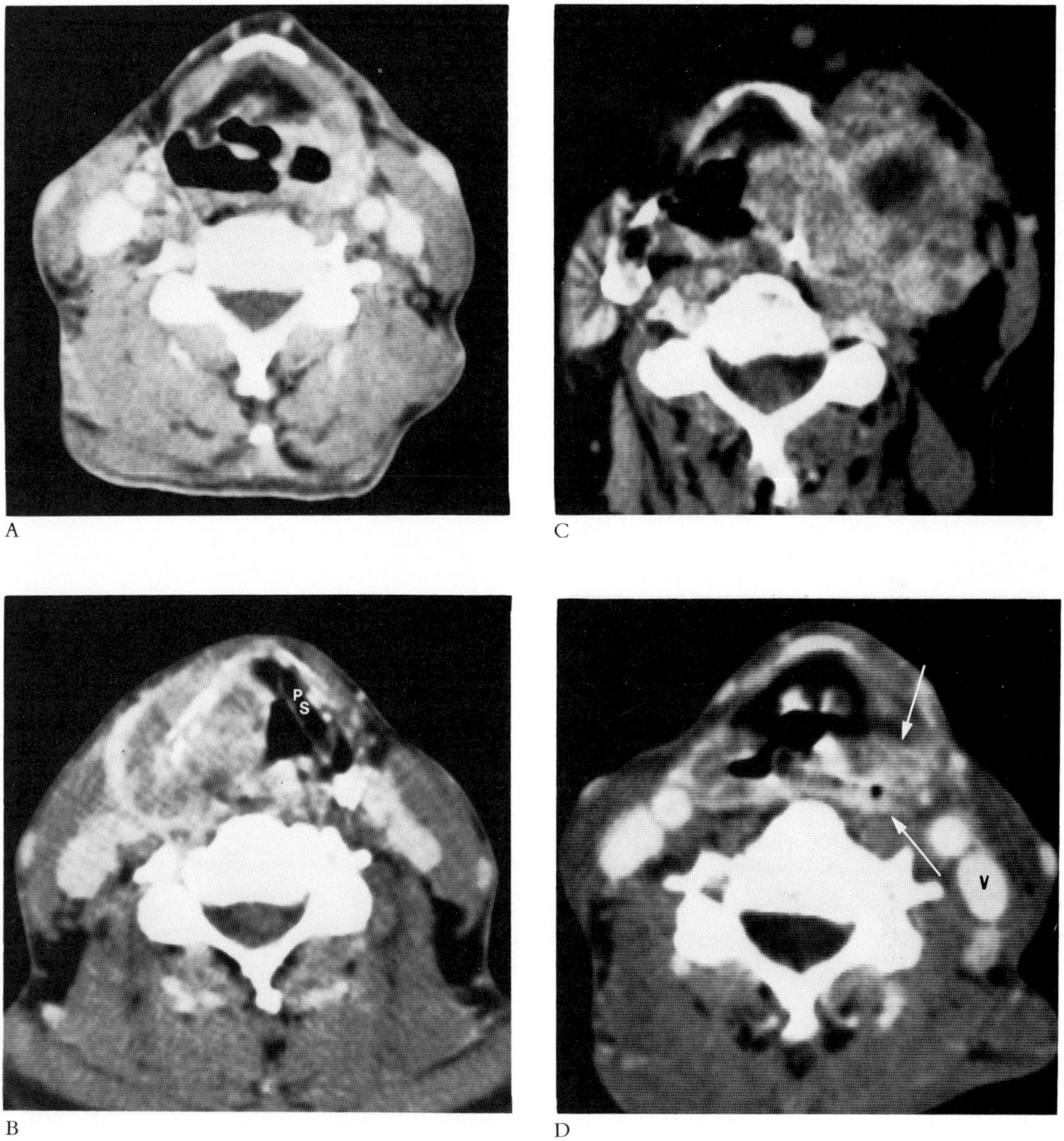

Figure 4-24. Pyriform sinus carcinomas (four different patients). A. Tumor presents as symmetric thickening of the left pyriform sinus. B. Right pyriform sinus mass grows out into the neck posterior to destroyed thyroid cartilage. *PS* = normal left paraglottic space. C. Left pyriform sinus carcinoma with adjacent necrotic matted neck nodes in patient presenting with a left neck mass (autopsy proven). D. Bilateral pyriform sinus carcinomas. Mass (*arrows*) fills the left sinus, and unsuspected second primary tumor is in the right sinus (autopsy proven). A metastatic node is posterior to the left internal jugular vein (*V*).

apices by mass effect or direct extension limit vocal cord mobility. Postcricoid tumors, with a higher incidence in women, account for approximately 20 percent of hypopharyngeal tumors. There is an association with the Plummer-Vinson syndrome. These tumors grow circumferentially and invade the cricoid cartilage and cricoarytenoid muscle. Posterior pharyngeal wall tumors spread superiorly and inferiorly to invade the tonsillar area and cervical esophagus respectively. Abundant lymphatics account for early spread to the jugulodigastric and retropharyngeal nodes. Postcricoid tumors may present with paratracheal and inferior deep cervical adenopathy.

CERVICAL ESOPHAGUS (Site 10)

Anatomy

The cervical esophagus extends from the cricopharyngeus muscle to the thoracic inlet. It lies directly behind and frequently bulges into the trachea, since the posterior tracheal wall is devoid of cartilage. Posterior to the cervical esophagus are the prevertebral muscles. The thyroid gland and common carotid arteries are lateral and anterior. Within the tracheoesophageal groove are the recurrent laryngeal nerve and inferior thyroid artery. At the thoracic inlet, the esophagus deviates slightly to the left and is in proximity to the thoracic duct.

Imaging

Barium Swallow

The barium swallow is frequently the initial procedure for evaluation of the cervical esophagus. Carcinomas of this region are stenotic and ulcerative (Figure 4-25A) with frequent tracheal fistulization.

Computed Tomography

CT demonstrates esophageal wall thickness, extension into adjacent structures, adenopathy, and cartilage invasion or destruction (Figure 4-25B).

Magnetic Resonance Imaging

MRI is best performed using surface coils in the axial and sagittal planes. The cricopharyngeus

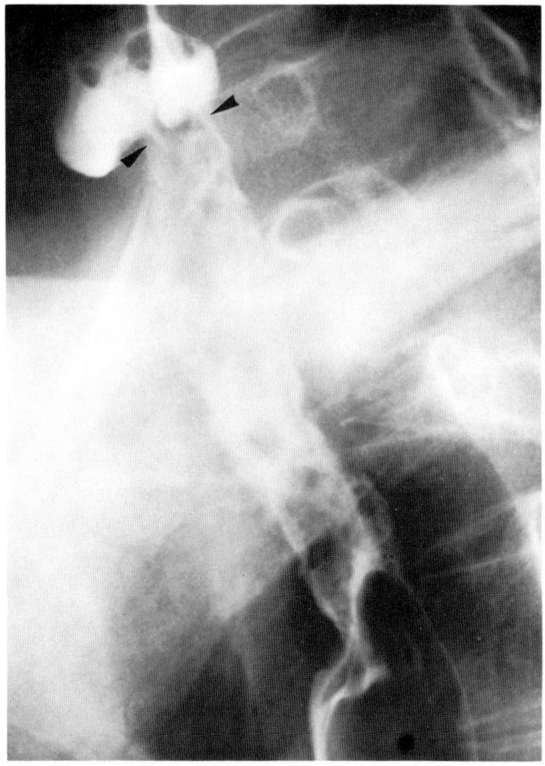

A

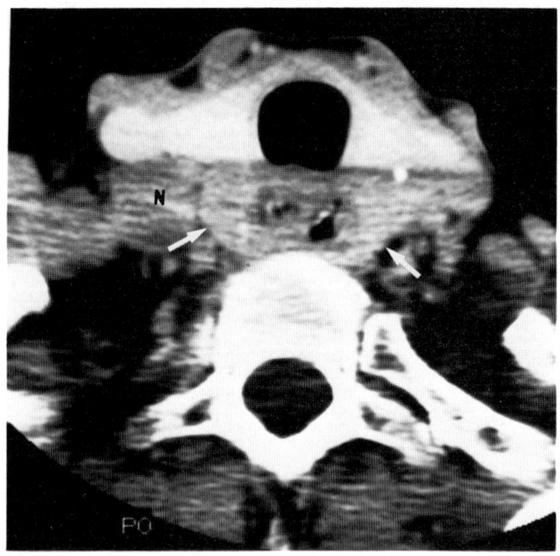

B

Figure 4-25. Squamous cell carcinoma of the cervical esophagus. A. Barium swallow shows a constricting ulcerated lesion extending from the level of the cricopharyngeus muscle (*arrowheads*) into the thorax. B. CT scan confirms the ulcerating mass (*arrows*) of the esophagus with extension into the soft tissues on the left and adjacent right-sided nodes (*N*).

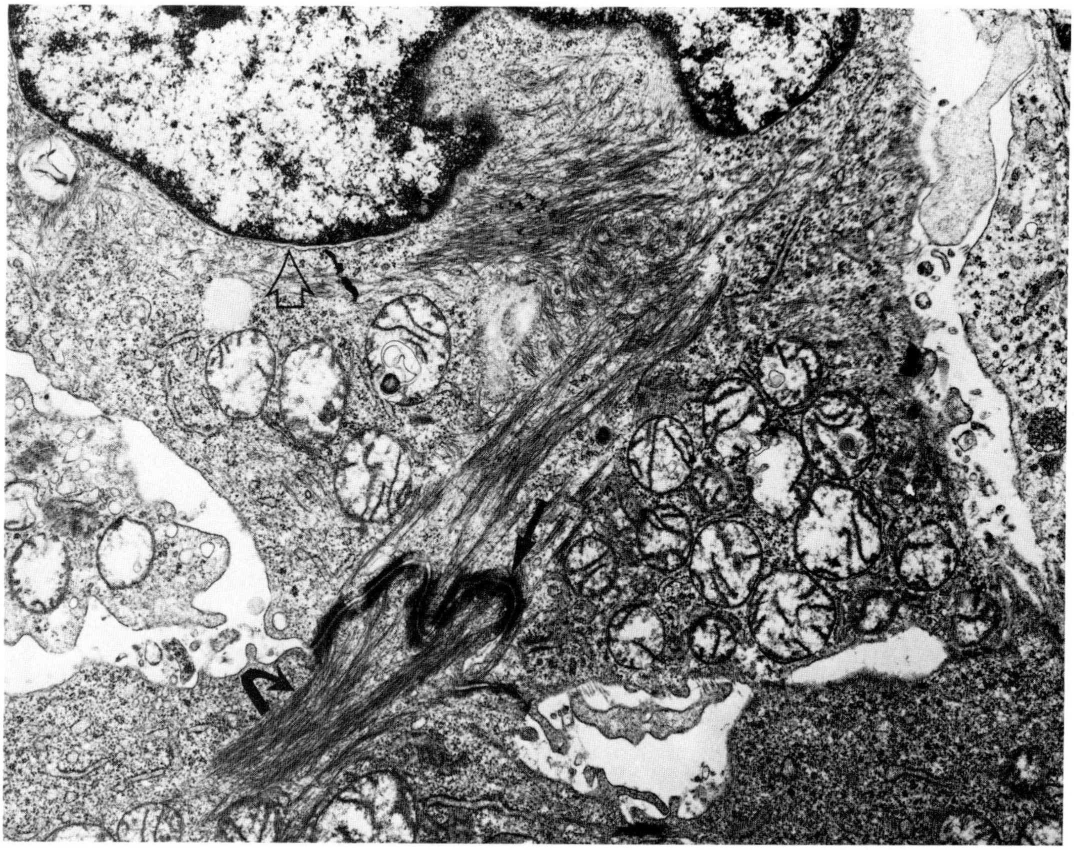

Figure 5-2. Squamous cell carcinoma (ultrastructure). Tonofilaments (*curved arrow*) of cytokeratin converge upon well-developed desmosomes (*solid arrow*). An enlarged and irregular nucleus (*open arrow*) is noted in the left upper hand corner.

Paranasal Sinuses and Nose (Site 2)
Relatively rare, the most frequent malignancy of the nasal cavity and paranasal sinuses is squamous cell carcinoma. They are found in the nasal vestibules, septum, and frontal, sphenoid, maxillary, and ethmoid sinuses [6].

Oral Cavity (Site 5)
Within the oral cavity, squamous cell carcinoma is the most common malignancy. Included are the buccal mucosa, gums (gingiva and alveolar mucosa), tongue, floor of the mouth, and palate [6,7].

Oropharynx (Site 6)
The following subsites are included in the oropharynx: soft palate, retromolar trigone, glossopalatine sulci, tonsillar beds, posterior faucial pillars, base of the tongue, valleculae, lateral and posterior pharyngeal walls, and the pharyngoepiglottic folds. The major subsites are the palatine arch, tonsils, and base of the tongue [7].

Hypopharynx (Site 7)
The hypopharynx extends from the superior margin of the epiglottis to the inferior border of the cricoid [8]. The pyriform sinus, postcricoid area, and pharyngeal wall also may be involved with squamous cell carcinoma.

Larynx (Site 8)
Squamous cell carcinoma of the larynx involves the supraglottis, glottis, and subglottis. The most common subsite is the glottis [9].

Table 5-1. Modified Jakobsson grading for squamous cancer

Parameters	Points 1	2	3	4
Tumor Itself				
Differentiation (keratin formation)	Much (50%)	Some (20–50%)	Little (5–20%)	None
Nuclear atypia	Few atypical cells (75% mature)	Moderate number atypical (50–75% mature)	Numerous atypical (25–50% mature)	Many atypical plus bizarre (0.25% mature)
Mitoses*	Occasional (0–1/HPF)	Moderate (2–3/HPF)	Many (4–5/HPF)	Numerous (6 or more/HPF)
Tumor-Host Relationship				
Pattern of invasion	Exophytic, with pushing border	Exophytic, with infiltrating border	Sessile, with infiltrating border	Dissociated cells
Vascular invasion	None	—	—	Present
Lymphoid response	Marked Continuous rim	Moderate Patchy	Slight Patchy	None —
Stage of invasion	CIS	Microinvasion	Superficial	Deep

*Average after counting all fields in the biopsy.
CIS = Carcinoma in situ; HPF = High-power field.
Source: Crissman JD, Gluckman J, Whiteley J, Quenelle D. Squamous cell carcinoma of the floor of the mouth. *Head Neck Surg* 3 : 2, 1980.

Cervical Esophagus (Site 10)
The American Joint Committee for Cancer Staging and End-Results Reporting divides the esophagus into three regions: cervical, mid-, and lower thoracic esophagus. The cervical esophagus extends from the pharyngoesophageal junction to the thoracic inlet (18 cm from the upper incisor teeth) [10]. Squamous cell carcinoma is the most common primary malignancy, representing approximately 8 percent of esophageal cancers. Tumors involving this area may cross from one boundary to another; that is, they may extend into the hypopharyngeal area and vice versa. Lymphatic drainage of the upper esophagus is to the paratracheal and inferior cervical nodes; approximately 10 percent of carcinomas of the cervical esophagus are associated with positive celiac nodes [11–13].

Verrucous Carcinoma

Verrucous carcinomas are low-grade squamous cell carcinomas that are found most commonly in the buccal sulcus and mandibular alveolar mucosa. They also are found on the maxillary alveolar mucosa, tongue tip, larynx, and nasal fossae. This indolent neoplasm presents clinically as a piled-up papillary mass with a micronodular surface. Histologically, it is characterized by a thickened squamous epithelial layer with bland nuclei. Cytologically, the cells do not appear malignant. There is an advancing margin of bulbous neoplasm with finger-like extensions of well-differentiated epithelium. Small cysts and epithelial pearls often are seen. Malignant features such as abnormal mitosis nuclear atypism and basement membrane disruption are rare. Actual microscopic invasion is not present. Usually a heavy inflammatory reaction consisting of lymphocytes and plasma cells is present [14,15].

Undifferentiated (Anaplastic) Carcinoma

Anaplastic carcinomas are devoid of squamous or glandular cells. Special staining procedures and immunocytochemical methods detect tumor markers (e.g., secretory material, keratin). A neoplasm devoid of tumor markers is classified as anaplastic or undifferentiated. Clinically, these neoplasms are aggressive and have a poor prognosis [16–18].

Adenocarcinoma

Adenocarcinomas originate from the mucous membranes of the minor salivary glands and other glands in the head and neck area. These neoplasms may arise from the nose, paranasal sinuses, larynx, trachea, and oral cavity. They commonly are found in the palate, buccal mucosa, tongue, floor of the mouth, and lips (Figure 5-3). Mucoepidermoid, adenoid cystic, and true adenocarcinomas are variants of glandular cancer that arise from structures in this area.

Mucoepidermoid Carcinoma

Histologically, true adenocarcinomas have glandular differentiation ranging from well-differentiated to undifferentiated patterns. When squamoid differentiation and mucous secretory cells coexist, the tumor is designated mucoepidermoid carcinoma (Figure 5-4).

Adenoid Cystic Carcinoma

Adenoid cystic carcinomas are distinctive in their histologic appearance. They are composed of basiloid cells with discrete acini containing eosinophilic material. Approximately 20 to 30 percent of tracheal adenocarcinomas are of this histology [19,20].

SPECIAL HEAD AND NECK PATHOLOGY

Salivary Gland Carcinoma (Site 3)

Salivary gland carcinomas are uncommon. Mucoepidermoid, acinic cell, and adenocystic carcinoma arising from pleomorphic adenoma

Figure 5-3. Adenocarcinoma. Well-differentiated acini are apparent. They mimic the mucosal lining of the parent organ.

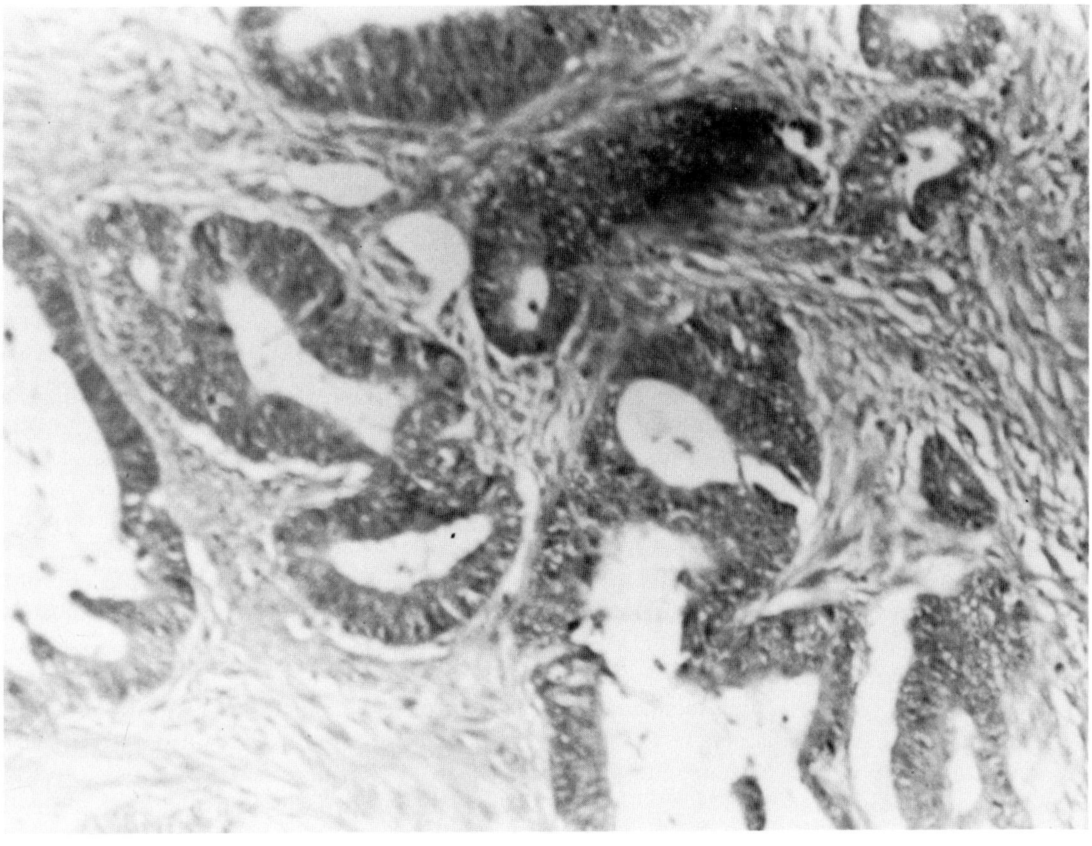

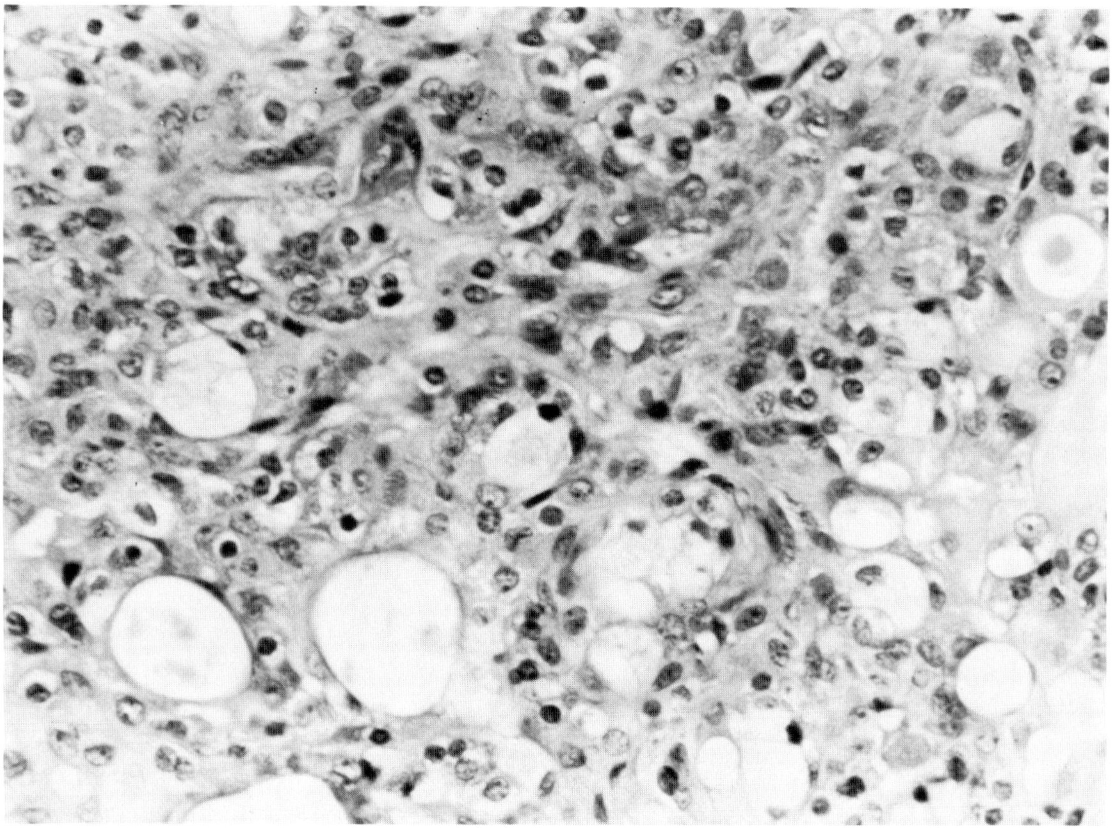

Figure 5-4. Mucoepidermoid carcinoma. Squamoid differentiation and mucous secretory cells coexist, as demonstrated in the photomicrograph.

are the common glandular malignancies. The uncommon forms are adenocarcinoma, squamous cell carcinoma, and undifferentiated carcinoma [21,22].

Most salivary gland carcinomas are found in the parotid gland. Carcinomas involving the submandibular gland represent approximately 10 percent of salivary gland tumors. The incidence of malignancy is higher in the submandibular gland than in the parotid gland. This is also true for malignancies involving the sublingual and minor salivary glands. Adenocarcinoma, adenoidcystic carcinoma, and anaplastic carcinoma are the major types of submandibular gland carcinomas [23–26].

Mucoepidermoid Carcinoma

Mucoepidermoid neoplasms, accounting for approximately 2 to 7 percent of salivary gland tumors, occur in the parotid glands and submandibular glands [21]. They also may arise in minor salivary glands, where they represent the second most common form of malignancy [21]. Grossly, these neoplasms are defined poorly and encapsulated incompletely. Histologically, the neoplasm presents as cords and sheets of squamous cells, mucus, and intermediate cells. The cells often have squamous features associated with small or large mucus-filled vacuoles that range from well-differentiated to less-differentiated areas. Periodic acid Schiff (PAS) and mucicarmine stains help confirm the presence of mucin. The clinical behavior is unpredictable and inconsistent with the histomorphology [18,21].

Acinic Cell Carcinoma and Adenoid Cystic Carcinomas

Acinic cell and adenoid cystic carcinomas are even less common. Acinic cell carcinomas represent 2 to 4 percent of parotid tumors. Grossly, this neoplasm is lobulated and appears encapsulated. They may present histologically as solid, microcystic, papillary cystic, or follicular growth patterns. The adenoid cystic carcinoma represents 2 to 6 percent of parotid tumors. It has poorly defined margins and may present histologically with a solid, tubular, or cribriform pattern [23].

Thyroid Carcinoma (Site 9)

Thyroid carcinomas are rare, representing only 0.4 percent of cancer deaths in the United States. There is an approximate female-to-male ratio of 2.3 : 1.0 [26]. Each anatomic subtype has its own distinctive biology and pathogenesis. The well-differentiated carcinomas include papillary adenocarcinoma, pure or mixed with a follicular pattern; pure follicular carcinoma; clear cell carcinoma; and oxyphil cell carcinoma. The poorly differentiated carcinomas are medullary carcinoma, undifferentiated carcinoma (with subtypes—small cell and giant cell), and epidermoid carcinoma [28].

Papillary Adenocarcinoma

Papillary adenocarcinomas range from microscopic foci in the thyroid gland or lymph nodes to nodules of 10 cm or more. Cystic spaces, sclerosis, and fronds (papillary excrescences) may be seen grossly. Histologically, the characteristic features include a complicated branching, tree-like pattern, "ground-glass" (Orphan Annie eye) appearance, grooved or cleared nuclei, and psammoma bodies. Metastases involve regional cervical lymph nodes and distant sites such as the lungs [29,30] (Figure 5-5).

Follicular Carcinoma

Follicular carcinoma, more aggressive than the papillary form, accounts for 25 percent of all thyroid cancers. Grossly, they usually are encapsulated and difficult to differentiate from benign neoplasms. Histologically, follicular carcinomas range widely in glandular formation and differentiation. Some share a trabecular pattern, whereas others have well-differentiated follicular carcinomas that range widely in glandular formation and differentiation. Some share a trabecular pattern, whereas others have well-differentiated follicles with colloid. Clear cell and oxyphil (Hürthle) variants have been described. There is an alteration in the clinical prognosis because of this particular histologic variation. Capsule and blood vessel invasion with metastasis differentiates these lesions from adenomas. Metastasis occurs commonly in lungs, bones, and in other distant sites [31–34] (Figure 5-6).

Medullary Carcinoma

Highly variable in appearance, medullary carcinoma is an infrequent malignancy. Derived from the parafollical (c) cells of neurosecretory origin, it belongs to the APUD family of tumors. Aside from a strong family history, the distinctive features are amyloid stroma and the ability to elaborate polypeptide products. Grossly, medullary carcinomas localize as discrete tumors in one lobe or numerous nodules infiltrating both lobes. They may spread outside of the thyroid capsule. The tumors are gritty and gray white to yellowish brown. Foci of hemorrhage and necrosis may be observed. These tumors, histologically, display an endocrine tumor-like pattern, having round to polygonal cells or spindle cells with a sarcomatoid appearance. Amyloid may be seen in the stroma, and cell nests may acquire a pseudopapillary configuration [35–35]. Ultrastructural studies usually confirm the presence of argyrophil-positive and argentaffin-positive neurosecretory granules. Immunoperoxidase techniques may demonstrate intracellular calcitonin [17].

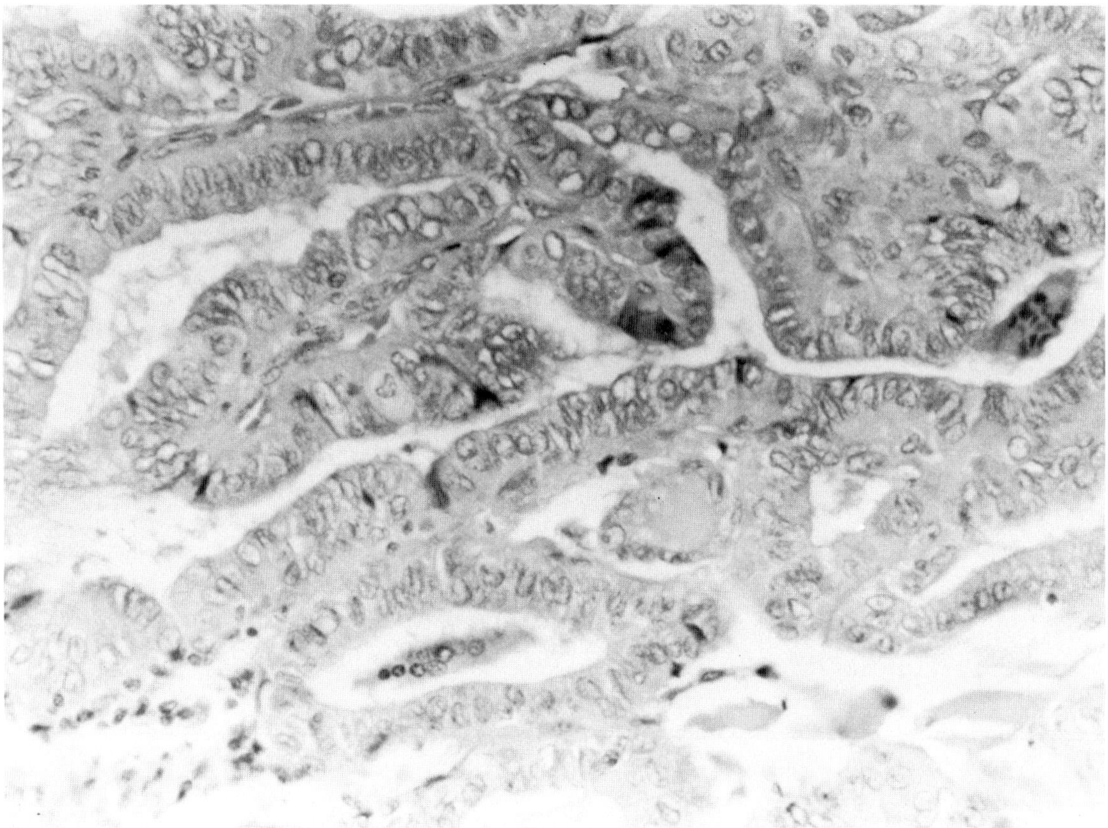

Figure 5-5. Papillary carcinoma of the thyroid gland. Papillary structures with fibrovascular cores are evident.

Undifferentiated Carcinoma

Approximately 10 to 15 percent of thyroid carcinomas are undifferentiated. These occur in the later ages (seventh and eighth decades) and include some of the most malignant neoplasms [37]. These neoplasms present grossly as bulky masses. Histologically, there are small-cell and giant-cell varieties. The giant cell variant has bizarre anaplastic cells with abnormal mitotic figures. The prognosis is poor.

Lymphomas

Cervical lymph nodes, followed by Waldeyer's ring, are the most frequent sites of head and neck lymphoma. The exact site of origin of Waldeyer's ring lymphoma (tonsils, nasopharynx, base of the tongue) often is difficult to determine [38]. The majority of extranodal lymphomas of the head and neck are the non-Hodgkin's type. Conversely, Hodgkin's lymphoma is rare in the extranodal sites.

Hodgkin's Lymphoma

Although Hodgkin's disease affects patients of all age groups, two peak periods occur: one during young adult life and the other in the elderly. Generally, men are affected more often than women in all age groups. The disease presents primarily in the supraclavicular and midcervical lymph nodes. Extranodal presentation is uncommon [39–41]. Histologic features of Hodgkin's disease vary according to the predominance or depletion of lymphocytes, Reed-Sternberg cells, "lacunar cells," mixture of lymphocytes, eosinophils, plasma cells and histiocytes, necrosis, and fibrosis (see Rye classification [Table 5-2]). The Reed-Sternberg cell is highly characteristic; however, it is not

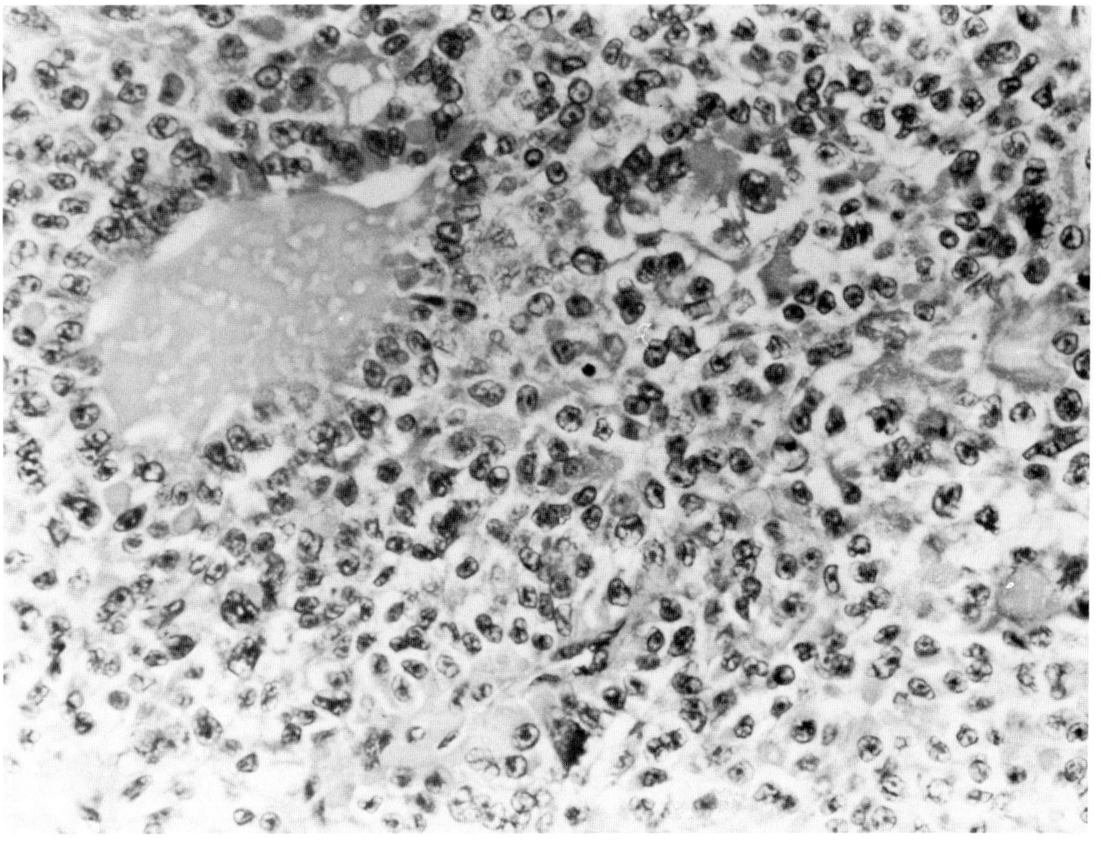

Figure 5-6. Follicular carcinoma of the thyroid gland. Moderately to poorly differentiated follicles are demonstrated. Capsular invasion is present in an adjacent area.

Table 5-2. Histologic features of Hodgkin's disease

Rye classification	*Pertinent histologic features*	*Relative prognosis*
Lymphocyte predominance	Many lymphocytes or a mixture of lymphocytes and histiocytes Few typical Reed-Sternberg cells Absence of necrosis and fibrosis	Most favorable
Nodular sclerosis	Nodules of lymphoreticular cells partially or completely separated by bands of collagen Many "lacunar cell" variants of Reed-Sternberg cells	Favorable
Mixed cellularity	Mixture of cells including lymphocytes, eosinophils, plasma cells, and histiocytes Many Reed-Sternberg cells Foci of necrosis and fibrosis	Guarded
Lymphocyte depletion	Many Reed-Sternberg cells and malignant histiocytes or abundant fibrosis and hypocellularity Few lymphocytes	Guarded

pathognomonic. It is also seen in benign lesions such as infectious mononucleosis, chronic lymphocytic leukemia, and Burkitt's lymphoma. The Rye classification of Hodgkin's disease is lymphocyte predominance, nodular sclerosis, mixed cellularity, and lymphocyte depletion. Hodgkin's disease must also be differentiated from immunoblastic or angioimmunoblastic lymphadenopathy and Lennert's lymphoma. Thus, it is necessary that adequate biopsies of tissues from the head and neck area are submitted for evaluation.

Non-Hodgkin's Lymphoma

The non-Hodgkin's lymphomas are a diverse group of malignant neoplasms that involve cervical lymph nodes. It is difficult to determine their frequency in extranodal sites of the head and neck area (Waldeyer's ring [Figure 5-7]) [38]. Over the years, the histopathologic classification of non-Hodgkin's lymphomas has been controversial [42]. The current classification was established by the National Cancer Institute Sponsored Study of Classifications on Non-Hodgkin's Lymphomas (Table 5-3) [43]. Histologic diagnosis of non-Hodgkin's lymphomas is predicated on cell type, cell morphology, sclerosis, histiocytes, plasmacytoid cells, epithelioid cells, and follicular architecture. Immunocytochemical methods are helpful in difficult cases [44–49].

Vascular Tumors

Paragangliomas

Paragangliomas are small-cell aggregations of neural crest origin that are associated with cranial nerves, their ganglia, and the ontogenetic

Figure 5-7. Non-Hodgkin's lymphoma. This photomicrograph represents large-cell lymphoma. Note the monotonous pattern of the lesion.

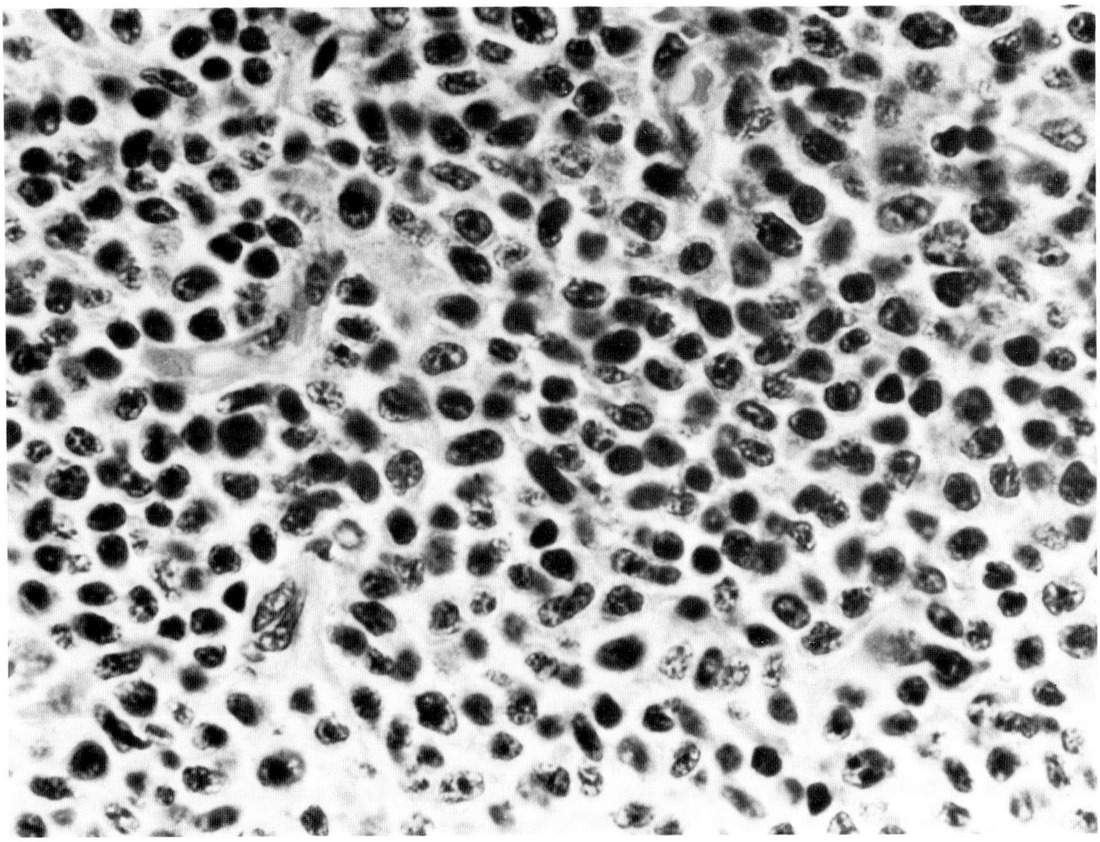

Table 5-3. Hodgkin's lymphoma: Working formulation versus Kiel classification

Working formulation	*Kiel equivalent or related terms*
Low grade	
Malignant lymphoma	ML lymphocytic, CLL
Small lymphocyte consistent with CLL plasmacytoid	ML lymphoplasmacytic, lymphoplasmacytoid
Malignant lymphoma, follicular	ML centroblastic-centrocytic (small), follicular + diffuse
Predominantly small cleaved–cell diffuse areas of sclerosis	
Malignant lymphoma, follicular	
Mixed, small cleaved– and large-cell diffuse areas of sclerosis	
Intermediate grade	
Malignant lymphoma, follicular	ML centroblastic-centrocytic (large), follicular + diffuse
Predominantly large cell	
Diffuse areas of sclerosis	
Malignant lymphoma, diffuse small cleaved–cell sclerosis	ML centrocytic (small)
Malignant lymphoma, diffuse	ML centroblastic-centrocytic (small), diffuse
Mixed, small- and large-cell sclerosis	ML lymphoplasmacytic/cytoid, polymorphic
Epithelioid cell component	
Malignant lymphoma, diffuse	
Large cell	ML centroblastic-centrocytic (large), diffuse
Cleaved cell	ML centrocytic (large)
Noncleaved cell	ML centroblastic
Sclerosis	
High grade	
Malignant lymphoma	
Large cell, immunoblastic	ML immunoblastic
Plasmacytoid	
Clear cell	T-zone lymphoma
Polymorphous	Lymphoepithelioid cell lymphoma
Epithelioid cell component	
Malignant lymphoma	ML lymphoblastic, convoluted cell type ML lymphoblastic, unclassified
Lymphoblastic	
Convoluted cell	
Nonconvoluted cell	
Malignant lymphoma	ML lymphoblastic, Burkitt type, and other B-lymphoblastic
Small noncleaved cell	
Burkitt's	
Follicular areas	
Miscellaneous	
Composite	
Mycosis fungoides	Mycosis fungoides
Histiocytic	
Extramedullary plasmacytoma	ML plasmacytic
Unclassifiable	
Other	

CLL = chronic lymphocyte lymphoma; ML = malignant lymphoma.

gill arches. There are several sites for these structures. Those associated with the head and neck are jugulotympanic paraganglioma (glomus jugulare), vagal paraganglioma (glomus vagale), and carotid body paraganglioma. Paragangliomas tend to be similar irrespective of their location. Grossly, most are ovoid or lobulated, rubbery, and partially encapsulated. They are gray, tan, or red, depending on their vascularity [50,51] (Figure 5-8). Histologically,

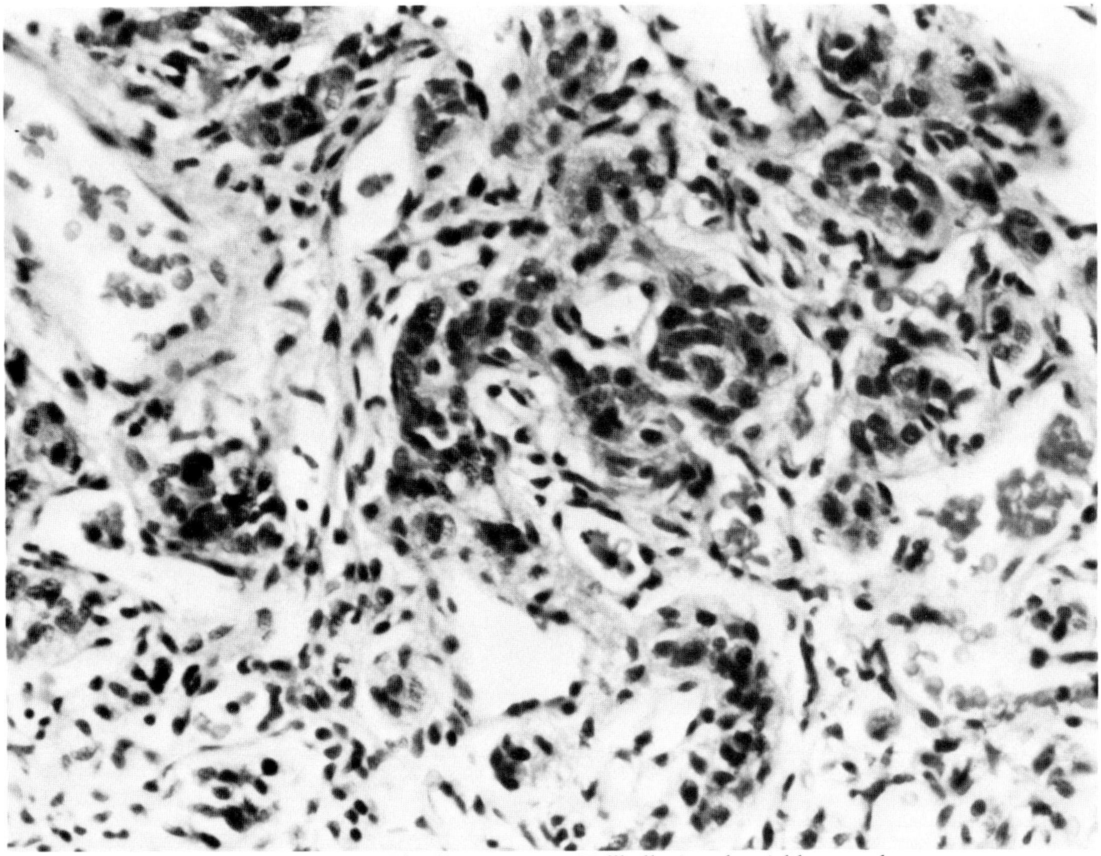

Figure 5-8. Paraganglioma. Organoid cell aggregates (Zellballen) and a richly vascular stroma are major features of this lesion.

they resemble normal paraganglion tissue. They are arranged in nests (Zellballen or cell balls) surrounded by a fine network of reticulin fibers containing many capillary-sized vessels. Brown to black cytoplasmic granules may be demonstrated by the Grimelius stain. Dense neurosecretory granules are demonstrated by electron microscopy. Malignancy is difficult to assess histologically; however, central necrosis of Zellballen, vascular invasion, and mitotic figures are useful in differentiating benign from malignant forms [50,51].

Jugulotympanic Paraganglioma (Glomus Jugulare)

The most common tumor of the middle ear, jugulotympanic paraganglioma is located in the lateral portion of the temporal bone [52]. Intracranial extension may occur in approximately 40 percent of cases. These tumors occur most often in middle-aged adults, with a female predominance of 2 : 1 to 5 : 1. The differential diagnosis includes aural polyp, meningioma, and metastatic carcinoma.

Vagal Paraganglioma (Glomus Vagale)

Vagal paragangliomas are rare and occur most often in the fourth to fifth decade of life, with a female predominance of 2.5 : 1.0. They present as a mass in the neck behind and deep to the mandible or just below the ganglion nodosum. Malignancy is rare but when present, metastasis may occur to the cervical lymph nodes, skull, vertebra, and pelvis.

Carotid Body Paraganglioma

Carotid body paraganglioma is the most common paraganglioma in the head and neck area.

It is most often unilateral but may occur bilaterally in 3 to 8 percent of cases. It is located on the medial aspect of the common carotid artery near its bifurcation [53]. There is no sexual predominance. This neoplasm must be differentiated from other lesions such as branchial cleft cyst, carotid artery aneurysm, lymphoma, and metastatic carcinoma.

DIAGNOSTIC MODALITIES

Biopsy

The biopsy is the most important diagnostic procedure in the evaluation of head and neck neoplasms. Therapy begins only with a definite diagnosis. There are basically four types of biopsies: excisional biopsy (removal of the entire lesion), incisional biopsy (partial removal of a lesion), needle biopsy (aspiration of a thin core of tissue), and fine-needle aspiration biopsy (aspiration of tissue cells for cytologic evaluation). Incisional and excisional biopsies are well-established diagnostic modalities. Needle biopsy and fine-needle aspiration with touch preparation (imprint) are relatively new [26].

The needle biopsy in head and neck oncology is somewhat controversial. Theoretically, it is acceptable for studying large and small lesions; however, one must be aware that the sample may not be representative of the entire lesion. Insufficient material may be obtained for accurate diagnosis. Special procedures such as electron microscopy and immunoperoxidase stains aid the pathologist in diagnosing ill-defined lesions. Needle biopsies may be difficult to interpret, especially when the pathologist relies upon histologic patterns.

Fine-needle aspiration biopsy is becoming more acceptable to both pathologists and clinicians. It has several advantages: (1) cost; (2) local anesthesia; (3) virtually pain free; (4) office procedure; (5) rapid interpretation (10–15 minutes); and (6) few complications. Fine-needle aspiration biopsy is useful for early diagnosis and follow-up [26].

Frozen Section

The frozen section is an acceptable and reliable procedure [54–55]. Although freeze artifacts are created, in most institutions it is approximately 97 to 98 percent accurate. Immediate histologic diagnosis helps surgical planning and often eliminates multiple or unnecessary surgery. When utilized wisely, the frozen section helps the surgeon to make immediate therapeutic decisions. Other indications are (1) differentiation between benign or malignant lesions; (2) determination of free surgical margins; (3) assurance that representative tissue for analysis has been removed; and (4) tissue identification such as vagus nerve, parathyroid gland, or ganglion cells. The limitations are basically inherent in the technique itself. With the introduction of the cryostat (an instrument with a chamber containing a microtome for sectioning frozen tissues), many of the problems associated with tissue artifacts have been solved. Sample selection by the surgeon and the inherent skill and training of the pathologist are necessary to eliminate false-positive and false-negative evaluations. Sampling error is an important cause for false-negative reports.

Electron Microscopy

Although it does not replace the light microscopy, electron microscopy is a diagnostic quality control. Generally, neoplastic cells tend to recapitulate their tissue of origin in some stage of their development. Observation of cellular organelles on the ultramicroscopic level, alone or in combination, often identifies the cells of origin (see Figure 5-2). Specifically, electron microscopy differentiates anaplastic or undifferentiated neoplasms and identifies metastatic neoplasms of unknown origin. It identifies such neoplasms as small-cell anaplastic carcinoma, Ewing's sarcoma, malignant lymphoma, and embryonal rhabdomyosarcoma [56].

One of the major limitations of electron microscopy is the inability to uniformly differentiate benign from malignant neoplasms, since organelles are found in the benign as well as the malignant cell. Errors in interpretation may result from sampling particularly large specimens. Often, poorly differentiated neoplasms defy classification even after extensive study. Electron microscopy is not a routine procedure to identify neoplasms that can be classified by simpler and less costly means.

ARMED FORCES INSTITUTE OF PATHOLOGY

The Armed Forces Institute of Pathology (AFIP) in Washington, D.C., is an excellent resource for difficult tissue consultations. The specimen should be processed and evaluated by the contributing hospital (pathologist) before a consultation is sought from the AFIP. This reduces the number of needless or unnecessary consultations. Often, second opinions on tissue diagnoses are requested by patients or physicians. The AFIP is the ideal institution for such consultation. Routine specimens are not submitted for consultation.

REFERENCES

1. Balogh K: The Head and Neck. In Rubin E, Farber J (eds): *Pathology*. New York: Lippincott, 1988. Pp 1260–1303.
2. Weiland LH: Nasopharyngeal Carcinoma. In Barnes L (ed): *Surgical Pathology of the Head and Neck*. New York: Marcel Dekker, 1985. Vol 1, pp 453–466.
3. Yeh S: A histological classification of carcinomas of the nasopharynx with a critical review as to the existence of lymphoepitheliomas. *Cancer* 15 : 895, 1962.
4. Ewing J: Lymphoepithelioma. *Am J Pathol* 5 : 99, 1929.
5. Batsakis JG: *Tumors of the Head and Neck: Clinical and Pathological Considerations* (2nd ed). Baltimore: Williams & Wilkins, 1982. Pp 144–186.
6. Batsakis JG: *Tumors of the Head and Neck: Clinical and Pathological Considerations* (2nd ed). Baltimore: Williams & Wilkins, 1982. Pp 144–186.
7. Odukoya O, et al: Squamous cell carcinoma of the oral cavity: A clinico-pathological study of 106 Nigerian cases. *J Maxillofac Surg* 14 : 267, 1986.
8. Thorek P: *Anatomy in Surgery* (3rd ed). New York: Springer-Verlag, 1985. Pp 223–236.
9. Kirchner JA: Two hundred laryngeal cancers: Patterns of growth and spread as seen in serial section. *Laryngoscope* 87 : 474, 1977.
10. American Joint Committee for Cancer Staging and End-Results Reporting: *Manual for Staging of Cancer*. Chicago: American Joint Committee, 1977. Pp 65–70.
11. Rosenberg JC, Schwade JG, Vaitkevicius VK: Cancer of the Esophagus. In DeVita VT Jr, Hellman S, Rosenberg A (eds): *Cancer Principles and Practice of Oncology*. Philadelphia: Lippincott, 1982. Pp 499–533.
12. Rogers EL, Goldkind L, Goldkins SF: Increasing frequency of esophageal cancer among black male veterans. *Cancer* 49 : 610, 1982.
13. Ezdinii EZ, et al: Chemotherapy of advanced esophageal cancer: Eastern Cooperative Oncology Group Experience. *Cancer* 46 : 2149. 1980.
14. Ackerman LV: Verrucous carcinoma of the oral cavity. *Surgery* 23 : 670, 1948.
15. Kraus FT, Perez-Messa C: Verrucous carcinoma: Clinical and pathologic study of 105 cases involving the oral cavity, larynx and genitalia. *Cancer* 19 : 26, 1966.
16. DeLellis RA: *Diagnostic Immunohistochemistry*. New York: Masson, 1981.
17. Taylor CR: Immunoperoxidase techniques: Theoretical and practical aspects. *Arch Pathol Lab Med* 102 : 113, 1978.
18. Taylor CR, Kledzik G: Immunohistologic techniques in surgical pathology: A spectrum of "new" special stains. *Hum Pathol* 12 : 590, 1981.
19. Acquarelli MJ, Ward NO, Hangos GW: Carcinoma of the trachea. *Ann Otol Rhinol Laryngol* 76 : 843, 1967.
20. Goldstein J: Primary carcinoma of the trachea: Report of two cases. *South Med J* 70 : 434, 1977.
21. Batsakis JG, et al: The pathology of head and neck tumors: Salivary glands—Part 2). *Head Neck Surg* 1 : 167, 1978.
22. Dardick I: Morphogenesis of salivary gland tumors: A prerequisite to improving classification. *Pathol Annu* 22(1) : 1, 1987.
23. Batsakis JG, Wozniak KJ, Regez JA: Acinous cell carcinoma: A histiogenetic hypothesis. *J Oral Surg* 35 : 904, 1977.
24. Goldblatt LI, Ellis GL: Salivary gland tumors of the tongue: Analysis of 55 new cases and review of the literature. *Cancer* 60 : 94, 1987.
25. Carvajal L, et al: Cystic adenoid carcinoma: A propos of 2 cases originating in salivary glands (English Abstract). *Med Cutan Iber Lat Am* 15 : 42, 1987.
26. Whitlatch SP: Psammoma bodies in fine needle aspiration biopsies in Acinic cell tumor (Letter). *Diagn Cytopathol* 2 : 268, 1986.
27. Silverberg E, Lubera J: Cancer statistics, 1987. *CA* 37 : 2, 1987.
28. Kapur MM, et al: Carcinoma of the thyroid: Differential behavior in solitary and multinodular tumors. *Br J Surg* 73 : 894, 1986.
29. Chen JK, Saw D: The grooved nucleus: A useful diagnostic criterion of papillary carcinoma of the thyroid. *Am J Surg Pathol* 10 : 672, 1986.
30. Bugis SP, et al: Diagnostic accuracy of fine needle aspiration biopsy versus frozen section in solitary thyroid nodules. *Am J Surg Pathol* 10 : 411, 1986.
31. Chen KT: Clear cell follicular adenoma of the thyroid. *J Surg Oncol* 34 : 170, 1987.

32. Livolsi VA: Mixed thyroid carcinoma: A real entity? *Lab Invest* 57 : 237, 1987.
33. Wang HH, Ducatman BS: Hurthle cell lesions in the thyroid (Letter). *Am J Clin Pathol* 88 : 122, 1987.
34. Arganini M, et al: Hurthle cell tumors: A twenty five year experience. *Surgery* 100 : 1108, 1986.
35. Glasgow SM, Beckman EN, Witkin M: Medullary carcinoma of the thyroid: Papillary and pseudopapillary patterns. *South Med J* 80 : 522, 1987.
36. Ordonez NG, Samaan NA: Medullary carcinoma of the thyroid metastatic to the skin: Report of two cases. *J Cutan Pathol* 14 : 251, 1987.
37. Robbins SL, Cotran RS, Kumar V: *Pathologic Basis of Disease* (3rd ed). Philadelphia: Saunders, 1984. Pp 1223–1224.
38. Saul SH, Kapadia SB: Secondary lymphoma of Waldeyer's ring: Natural history and association with prior extranodal disease. *Am J Otolaryngol* 7 : 34, 1986.
39. O'Reilly BJ, Kershaw JB: Hodgkin's disease of the nasopharynx. *J Laryngol Otol* 101 : 506, 1987.
40. Smith P, et al: Primary Hodgkin's disease of the thyroid. *J Med Assoc Ga* 75 : 538, 1986.
41. Baden E, et al: Hodgkin's lymphoma of the oropharyngeal region: Report of four cases and diagnostic value of monoclonal antibodies associated with Reed-Sternberg cells. *Oral Surg* 64 : 88, 1987.
42. Harris NL: Lymphoma 1987: An interim approach to diagnosis and classification. *Pathol Annu* 22 (pt 2) : 1, 1987.
43. National Cancer Institute sponsored study of classifications of non-Hodgkin's lymphomas: Summary and description of a working formulation for clinical usage. *Cancer* 49 : 211, 1982.
44. Henry K: National Cancer Institute retrospective study of the non-Hodgkin's lymphomas (Abstract). BNLI Report No. 7. *Clin Radiol* 32 : 499, 1981.
45. Makepeace AR, Fermont DC, Bennett HMH: Non-Hodgkin's lymphoma of the tonsil: Experience of treatment over a 27 year period. *J Laryngol Otol* 101 : 1151, 1987.
46. Nash JR, et al: Non-Hodgkin's lymphoma of the head and neck: Prognostic factors. *Clin Otolaryngol* 12 : 203, 1987.
47. Ellison DJ, et al: Mitotic counts in follicular lymphomas. *Hum Pathol* 18 : 502, 1987.
48. Gospodarowicz MK, et al: Patterns of disease in localized extranodal lymphomas. *J Clin Oncol* 5 : 875, 1987.
49. Manoharan A, Smart RC, Pitney WR: Primary extranodal non-Hodgkin's lymphoma. *Pathology* 18 : 413, 1986.
50. Glenner GG, Grimley PM: Tumors of the Extra Adrenal Paraganglion System (including chemoreceptors). In: *Atlas of Tumor Pathology*. Series 2, Fascicle 9. Washington, DC: Armed Forces Institute of Pathology, 1974.
51. Lack EE, et al: Paragangliomas of the head and neck region: A clinical study of 69 patients. *Cancer* 39 : 397, 1977.
52. Basma NJ, Robin PE: Glomus jugulare tumor masquerading as idiopathic facial nerve palsy. *J Laryngol Otol* 101 : 605, 1987.
53. Hana GA, Ali MH: Chemodectoma of the larynx. *J Laryngol Otol* 100 : 1081, 1986.
54. Saltzstein SL, Nahum AM: Frozen section diagnosis: Accuracy and errors, uses and abuses. *Laryngoscope* 83 : 1128, 1973.
55. Kovi, J: *Frozen Section in Surgical Pathology: An Atlas*. Boca Raton, FL: CRC, 1983. Vol I, pp 1–10.
56. Wheelis RF, Hammer SP, Yarington CT: The ultra structural diagnosis of tumors of the head and neck. *Laryngoscope* 89 : 234, 1979.

6

Staging

ERNEST M. MYERS

KEY CONCEPTS

TNM System; Stage; Mapping; Prognosis

MILESTONES

1902	Head and Neck Lymphatics	Polya
1942	Treatise on the Lymphatic System	Drinker
1944	Head and Neck Cancer and Cervical Metastasis	Martin
1955	"Surgical Pathology of the Larynx"	Ogura
1976	International Classification of Diseases for Oncology	World Health Organization
1977	Manual for Staging of Cancer	AJC
1980	"Surgical Pathology of the Larynx and Hypopharynx"	Sessions
1985	Staging and Multifactoral Analysis	Jacobs et al.
1987	Cervical Lymph Node Metastasis and Prognosis	Richard et al.
1989	"Surgical Pathology of the Oral Cavity and Oropharynx"	Sessions et al.

TNM SYSTEM

Staging is the succinct description of a tumor in regard to its origin and spread. The accepted format is the TNM classification: T, primary tumor; N, local or regional metastasis; and M, distant spread or metastasis. Within each division, increasing involvement is categorized by the combination of the capital letter with a numerical suffix (Table 6-1).

Classification

As the primary tumor increases in size and involvement, the following designations appear:

T_0—no clinical tumor
T_1, T_2, T_3, T_4—ascending size increase

Regional lymph node involvement is similarly described:

N_0—no clinical involvement
N_1, N_2, N_3—ascending degrees of nodal involvement

Distant metastasis is designated as follows:

M_0—no observable distant metastasis
M_1, etc.—ascending degrees of distant metastatic involvement (sites specified)

Stage

Staging is the grouping of more than one TNM classification. The stages generally are as follows (Figure 6-1):

Stage I: T_1, N_0, M_0
Stage II: T_2, N_0, M_0
Stage III: $T_3N_0M_0$; T_1, T_2, or T_3 plus N_1
Stage IV: T_4N_0;T_4N_1; any T plus N_2M_0, any T plus N_3M_0; any T, any N plus M_1

Table 6-1. Staging essentials

Complete history
Comprehensive physical examination
Performance status assessment
Indirect nasopharyngoscopy and laryngoscopy
Chest x-ray
Multichemistry screening
Computed tomography (CT) scan(s) or magnetic resonance imaging (MRI)
Panendoscopy and biopsy

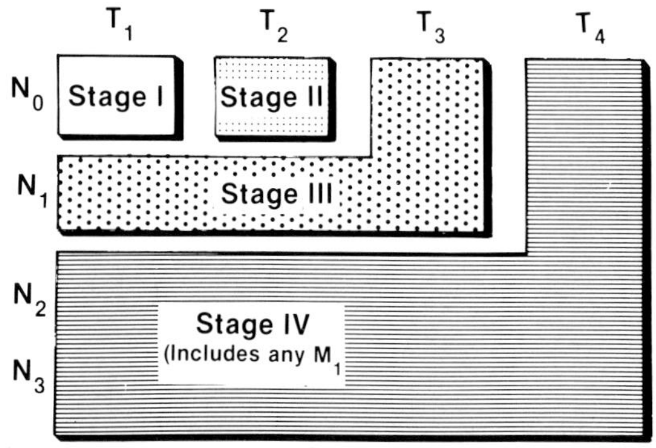

Figure 6-1. General staging guidelines.

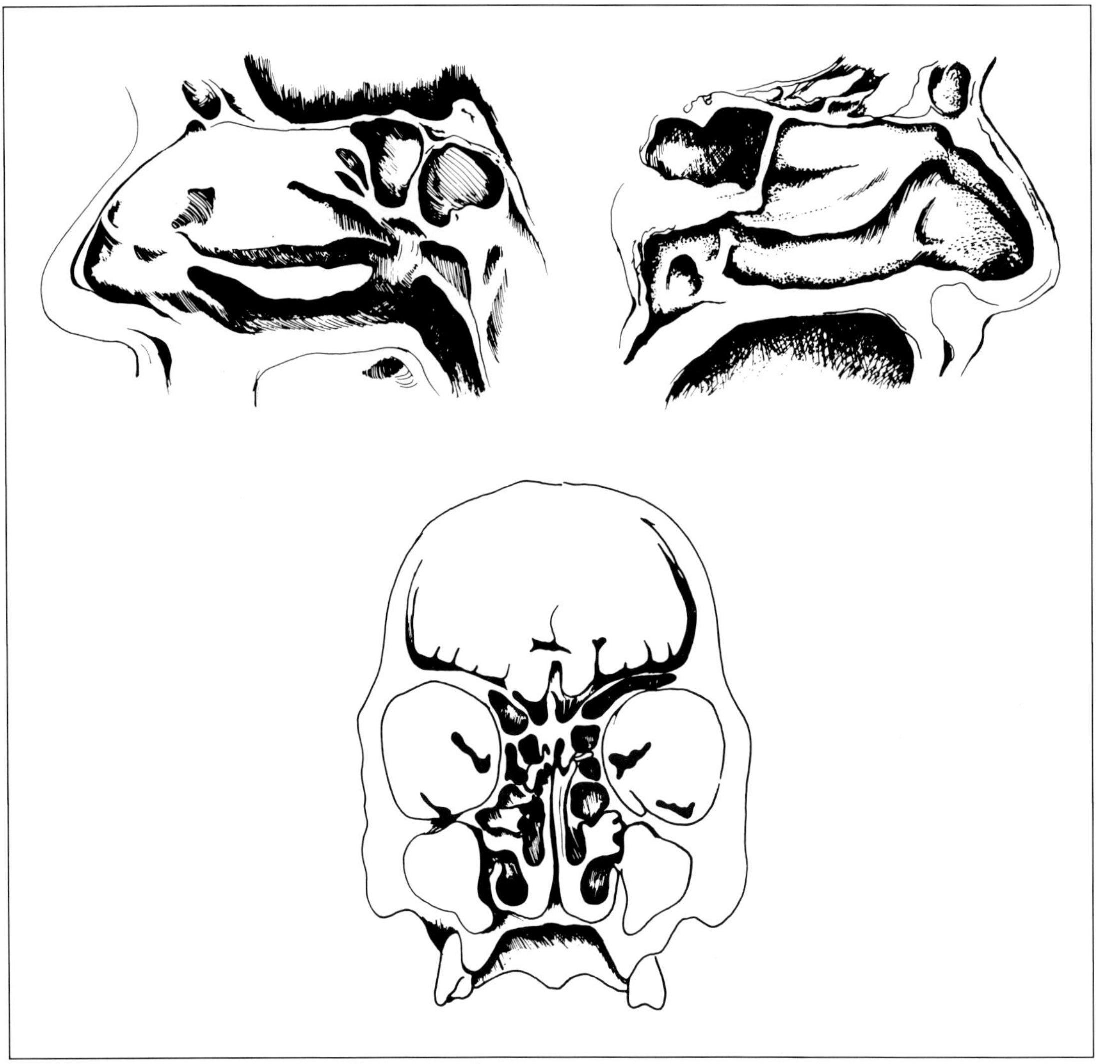

Figure 6-2. Map of the paranasal sinuses and nose.

The TNM classification and stage are abbreviations that enable oncologists to communicate, plan, and monitor therapy. There is a direct correlation with prognosis: as the classifications are ascended, prognosis worsens. In addition, there is a general relationship with pathogenesis. Finally, the TNM system provides a means of comparing and contrasting treatment plans [1].

Sites and Subsites

Unlike many areas of the body, the complex anatomy of the head and neck dictates the adaptation of the TNM format to a variety of specific anatomic sites (see Chapter 1). The rationale is that tumors originating from each site have very different clinical behaviors. In essence, although there are 10 primary sites, 4 of these primary sites have secondary and tertiary subsites, resulting in a total of 50 potential primary head and neck sites. Each site has a characteristic clinical presentation and prognosis. Although this seems imposing, accurate staging has profound therapeutic and prognostic implications. Thus, it is imperative that the tumor be located precisely [2].

Assessment

Classically, the TNM system was a clinical format whose foundations were physical diagnosis and general diagnostic modalities. However, due to the complexity of head and neck oncology, at Howard University Cancer Center, the complete spectrum of diagnostic modalities are utilized. For example, the correlation of plain roentgenographs, computed tomography (CT), nuclear scans, and magnetic resonance imaging (MRI) greatly increases information. Inclusion of all pertinent data results in greater accuracy, and a more precise, logical treatment plan. Heretofore, the reliance on a strict clinical format has resulted in understaging. Therefore, *all* appropriate diagnostic modalities are utilized in formulating a final TNM classification [3–5].

Limitations

Several authors challenge the usefulness of the TNM system [6]. Retrospective computer analysis of stage II and stage III laryngeal cancers, for example, have uncovered underemphasized prognostic variables [6]. However, with rare exceptions, few critics suggest specific measures to improve the system [7]. For now, this is the best we have to offer. Hopefully, in the future, retrospective and prospective computer analysis of large cooperative studies will modify, replace, or perfect the system [8].

MAPPING

A map is invaluable for describing and monitoring therapeutic responses (Figures 6-2, 6-3, and 6-4). Staging and mapping are performed usually after biopsy or panendoscopy (see Table 6-1). Precise mapping and staging are the foundations of treatment planning (see Chapter 7). The correlation of physical examination, diagnostic radiology, and panendoscopy enables the head and neck oncologist to map the lesion accurately. Tatoos are useful for marking lesions, particularly if preoperative radiation or chemotherapy is part of the treatment plan. If anything, the oncologist should err on the side of overstaging, since there is a natural tendency to understage. It is well-known that understaging results in inappropriate treatment and ultimately affects prognosis. Therefore, only the senior head and neck oncologist should map and stage lesions.

Sinuses and Nose (Site 2)

Sinuses

Tumors arising in the sphenoid, ethmoid, and frontal sinuses are not staged. Currently, only tumors of the maxillary sinus are staged (Table 6-2; Figures 6-5 and 6-6). Hopefully, further studies will result in the staging of cancers of the nasal cavity and ethmoid sinuses [9].

Nose

The roughly cylindrical area of the nose includes the septum (medially), turbinates (laterally),

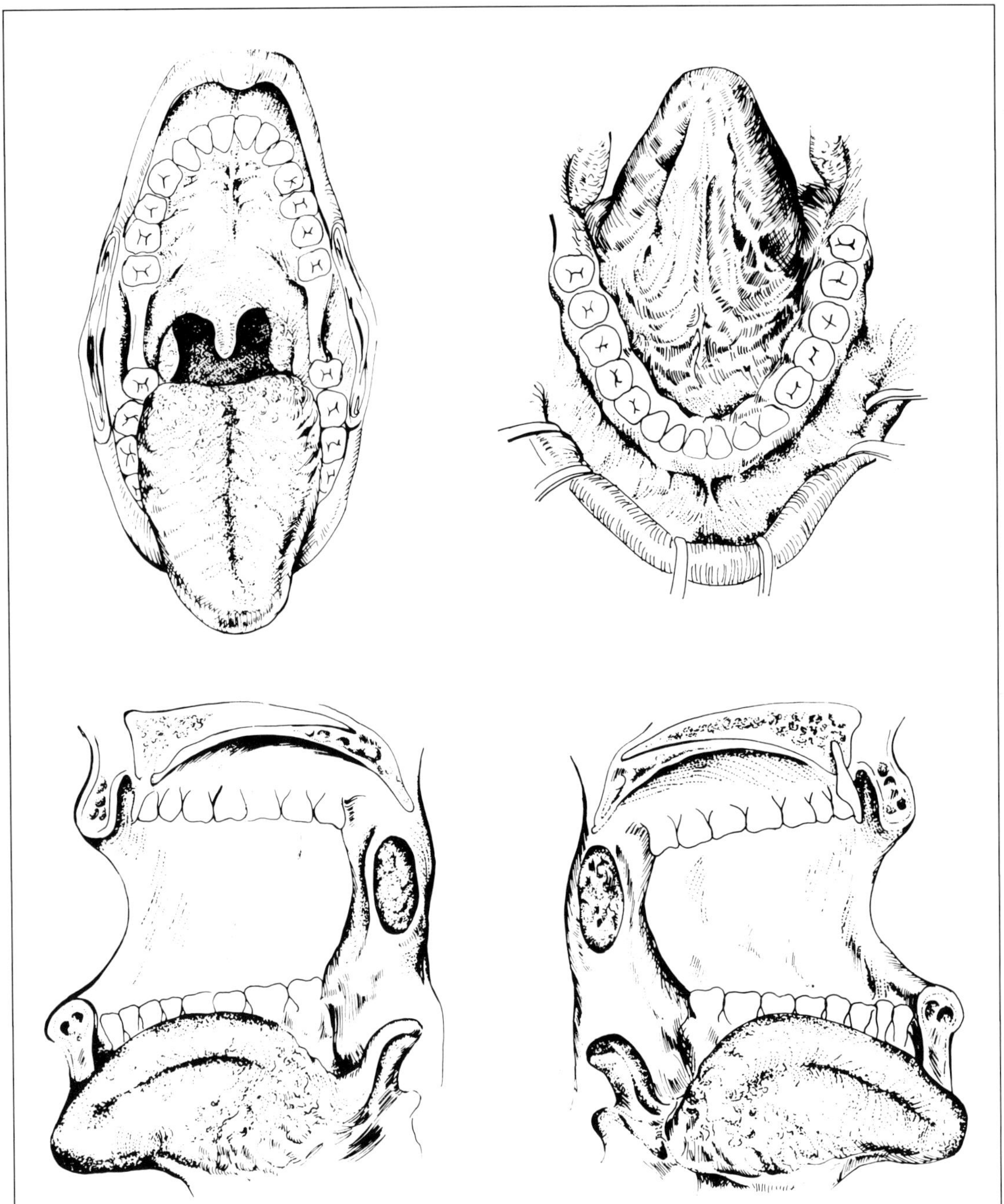

Figure 6-3. Map of the oral cavity and oropharynx.

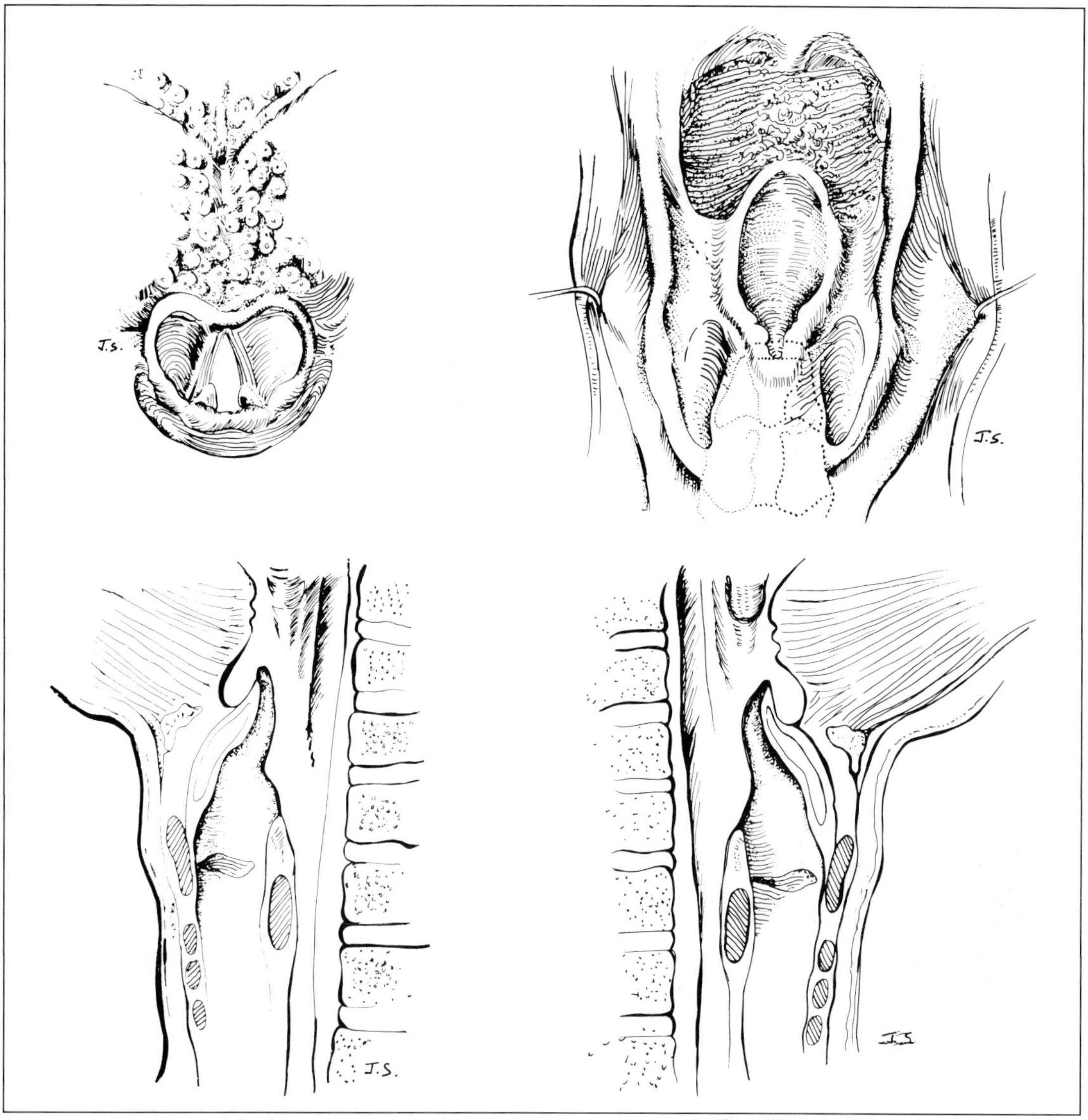

Figure 6-4. Map of the hypopharynx and larynx.

vestibule (anteriorly), and choanae (posteriorly). Tumors in this site are rare and may be confused with maxillary and ethmoid sinus malignancies.

Salivary Glands (Site 3)

The major salivary glands are the parotid, submandibular, and sublingual glands. Most neoplasms are found in the parotid and submandibular glands [10]. Those arising from the sublingual glands are often confused with floor of the mouth malignancies (Table 6-3).

Lips (Site 4)

The lips, extensions of the oral cavity, project outwardly from the mucocutaneous junction and the commissures (Figure 6-7). Most classifications include this site with the oral cavity. However, since tumors in this site have a unique pathogenesis and prognosis (Table 6-4), they are classified separately.

Table 6-2. Paranasal sinuses and nose (Site 2): maxillary sinus*

Classification	*Description*
T_1	Tumor confined to the infrastructure without bony erosion or destruction
T_2	Tumor erosion or bony destruction (hard palate; nasal wall)
T_3	Tumor invading the cheek, orbit, anterior ethmoid sinuses, or posterior wall
T_4	Massive tumor with invasion of orbit, cribiform plate, posterior ethmoids, sphenoid, nasopharynx, pterygoid plates, or skull base

*Ohngren's line, a theoretic plane joining the medial canthus of the eye with angle of the mandible, divides the maxillary antrum into anterior/inferior (the infrastructure) and superior/posterior (the suprastructure) portions.
Source: Adapted from Beahrs OH, et al (eds): *Manual for Staging of Cancer* (3rd ed). Philadelphia: Lippincott, 1988.

Table 6-3. Salivary glands (Site 3)*

Classification	*Description*
T_1	Tumor less than 2 cm in greatest diameter
T_2	Tumor greater than 2 cm but less than 4 cm in greatest diameter
T_3	Tumor greater than 4 cm but less than 6 cm in greatest diameter
T_4	Tumor greater than 6 cm

*All categories are subdivided into (a), no local extension, or (b), local extension.
Source: Adapted from Beahrs OH, et al (eds): *Manual for Staging of Cancer* (3rd ed). Philadelphia: Lippincott, 1988.

Figure 6-5. CT scan, paranasal sinuses. A $T_4N_1M_0$ carcinoma of the left maxilla presented with gingiva-buccal and palatal invasion.

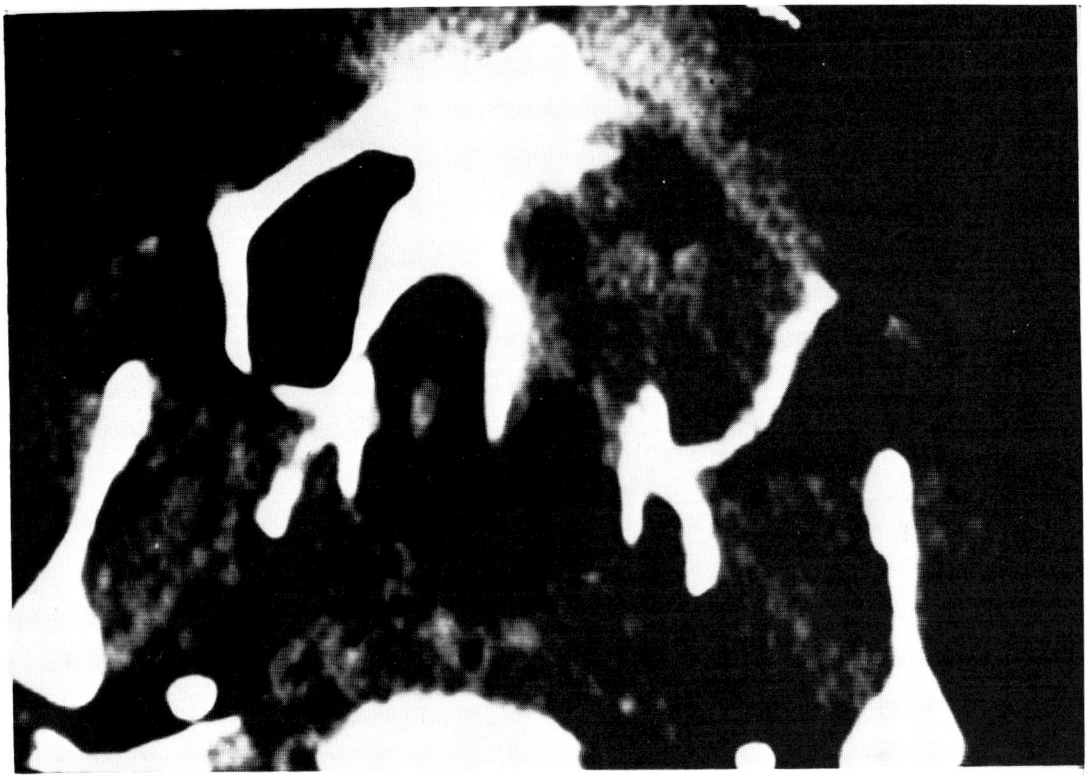

Table 6-4. Lips (Site 4)

Classification	*Description*
T_1	Tumor less than 2 cm in size
T_2	Tumor greater than 2 cm but less than 4 cm
T_3	Tumor greater than 4 cm
T_4	Deep invasion of bone and muscle

Source: Adapted from Schuller DE, Skin DW, Metch MS: Analysis of treatment failure patterns. *Arch Otolaryngol Head Neck Surg* 115 : 834, 1989.

Oral Cavity (Site 5)

The oral cavity consists of seven subsites [11]. Anatomically, it extends from the lips to the circumvallate papillae (Table 6-5). The subsites are floor of the mouth, mobile (anterior) tongue, alveolar arches, hard palate, retromolar trigone, and buccal mucosa.

Floor of the Mouth

The floor of the mouth, a crescent-shaped space overlying the mylohyoid and hyoglossus muscles, extends from the lingual surface of the lower alveolar ridge to the undersurface of the tongue (Figure 6-8). The posterior boundary is the anterior tonsillar pillar; the anterior boundary is the lower lip. Divided into two sides by the frenulum, it includes the submandibular and sublingual ostia.

Figure 6-6. A and B. Soft-tissue CT scans show extensive soft-tissue and bone invasion associated with this $T_4N_0M_0$ carcinoma of the left maxilla. C and D. Bone windows graphically illustrate anterolateral maxillary and palatal invasion.

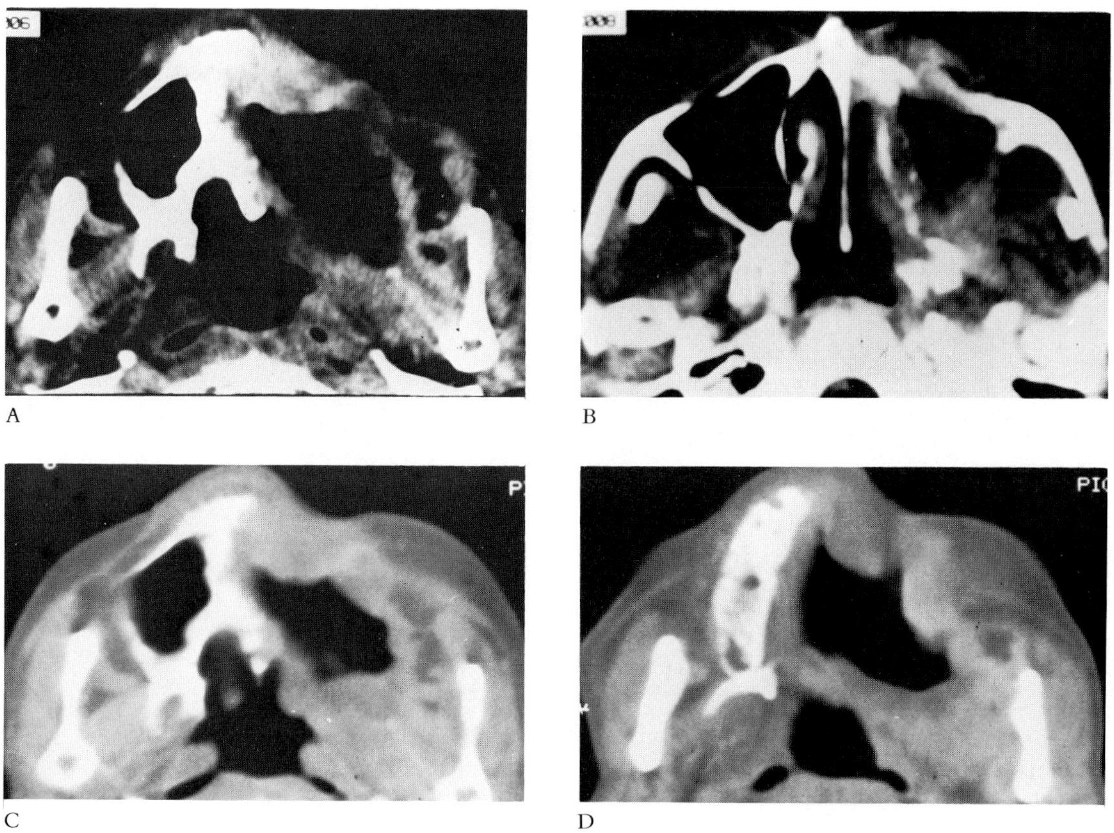

A B C D

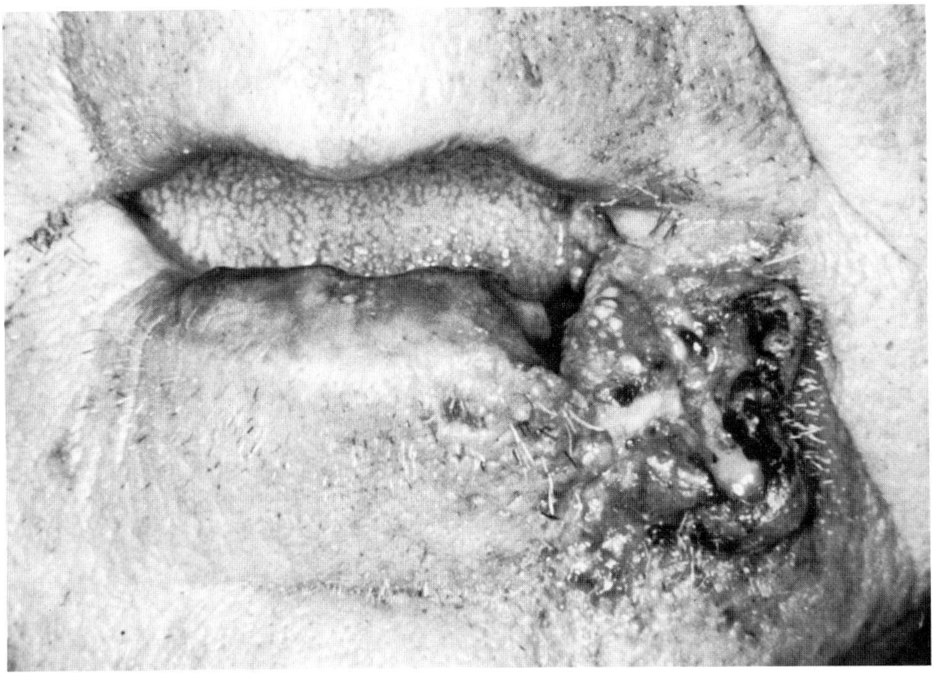

Figure 6-7. $T_3N_0M_0$ (stage III) squamous cell carcinoma of the lower lip with involvement of the left commissure.

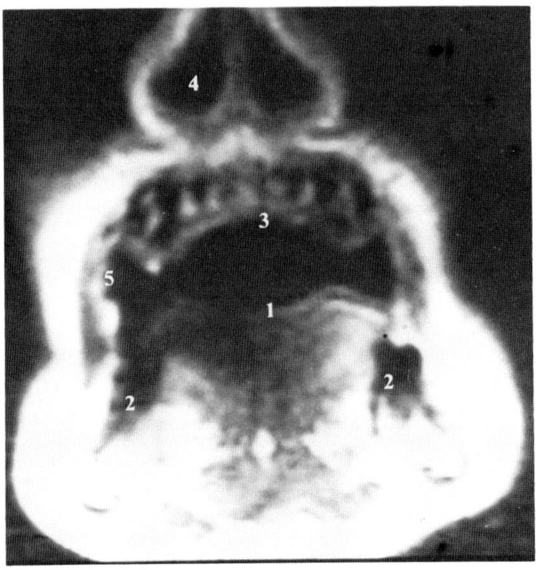

A

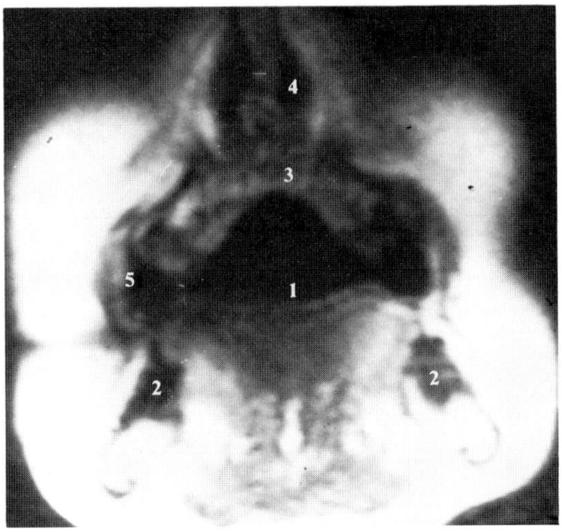

B

Figure 6-8. MRI, coronal views of the face and anterior floor of the mouth. *1*-tongue; *2*-floor of the mouth; *3*-alveolar process; *4*-nasal apertures; *5*-buccal mucosa.

Table 6-5. Oral cavity (Site 5)

Classification	*Description*
T_1	Tumor 2 cm or less in greatest diameter
T_2	Tumor greater than 2 cm but less than 4 cm in greatest diameter
T_3	Tumor greater than 4 cm in greatest diameter
T_4	Massive tumor involving or invading adjacent structures (e.g., tongue, bone, muscle)

Source: Adapted from Beahrs OH, et al (eds): *Manual for Staging of Cancer* (3rd ed). Philadelphia: Lippincott, 1988.

Table 6-6. Nasopharynx (Site 1)

Classification	*Description*
T_1	Tumor confined to one subsite
T_2	Tumor involving two subsites (posterosuperior and lateral walls)
T_3	Tumor extending into the nasal cavity or oropharynx
T_4	Skull base invasion, cranial nerve involvement, or both

Source: Adapted from Beahrs OH, et al (eds): *Manual for Staging of Cancer* (3rd ed). Philadelphia: Lippincott, 1988.

Table 6-7. Nasopharynx (Site 1): 1988 proposal

	Score	
Characteristics	*Yes*	*No*
Seven or more symptoms	+1	0
Lower neck nodes	+1	0
WHO type 1*	+1	0
Extensive tumor	+0.5	0
Symptoms < 2 months	−0.5	0
Stage A	Score < 0	
Stage B	0 to 0.99	
Stage C	1.00 to 1.99	
Stage D	≥ 2.00	

*WHO (World Health Organization):
WHO 1: squamous cell carcinoma.
WHO 2: nonkeratinizing carcinoma.
WHO 3: undifferentiated carcinoma.

Source: Adapted from Neel HB, Taylor WF: New staging system for nasopharyngeal carcinoma. *Arch Otolaryngol Head Neck Surg* 115 : 1293, 1989.

Anterior Two-Thirds of the Tongue

The anterior tongue extends from the circumvallate papillae to the floor of the mouth. It includes the tip, lateral borders, dorsum, and undersurface (nonvillous surface).

Upper Alveolar Ridge

The maxillary alveolar process includes the mucosal attachment of the buccal gutter to the hard palate. Its posterior margin is the pterygopalatine arch.

Hard Palate

The hard palate lies between the upper alveolar ridges and the mucous membrane covering the palatine process of the maxilla (Figure 6-9). It extends from the inner surface of the superior alveolar ridge to the posterior edge of the palatine bone.

Lower Alveolar Ridge

The lower alveolar ridge is composed of the mandibular alveolar process of the mandible and its overlying mucosa (Figure 6-10). It spans the buccal gutter to the free mucosa of the floor of the mouth. Anteriorly, it begins from the floor of the mouth mucosa and ends, posteriorly, at the ascending ramus of the mandible.

Retromolar Trigone

The retromolar trigone, a triangular area of mucosa, overlies the ascending ramus of the mandible from the third molar to the maxillary tuberosity.

Buccal Mucosa

The buccal mucosa is the lining of the inner surface of the cheeks and lips to the pterygomandibular raphe.

Pharynx (Sites 1, 6, and 7)

The pharynx is divided into three primary sites: nasopharynx, oropharynx, and hypopharynx. Each is divided into subsites.

Nasopharynx (Site 1)

The nasopharynx extends from the choanae to the base of the skull and slopes laterally and downwardly to the posterior pharyngeal wall

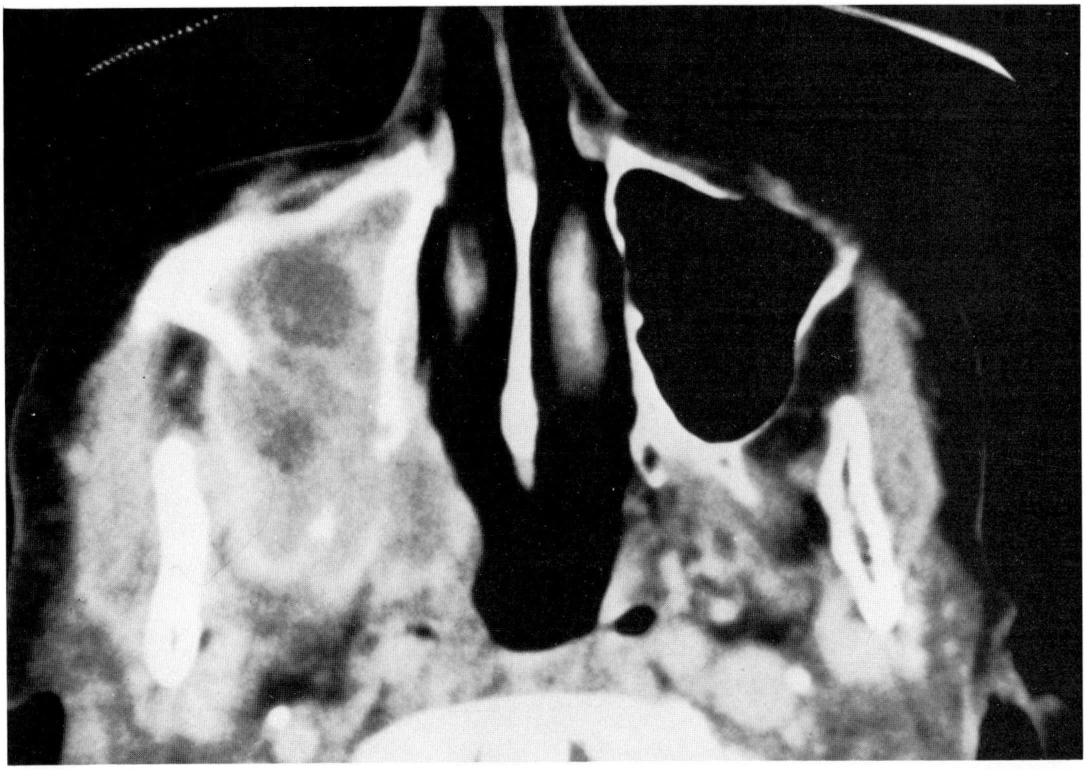

A

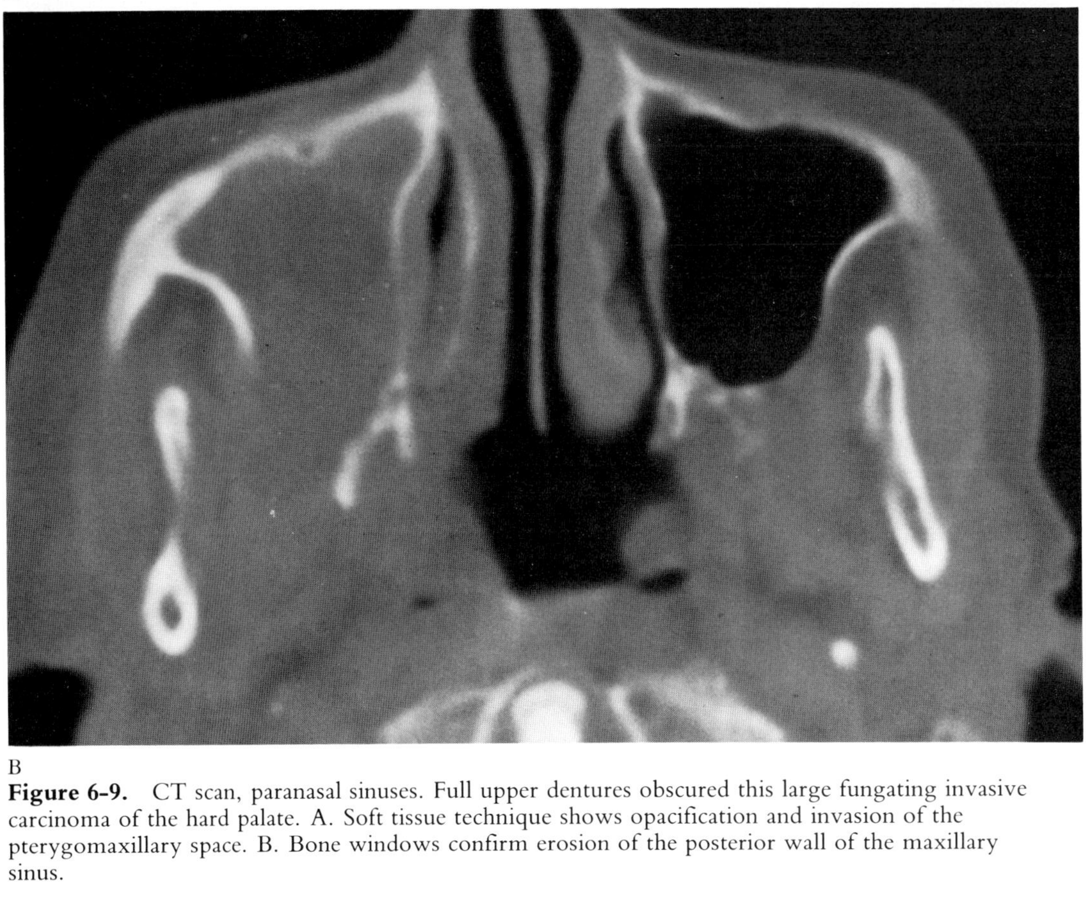

B

Figure 6-9. CT scan, paranasal sinuses. Full upper dentures obscured this large fungating invasive carcinoma of the hard palate. A. Soft tissue technique shows opacification and invasion of the pterygomaxillary space. B. Bone windows confirm erosion of the posterior wall of the maxillary sinus.

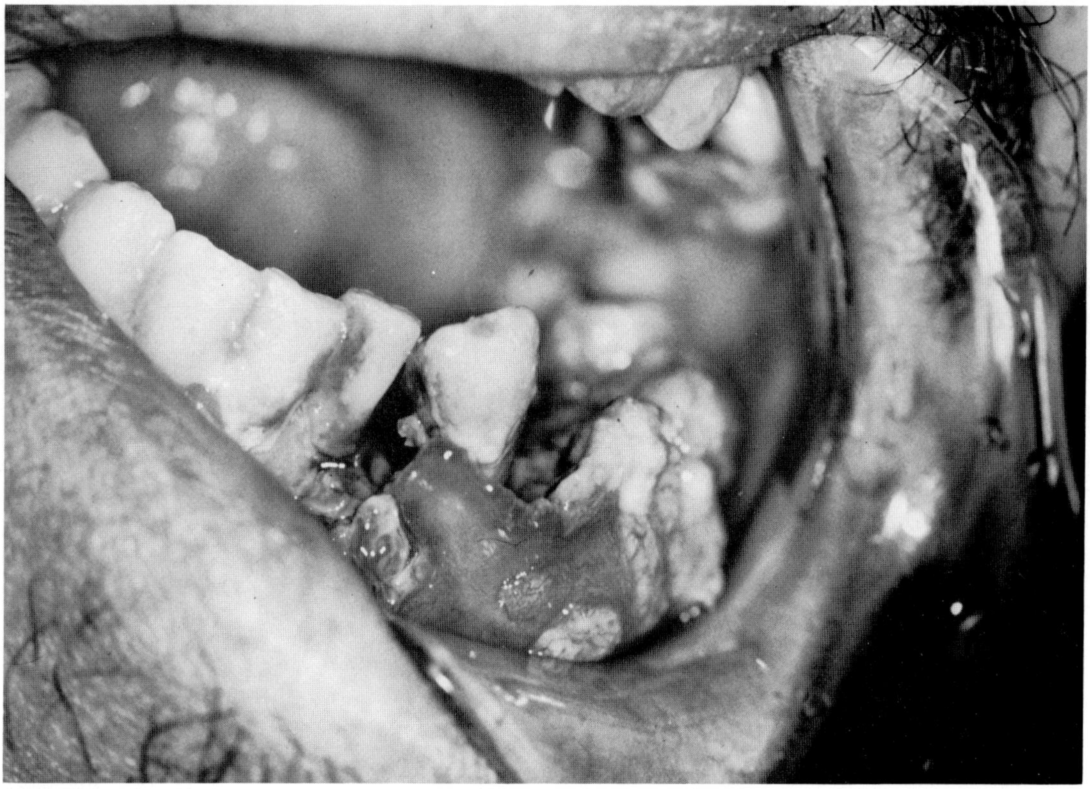

Figure 6-10. T_4N_1 (stage IV) squamous cell carcinoma of the left alveolar process with extensive mandibular invasion and a small left submandibular node.

(Tables 6-6 and 6-7). The lateral wall is composed of the torus tubarius, eustachian tube, and Rosenmüller's fossa. The inferior boundary is the horizontal plane extended from the hard palate [8].

Oropharynx (Site 6)

The oropharynx includes the area posterior from the hard palate to the hyoid bone (Table 6-8; Figures 6-11 through 6-14). Continuous with the oral cavity, it encompasses the faucial arches, soft palate, uvula, tonsillar pillars, and base of the tongue. Its anterior margin is the junction of the hard and soft palate, tonsillar pillars, and circumvallate papillae. It includes the base of the tongue, from the circumvallate papillae to the epiglottis (vallecula), the pharyngoepiglottic, and glossoepiglottic folds. The lateral walls emerge into the tonsils and tonsillar fossae [12].

Table 6-8. Oropharynx (Site 6)

Classification	*Description*
T_1	Tumor 2 cm or less in greatest diameter
T_2	Tumor greater than 2 cm but less than 4 cm in its greatest diameter
T_3	Tumor greater than 4 cm in its greatest diameter
T_4	Massive tumor with invasion of bone, soft tissues of the neck, or deep musculature of tongue

Source: Adapted from Beahrs OH, et al (eds): *Manual for Staging of Cancer* (3rd ed). Philadelphia: Lippincott, 1988.

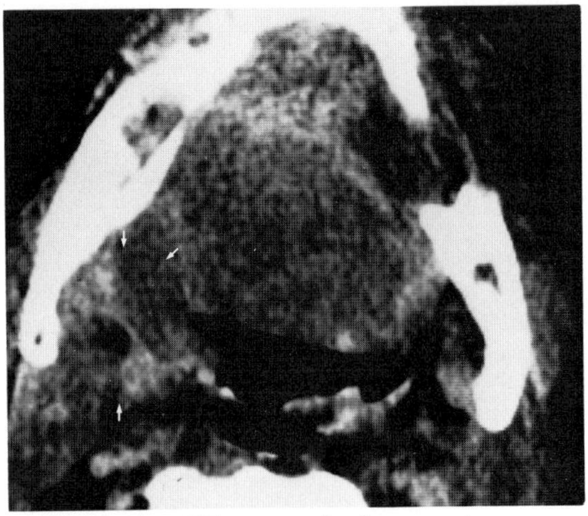

Figure 6-11. CT scan, neck. An extensive $T_4N_1M_0$ carcinoma of the left tonsil involves most of the posterior and mobile tongue.

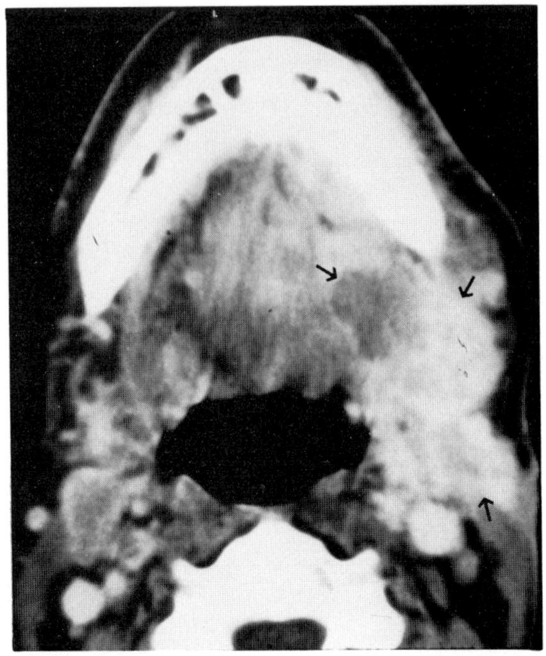

A

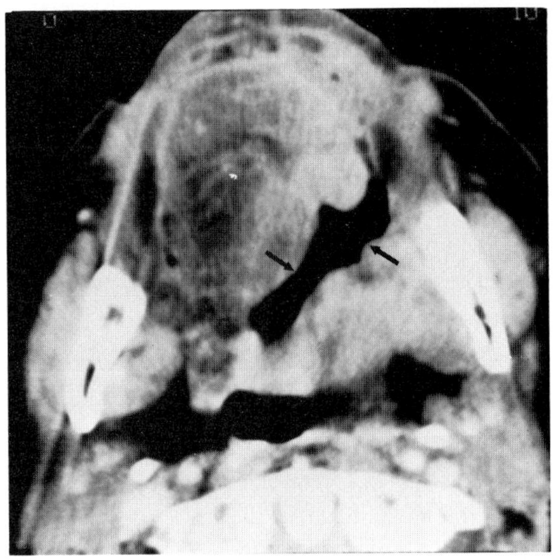

B

Figure 6-12. CT scan, neck (mandible to thoracic inlet). A. This 66-year-old man presented with a large $T_4N_3M_0$ carcinoma of the left tonsil with base of tongue and bilateral cervical metastases. B. The primary tumor invades the base of the tongue, crosses the midline, and creates a furrow (*arrows*). C. The right and left submandibular triangles as well as the carotid sheath (*left*) are involved. D. Extensive left midcervical metastasis with associated laryngeal displacement. E. The inferior boundary of the left midcervical metastasis demonstrates multiple nodes; one shows ring enhancement (*arrow*).

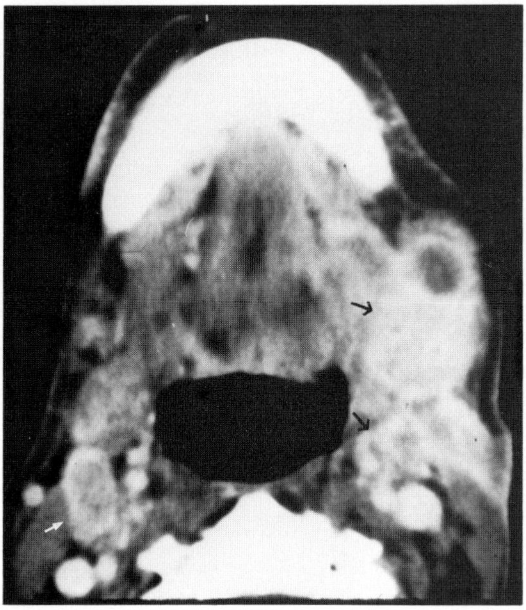

C

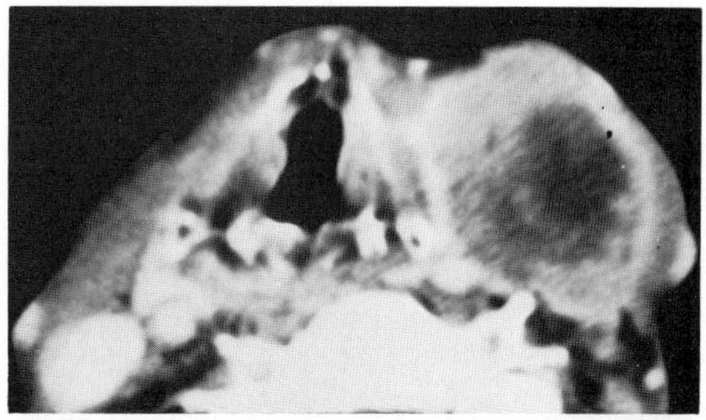

D

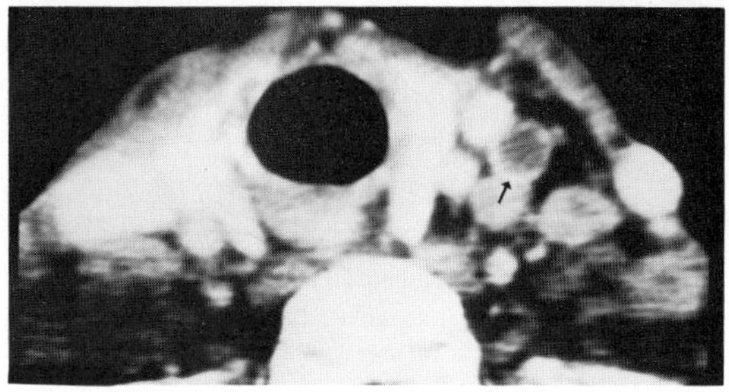

E

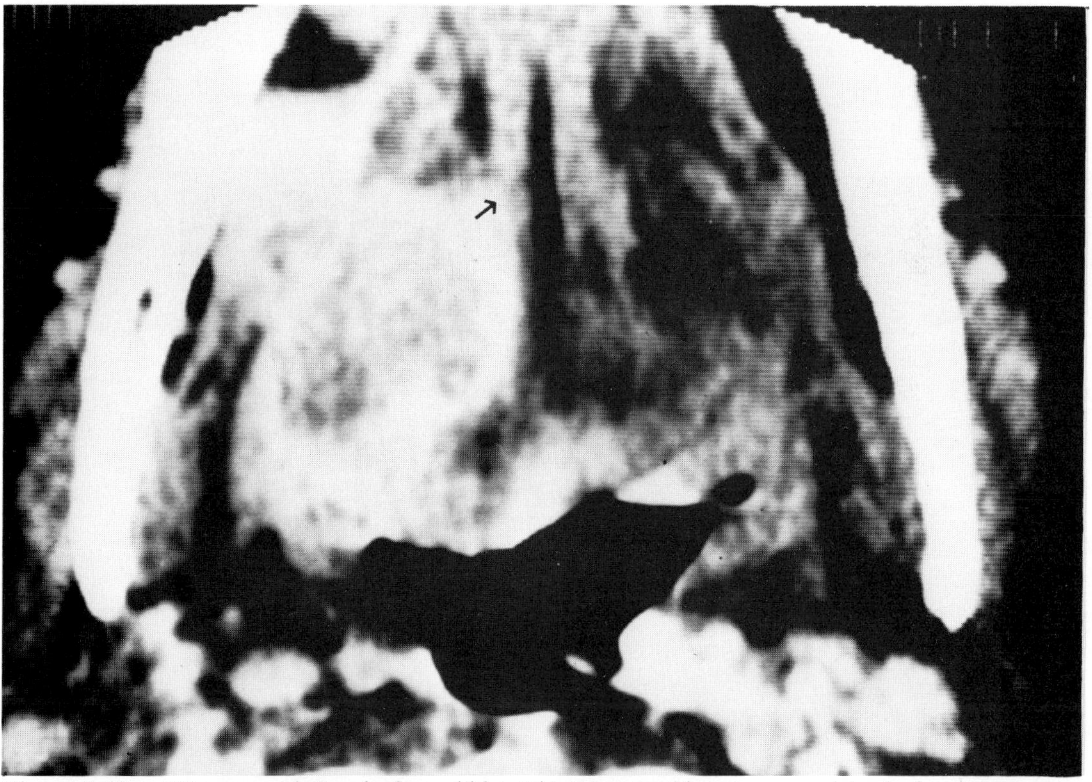

Figure 6-13. CT scan, neck (level of mandible). This 74-year-old patient complained of a persistent right-sided sore throat and halitosis. Indirect laryngoscopy demonstrated a large exophytic (*right*) base of tongue lesion. Note the invasion and displacement of the genioglossus (*arrow*).

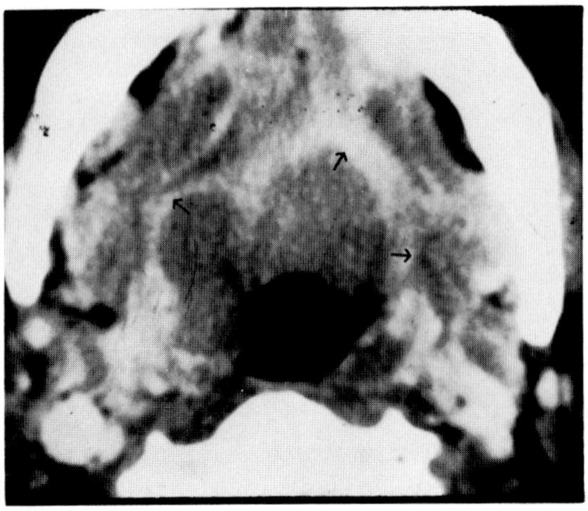

A

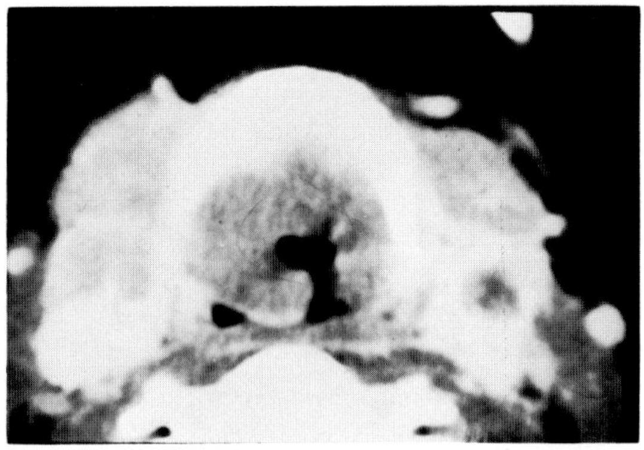

B

Figure 6-14. CT scan, neck: (A) level of mandible; (B) level of hyoid bone. Unremitting sore throat unresponsive to antibiotics was the presentation of this extensive base of tongue carcinoma (A) with bilateral cervical metastases and airway compromise (B).

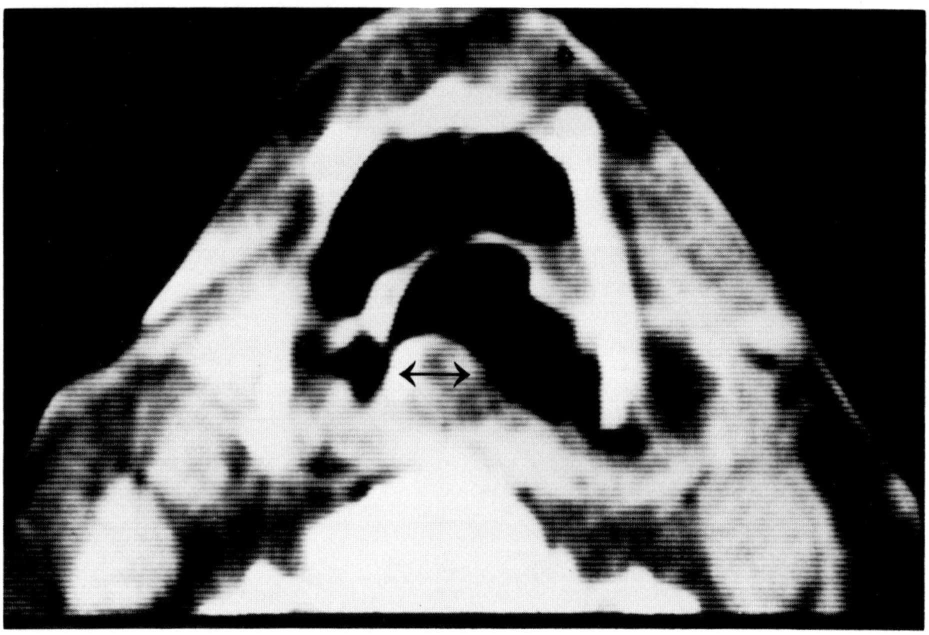

Figure 6-15. CT scan, neck (level of epiglottis). A large posterior pharyngeal wall carcinoma with some associated hypopharyngeal dilatation.

Hypopharynx (Site 7)

The hypopharynx extends from the plane of the hyoid bone superiorly to the plane of the lower border of the cricoid cartilage inferiorly (Table 6-9, Figures 6-15 and 6-16). It consists of three subsites: the pyriform sinus, the posterior surface of the larynx (postcricoid area), and the lower posterior pharyngeal wall.

Larynx (Site 8)

The anterior border of the larynx includes the epiglottis (lingual surface), thyrohyoid membrane, anterior commissure, anterior wall of the subglottis, cricothyroid membrane, and the anterior arch of the cricoid (Table 6-10) [13].

The posterior and lateral border consists of the aryepiglottic folds, arytenoids, interarytenoid space, and cricoid cartilage. The superior and lateral limit is the tip and lateral border of the epiglottis. The inferior extent is a plane passing through the inferior edge of the cricoid cartilage.

Table 6-9. Hypopharynx (Site 7)

Classification	*Description*
T_1	Tumor confined to one subsite
T_2	Extension to adjacent region or subsite without fixation of hemilarynx
T_3	Extension to adjacent region or subsite with fixation of hemilarynx (cord paralysis)
T_4	Invasion of adjacent cartilage or soft tissues

Source: Adapted from Beahrs OH, et al (eds): *Manual for Staging of Cancer* (3rd ed). Philadelphia: Lippincott, 1988.

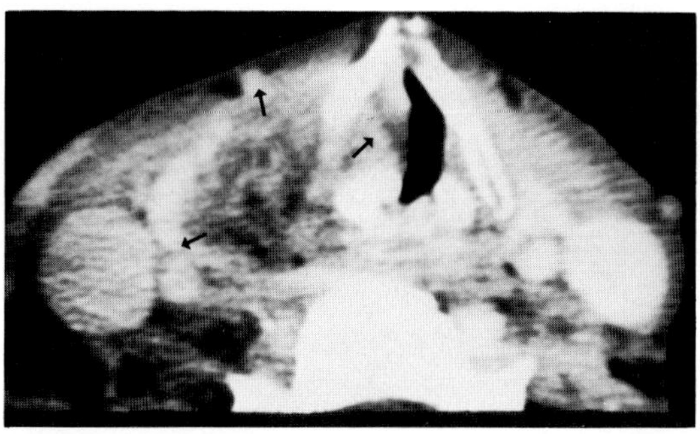

A

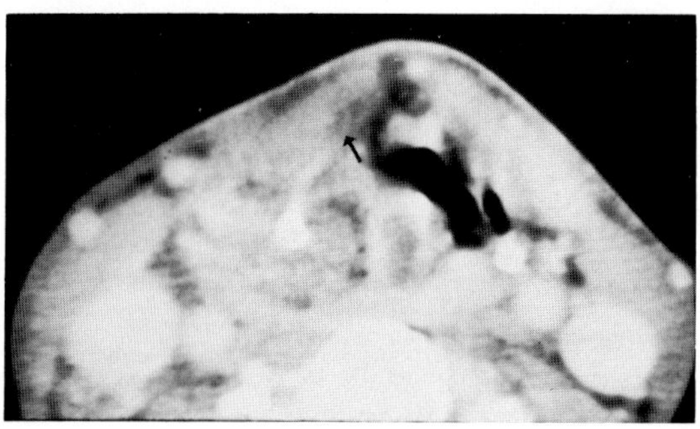

B

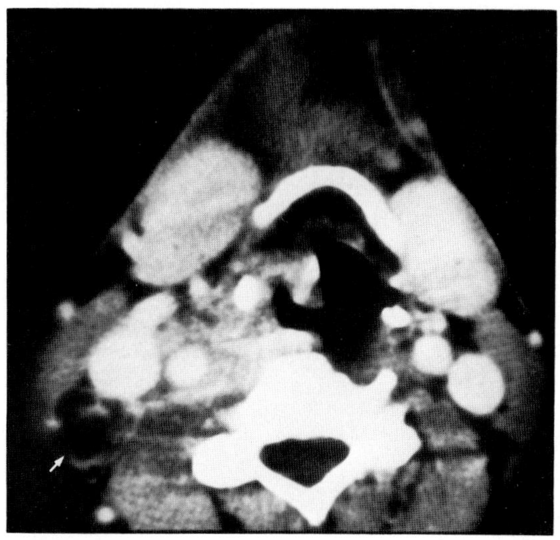

C

Figure 6-16. CT scan, neck: (A, B) level of larynx; (C) level of hyoid bone. A and B. $T_4N_1M_0$ carcinoma of the hypopharynx with base of tongue and thyroid cartilage invasion associated with airway compromise. C. Deep cervical metastasis, arrow (right).

Table 6-10. Larynx (Site 8)

Subsite	*Classification*	*Description*
Supraglottis	T_1	Tumor confined to the subsite with normal mobility
	T_2	Tumor involving more than one subsite (glottis) without fixation
	T_3	Tumor limited to larynx with fixation or extension to postcricoid area, medial wall of pyriform sinus, or preepiglottic space
	T_4	Massive tumor extending beyond the larynx to involve oropharynx, soft tissues of neck, or destruction of thyroid cartilage
Glottis	T_1	Tumor confined to vocal cords with normal mobility, including involvement of anterior or posterior commissures
	T_2	Supraglottic or subglottic extension with normal or impaired cord mobility
	T_3	Tumor confined to the larynx with cord fixation
	T_4	Massive tumor with thyroid cartilage destruction, or extension beyond the larynx
Subglottis	T_1	Tumor confined to the subglottis
	T_2	Tumor extension to vocal cords with normal or impaired cord mobility
	T_3	Tumor confined to the subsite with cord fixation
	T_4	Massive tumor with cartilage destruction or extension beyond the larynx

Source: Adapted from Beahrs OH, et al (eds): *Manual for Staging of Cancer* (3rd ed). Philadelphia: Lippincott, 1988.

Thyroid and Parathyroids (Site 9)

The thyroid is a shield-shaped gland located in the suprasternal or visceral triangle of the anterior carotid triangle (Table 6-11, Figures 6-17 and 6-18). Normally, it is difficult to palpate; most tumors present as a palpable asymmetry.

The parathyroids are too small to be distinguished from the thyroid gland. Parathyroid tumors are usually confused with thyroid neoplasms.

Esophagus (Site 10)

The cervical esophagus spans the cricopharyngeus (upper sphincter) to the thoracic inlet. Tumors in this site are rare and may be confused with advanced thyroid, hypopharyngeal, or laryngeal malignancies. Staging is based on basic esophageal anatomy; T_1, lamina propria or submucosa; T_2, muscularis propria; T_3, adventia; and T_4, invasion of adjacent structures.

PROGNOSIS

Staging does not imply that head and neck cancers are progressional. Although most head and neck cancers grow predictably, many variations exist [14,15]. In reality, prognosis is modified by pathology and pathogenesis (see Chapters 1 and 5).

Primary Tumor

Size

Oral Cavity

With few exceptions, regional metastasis is directly proportional to the size of the primary tumor.

Nasopharynx, Base of the Tongue, and Hypopharynx

A local metastasis may be the only sign of a small, even microscopic primary tumor (see Chapter 2).

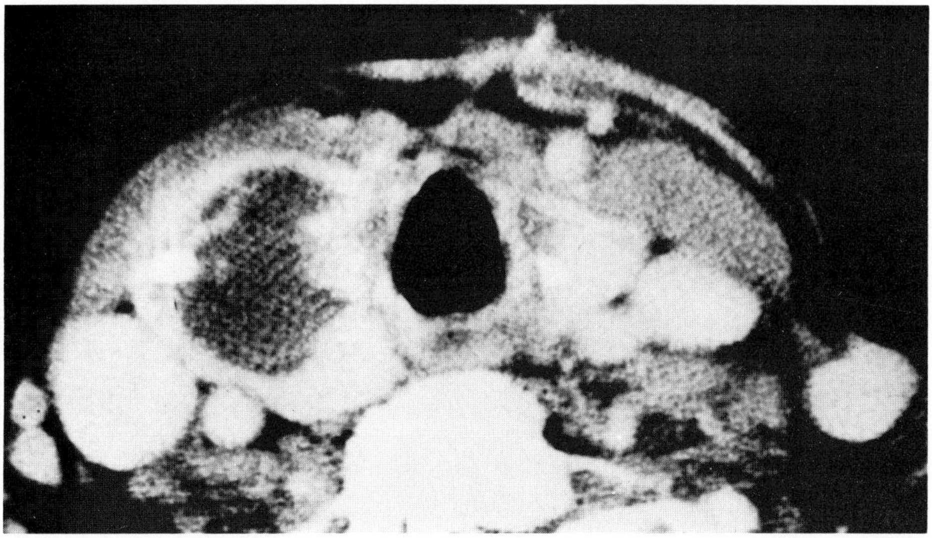

A

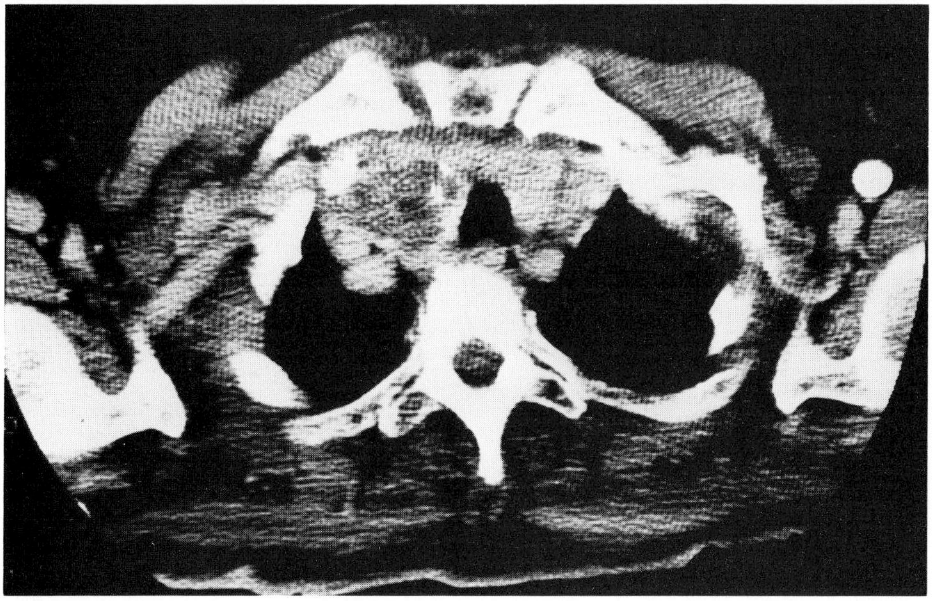

B

Figure 6-17. CT scan, neck. A. A senile 84-year-old patient refused fine-needle aspiration of this large right thyroid mass. B. Chest CT documents superior and anterior mediastinal involvement.

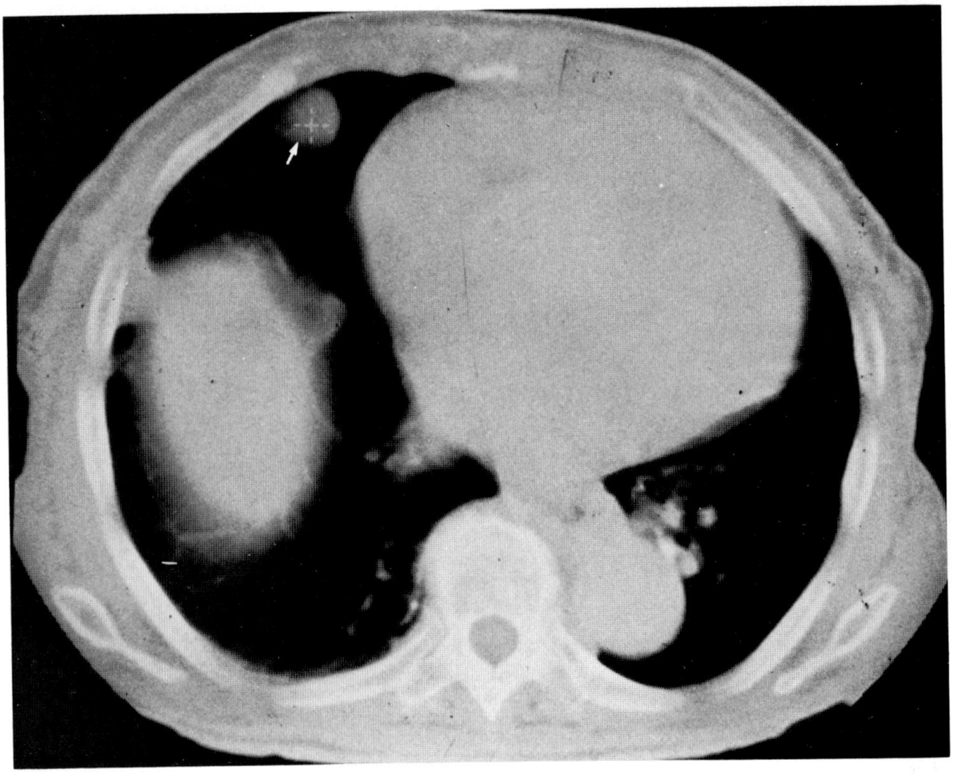

C
Figure 6-17. CT, chest. C. Lung metastasis.

Figure 6-18. A. Initially presenting with impending upper airway obstruction, this 58-year-old woman was found to have right true vocal cord paralysis, left true vocal cord paresis, and left thyroid mass. The CT scan shows a homogeneous left thyroid mass (arrows). B. Thyroid scan (iodine) confirmed a large "cold" mass in the left lobe. Follicular carcinoma was found on fine-needle biopsy.

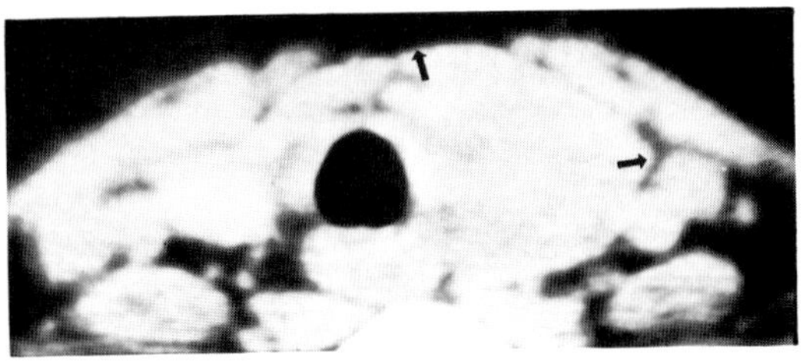

A

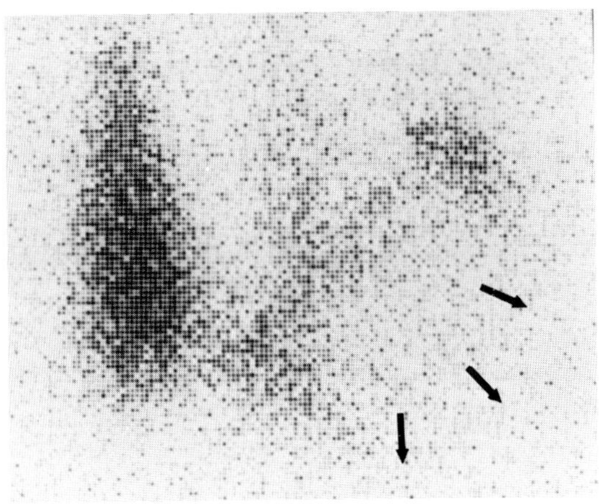

B

Table 6-11. Thyroid and parathyroids (Site 9)*

Classification	*Description*
T_1	Tumor, confined to gland, less than 1 cm in greatest diameter
T_2	Tumor, confined to gland, greater than 1 cm but less than 4 cm
T_3	Tumor, confined to gland, greater than 4 cm
T_4	Tumor, of any size, beyond the gland

*Separate stage groupings are recommended for each histologic type of thyroid carcinoma.
Source: Adapted from Beahrs OH, et al (eds): *Manual for Staging of Cancer* (3rd ed). Philadelphia: Lippincott, 1988.

Location

Squamous cell carcinoma in the base of the tongue has a decidedly worse prognosis than squamous cell carcinoma of the anterior tongue.

Metastasis

The presence of regional or distant metastasis, regardless of primary size, is associated with poor prognosis (Table 6-12; Figure 6-19) [16].

Location

Posterior triangle or level V metastasis, aside from nasopharyngeal carcinoma, is associated with a poor prognosis [17].

Extracapsular Spread

Lymph nodes, regardless of location, with capsular rupture are associated with the poorest prognosis (Figure 6-20) [18]

Table 6-12. Metastasis

Source	*Classification*	*Description*
Cervical (Regional) (N)	N_0	No positive node(s)
	N_1	Single ipsilateral node less than 3 cm in greatest diameter
	N_2	Single ipsilateral node 3–6 cm in diameter or multiple ipsilateral nodes, none greater than 6 cm; homolateral nodes, none over 6 cm in diameter
	N_{2a}	Single ipsilateral node 3–6 cm in greatest diameter
	N_{2b}	Multiple ipsilateral nodes, less than 6 cm in greatest diameter
	N_{2c}	Bilateral or contralateral nodes less than 6 cm in greatest diameter
	N_3	Massive ipsilateral bilateral or contralateral node(s) greater than 6 cm
Distant (M)	M_x	Metastasis unknown
	M_0	No (known) distant metastasis
	M_1	Distant metastasis; specify site(s)

Source: Adapted from Beahrs OH, et al (eds): *Manual for Staging of Cancer* (3rd ed). Philadelphia: Lippincott, 1988.

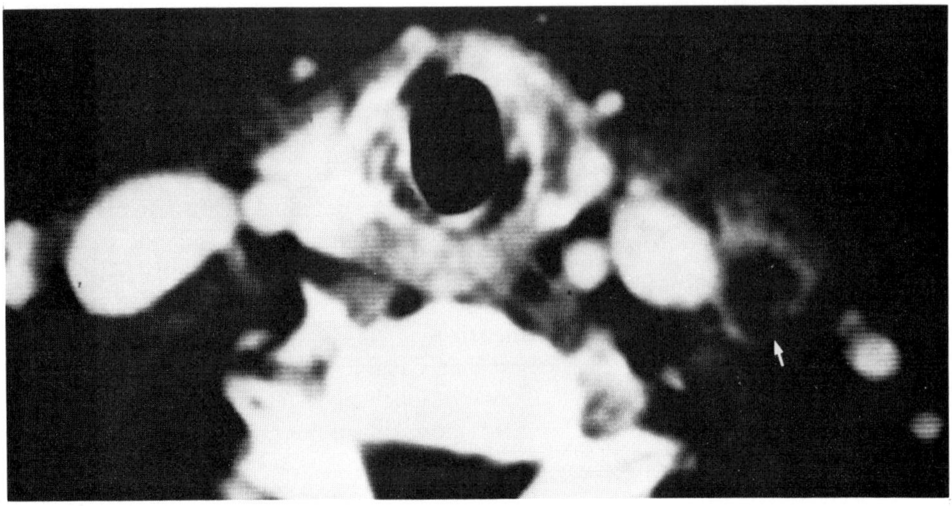

Figure 6-19. CT scan, neck (level of cricoid cartilage). Somewhat atypical, this ring-enhanced lymph node metastasis is secondary to a carcinoma of the larynx (arrow).

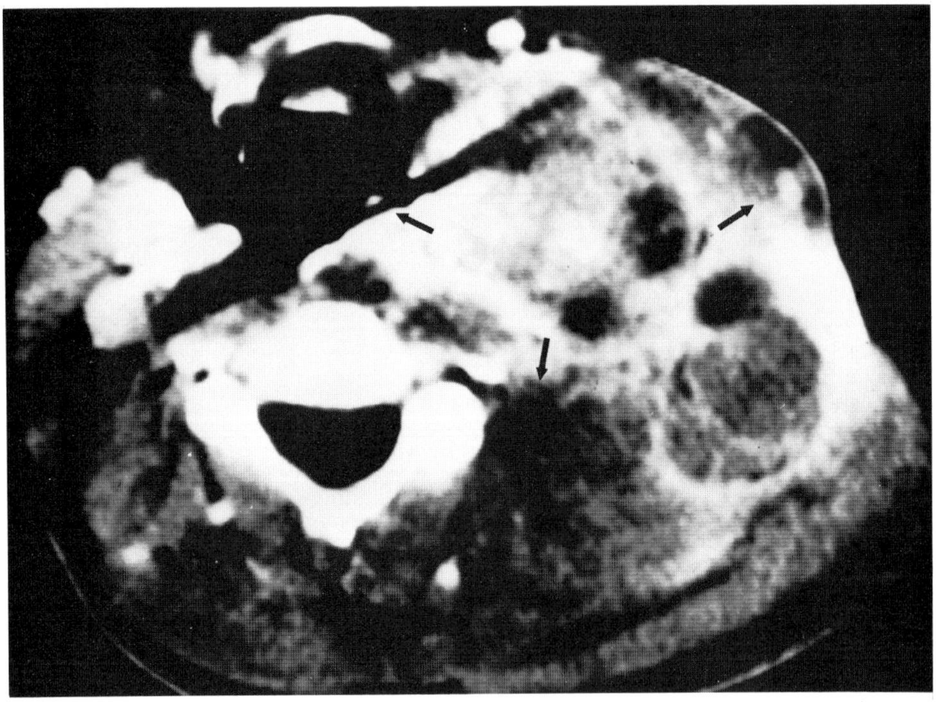

Figure 6-20. CT scan, neck (level of hypopharynx). Despite aggressive preoperative chemotherapy and radiation therapy, this semi-fixed neck mass invaded the deep cervical musculature and carotid sheath.

REFERENCES

1. Beahrs OH, et al. (eds): *Manual for Staging of Cancer* (3rd ed). Philadelphia: Lippincott, 1988.
2. Schuller DE, Skin DW, Metch MS: Analysis of treatment failure patterns. *Arch Otolaryngol Head Neck Surg* 115 : 834, 1989.
3. Sulfaro S, et al: T staging of the laryngohypopharyngeal carcinoma. *Arch Otolaryngol Head Neck Surg* 115 : 613, 1989.
4. Baatenburg de Jong RJ, et al: Metastatic neck disease: Palpation vs ultrasound examination. *Arch Otolaryngol Head Neck Surg* 115 : 689, 1989.
5. Close LG, et al: Computed tomographic evaluation of regional lymph node involvement in cancer of the oral cavity and oropharynx. *Head Neck Surg* 11(4) : 309, 1989.
6. Jacobs JR, Spitznagel EL, Sessions DG: Staging parameters for cancers of head and neck: A multifactoral analysis. *Laryngoscope* 95 : 1378, 1985.
7. Davis RK: Prognostic variables in head and neck cancer: Symposium on squamous cell cancer of head and neck. *Otolaryn Clin North Am* 18(3) : 411, 1985.
8. Neel HB, Taylor WF: New staging system for nasopharyngeal carcinoma. *Arch Otolaryngol Head Neck Surg* 115 : 1293, 1989.
9. Spiro JD, Soo KC, Spiro RH: Squamous carcinoma of the nasal cavity and paranasal sinuses. *Am J Surg* 158 : 328, 1989.
10. Spiro RM, et al: Carcinoma of the major salivary glands: Recent trends. *Arch Otolaryngol Head Neck Surg* 115 : 316, 1989.
11. Spiro RH, Spiro JD, Strong E: Surgical approach to squamous carcinoma confined to the tongue and the floor of the mouth. *Head Neck Surg* 9 : 27, 1986.
12. Mizono GS, Diaz RF, Fu K: Carcinoma of the tonsillar region. *Laryngoscope* 96 : 240, 1986.
13. Eiband JD, et al: Prognostic factors in squamous cell carcinoma of the larynx. *Am J Surg* 158 : 314, 1989.
14. Ogura JH, et al: Long-term therapeutic results—cancer of the larynx and hypopharynx: Preliminary report. *Laryngoscope* 85 : 1746, 1975.
15. Hong WK, et al: Patterns of relapse in locally advanced head and neck cancer patients who achieve complete remission after combined modality therapy. *Cancer* 56(6):1242, 1985.
16. Jesse JH, Lindberg SD: The efficacy of combining radiation therapy with surgical procedure in patients with cervical metastasis from squamous cancer of the oropharynx and hypopharynx. *Cancer* 35 : 1163, 1975.
17. Sessions DG: Surgical pathology of cancer of the larynx and hypopharynx. *Laryngoscope* 90 : 557, 1980.
18. Johnson JT, et al: Cervical lymph node metastasis. *Arch Otolaryngol* 111 : 534, 1985.

II

TREATMENT

7

Planning

ERNEST M. MYERS

KEY CONCEPTS

Patient Assessment; Doctor-Patient Relationship; Tumor Board; Tumor Registry; Informed Consent; Ethics

MILESTONES

1976	Natural Death Act	California
1982	Power of Attorney (Medical)	Pennsylvania
1981	Natural Death Act	District of Columbia
1983	President's Commission for the Study of Ethical Problems in Medicine and Behavioral Research	District of Columbia
1984	Designated Proxy for Incompetent Patients	California
1985	Living Will Act	Maryland

PATIENT ASSESSMENT

The ultimate goal of head and neck oncology is disease ablation and rehabilitation to the highest physiologic and psychological state. The ideal cure has minimal functional and structural impairment. In reality, the ideal is compromised by severe problems that impact on treatment planning (Table 7-1). Malnutrition, chronic obstructive lung disease, diabetes mellitus, and cardiovascular disease, singularly or collectively, alter the best treatment plans. Multimodality treatment such as chemotherapy, surgery, and radiotherapy requires stable patients. Patients must be capable of withstanding aggressive therapy and the side effects of powerful medications. In addition, they must endure uncomfortable instrumentation and an imposing hospital environment. Today, with a team composed of key specialists, many marginal and unstable patients are able to withstand the rigors of modern oncology.

Problem List

The result of an in-depth assessment is a problem list. Such a list encompasses all past and current problems that may impact on treatment and rehabilitation. The problems are divided into active (current) and inactive (resolved) problems (Figure 7-1). For completeness, psychological, social, and economic problems also are included. In short, this is a complete patient inventory, whose constant reappraisal ensures that the attending and consulting physicians render appropriate continuity of care.

THE DOCTOR-PATIENT RELATIONSHIP

The qualities personified throughout the doctor-patient relationship are compassion, commitment, and competence.

Table 7-1. Patient assessment

Historical data
Age
Sex
Race/ethnic group
Occupation
Habits
Education
Past medical history
Physiologic data
Nutrition
Active medical problems
Performance status (ECOG scale)
Normal activity
Symptomatic but ambulatory
Needs assistance—50% ambulatory
Needs nursing care—bedridden
Psychosocial support
Family
Spouse
Employer
Finances
Insight and acceptance

Compassion

Compassion is sympathy coupled with the desire to alleviate another's distress. Today, it often remains in the background as physicians strive for technical excellence; however, it is as important as clinical skills. Compassion determines whether these skills are utilized with lofty aims. The compassionate physician understands the physical and psychological impact of suffering on the patient. In short, the true physician identifies with the patient.

Commitment

Although today's trend is depersonalized medical care, the nature of head and neck cancer fosters an intense doctor-patient relationship. Cancer evokes strong emotions. The impact of head and neck cancer, with its potential for the abrupt alteration of body image, is perhaps the most devastating of all. The need for treatment, extending over weeks and months, requires understanding and empathy from all physicians, especially the attending physician. Regardless of whether the responsible physician is an internist or surgeon, an intense one-on-one relationship naturally develops. From diagnosis, to treatment, throughout rehabilitation, this relationship spans months and perhaps years. It is based on mutual respect and trust. Anything less is counterproductive [1].

Competence

From the first encounter, the patient has an obvious disadvantage. The physician's competence is known only by testimony and reputation. Patients hope and assume their complaint will be handled with skill and dispatch. Nowhere is competence more necessary than in oncology. The oncologist must be current, well-versed, and receptive to new skills. Modern oncology changes rapidly and therefore requires physicians and ancilliary personnel who adapt and improve over time.

TUMOR BOARD

Head and neck oncology is too complex for one physician to manage comprehensively [2, 3]. Effective treatment requires the coordination of multiple services and specialists. Therefore, an interdisciplinary team or tumor board is recommended.

Goals and Composition

The board includes physicians, allied health professionals, and other ancillary personnel. Its goals are (1) early diagnosis, (2) proper treatment, (3) rehabilitation, and (4) follow-up. An effective head and neck tumor board consists of an otolaryngologist, surgical oncologist, radiation oncologist, medical oncologist, plastic surgeon, oral surgeon, radiologist, psychologist, rehabilitation nurse, speech pathologist, audiologist, and social worker. The absence of any of these elements reduces it effectiveness significantly. Furthermore, each board member should be a compatible and effective communicator. Comfortable with their defined responsibilities, the members must understand and respect each other's role. Finally, the board proceedings should be conducted in a professional and objective manner.

Conduct of Proceedings

The minimum requirements are (1) history of the present illness, (2) physical findings, (3) per-

Problem Number	Date Onset	Date Entered	Active Problems	Date Resolved
1				
2				
3				
4				
5				
6				
7				
			Inactive Problems (Resolved Prior to Admission)	
1				
2				
3				
4				
5				
6				
7				

PATIENT IDENTIFICATION
HUH-410

NUR 312-25-0376

Figure 7-1. Patient problem list.

tinent laboratory data, (4) pathologic diagnosis, and (5) stage. For maximal effectiveness the board should have available pertinent computed tomography (CT) or magnetic resonance imaging (MRI) scans. Both the attending physician and the patient should be present. This is an ideal forum for introducing the patient to the various specialists. In addition to defusing stress, it is the first step toward informed consent. This is extremely helpful when experimental or investigational options are being considered.

Documentation

Minutes

A summary for every patient is recorded and filed. The findings and recommendations are stated clearly. A sign-in sheet is provided for each board participant. Such a basic format allows the board to follow many patients. It also satisfies Continuing Medical Education and Residency Review Committee requirements.

Photography

Whenever possible, unusual or complicated cases are documented photographically. The recommended basic equipment is (1) 35-mm SLR camera, (2) self-contained right flash, (3) 50- or 100-mm macro lens, and (4) 64 or 100 ASA color slide film. Preoperative and intraoperative slides are excellent documentation and teaching aids. They are especially helpful for follow-up. Slides enliven the meetings and create ongoing interest. Finally, they are a major contribution to teaching files and possible peer review publications.

TUMOR REGISTRY

A registry formalizes long-term documentation and follow-up; it is a natural evolution from the tumor board. Nationally, such registries are encouraged by the American College of Surgeons for malignancy tabulation and active ongoing follow-up.

Computers

Although an effective tumor registry can begin with a simple filing system, computerized records are invaluable. A modern flexible system accomplishes several goals: (1) case tabulation; (2) instantaneous retrieval; (3) correlation of treatment, stage, and prognosis; and (4) statistical analysis. The last is invaluable for perspective or retrospective case review.

Automated Imaging

Automated imaging combines photocopying and computerization. This allows handwritten records, photographs, and slides to be stored and retrieved. Such a system has exciting teaching and clinical research possibilities.

INFORMED CONSENT

In 1981, the President's Commission for the Study of Ethical Problems in Medicine and Behavioral Research was created. This commission upheld two fundamental concepts: patient well-being and self-determination. The commission emphasized voluntary decisions by competent patients, only after full disclosure of the pertinent facts. Withholding no unpleasant information, the physician must present options, benefits, and risks. A valid consent is a shared decision based on the patient's active participation [4]. This active participation is preceded by effective physician communication of all the facts. Only after full disclosure are competent adults entitled to accept or reject care based on their own personal values and goals [5]. To safeguard this right, the physician must communicate clearly the disease concept, pathogenesis, and the pros and cons of the proposed treatment. In short, the commission reaffirmed the ethics and legality of informed consent.

Bias

Physician bias is rarely discussed [6]. However, in reality, there are several apparent sources: remuneration, protocol commitment, and personal values (philosophy, religion). Unconsciously, the physician may minimize possible complications and maximize the benefits of a particular therapy. Many physicians tend to value prolongation of life, whereas patients may be concerned with the quality of life. The open appraisal of personal biases coupled with sensitive communication allows for a more honest recommendation.

Guidelines

What is the appropriate information necessary to allow a patient to make an informed decision? Should the physician urge acceptance of the prescribed therapy? If so, how strongly? When does the persuasion become coercion? Is the preservation of life the supreme goal? Does the quality of life have relevance? If so, how much? Who decides and how?[6].

The management of head and neck cancer often has grim consequences in regard to dysfunction and disfigurement. Many times the benefits of medical treatment are unpredictable. Some of the consequences of treatment are as follows: drooling, dysphonia, aphonia, xerostomia, dental extractions, pain, and tracheostomy. Ultimately, these may lead to social rejection and death.

According to McGraw [7], optimal medical care requires adherence to four conditions:

1. What is wrong must truly be understood. Often this means that the patient's original complaints must be rephrased.
2. There must be an agreement between the doctor and the patient as to what is wrong.
3. What must be done must be arrived at by considering the patient's life as a whole.
4. There must be an agreement between the doctor and the patient as to what is to be done and why. In any case, this decision is obviously the patient's. The doctor makes available his knowledge and skill to the patient, who makes the decision.

Consent Terminology

The Howard Cancer Center utilizes several consent forms (Figures 7-2, 7-3, and 7-4). The following passages illustrate key items included in these consents.

Alternatives

"The possible alternatives to the proposed therapy are. . . ." The patient is given all of the feasible alternatives. The pros and cons of each are presented and discussed. This item is a basic foundation of informed consent.

Risks

"I have been made aware of certain risks and consequences that are associated with the proposed procedure. I understand that the explanation of the risks and consequences is not exhaustive and that other, more remote side effects may arise." All common and uncommon risks are discussed openly. The patient is given every opportunity to consent or reject the proposed procedure. Patients are not "sold" or pressured to accept any therapy or procedure.

Guarantee

"No guarantee or assurance has been given by anyone, as to the results that may be obtained." This is self-explanatory, but many malpractice suits have been filed because guarantees were implied or perceived to be implied.

Acknowledgment

"I acknowledge that I have read this document in its entirety and that I fully understand it and that all blank spaces have either been completed or crossed off prior to my signing." This statement reaffirms complete understanding and literacy. If the patient is illiterate or English is not the primary language, the consent is co-signed by a proxy who fully understands and explains the consent to the patient. The same situation applies to the incompetent or unconscious patient. The proxy (e.g., relative, spouse) is invaluable during counseling and the discussion of the permit.

Comatose Patients

When a patient is comatose, vital decisions are approved by a proxy, that is, next of kin, the court, or an ethics committee. Without a proxy, the comatose patient is restricted only to the basic hospital resources. The physician provides care or performs invasive procedures only after proxy approval.

Incompetent and Illiterate Patients

Only a proxy can legitimize an incompetent or illiterate patient's consent [8]. In the absence of next of kin, the court appoints a surrogate. In an emergency, two nonattending physicians may approve procedures or operations, but only

Patient ______________________ Date: ____________ Time: ________ A.M.; ________ P.M.

1. I hereby authorize Dr. ______________________ and such assistants as may be selected by him, to perform upon:

____

(State name of patient or myself)

The following procedure(s) ______________________

(State nature of procedure(s) to be performed)

____

which appear indicated by the diagnostic studies already performed.

2. I consent to the adminstration of whatever type of anesthesia is deemed necessary and desirable by the attending anesthesiologist for the surgical procedure(s) contemplated. I understand that the maintenance of an open airway is of primary importance and that the maintenance of an open airway may necessitate instrumentation within the mouth which might unavoidably result in dental damage and/or irritation of the nose and throat.

3. I acknowledge that I have been informed that I or my surgeon may select an anesthesiologist other than the attending anesthesiologist.

4. The procedure(s) listed in Paragraph 1 have been explained to me by Dr. ____________ and the nature and purpose of the operation, possible alternative methods of treatment, the risks involved, and the possibility of complications have been explained to me. No guarantee or assurance has been given by anyone, as to the results that may be obtained.

5. It has been explained to me that, during the course of the operation, unforeseen conditions may be revealed that necessitate an extension of the original procedure(s) or different procedure(s) than those set forth in Paragraph 1. I t. erefore authorize and request that the above named surgeon and his assistants perform such surgical procedures as are necessai and desirable in the exercise of professional judgment. The authority granted under this paragraph shall extend to remedying all conditions that require treatment and are not known to Dr. ____________ or the attending anesthesiologist at the time the operation is commenced.

I consent to the photographing of the tissue specimens, operations and procedures to be performed for medical, scientific or educational purposes, provided my identity is not revealed by the pictures or by descriptive texts accompanying them.

6. For the purpose of advancing medical knowledge, I consent to the admittance of medical students and other observers, in accordance with ordinary practices of this medical facility, to the use of closed-circuit television, the taking of photographs (including motion pictures), and the preparation of drawings and similar illustrative graphic material, and I also consent to the use of such photographs and other materials for scientific purposes.

7. I consent to the disposal by authorities of the above-named medical facility of any tissues or parts which it may . ? necessary to remove. ☐ Yes ☐ No

(If "NO" is checked, please fill in "a")

a. I agree to dispose of the tissues within ______ hours. (It must be within 72 hours as stated by the physician.)

______________________ Witness

______________________ Signature of Patient

If the patient is unable to sign or is a minor, complete the following:

Patient is a minor ______ years of age and/or is unable to sign because ______________________

______________________ Witness

______________________ Closest relative or legal guardian

______________________ Physician's Signature

PRO 439 001 9/80 Rev. HUH-175

Figure 7-2. Consent for medical or surgical procedure.

1. Induction chemotherapy with Cis-platinum and 5 Day Infusional Therapy of 5-Fluorouracil for Advanced (Stage III or IV) Head and Neck Cancer.

Site: ____________________

Procedures:

a. Cis-platinum by vein

b. 5-Fluorouracil by vein for 5 days

c. Repeat a & b every three weeks for 3 courses

d. Surgery and/or radiation after completion of chemotherapy.

You have advanced cancer of the head and neck region. Your disease is too advanced to expect that you can be cured with surgery alone, radiation alone, or combined surgery and radiation. We are interested in determining whether giving chemotherapy first to shrink the tumor will make the cancer small enough for operation and/or more treatable with radiation. The drugs you will receive will be cis-platinum and 5-fluorouracil. The drugs will be given by vein. After completion of chemotherapy you will then be re-evaluated for operation followed by radiation or if inoperable given radiation and re-evaluated again for operation.

Cis-platinum is a drug which can produce decreased blood counts or kidney failure. Kidney failure is almost always prevented by giving a drug (mannitol) which you will receive when you receive cis-platinum. Some patients can develop deafness from the drug. 5-fluorouracil can cause a decrease in blood counts and sores in mouth. The 5-fluorouracil will be given for 24 hours for 5 days by vein and will require hospitalization for this therapy. Both drugs will cause nausea and vomiting. We will give you medication to prevent or decrease nausea and vomiting. You will be monitored closely for these side effects, but if they occur, they could be serious and life threatening.

In order to reduce your chances of developing the toxicities discussed above as well as reducing your chances of developing another cancer, we strongly urge you to stop smoking (or using tobacco in any form) and to stop drinking alcoholic beverages (beer, whiskey, wine). For you to continue to smoke and drink alcohol increases your chances of doing poorly on this experimental program. We also suggest that you pay attention to nutrition by eating more good foods as your doctor will explain to you.

A

Figure 7-3. Consent for investigative procedures.

We do not know if there is any advantage for you to be treated in this way. Some evidence suggests that the program is safe under medical supervision and has a good chance of improving your chances for cure as compared to standard treatment with radiation or surgery alone. As an alternative, you could be offered radiation therapy, surgery, chemotherapy, or supportive care.

The investigators will do everything possible to prevent or reduce discomfort and risk, but is is not possible to predict everything that might occur. If you have unexpected discomfort or think something unusual or unexpected is occurring you should contact:

M.D. at (202)

Your confidentiality will be maintained and reference to you will be as patient number or hospital number in reporting data.

In the event of any injury resulting from any research procedure, acute medical care will be provided, but no Federal, District of Columbia Government or Howard University funds will be available for compensation.

Anyone who agrees to participate in this research may change his/her mind at any time. Refusal to participate or to continue to participate will not harm your relationship with your physician, the hospital, or those doing the research. They will do the best they can for you whether or not you participate in this research.

You have read the preceding description of this investigation, and you freely give your consent to participate. You understand that you have the right to ask questions at any time and refuse to continue if you so desire. You will receive no payment for your participation.

I acknowledge that I have received a copy of this consent form.

signed (Patient or Relative - specify) Date

signed (Witness) Date

signed (Witness) Date

If you have questions at any time that you would like to discuss with someone other than the investigators on this project, please call the Office of the Executive Secretary, Institutional Review Board at 636-

B

Figure 7-3. (continued)

NAME: ______________________
ADDRESS: ______________________
AGE: ____________ SEX: ____________
HOSPITAL NO : ______________________
RADIATION NO.: ______________________

Patient ______________________ **Date** __________

Time __________ **A.M.** __________ **P.M.**

1. I, (or ______________ for ______________) hereby authorize Dr. ______________ and/or such assistants as may be selected by him to administer a series of radiation therapy treatment to ______________ (myself/the patient).

2. The nature and purpose of the treatments have been explained to me by Dr. ______________
I understand that the radiation therapy treatments are being used to treat me for ______________
(name of disease)
and that the treatments will be directed at ______________
(area encompassed by portals)
Small tattoos may be placed on my skin to permanently identify the boundaries of the treatment beam.

3. The possible alternatives to radiation therapy are: ______________
(describe alternative methods of treatment)
____

4. I have been made aware of certain risks and consequences that are associated with the radiation therapy. These are:
____
(describe risks and consequences)
____
____
____

5. I understand that the explanation of the risks and consequences is not exhaustive and that other, more remote side effects may arise, i.e. treatment related cancer. I have been advised that additional remote risks and consequances will be explained to me upon request.

I acknowledge that I have received no guarantee concerning the radiation therapy to which I am consenting.

I acknowledge that I have been given the opportunity to ask questions concerning the radiation therapy and its risks and consequences and my questions, if any, have been answered to my satisfaction.

6. I acknowledge that I have read this document in its entirety and that I fully understand it, and that all blank spaces have either been completed or crossed off prior to my signing.

______________ ______________
Witness *Signature of Patient*

If patient is unable to sign or is a minor, complete the following:)

Patient (is a minor ________ years of age) is unable to sign because ______________
____

______________ ______________
Witness *Closest Relative or Legal Guardian*

Figure 7-4. Consent for radiation oncology treatment.

as a last resort. If there is any question of competency, a psychiatrist documents the patient's mental status and psychiatric state. Family members or friends can assist in providing information about a patient's mental condition and decision-making capabilities. Although the family should be involved with most major decisions, there is a fine line between such involvement and patient privacy.

Ultimate Responsibility

Even when both physician and patient are compatible and comfortable with each other, substantial barriers still exist (Figure 7-5). One major barrier is the effective communication of vital medical information into clear, understandable language. The translation of medical terminology into layman's terms is a universal problem. The foundation of informed consent is clarity; therefore, the abstract must be converted into the concrete. More importantly, the explanation must be delivered without any hint of condescension (See Appendix).

Today, health care is often delivered in a fragmented fashion. Such an atmosphere fosters the perception of a fragmentation of responsibility. To dispel this perception, there must be a readily designated attending physician or surgeon for each patient. Although care is delegated to assistants, one individual is always responsible for communicating to the patient. Therefore, the informed consent is ultimately the attending physician's responsibility.

Figure 7-5. Consent dynamics. 1. See Table 7-1. 2. See Chapter 5. 3. See Chapter 6. 4. Plan A, the best option as proposed by the tumor board. 5. Next of kin, power of attorney, court, etc.

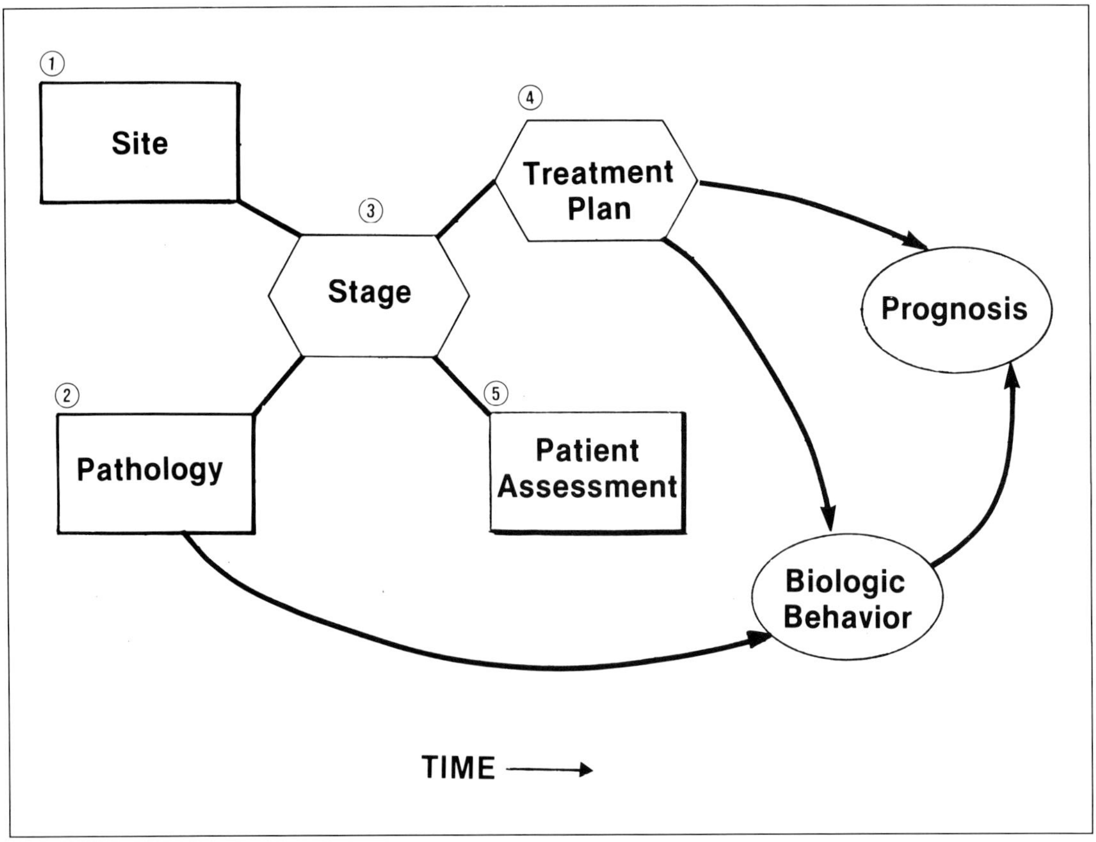

THE PLANNING PROCESS

Planning Variables

The treatment of head and neck cancer changes constantly (Table 7-2). Given this state of flux, therapy requires detailed assessment, not only of the cancer, but also of the patient's psychological makeup, goals, and personal needs (Figure 7-6). A knowledgeable tumor board must have the collective wisdom to choose the optimal plan for each patient. This plan comprises three variable factors: tumor, patient, and physician. Tumor factors are discussed in detail in Chapters 1 and 5. Procrastination is the primary adverse patient factor (see Chapter 19); it delays diagnosis, treatment, and ultimately affects prognosis. For multiple reasons (personal, cultural, or social), many patients seek attention late and are first encountered with well-advanced disease. Physician factors, although not discussed openly, are also a source of delay; too often patients are treated for weeks or months for the subtle symptoms of head and neck malignancy before the diagnosis is made (see Chapter 2).

Staging

Accurate staging is the foundation of basic planning (Tables 7-3 and 7-4; see also Chapter 6). Aside from staging, other variables may alter plans (i.e., tumor histology, the patient's preference, past medical history).

Radicality

Treatment is recommended after the analysis of tumor aggressiveness, morbidity, mortality, and prognosis [3]. It is well-known that the best chance for cure is the first time the cancer is treated. Thus, if indicated, radicality must be considered. Modern reconstructive techniques allow the surgeon to decrease disfigurement and maintain function. However, as the probability of cure decreases, radicality may or may not be justified. There are obvious dilemmas: a conservative approach may lead to recurrence, whereas a more radical approach may lead to increased morbidity or mortality. There is a fine line between the two philosophies. When the incidence of mortality approaches morbidity, that particular treatment option is discarded. If cure is unlikely, palliation or conservative treatment is recommended.

New Malignancy

For new malignancies, the general scheme as presented in Table 7-3 is recommended. Since treatment planning is predicated largely on stage, the following guidelines are presented.

Stage I

Single-modality treatment is advocated for stage I. When the incidence of secondary or metachronous primary cancers is high, surgery is advocated. Thus, radiotherapy is reserved for possible future malignancies. However, if the site and pathology so indicate, radiotherapy is chosen as the first modality.

Stage II

Depending on the site, stage II patients are treated with surgery and radiotherapy. Whenever possible, post-operative radiation is given within 4 to 6 weeks of surgery.

Stages III and IV

Patients with stage III or IV cancer are candidates for triple-modality treatment, with chemotherapy preceding surgery and radiotherapy. The need for rehabilitation is almost universal, since the probability of functional disability is high.

Option 1: Induction Chemotherapy, Surgery, and Radiotherapy

This is the most vigorous and time-consuming treatment option. The preliminary results of this protocol (see Chapter 8) are very encouraging. However, triple-modality treatment is considered investigational and requires a minimum of 20 weeks to complete, assuming that there are no treatment breaks or complications.

Option 2: Surgery, Followed by Radiotherapy

Less desirable then option 1, this treatment is reserved for those patients who are not chemotherapy candidates. Again, depending on the site, the prospects for cure remains high.

Table 7-2. Treatment modalities

Modality	*Indications*	*Contraindications*	*Advantages*	*Disadvantages*
Chemotherapy	Radiation failures Surgical failures Poor surgical risks Persistent or recurrent disease	Renal failure Respiratory failure	Systemic disease Repeatable Cost-effective Availability	Morbid and mortal side effects Large anoxic or avascular tumors Patient compliance
Radiotherapy	Positive surgical margins Surgical failures Synchronous head and neck carcinomas	Large anoxic tumors Hostile or uncooperative patients	Large treatment area Preservation of function Low morbidity and mortality Outpatient milieu	Xerostomia Anorexia Nonrepeatable Tumor radioresistance Inconsistent availability Patient compliance
Surgery	Radiation failures (local disease) Chemotherapy failures Small localized disease	Distant metastasis Renal failure Hepatic failure Coagulopathy Poor respiratory reserve Recent myocardial infarction Malnutrition	Ablation of large anoxic tumors (local) Immediate pathologic analysis Availability	Diffuse, microscopic disease Physiologic dysfunction Disfigurement Morbid and mortal complications Costs

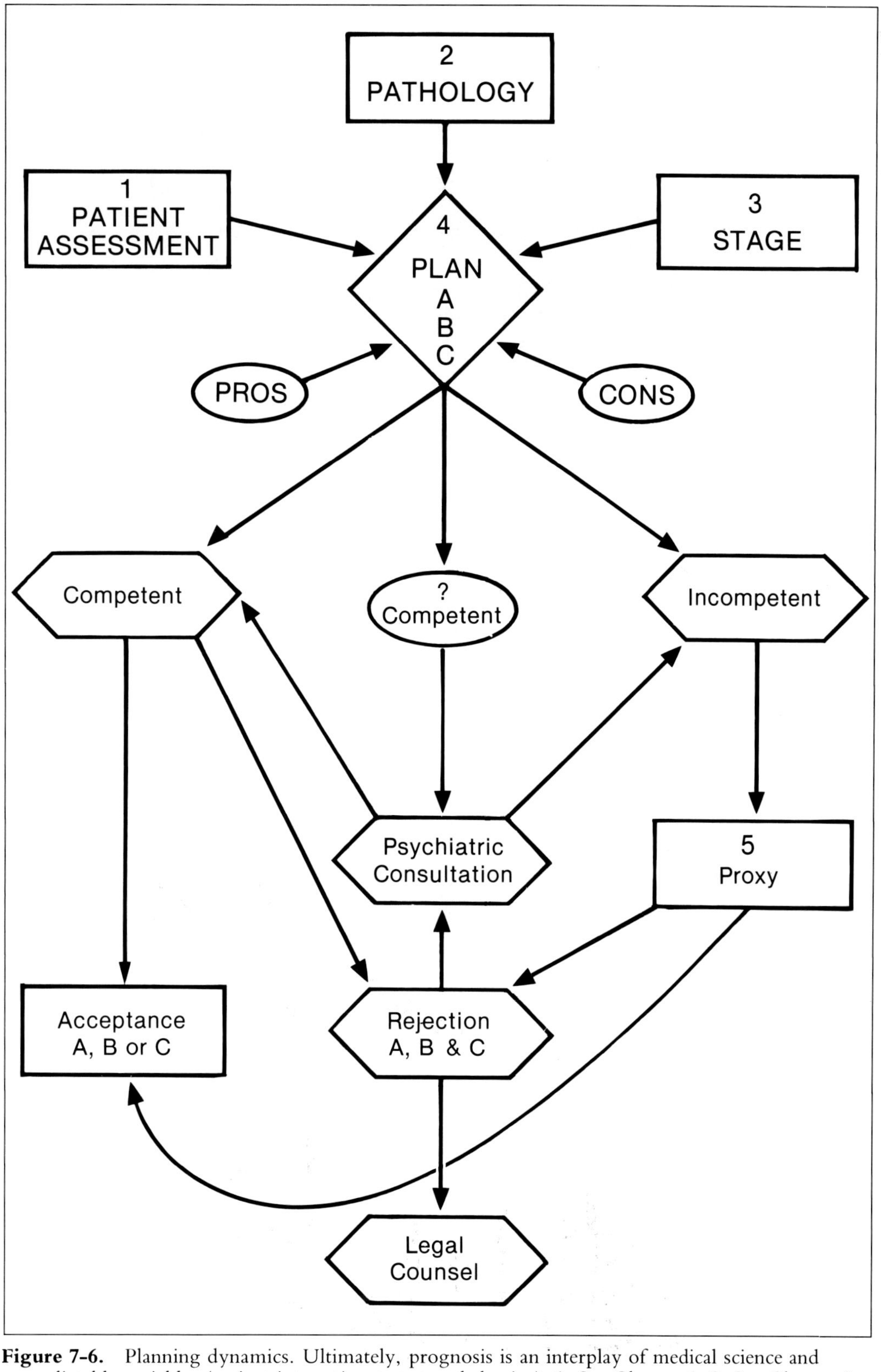

Figure 7-6. Planning dynamics. Ultimately, prognosis is an interplay of medical science and unpredictable variables (patient interaction to tumor behavior). 1. See Chapter 1. 2. See Chapter 5. 3. See Chapter 6. 4. See Chapter 7. 5. See Chapters 2, 12, and 22.

Table 7-3. Planning: site versus stage

Site	*Stage I*	*Stage II*	*Stage III*	*Stage IV*
1. Nasopharynx	Radiotherapy	Radiotherapy	Radiotherapy Surgery	Triple-modality therapy
2. Paranasal sinuses Nose	Surgery	Surgery Radiotherapy	Triple-modality therapy	Triple-modality therapy
3. Salivary glands	Surgery	Surgery	Surgery Radiotherapy	Surgery Radiotherapy
4. Lips	Surgery Radiotherapy	Surgery Radiotherapy	Triple-modality therapy	Triple-modality therapy
5. Oropharynx	Radiotherapy Surgery	Surgery Radiotherapy	Triple-modality therapy	Triple-modality therapy
6. Oral cavity	Surgery Radiotherapy	Surgery Radiotherapy	Triple-modality therapy	Triple-modality therapy
7. Hypopharynx	Surgery Radiotherapy	Surgery Radiotherapy	Triple-modality therapy	Triple-modality therapy
8. Larynx	Laser Surgery Radiotherapy	Surgery Radiotherapy	Triple-modality therapy	Triple-modality therapy
9. Thyroid/parathyroids	Surgery	Surgery	Surgery Radioactive iodine Radiotherapy	Chemotherapy Radiotherapy
10. Cervical esophagus	Surgery Radiotherapy	Surgery Radiotherapy	Laser Triple-modality therapy	Laser Triple-modality therapy

Table 7-4. Stage versus treatment options

Presentation	Stages I & II: Option A	A′	Stages III & IV: A	B	C	D
Initial	Surgery	Radiotherapy (full-course)	Triple-modality therapy	Surgery Radiotherapy (post-op)	Chemotherapy Radiotherapy	Radiotherapy
Recurrence or persistence	Radiotherapy (post-op)	Surgery	Surgery (+/−) Radiotherapy (+/−) Chemotherapy	Surgery (+/−) Radiotherapy (+/−) Chemotherapy	Chemotherapy	Surgery (+/−)
End-stage	Not applicable	Not applicable	Chemotherapy	Chemotherapy	Chemotherapy	Chemotherapy

A, A′ } First option.
B Second option.
C Third option.
D Fourth option.

Option 3: Induction Chemotherapy and Radiotherapy
This option is an alternative for patients who are either medically unfit or who refuse surgery [9]. This protocol is especially effective when the patient has a complete chemotherapeutic response.

Option 4: Full-Course Radiotherapy
This protocol is indicated for patients unfit for surgery or chemotherapy. Although usually palliative, there is the remote possibility for cure, depending on the site.

Recurrent Malignancy

Restaging is the initial planning step with recurrent malignancy [10, 11]. Patients fail either at the primary, regional, or distant sites. From three basic failures there emerge seven possible patterns (Figure 7-7). When failure occurs, the planning process is repeated, although altered by prior therapy (Table 7-5): previous modalities such as full-course radiotherapy may be exhausted and unavailable (Figure 7-8).

Stage Analysis of Salvage Treatment

Stage I/II
If the patient is fortunate, stage I or II recurrences have acceptable salvage rates. Whether

Figure 7-7. Venn diagram: failure pathways.

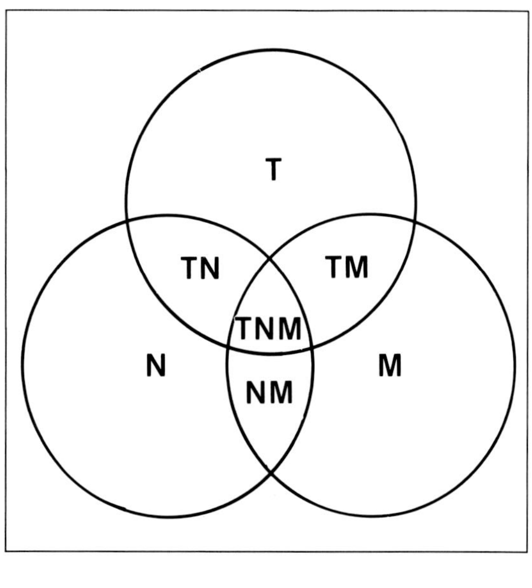

Table 7-5. Failure patterns versus salvage treatment

Failure	Salvage: Surgery	Radiation	Chemotherapy
T	Yes/no	Yes/no	Yes/no
N	Yes/no	Yes/no	Yes/no
M	Yes/no	Yes/no	Yes/no
TN	Yes	Yes/no	Yes/no
TNM	No	Yes/no	Yes/no
NM	No	Yes/no	Yes
M	Yes/no	Yes/no	Yes

surgery or radiation was the initial modality dictates the recommended salvage modality [12–14]. Unlike new malignancy planning, recurrences almost always require some form of rehabilitation and extended care.

Stage III/IV

Since the prospects for cure are dismal in stage III or IV, treatment is almost always palliative. Chemotherapy plays a central role; indeed, it may be the only available treatment. Depending on circumstances, no treatment and intense supportive care are also options (see Chapter 20). Having exhausted all available treatments, many terminally ill patients present difficult ethical dilemmas.

Figure 7-8. Treatment: recurrent carcinoma. As time passes, the need for supportive care increases inversely as the therapeutic options diminish.

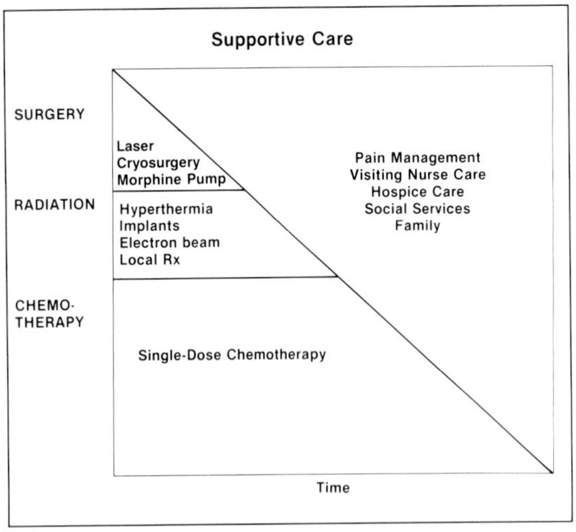

ETHICS

One may define ethics as human action governed by moral principles [15]. Given such a broad definition, ethical principles certainly are intertwined with medicine. Specifically, medical ethics cluster in five pivotal areas: patient autonomy, euthanasia, human research, resource allocation, and the impact of technology on the art of medicine. Several areas have been discussed previously; however, the following analysis provides additional insight.

Confidentiality

Confidentiality is implicit between doctor and patient. This basic Hippocratic tenet is preserved easily in the private office, but it is difficult to safeguard in the hospital or clinic [16]. The proliferation of computer terminals linked to medical records and hospital laboratories makes recall all too easy. A byproduct of easy access is the erosion of confidentiality. Few hospitals restrict information access; thus the privacy of all patients is fragile and at risk. Physicians, physicians-in-training, and ancillary personnel must be alert and strive to preserve patient confidentiality.

Computers

Computer access should be restricted. The following is recommended: (1) secure and limit access, (2) be suspicious of unauthorized persons on nursing units, and (3) periodically change the access codes.

Charts

Especially in teaching hospitals, charts are too accessible. Medical students, residents, respi-

DECLARATION

Declaration made this _______ day of ______________________(month, year). I ________________________________, being of sound mind, willfully and voluntarily make known my desires that my dying shall not be artificially prolonged under the circumstances set forth below, do declare:

If at any time I should have an incurable injury, disease, or illness certified to be a terminal condition by two (2) physicians who have personally examined me, one (1) of whom shall be my attending physician, and the physicians have determined that my death will occur whether or not life-sustaining procedures are utilized and where the application of life-sustaining procedures would serve only to artificially prolong the dying process, I direct that such procedures be withheld or withdrawn, and that I be permitted to die naturally with only the administration of medication or the performance of any medical procedure deemed necessary to provide me with comfort, care or to alleviate pain.

In the absence of my ability to give directions regarding the use of such life-sustaining procedures, it is my intention that this declaration shall be honored by my family and physician(s) as the final expression of my legal right to refuse medical or surgical treatment and accept the consequences from such refusal.

I understand the full import of this declaration and I am emotionally and mentally competent to make this declaration.

Signed ______________________________

Address ______________________________

____

I believe the declarant to be of sound mind. I did not sign the declarant's signature above for or at the direction of the declarant. I am at least eighteen (18) years of age and am not related to the declarant by blood or marriage, entitled to any portion of the estate of the declarant according to the laws of intestate succession of the District of Columbia or under any will of declarant or codicil thereto, or directly financially responsible for declarant's medical care. I am not the declarant's attending physician, an employee of the attending physician, or an employee of the health facility in which the declarant is a patient.

Witness ______________________________

Witness ______________________________

Figure 7-9. Living will.

ratory therapists, nursing students, in fact everyone, can leisurely peruse the charts. One possible safeguard is the separation of the history from the progress notes. This gives access of the more confidential portions to the attending physicians and nurses. A model for this is found in some psychiatric wards.

Public Forums

Elevators, hallways, and the cafeteria are inappropriate places for the discussion of patient maladies. Information overheard by relatives is devastating, and the possibility of medical litigation is very real. Everyone on the nursing unit should be identified and monitored. Finally, these measures should not be confused with secrecy, but as safeguards of Hippocratic ideals.

Resuscitation

One presumes resuscitation for any patient in the event of an unexpected arrest [17]. Despite well-planned and sophisticated efforts, at times we fail. If our best is not good enough, what then? In general, a physician is obligated to sustain life. However, a competent patient is entitled to forego cardiopulmonary resuscitation. Moreover, physicians have a duty to assess whether a patient is a resuscitation candidate [18]. If a patient is terminal, the decision not to resuscitate, with the consent of the patient or proxy, is an ethical justification.

The following "no code" guidelines are recommended: (1) documented central nervous system death (by electroencephalogram); (2) irreversible coma associated with incurable disease; (3) unrelenting pain and suffering with dismal prospects for cure; (4) exhaustion of medical therapy for either cure or palliation; and (5) patient or family consent. Once the "no code" status is sanctioned and witnessed, it is written clearly in the chart by the attending physician. This alerts all concerned and prevents needless resuscitation.

Euthanasia

Self-Determination

Only a competent and informed patient can refuse life support [15]. Some are willing to prolong their lives, even if the ultimate fate is pain and discomfort. Others give up without a whimper when confronted with long, involved treatment options. In each case, ethics and the law support competent patients who decline life-sustaining treatment and or any medical intervention. When a competent patient refuses treatment, the physician, after adequate counseling, quietly withholds further treatment [19]. Forced therapy violates self-determination.

Ethics Committee

In short, the physician preserves life but recognizes the patient's right to refuse treatment, including any that sustains life (Figure 7-9). Obviously, these are difficult decisions for both physician and patient. Therefore, many hospitals have established committees to review matters involving medical ethics [20–22]. These committees provide valuable guidelines to safeguard both patient desires and institutional responsibilities. Once the decision to forego "heroic measures" has been made by all parties, the patient is not abandoned. Even in terminal situations, excellent supportive care is rendered without exception.

REFERENCES

1. Arnold RM, Povar GJ, Howell JD: The humanities, humanistic behavior and the humane physician. *Ann Intern Med* 106 : 313, 1987.
2. Ingelfinger F: Arrogance. *N Engl J Med* 304 : 1507, 1980.
3. Goepfert H: Are we making progress? *Arch Otolaryngol* 110 : 562, 1984.
4. Anderson AD: The reality of restorative care in Harlem's municipal hospital: The patient as a therapeutic agent. *Arch Phys Med Rehabil* 56(48) : 9, 1975.
5. Hawkins C: *Mishap or Malpractice*. Boston: Blackwell, 1985.
6. Frank HA, Davidson TM: Ethical dilemmas in head and neck cancer. *Head Neck Surg* 11(1) : 22, 1989.
7. McGraw J: *Ferment in Medicine*. Philadelphia: Saunders, 1960.
8. Stembrook R, Lo B: Decision making for incompetent patients by designated proxy: California's new law. *N Engl J Med* 210 : 1598, 1984.
9. Rubin P, Carter S: Combination radiation therapy and chemotherapy: A logical basis for their use. *Cancer* 26 : 274, 1976.
10. DeSanto LW: T_3 glottic cancer: Options and consequences of the options. *Laryngoscope* 94 : 1311, 1984.
11. Rubin, P: A unified classification of tumors: An oncotaxonnary with symbols. *Cancer* 31 : 963, 1973.
12. Emami B, Bignardi M, Devineni VR. Reirradiation of recurrent head and neck cancers. *Laryngoscope* 97 : 85, 1987.
13. Davis RK, et al: Prognostic indicators in head and neck cancer patients receiving combined therapy. *Arch Otolaryngol Head Neck Surg* 115 : 1443, 1989.
14. Schuller DE, Stein DW, Metch B: Analysis of treatment failure patterns: A Southwest Oncology Group Study. *Arch Otolaryngol Head Neck Surg* 115 : 834, 1989.
15. Walker B: Ethics in health services and medical care. *J Natl Med Assoc* 81 : 13, 1988.

16. Siegler, M: Confidentiality in medicine: A decrepit concept. *N Engl J Med* 307 : 1518, 1982.
17. Fox M, Lipton HL: The decision to perform cardiopulmonary resuscitation in the hospital. *N Engl J Med* 309 : 607, 1983.
18. Newton RC, Miles TP: The need for a do not resuscitate policy in a public city hospital. *J Natl Med Assoc* 80 : 1057, 1988.
19. Cassel EJ: The nature of suffering and the goals of medicine. *N Engl J Med* 306 : 639, 1982.
20. Rachels J: *The End of Life: Euthanasia and Morality*. New York: Oxford University Press, 1981.
21. Pellegrino ED, Thomasina DC: *A Philosophical Basis of Medical Practice*. New York: Oxford University Press, 1981.
22. President's Commission for the Study of Ethical Problems in Medicine and Biomedical and Behavioral Research: *Decisions to Forego Life Sustaining Treatment*. Washington, DC: Government Printing Office, 1983.

LAYMAN'S HEAD AND NECK GLOSSARY

Angiogram X-ray of the veins and arteries; they are usually injected with a material to highlight their patterns.

Arrest Loss of breathing and/or heartbeat.

Aspiration Regurgitated or swallowed fluid in the tracheobronchial tree; usually causes a pneumonia.

Autopsy Analysis of the body organs to determine disease and the events causing death.

Biopsy To take a small piece of tissue.

Cancer Malignant tumor.

Carotidectomy Removal of the largest artery in the neck; this may result in a stroke.

Chemotherapy Treatment of cancer by drugs.

Consent Written permission to perform a procedure or procedures.

Consultation Request for a conference with another physician, usually a specialist.

CT or CAT Scan Computed tomography scan, a computer x-ray.

CVA Cerebrovascular accident; stroke.

Esophagostomy Hole in food passage (in the neck) for feeding.

Fistula Poor healing that has resulted in a hole from the inside to the outside.

Flap Tissue, usually skin from the shoulder, chest, or back, to fill in a hole or defect (usually the result of surgery).

Gastrostomy Hole in the stomach for feeding.

Glossectomy *Partial*—removal of a portion of the tongue.
Total—removal of the entire tongue.

Hospice Hospital for dying patients.

ICU Intensive care unit.

Laryngectomy *Total*—removal of the entire voice box with complete loss of voice.
Hemi—Removal of lateral half of the voice box without loss of voice.
Subtotal supraglottic laryngectomy—removal of the upper half of the voice box without loss of voice.

LAYMAN'S HEAD AND NECK GLOSSARY *Continued*

	Partial laryngopharyngectomy—removal of a portion of the food passage and voice box without loss of voice.
Medical oncologist	Specialist who treats cancer with drugs.
Metastasis	Spread of cancer.
Mandibulectomy	Removal of the jaw. *Hemi*—removal of half of the jaw. *Partial*—removal of part of the jaw.
Maxillectomy	Removal of the large facial bone and sinus beneath the eye.
Myocutaneous flap	Skin *and* muscle from the shoulder, chest, or back to fill in a surgical defect.
Neck dissection	Removal of the large vein, fat, and glands in the neck. *Radical*—as above, plus the large muscle in the neck, tissue under the jaw, and nerve to the shoulder. *Modified*—preservation of the large muscle in the neck, tissue under the jaw, or the nerve to the shoulder.
Necrosis	Dead tissue.
Oncologist	Cancer specialist.
Panendoscopy	Looking behind the nose into the food and breathing passages and into the voice box (there are no external incisions).
Pneumonia	Infection and/or inflammation of the lungs.
Radiotherapist	Specialist who treats cancer with radioactive rays or particles.
Radiotherapy	Treatment of cancer by radioactive rays or particles.
Skin graft	Thin slice of skin, usually from the thigh, to cover an exposed surface.
Surgical oncologist	Specialist who treats cancer with surgical techniques.
Tracheostomy	Permanent hole in windpipe for breathing.
Tracheotomy	Temporary hole in windpipe for breathing.
Tumor board	Conference of medical specialists who treat cancer.

8

Chemotherapy

ROBERT M. WHITE, JR.

KEY CONCEPTS

Medical Assessment; Patient Selection; Prognostic Factors; Cytotoxic Agents; Toxicity

MILESTONES

1 A.D.	Colchicine	Discorides
1865	Arsenic for Leukemia	Lissauer
1898	First Alkylating Agent	Ehrlich
1912	Benzol for Chronic Myelogenous Leukemia	Koranzi
1946	Urethane for Chronic Myelogenous Leukemia	Waddow
1947	Folate for Solid Tumors and Leukemia	Farber
1949	Methotrexate	
1956	Gestational Trophoblastic Neoplasms, Cure with Methotexate	Li
1957	5-Fluorouracil	Heidelberger
1960	Wilms' Tumor Cure with Radiation and Chemotherapy	
1964	Acute Lymphocytic Leukemia Remission with Vincristine and Prednisone	
1964	Burkitt's Lymphoma Cure	
1965	Cisplatin	Rosenberg
1966	Bleomycin	Japan
1970	MOPP Reported to Cure Advanced Hodgkin's Disease	
1973	Effective Chemotherapy for Rhabdomyosarcoma	
1975	Induction Head and Neck Chemotherapy	
1975–76	Combination Chemotherapy Cure of Testicular Carcinoma	
1976	Effective Adjuvant Chemotherapy for Breast Carcinoma	
1977	Chemotherapeutic Cure of Childhood Ovarian Carcinoma	

In 1990, approximately 43,000 new cases of squamous cell carcinoma of the head and neck were diagnosed in the United States. There were 13,000 disease-related deaths [1]. The excessive use of tobacco and alcohol is the main cause [2]. Thus, patient management comprises treatment not only of the cancer but also of the medical complications of a consumptive life-style.

MEDICAL ASSESSMENT

Table 8-1 summarizes the medical problems found singly or in combination with head and neck cancer [3–6]. The medical consequences of these problems are considered before attributing a chief complaint to metastatic disease or a paraneoplastic syndrome. Special attention is focused on the cessation of tobacco and alcohol use and the improvement of nutrition. The medical problems are managed in the usual manner except that beta blockers are avoided in hypertensive patients to prevent pulmonary complications and sedatives are introduced early in alcoholics to prevent alcohol withdrawal syndrome.

Table 8-1. Coexisting illness

Malnutrition
Weight loss
Vitamin deficiencies
Electrolyte imbalance
Cardiovascular system
Atherosclerotic cardiovascular disease
Hypertension
Respiratory system
Aspiration pneumonia
Airway obstruction (secondary to tumor)
Chronic obstructive pulmonary disease
Gastrointestinal system
Poor oral hygiene
Cirrhosis
Pancreatic insufficiency
Gastrointestinal bleeding
Hematopoietic system: anemia
Folate deficiency
Vitamin B_{12} deficiency
Iron deficiency
Coagulopathy
Endocrine system: diabetes mellitus
Alcoholism
Alcohol withdrawal syndrome
Second neoplasms
Head and neck
Esophagus
Lung
Colon and rectum

DIAGNOSIS

Every effort is made to confirm pathologically the diagnosis of squamous cell carcinoma and its anatomic site of origin (see Chapter 5). Electron microscopy, histochemistry, and immunologic procedures aid in this process. Occasionally, these techniques clarify the diagnosis of an anaplastic or undifferentiated carcinoma biopsied from a cervical node, whose differential diagnosis includes poorly differentiated squamous cell carcinoma, large-cell lymphoma, melanoma, or poorly differentiated adenocarcinoma [7]. Chemotherapy is withheld until a precise diagnosis is obtained.

PATIENT SELECTION

Not all patients are candidates for chemotherapy. Patients are considered for investigational chemotherapy, alone or as a component of multimodality therapy. In general, chemotherapy is reserved, inductively, for stage III and stage IV patients and for radiation or surgery failures.

Recurrent Disease

Chemotherapy for patients who have early or advanced disease treated previously with surgery or radiation but who now have recurrent local (common) or distant disease (uncommon) is palliative. Careful selection and administration of cytotoxic agents are a necessity, since prior therapies (surgery and radiation) disrupt the vascular supply, resulting in poor response rates (<30%) with single-agent or combination chemotherapy. Furthermore, these patients have higher chemotherapy toxicities due to damage from previous therapies, poor performance status, and weight loss. Therefore, bedridden patients, patients who have lost greater than 10 percent of their body weight, and patients who are not able to comply with follow-up are not good chemotherapy candidates [3, 8].

Advanced Disease (Untreated)

Patients with stage III or IV disease who have not received any prior treatment appear to benefit most from chemotherapy, since they have an undisturbed vascular supply. Also they tend

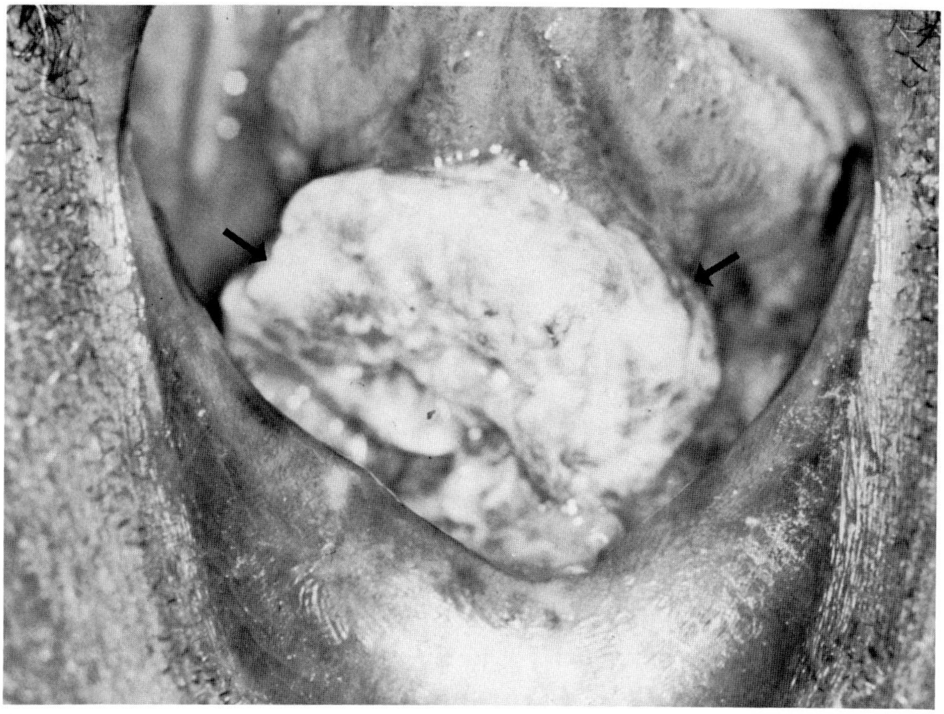

A

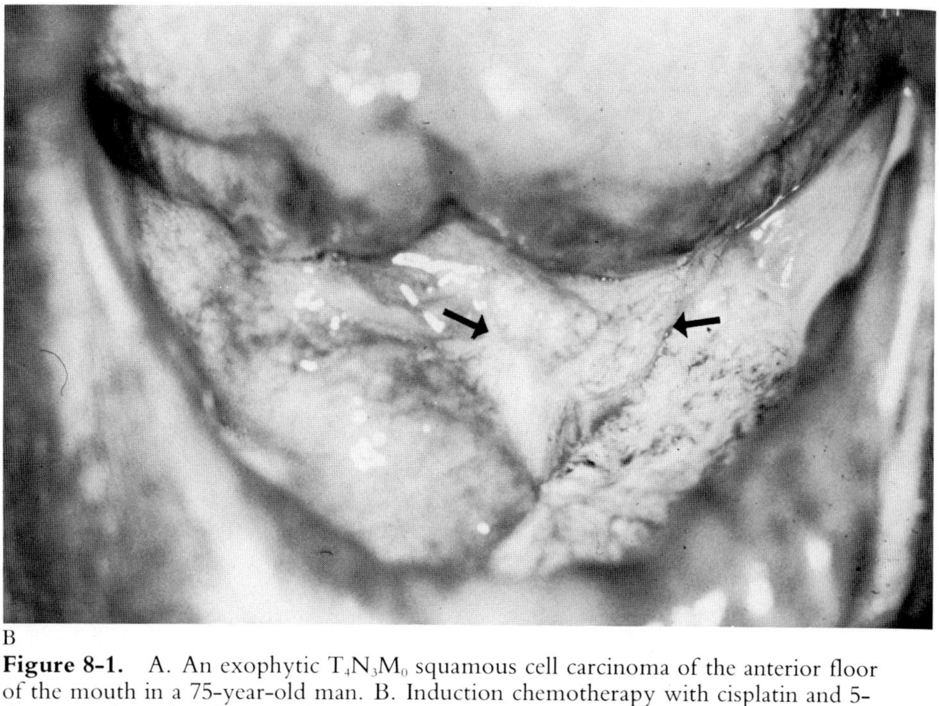

B

Figure 8-1. A. An exophytic $T_4N_3M_0$ squamous cell carcinoma of the anterior floor of the mouth in a 75-year-old man. B. Induction chemotherapy with cisplatin and 5-fluorouracil produced a partial response after three courses of therapy. An early response was observed prior to the second course of therapy.

to have a better performance and nutritional status, allowing them to tolerate more intensive chemotherapeutic regimens [8].

EVALUATION OF RESPONSE

Because of chemotherapy's severe, life-threatening toxicity, the extent of disease is assessed before treatment and monitored throughout the treatment course. This assessment includes physical examination, endoscopy, and computed tomography (CT) scan (primary and nodal disease). Perpendicular measurements of disease are made and compared pre- and post-chemotherapy. Careful monitoring is necessary to justify the continuation of these toxic drugs (Figures 8-1, 8-2, and 8-3).

Guidelines

Complete response: disappearance of all disease as documented by physical examination, endoscopy, CT scan, and the absence of cancer in any surgical specimen. The physical evidence of a response must endure at least 4 weeks.

Partial response: decrease by at least 50 percent (in the product of the longest perpendicular diameters of measurable disease), no new lesions, and residual cancer in any surgical specimen from a patient clinically assessed to have a complete response.

Minimal response: decrease in all disease by 25 to 50 percent (in the product of the longest perpendicular diameters of measurable lesions).

Figure 8-2. A. A large exophytic metastatic squamous cell carcinoma in a 54-year-old man. B. After three courses of cisplatin, the tumor almost disappeared completely.

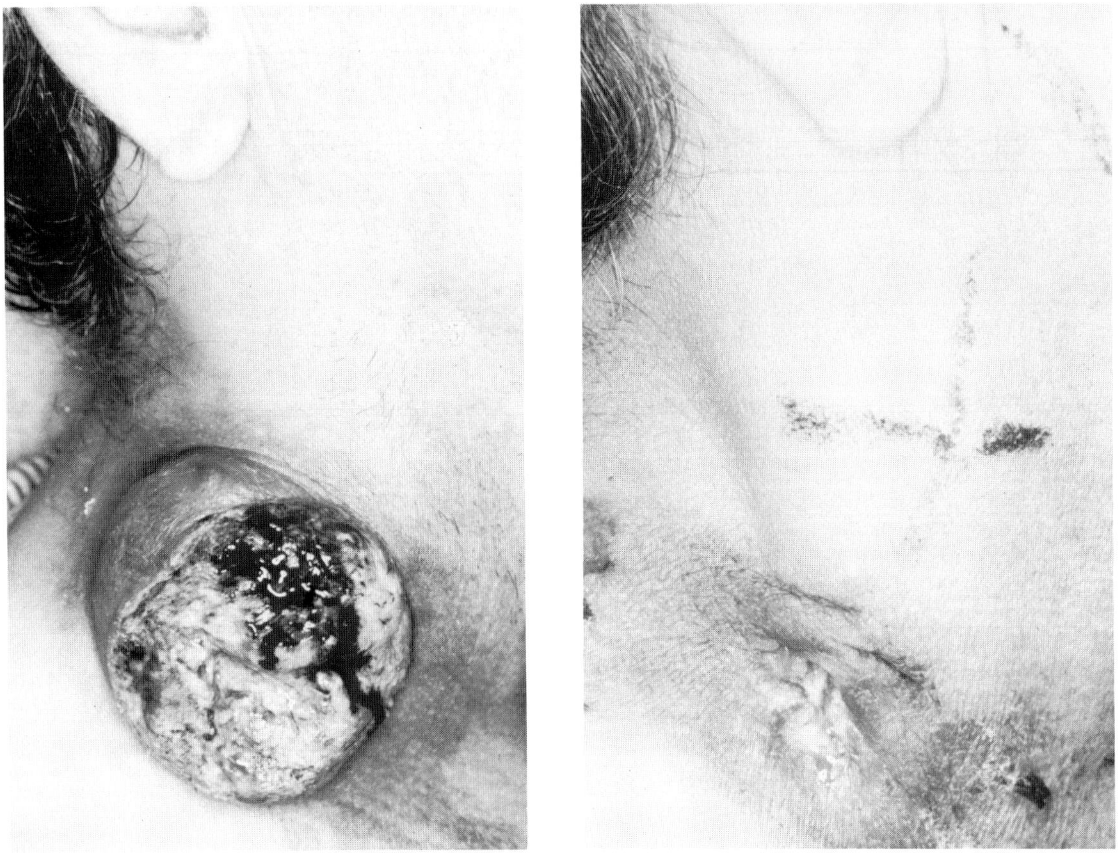

A B

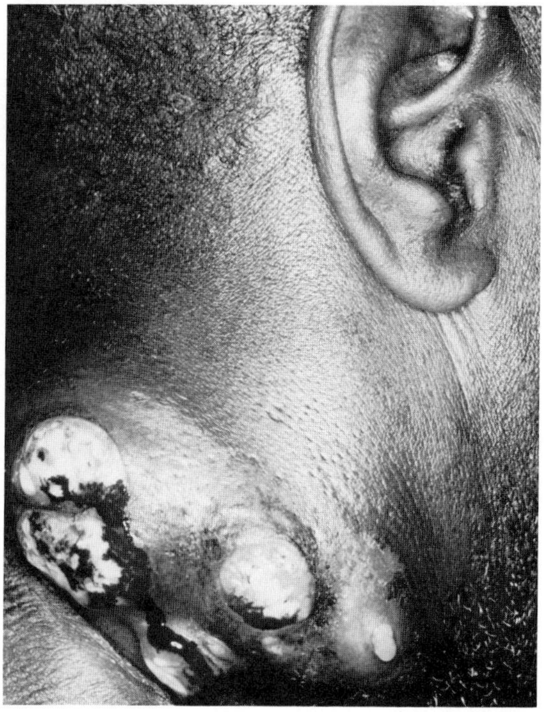

A

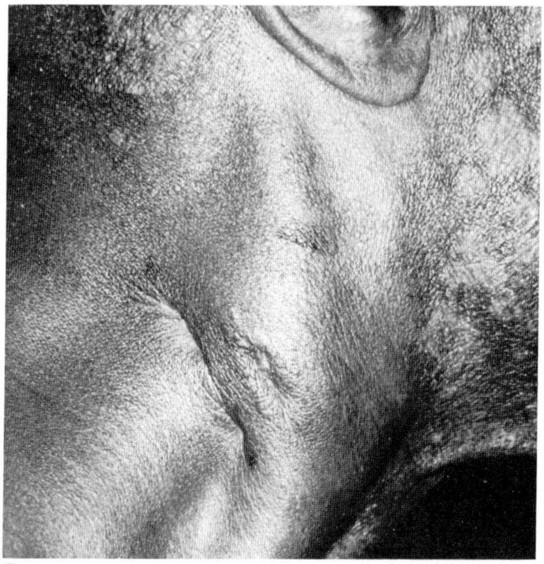

B

Figure 8-3. A. A 59-year-old man with $T_4N_3M_0$ squamous cell carcinoma of the larynx that presented with a bleeding, ulcerated neck mass and stridor. B. A partial response is documented; bleeding and stridor improved within 3 days of initiating treatment with cisplatin and 5-fluorouracil.

No response: none of the above, progression of disease or clinical deterioration (weight loss, symptoms, or performance score) [9].

Prognostic Factors

Performance Status

Performance status assesses the degree of debility from the cancer or the concurrent illnesses (Tables 8-2 and 8-3). Patients who are Eastern Cooperative Oncology Group (ECOG) performance status 0 to 2 respond better to chemotherapy with fewer toxicities, particularly patients with recurrent disease. Patients who are performance status 3 to 4 seldom respond and have frequent chemotherapy toxicities [10].

Weight Loss

Patients who have had a greater than 10-percent loss of body weight do not respond as well as patients who maintain their nutrition (see Chapter 21) [10]. Many head and neck cancer patients are malnourished due to alcoholism or dysphagia. Chronic alcoholism predisposes patients to multiple vitamin, mineral (Mg^{2+}, Ca^{2+}), and electrolyte (K^+) deficiencies [3].

Table 8-2. Performance status (ECOG)*

Grade	*Description*
0	Ambulatory; asymptomatic
1	Ambulatory; symptomatic (e.g., painful nodal disease, dyspnea from laryngeal obstruction, aspiration from hypopharyngeal disease, painful tonsillar mass)
2	Less than 50% of wakeful hours in bed
3	Greater than 50% of wakeful hours in bed
4	Bedridden

*Eastern Cooperative Oncology Group.

Table 8-3. Prognostic factors

Performance status
Weight loss
Prior therapy (chemotherapy, radiation, surgery)
Extent of disease (tumor or nodal stage)
Timing of chemotherapy (induction versus salvage)

Prior Therapy

Patients with prior surgery, radiation, or chemotherapy respond poorly. Previous surgery or radiation alters vascularity. Chemotherapy is not delivered easily to fibrotic or poorly vascularized areas. Palliative chemotherapy is ineffective, probably secondary to a resistant clone of malignant cells (see Chapter 1) [8].

Extent of Disease

The tumor volume (primary and nodal) inversely affects response to chemotherapy; that is, patients with the least disease respond the best [11, 12].

Timing of Chemotherapy

Induction chemotherapy has response rates double those obtained in patients with prior surgery or radiation. Complete response rates of 10 to 50 percent in previously untreated patients are common [8, 12].

CYTOTOXIC AGENTS

Agent selection is based on patient assessment in relation to drug toxicity (Table 8-4). For example, a patient with severe chronic obstructive pulmonary disease is not a good candidate for bleomycin. Similarly, patients with renal insufficiency are not candidates for methotrexate or cisplatinum. Finally, intensive combination chemotherapy in debilitated patients with poor performance status is discouraged [3, 8, 11, 13, 14]. Figure 8-4 illustrates the cell cycle and the sites of action of the cytotoxic agents [15].

Methotrexate

Site of Action

Methotrexate is an S-phase specific inhibitor of dihydrofolate reductase, blocking the synthesis of DNA and RNA.

Dosage

Weekly doses of 40 to 60 mg/m^2 IV are administered safely to patients with recurrent disease.

Toxicity

The toxicities include mucositis, diarrhea (hemorrhagic enteritis), nausea and vomiting,

Table 8-4. Head and neck chemotherapy

Family	*Drug*	*Action*	*Site of Action*	*Dosage**	*Side effects*
Antimetabolites	Methotrexate	Inhibits dihydrofolate reductase Inhibits DNA and purine synthesis	S-phase	40–60 mg/m^2/wk	Myelosuppression, mucositis, renal tubular necrosis, hepatic fibrosis, pneumonitis
	5-Fluorouracil	Thymidylate synthesis inhibition	S-phase	600 mg/m^2/wk (bolus)	Myelosuppression (bolus), gastrointestinal (continuous infusion), myocardial ischemia, acute cerebellar syndrome
		RNA synthesis inhibition		1000 mg/m^2/24 hr for 5 days	
Miscellaneous	Cisplatin	DNA base cross-links	G_1	80–120 mg/m^2 every 3 wk	Nephrotoxicity, vomiting, ototoxicity, electrolyte imbalance, neuropathy
	Vincristine	Mitotic spindle toxin	M-phase	1–2 mg/m^2	Peripheral neuropathy, constipation, cranial nerve palsy, alopecia
Antibiotics	Bleomycin	Cleaves DNA strands by free radicals	G-phase Early S-phase	1–15 units/m^2/wk	Mucositis, rash, stomatitis, pulmonary fibrosis, fever, chills

*See text for combination therapy dosages.

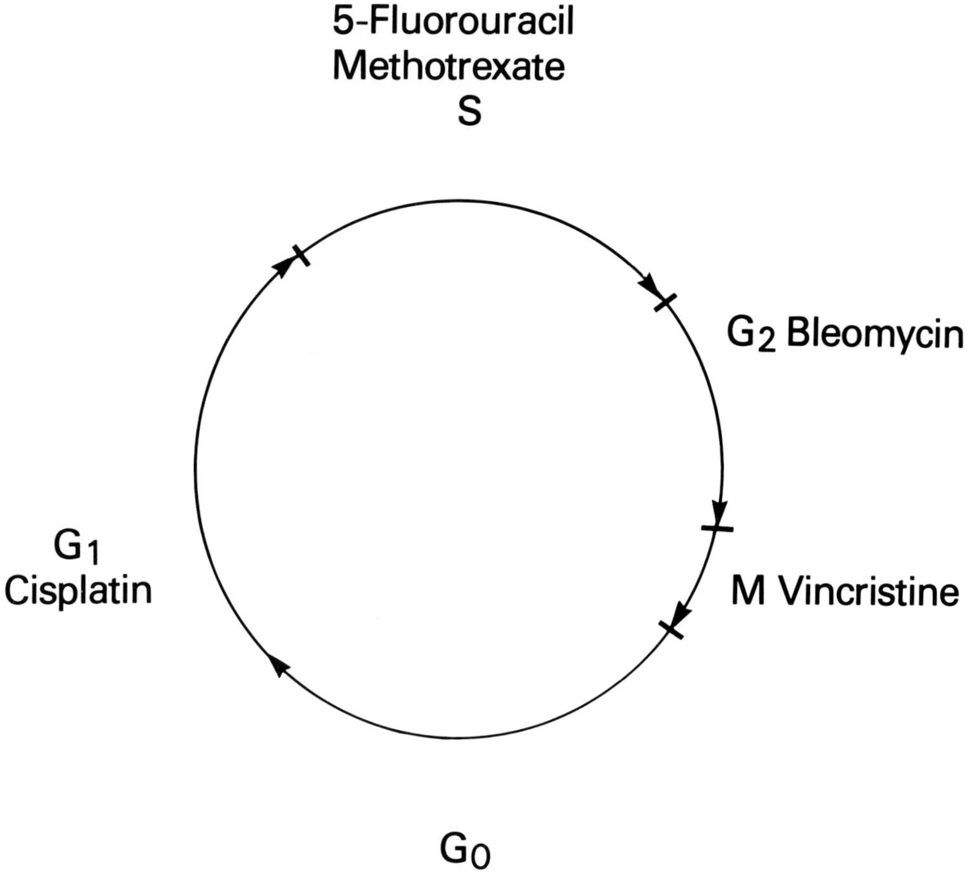

G_0	Long-term quiescent phase
G_1	Nondividing, postmitotic, metabolic (RNA & protein synthesis), preDNA synthesis
S	DNA synthesis phase
G_2	Postsynthetic, premitotic phase
M	Mitosis

Figure 8-4. The cell cycle. This is a schematic representation of DNA/RNA synthesis and mitosis. Note that the various chemotherapeutic agents are effective at specific sites in this dynamic process.

intestinal perforation, severe leukopenia, thrombocytopenia, hepatic fibrosis, renal tubular necrosis, third-space accumulation (and resultant prolongation of toxicity), pneumonitis, and alopecia.

Avoidance of Toxicity

Toxicity is prevented by adequate hydration, urine alkalinization for high-dose methotrexate (intravenous or oral bicarbonate, acetazolamide), leucovorin rescue for moderate- to high-dose methotrexate, drainage of third-space fluid collections (pleural effusions, ascites), and withholding therapy in patients with renal insufficiency.

Bleomycin

Site of Action

Bleomycin is a G_2-phase specific drug that causes DNA breakage in susceptible malignant cells. It also has effects in late G_1, early S, and M phases.

Dosage

The drug is administered usually in combination with other cytotoxic agents at doses of 1 to 15 units/m^2 IV weekly. Prior to administering the full dose, a test dose of 1 unit is given and the patient observed for hypotension. A maximum total dose of 400 units is given safely.

Toxicity

These include pulmonary fibrosis (insidious dyspnea, rales, basilar fibrosis, reduced diffusion capacity of carbon monoxide), alopecia, hyperpigmentation, erythroderma, desquamation of hands and feet, postinjection fever and chills, cardiopulmonary arrest, and stomatitis.

Avoidance of Toxicity

Toxicity is diminished by withholding the drug in patients over the age of 70 or in patients who have pulmonary disease, previous chest radiation, or renal insufficiency. A 40-percent drop in the predicted carbon monoxide diffusion capacity necessitates drug discontinuation. Patients treated with this drug should receive minimal FIO_2 (30%) during anesthesia to prevent progressive, life-threatening pulmonary fibrosis and pneumonitis.

5-Fluorouracil

Site of Action

5-Fluorouracil (5-FU), S-phase specific, inhibits thymidylate synthetase and the formation of deoxythymidine triphosphate (DNA). 5-FU also forms a ribose-triphosphate (5-FUTP), producing fraudulent RNA.

Dosage

Weekly bolus doses of 600 mg/m^2 IV are administered. A dosage of 1000 mg/m^2 continuously over 24 hours for 5 consecutive days (repeated every 3–4 weeks) theoretically is more effective and has fewer life-threatening toxicities.

Toxicity

The toxicities depend on the mode of delivery: myelosuppression (leukopenia and thrombocytopenia) and mucositis from bolus administration; mucositis, diarrhea, and gastrointestinal ulceration by continuous intravenous infusion. The general toxicities are nausea and vomiting, alopecia, dermatitis, hyperpigmentation, and cerebellar ataxia (high doses).

Avoidance of Toxicity

Myelosuppression is diminished with daily coadministration of allopurinol (300 mg PO). Good oral hygiene and gargling with 1 teaspoon of baking soda in 8 ounces of warm water frequently reduces the incidence and relieves impending mucositis. One part hydrogen peroxide to 2 parts water is also a good gargle.

Cisplatin (Cis-diamminedichloroplatinum)

Site of Action

Cisplatin cross-links DNA by formation of covalent bonds. It is nonspecific in its actions on the cell cycle although G_1 is most sensitive.

Dosage
Doses of 80 to 120 mg/m^2 IV every 3 weeks are given safely.

Toxicity
The main toxicities include renal failure, electrolyte imbalance (hypomagnesemia, hypocalcemia, and hypokalemia), and severe nausea and vomiting. Cisplatin also causes myelosuppression (leukopenia, anemia, and thrombocytopenia), high-frequency ototoxicity (see Chapter 27), and peripheral neuropathy.

Avoidance of Toxicity
Renal toxicity is prevented by osmotic diuresis and drug administration in hypertonic saline. For example, after 2 liters of 5% dextrose in one-half normal saline with 40 mEq/liter of potassium chloride is infused over 12 hours, 12.5 gm of mannitol is administered just prior to cisplatin. The cisplatin is infused in 250 ml of 3% saline over 30 minutes, followed by an additional 25 gm of mannitol in 1 liter of 5% dextrose in one-half normal saline infused over 4 hours.

Antiemesis is accomplished with metoclopramide (Reglan), 2 to 3 mg/kg IV ½ hour prior to and 1½ hours after cisplatin. Additional doses every 2 to 3 hours up to 12 hours after cisplatin control emesis. Diphenhydramine (Benadryl), 50 mg IV, plus dexamethasone (Decadron), 20 mg IV, with the first dose of metoclopramide aids antiemesis and reduces metoclopramide's extrapyramidal toxicity. Patients who cannot tolerate metoclopramide are medicated with droperidol, 7.5–10.0 mg IM, plus diphenhydramine, 50 mg IV, plus dexamethasone, 20 mg IV, 30 minutes prior to cisplatin. The droperidol (Inapsine) is repeated 4 hours and the diphenhydramine 6 hours after cisplatin. Prochloperazine (Compazine), 10 mg PO or IM every 4 to 6 hours, is an acceptable antiemetic for the other described agents.

These patients are at risk from nutritional hypomagnesemia as well as cisplatin-associated depletion. Monitoring serum magnesium levels prior to cisplatin with appropriate supplementation with magnesium sulfate, 1 gm IM in each buttock, avoids complications. Additional supplementation is accomplished with oral magnesium oxide.

Vincristine

Site of Action
Vincristine binds tubulin, causing depolymerization and reduced formation of the microtubular apparatus of the mitotic spindle. The drug is mitosis phase specific.

Dosage
Doses of 1–2 mg/m^2 (maximum dose of 2 mg) are given weekly.

Toxicity
The major toxicity is dose-related peripheral neuropathy manifesting as reduced deep tendon reflexes, extremity paresthesias, cranial nerve palsies, constipation, and weakness of foot dorsiflexors and wrist extensors. The drug also causes alopecia, rarely leukopenia, and soft-tissue necrosis (intravenous extravasation). Some patients develop inappropriate antidiuretic hormone syndrome.

Avoidance of Toxicity
Neurologic toxicity is alleviated by dosage reduction or omission. Patients with pretreatment neurologic problems, such as alcoholic or diabetic neuropathies, are at increased risk of neurotoxicity. The addition of cathartics reduces constipation.

Combination Therapy
In general, combination chemotherapy works best in previously untreated patients. These candidates have a high complete response rate and minimal toxicity [6]. However, in previously treated patients, the overall response rate is low, 25 to 35 percent, and toxicity increases markedly. For these patients, combination chemotherapy offers no advantage over weekly, single-agent methotraxate for palliation. Figure 8-5 illustrates the decisions made in these patients.

1. Cisplatin (100 mg/m^2) IV on day 1 followed by 5-FU (1000 mg/m^2 per day) continuously

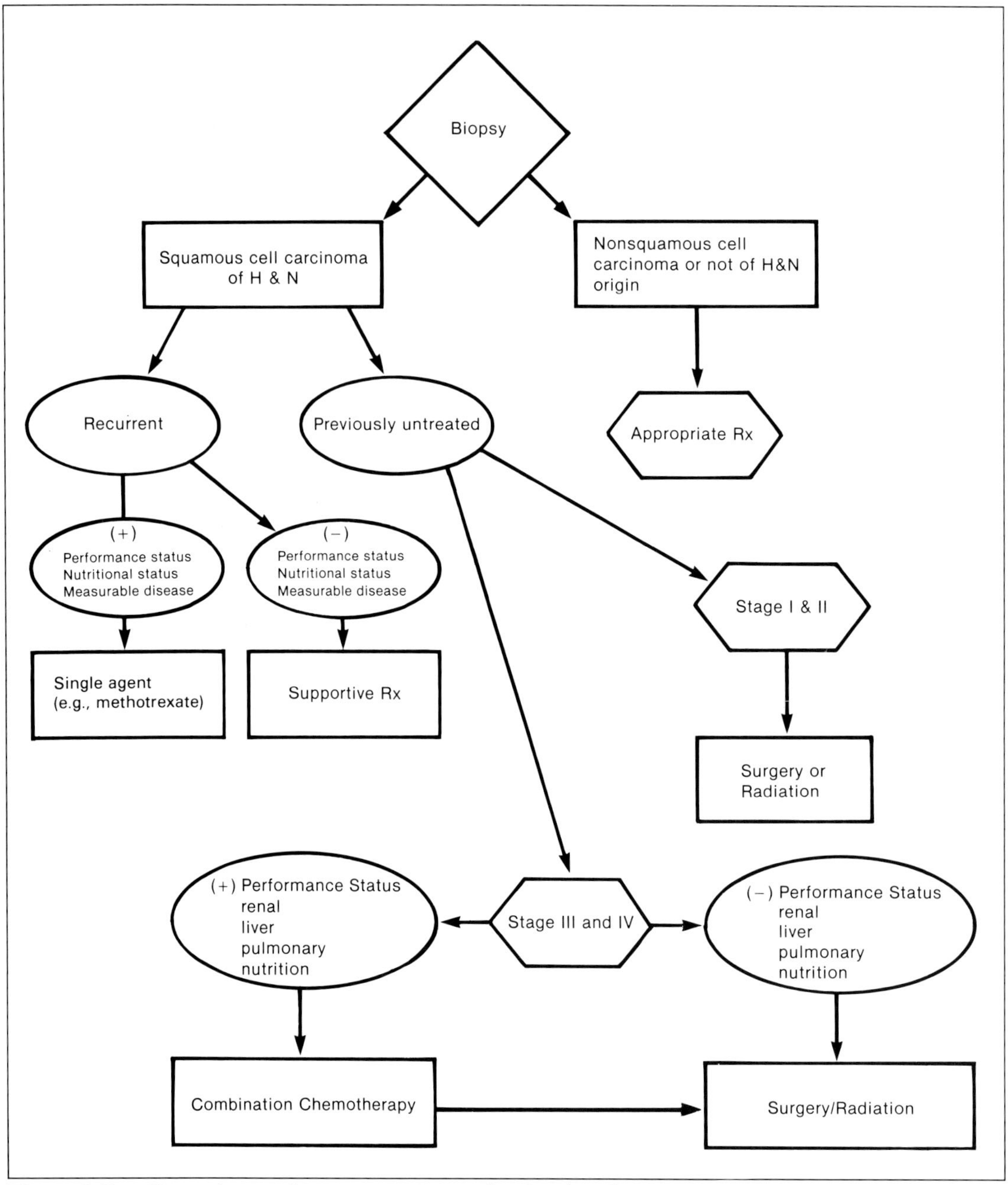

Figure 8-5. Chemotherapy dynamics. *H & N* = head and neck.

by infusion for 5 consecutive days is one regimen that is repeated every 3 weeks. Several studies have reported an 83- to 93-percent total response rate and a 20- to 54-percent complete response rate in previously untreated patients [17–19].

2. Methotrexate (40 mg/m^2) IV on days 1 and 15, bleomycin (10 units) IV on days 1, 7, and 15, and cisplatin (50 mg/m^2) IV on day 3 is repeated every 3 weeks. This regimen has an estimated 70-percent total response rate and a 20-percent complete response rate as primary therapy [19].
3. The following regimen is repeated every 2 weeks: methotrexate (200 mg/m^2) IV over 1 hour followed in 2 hours by 5-FU (600

mg/m^2) IV over 2 hours; and 24 hours from the start of therapy, leucovorin (10 mg/m^2) IV every 6 hours for 6 doses. The objective response rate is 70 percent with a complete response rate of 19 percent in previously untreated patients [20]. However, controlled, randomized trials comparing sequential methotrexate followed by 5-FU with the reverse sequence (5-FU, methotrexate) fail to demonstrate an advantage in response rate or survival for patients receiving the methotrexate followed by 5-FU [22–24]. These trials demonstrate greater myelosuppression and gastrointestinal toxicity with the methotrexate followed by 5-FU. In an animal model, when a nontoxic dose of 5-FU is followed by methotrexate, the toxicities associated with methotrexate (myelosuppression and gastrointestinal disturbances) are virtually eliminated [24, 25]. This alternative approach may show promise in patients when after a priming dose of 5-FU, escalating doses of methotrexate are administered without toxicity but significant antineoplastic activity is retained.

4. Cisplatin (80 mg/m^2) IV on day 1 over 24 hours, vincristine (1 mg/m^2) IV on day 3, and bleomycin (15 units/day) is given by continuous infusion for 4 days. This regimen has a total response rate of 67 percent and a complete response rate of 5 percent as primary therapy [26].

Finally, randomized controlled trials of induction chemotherapy followed by local therapy (surgery and/or radiation) versus local therapy alone fail to demonstrate better survival with the addition of induction chemotherapy over local therapy alone [27, 28]. Presently, induction chemotherapy for advanced head and neck cancer remains experimental.

REFERENCES

1. Silverberg E, Boring CC, Squires TS: Cancer Statistics, 1990. *CA* 40 : 9–26, 1990.
2. Decker J, Goldstein JC: Current concepts in otolaryngology: Risk factors in head and neck cancer. *N Engl J Med* 306 : 1151, 1982.
3. Al-Sarraf M: Head and neck cancer: Chemotherapy concepts. *Semin Oncol* 15 : 70, 1988.
4. Spaulding M, et al: Induction therapy in head and neck cancer: A comparison of two regimens. *Cancer* 57 : 1110, 1986.
5. Spaulding M: Adjuvant chemotherapy in advanced head and neck tumors. *Laryngoscope* 94 : 476, 1984.
6. Bosl GJ: Adjuvant chemotherapy in the management of stage III and IV tumors of the head and neck. *CA* 33 : 139, 1983.
7. Kempson RL, Hendrickson MR: The Impact of Pathology on Cancer Treatment. In Carter SK, Glatstein G, Livingston RB (eds), *Principles of Cancer Treatment*. New York: McGraw-Hill, 1982. Pp 26–33.
8. Hong WK, Bromer R: Current concepts: Chemotherapy in head and neck cancer. *N Engl J Med* 308 : 75, 1983.
9. Glick JH, Zehngebot LM, Taylor SG: Chemotherapy for squamous cell carcinoma of the head and neck: A progress report. *Am J Otolaryngol* 1 : 306, 1980.
10. Amer MH, Al-Sarraf M, Vaitkevicius V: Factors that affect response to chemotherapy and survival of patients with advanced head and neck cancer. *Cancer* 43 : 2202, 1979.
11. Wolf GT, Makuch RW, Baker SR: Predictive factors for tumor response to preoperative chemotherapy in patients and head and neck squamous carcinoma: The head and neck contracts program. *Cancer* 54 : 2869, 1984
12. Ervin TJ, Clark JR, Weischselbaum RR: Multidisciplinary treatment of advanced squamous carcinoma of the head and neck. *Semin Oncol* 12: 72, 1985.
13. Krakoff IH: Cancer chemotherapeutic agents. *CA* 37 : 93, 1987.
14. Wittes RE: Chemotherapy of head and neck cancer. *Otolaryngol Clin North Am* 13 : 515, 1980.
15. Gussack GS, Brantley BA, Farmer JC: Biology of tumors and head and neck cancer chemotherapy, *Laryngoscope* 94 : 1181, 1984.
16. Kies MS, et al: Analysis of complete responders after initial treatment with chemotherapy in head and neck cancer. *Laryngol Head Neck Surg* 93 : 199, 1985.
17. Rooney M, Kish J, Jacobs J, et al: Improved complete response rate and survival in advanced head and neck cancer after three-course induction therapy with 120-hour 5-FU infusion and cisplatin. *Cancer* 55 : 1123, 1985.
18. Dasmahapatra KS, et al: A prospective evaluation of 5-fluorouracil plus cisplatin in advanced squamous cell cancer of the head and neck. *J Clin Oncol* 3 : 1486, 1985.
19. Kuten A, et al: Multidrug chemotherapy using bleomycin, methotrexate and cisplatin alone or combined with radiotherapy in advanced head and neck cancer. *Cancer Treat Rep* 67 : 573, 1983.
20. Ringborg U, et al: Sequential methotrexate–5-

fluorouracil treatment of squamous cell carcinoma of the head and neck. *Cancer* 52 : 971, 1983.
21. Browman GP, et al: Prospective randomized trial of one-hour sequential versus simultaneous methotrexate plus 5-fluorouracil in advanced and recurrent squamous cell head and neck cancer. *J Clin Oncol* 1 : 787, 1983.
22. Coates AS, et al: Combination therapy with methotrexate and 5-fluorouracil: A prospective randomized clinical trial of order of administration. *J Clin Oncol* 2 : 756, 1984.
23. Browman GP, et al: Methotrexate/fluorouracil scheduling influences normal tissue toxicity but not antitumor effects in patients with squamous cell head and neck cancer: Results from a randomized trial. *J Clin Oncol* 6 : 963, 1988.
24. Robbins TJ, et al: Modulation of high dose methotrexate toxicity by a non-toxic level of 5-fluorouracil. *Toxicology* 41 : 61, 1986.
25. Robbin TJ, Bowen D: Toxicity, pathological effects and antineoplastic activity of a non-toxic dose of 5-fluorouracil in combination with methotrexate. *Anticancer Res* 8 : 43, 1988.
26. Amrein PC, Fingest H, Weitzman SA: Cisplatin-vincristine-bleomycin therapy in squamous cell carcinoma of the head and neck. *J Clin Oncol* 1 : 421, 1983.
27. Tannock IF, Browman G: Lack of evidence for a role of chemotherapy in the routine management of locally advanced head and neck cancer. *J Clin Oncol* 4 : 1121, 1986.
28. Taylor SG: Editorial: Why has so much chemotherapy done so little in head and neck cancer? *J Clin Oncol* 5 : 1, 1987.

9

Radiotherapy

EBRAHIM ASHAYERI AND JoANN COLLIER-MANNING

KEY CONCEPTS

Radiation Biology; Preoperative Radiation; Postoperative Radiation; Intraoperative Radiation; New Horizons

MILESTONES

2000 B.C.	Hyperthermia	Ramagana
1896	X-Rays	Roentgen
	Pharyngeal Cancer Irradiation	Wright
1898	Radium	Curies
1899	Basal Cell (Nose) Irradiation	Sjögren
1902	Laryngeal Cancer Irradiation	Scheppegie
	Pastille Radiometer	Holznecht
1903	Radium for Head and Neck Cancer	Abbé
1908	Radium Applicators	Dominic
1919	Fractionation	Contald
1927	Dosimetry	Mackee
1933	Elective Neck Irradiation (Cancer of the Lip)	Widmann
1952	Oxygen Effect	Read
1956	Mammalian Radiation Biology	Pack, Marcus
1976	Intraoperative Irradiation (Howard University Hospital)	Henschke, Goldson

After the discovery of x-rays and radioactive substances, a variety of benign and malignant conditions were treated utilizing radiation. At first, radiotherapy was utilized empirically with little or minimal understanding of its effects or efficacy [1]. With the exception of cancers of the cervix and the upper aerodigestive system, only unresectable tumors were referred for irradiation in the 1920s and 1930s. Inoperable tumors such as advanced primary tumors of the breast, parotid, and rectum and soft-tissue sarcomas were treated with radiotherapy. The energy and doses were low (200 kV) and often did not produce significant regression. Therefore, many tumors were misclassified as radioresistant [2]. In its infancy, there was no dependable method of tissue dosimetry available, and the basics of radiation biology and dose-time relationships were not understood. It was only after 1952 [3] and 1956 [4] that the two most important factors determining curability were described: the percentage of hypoxic malignant cells and the number of clonogenic cells.

RADIATION BIOLOGY

Radiation biology, the basis of clinical radiotherapy, is the quantitative and qualitative effects of radiation upon cell death, repair, and replication in normal and neoplastic tissue. Radiation produces nonviable cells. A çell is considered nonviable if mitosis is arrested and it loses its proliferative capacity. A nonviable cell may exist for a prolonged period and may even go through several division cycles before lysis. Rapidly dividing cells lyse more readily after irradiation when compared to slowly dividing cells. Ultimately, cell death is dependent on radiation dose and duration [4].

Dose-Response Curves

Slope

Cell death following irradiation is an exponential function of dose: a specified dose kills a constant irradiated cell fraction [4]. A typical dose-response curve plots the log of cell survival against radiation dosage (Figure 9-1). The slope of the curve varies with cell radiosensitivity, environment, radiation type, method of administration, and the biologic state of the cells [5,6]. The curve has a characteristic "shoulder" followed by a straight line. The more resistant the cells, the broader the shoulder and the less steep the slope.

Figure 9-1. Dose-response curve.

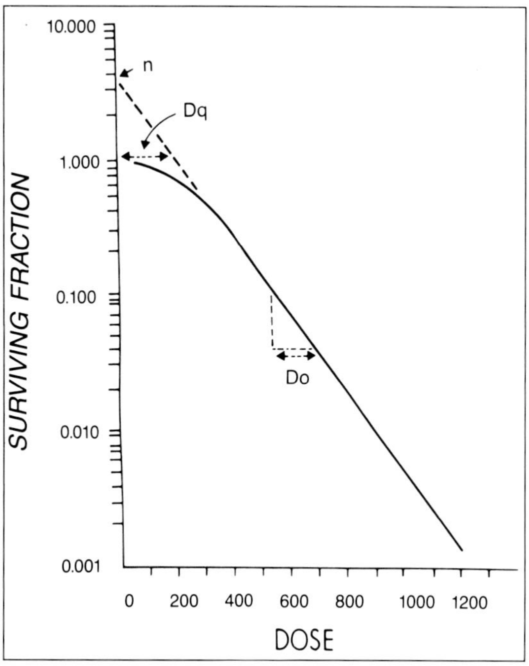

Shoulder

The shoulder represents accumulated cellular damage and subsequent repair (Elkind recovery).

A popular theory of radiation effect is the multiple-target model. Cells contain critical structures or targets that are essential for reproduction. These targets generally are accepted as DNA molecules within genes. Radiation-induced damage to a DNA molecule (target) may trigger a sequence of serious cellular changes. However, singular DNA damage is repaired rapidly. In mammalian cells, multiple targets must be hit almost simultaneously to affect reproduction. This contrasts with bacteria or haploid cells that require only one hit. In short, the shoulder of the mammalian cell dose-response curve is a graphic demonstration of sublethal and reparable damage to critical targets.

The number of critical targets in the cell dictates the shape of the shoulder. If the slope is extrapolated to the point of intersection with the ordinate (Figure 9-1), the length of the ordinate between the 100-percent survival point and the intersection is called the extrapolation number (n). This is the average number of critical targets in each cell. Physiologic conditions of the cell, oxygenation, phase of mitotic cell cycle, and other unknown factors alter the n.

Q-Factor

Irradiation of multiple cells in contact demonstrate a larger n than the same cells irradiated singly. Alper [7] has discussed the limitation of the repair process or presence of a material (Q-factor) that is depleted in the process of repair. Diffusion of such a factor from one cell to an adjacent cell might explain the above discrepancy. According to the cell survival curve, larger tumor cell volume requires higher radiation doses for eradication, which may lead to the assumption that a certain minimal number of cells is essential for tumor viability. The curve demonstrates that most mammalian cells are capable of recovering from a substantial radiation-induced injury in a few hours.

Oxygen Effect

Oxygen Enhancement Ratio

The oxygen effect on irradiated cells was observed as early as 1921 and was first described quantitatively in vegetable seeds by Gray and Read in 1952 [3]. Mammalian cells under hypoxic and aerated conditions result in similar survival curves (Figure 9-2). Under hypoxic conditions, the radiation dose for sparsely ionizing radiations (x-ray and gamma rays) produces similar biologic effects that are three times that of oxygenated conditions. The dose ratio (hypoxic versus oxygenated condition) resulting in the same biologic effect is called the oxygen enhancement ratio (OER). This is the same for all survival levels. For densely ionizing radiation (alpha particles), oxygen has no effect on the survival curve. The OER is 1.0, and the shoulder is absent in the survival curve. Neutron beams (intermediate ionizing radiation) has an OER of approximately 1.6 (Figure 9-2).

Concentration

Theoretically, oxygen must be present for radiation absorption in tissues. Delays longer than a few milliseconds neutralize the oxygen effect. The dose-modifying effect of oxygen depends on its concentration in tissue. Most sensitization occurs as oxygen concentration increases from 0 to 300 mm Hg, and it plateaus when the oxygen concentration characteristic of air is attained. Therefore, concentrations approaching pure oxygen have little effect (Figure 9-3) [5–7].

Dose Versus Volume

Large Tumors

An exponential relationship exists between dose and the surviving fraction. Large tumors have other associated variables such as increased vascularity, inflammation, necrosis, hypoxia, intercellular contact, and growth that decrease

Figure 9-2. Survival cure. *OER* = oxygen enhancement ratio.

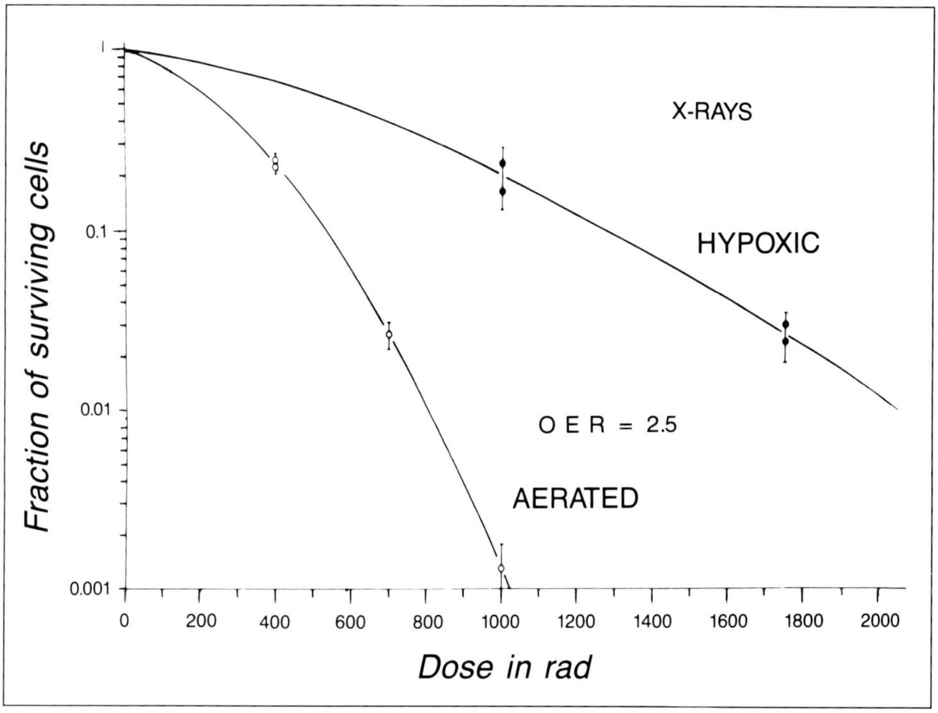

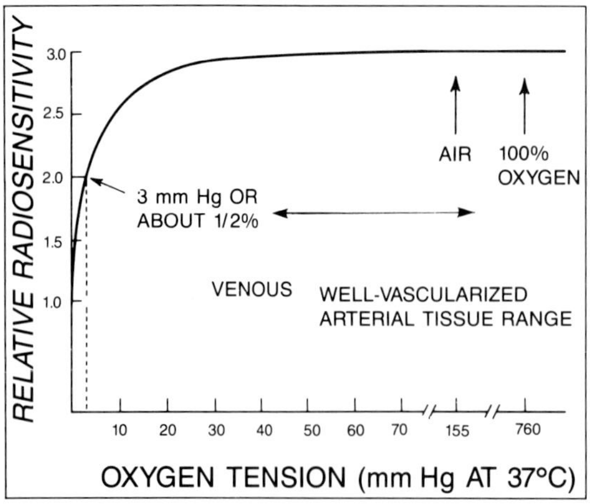

Figure 9-3. Oxygen effect.

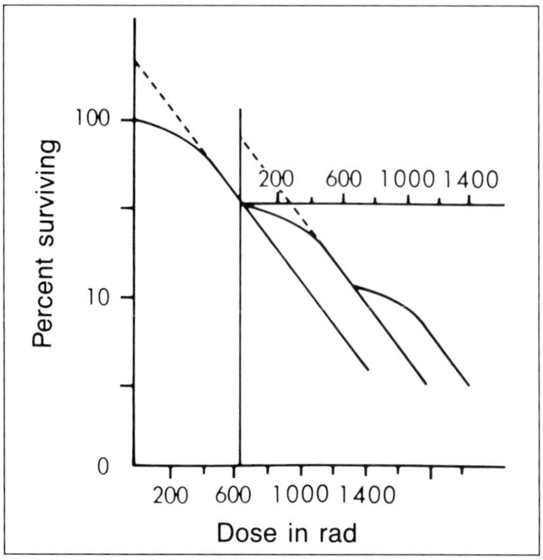

Figure 9-4. Fractionation.

sensitivity. Thus, higher doses are required for large tumor eradication.

Tolerance

As the irradiated volume increases, even with fractionation, tolerance decreases. This is the greatest limitation of radiotherapy for the treatment of cancers. Without the limitation of normal tissue tolerance, all cancers potentially are curable by radiation.

Fractionation

Radiation, delivered in increments or fractions over a period of hours or days, usually, but not always, results in reproduction of the "shoulder" and reduced biologic effects (Figure 9-4). Tissue recovery occurs in less than 24 hours. The dependency of biologic effectiveness on fractionation is called the dose-time relationship. Cell recovery (Elkind recovery) between increments is responsible for this reduced effect [1].

Cells exposed to fractionated irradiation grow, but more slowly. Despite reduced efficiency, superior treatment results are achieved with fractionation. This occurs theoretically, because of different recovery rates between different cell types. In vivo and in vitro studies show no survival curve differences between cancerous and normal cells. However, there is a difference in normal tissue regeneration and the rate of radiation-induced changes. Radiation-induced cell death initiates a "homeostatic stimulus" that triggers a feedback mechanism to activate reparation. Malignant cells usually are less sensitive to this stimulus. Fractionation permits reparation of all cells and, to a lesser extent, cancer cells. Associated with tumor shrinkage during fractionation is the reoxygenation of remaining cells. Fractionation has the following advantages (Table 9-1):

1. Any tumor with radius greater than 200 μ contains a necrotic center. Regardless of the size of the necrotic center, the viable tumor cell thickness essentially remains constant at 100 to 180 μ. After initial fractionation, well-oxygenated cells are killed with a reduction in absolute number of cells. If the available oxygen remains unchanged, the oxygen concentration per remaining cells increases and results in a reduction of hypoxic cells. Previously compressed blood vessels secondary to tumor growth are decompressed, thus improving the oxygenation of the remaining tumor. Vascular damage secondary to irradiation changes capillary permeability, blood flow, local thrombosis, hemorrhage, and eventually vascular occlusion. These critical radiation changes are enhanced by fractionation.

Table 9-1. The efficacy of fractionation

Four "R"s of radiation therapy	
Repair (intracellular)	Elkind recovery from substantial radiation injury occurs within the first 24 hours. There is no systemic difference in the survival curves of cancer cells and normal cells.
Repopulation	Through regeneration of the stem cells, there is a resumption of mitosis between fractions. There is little or no homeostatic stimulation of tumor regrowth following radiation-induced cell killing.
Reoxygenation	Hypoxic cells irradiated by sparsely ionizing radiations require three times higher doses than aerated cells (OER). After each fraction, cells in well-oxygenated layers of the tumor are killed and cleared from the area. The tumor shrinks and results in a relative increase in vascularity and decrease in hypoxic cells. This repeats with each fraction.
Radiation synchrony (redistribution)	The cells in the most sensitive stage of the cell cycle are killed in large numbers, producing a viable population with a synchronous cell cycle.

2. Because of differential recovery rates between normal and neoplastic tissues, epidermis and bowel mucosa recover much more rapidly than the squamous cell carcinoma and adenocarcinoma respectively. This difference is exploited by fractionation.
3. Correction of hemorrhage, infection, and nutrition during fractionation improves the patient's tolerance throughout the remaining treatment course.
4. A high single fraction, although effective, is uncomfortable, dangerous, and even fatal.

COMBINED TREATMENT

Cancer control depends on tumor size, local extension, and treatment. Due to the limitations of both surgery and radiotherapy, the need for combined therapy is clear (see Chapter 7). Subclinical cancer foci are eradicated readily by irradiation, whereas bulky tumors are less susceptible to irradiation. However, residual subclinical malignant cells after massive surgical resections may result in local failure. The basic assumption is that combined treatment should increase local-regional control [8–12].

The following combinations commonly are used for surgery and irradiation in the same anatomic site (Table 9-2):

1. Preoperative radiotherapy.
2. Postoperative radiotherapy.
3. Sandwich technique.

Preoperative Radiotherapy

While preoperative irradiation must encompass the undetected, finger-like tumor extensions, transected tumor or positive surgical margins are less than adequate surgery. Preoperative radiotherapy is contraindicated for unresectable or metastatic disease.

Postoperative Radiotherapy

When the tumor boundaries are unclear preoperatively, surgery may spill cells and leave residual disease. Transected tumors or positive surgical margins are less than adequate surgery.

Goals

1. Ablation: sterilization of gross residual cancer.
2. Prophylaxis: attenuation of spilled cells.
3. Reduction: decreased tumor burden, requiring smaller radiation dose.
4. Precision: accurate evaluation of tumor boundaries.

Dose

In the presence of gross residual disease, higher cancercidal doses dictated by cell type and volume are required, along with the expected inherited risks. However, for suspected micro-

Table 9-2. Combined treatment

Regimen	*Advantages*	*Disadvantages*	*Timing*	*Treatment*
Preoperative radiotherapy	1. Increased resectability 2. Decreased tumor seeding 3. Decreased iatrogenic metastases	1. Surgery delay 2. Occult distant metastasis 3. Patient refusal for further treatment 4. Compromised surgical margins	Surgery is recommended 3–6 weeks post-therapy	4500–5500 cGy in 4½–5½ weeks
Postoperative radiotherapy	1. Ablation of gross residual disease 2. Prophylaxis following close surgical margins 3. Decreased tumor burden 4. Accurate tumor location	1. Disturbed margins, vascularity, and lymphatics 2. Higher treatment volume 3. Increased susceptibility to radiation damage	Allowance for complete wound healing, but no greater than 3 months following surgery	5000–5500 cGy in 5–5½ weeks

scopic disease, doses in the range of 5000 to 5500 cGy in 5 to 5½ weeks are recommended.

Timing

For postoperative irradiation, complete wound healing must be achieved; delayed healing or wound dehiscence complicates treatment. However, prolonged intervals of more than 3 months between surgery and irradiation can result in increased local recurrence.

Disadvantages

1. Disturbed tumor boundaries, anatomy, and blood flow require higher irradiation doses.
2. A larger treatment volume must encompass the entire surgical field to include possible spilled cancer cells.
3. Postoperative connective tissue is more susceptible to radiation damage.
4. Usually cancers treated by surgery are less radiosensitive and require very high doses of radiation.
5. Advanced disease is more common in patients referred for postoperative irradiation.

A review of these observations and assumptions should not discourage administration of postoperative radiotherapy. Its curative benefits have been proved repeatedly in the treatment of cancers of the skin, head and neck, breast, pelvic organs, testicle, Wilms' tumors, and gastric lymphomas.

Sandwich Technique

The delivery of preoperative irradiation to a larger volume supplemented by postoperative treatment to a smaller field (boost) is called sandwich technique. This is justified for persistent post-surgical disease.

NASOPHARYNX (Site 1)

Nasopharyngeal cancer has a predilection for southern Chinese inside and outside China. The close association of herpesvirus, Epstein-Barr virus (EBV), and nasopharyngeal carcinoma, independent of geography, has created much interest in the relationship of viruses and malignancy [12,13]. The treatment of choice is irradiation; therefore the radiotherapist assumes the primary management of this disease. Treatment prognosis and survival are dependent on stage, histopathology, and the quality of radiation (see Chapters 4, 5 and 6).

Patterns of Spread

Treatment strategy and portals are dictated by primary location, local spread, and regional metastasis. Local extension to surrounding structures is present in most cases on initial presentation. The most common contiguous sites are the oropharynx, skull base, tonsil, and cranial nerves [14]. Ninety percent of the patients have lymph node metastasis with a very high incidence of bilateral, posterior cervical and supraclavicular involvement [15,16].

Treatment

Approach

Despite the high incidence of contiguous spread, the nasopharynx is a silent area with few symptoms (see Chapter 2). Local recurrence, without neck node or distant metastases, varies from 20 to 35 percent [17,18] to 64 to 74 percent [16,19].

Planning

Due to the cryptic nature of nasopharyngeal carcinoma, a generous treatment volume is necessary [17,20–23]. The portals encompass the skull base, suprasellar area, anterior occipital bone, posterior nasal cavity, orbit, maxillary sinus, tonsillar fossa, and the retropharyngeal and posterior cervical nodes. Bilaterally, the deep cervical nodes, anterior and posterior, must be treated. For clinically negative necks, 5000 to 5500 cGy is adequate. However, for clinically positive necks, the dose is increased to 6000 cGy, using electron or photon beams (anteroposterior ports with spinal cord blocking). Residual disease is boosted with 1000 to 2000 cGy to the primary site only [24].

Doses 6500 to 7000 cGy over 6½ to 8 weeks are required for adequate treatment. Larger primary lesions may require higher doses and volumes. To avoid prohibitive brain stem, skull base, and hypothalamic complications, higher doses are given with intracavitary irradiation or interstitial implants.

Technique

Refined treatment—external beam, intracavitary, and interstitial irradiation—has resulted in a remarkable decrease of potential complications while increasing local and regional control. Treatment volume is based on physical examination (including a complete neurologic examination), nasopharyngoscopy, and most importantly computed tomography (CT) or magnetic resonance imaging (MRI) scans. Inactive tumor markers enhance dosage accuracy [14,23].

Three-field (two lateral opposing and single anterior) and four-field (two lateral opposing and two anterior facial fields) techniques are used. For most cases, the three-field technique is adequate, especially in advanced disease with anterior extension.

Recurrence

More than half the patients die from local recurrence without neck nodes or distant metastases. The interval between initial treatment and recurrence varies from 2 years (squamous cell carcinoma) to more than 5 years (lymphoepitheliomas). The diagnosis of recurrent disease is difficult and relies on a high index of suspicion. Persistent headache and cranioneuropathies are the most common complaints of recurrent disease. Five-year survival rates of 41 percent, and 10-year survival rates of 25 percent have been reported [25].

Complications

Hypopituitarism, hypothyroidism, transient central nervous system syndrome, radiation myelitis, trismus, ninth through twelfth cranial nerve palsy, optic neuritis, radiation retinopathy, and brain necrosis are documented. Caution must be exercised to differentiate between recurrences versus radiation complications.

Results

Although recent protocols from the People's Republic of China are more encouraging, the overall 5-year survival rate for treated nasopharyngeal carcinoma averages 30 percent for squamous cell carcinoma, 43 percent for lymphoepithelioma, and 57 percent for lymphoma. A 5-year survival rate of 55 percent in patients with N_0 disease deteriorates to 40 percent in N_1 or N_2 disease and 23 percent in N_3. Skull base and cranial nerve involvement (I–VI) have a 24-percent 5-year survival rate.

PARANASAL SINUSES (Site 2)

Most paranasal sinus carcinomas are advanced locally when first diagnosed, yet up to 30 percent of the patients are cured by a combination of surgery and radiotherapy (see Chapters 4 and 5). Greater than 50 percent of early-stage patients have no evidence of disease (NED) at 3 years [26]. With the exception of T_1 lesions involving the mucosa (treated by surgery alone), radiotherapy is given preoperatively or postoperatively for cure or alone for palliation.

Pattern of Spread

The extent of the tumor and the particular sinus are the main considerations for treatment planning. Many tumors are resectable with acceptable functional results (see Chapter 13). Radiation therapy (preoperatively or postoperatively), even in the presence of negative margins, is recommended.

Treatment

Technique

Preoperative Therapy

Fletcher [27] recommends preoperative radiation for younger patients in reasonably good health and postoperative radiation for most patients, especially those over 70 years of age, in negative nitrogen balance, or with a history of recent weight loss (Table 9-3).

Postoperative Therapy

Most radiotherapists recommend postoperative radiotherapy 4 weeks after surgery, despite negative pathologic margins. The dose ranges from 5000 cGy in 5 weeks to 6000 cGy in 6 weeks. Because these lesions tend to spread submucosally to other sinuses, all ipsilateral paranasal sinuses are included in the treatment field.

Neck Disease

The neck is irradiated after neck dissection for positive disease (see Chapters 3 and 16). Lymph node metastasis occurs in 20 percent of overall cases, although the higher the T category, the greater the risk [26]. Because of this relatively low risk of involvement, Wang [26] does not recommend elective neck irradiation or routine neck dissection for negative necks. Fletcher [27], however, recommends elective neck irradiation of at least the upper neck nodes in T_3 and T_4 lesions. The submandibular, subdigastric, and upper posterior cervical triangle lymph nodes (levels I and II) can be involved with maxillary and ethmoid sinus malignancies.

Massive or Inoperable Disease

Massive disease involving the orbit is best treated by exenteration. However, disease that has spread to the nasopharynx, skull base, pterygoid fossa, or distant sites is unresectable and is treated palliatively to 6000 cGy [28].

For some inoperable lesions, radiation reduces the tumor for possible resection. A dose of 6000 cGy in 6 weeks is given, followed by a postoperative boost for residual disease. The delay between radiation and surgery is 1 week for every 1000 cGy delivered.

Recurrence

Physical examination, a careful history, and baseline CT or MRI scans are critical for detect-

Table 9-3. Radiotherapy of the paranasal sinuses (site 2)*

Subsite	*Technique*
Maxillary sinus	Postoperative radiotherapy including maxilla, nasal cavity, ethmoid sinuses, nasopharynx, pterygopalatine fossa ± orbit: 1. Anterior field ± one or two lateral fields (electron beam to frontal lobes) 2. Eye shield with 5-degree tilt of anterior portal 3. Opposing lateral fields with wedges, 5- to 10-degree tilt posteriorly
Ethmoid sinus	1. 6500–7500 cGy, 6½–7½ weeks with cone down field after 6000 2. Preoperative or full-course radiotherapy preferred 3. Postoperative radiotherapy if feasible: a. Field similar to those of maxillary sinuses b. Extension of superior field 1–3 cm above the base of the skull

*For frontal and sphenoid sinuses, see Ethmoid Sinus.

ing recurrence. Aggressive treatment with second-line treatment may save some patients.

Complications

The early complications include nasal synechiae, conjunctivitis, sinusitis, and xerophthalmia. The late complications are otitis media, decrease or loss of vision, cataracts, osteoradionecrosis, and rarely Lhermitte's sign. Eye complications are the most frequent and devastating complications [28].

Results

The Massachusetts General Hospital reviewed 100 cases of paranasal sinus carcinoma from 1960 to 1978. Sixty-seven patients had maxillary sinus disease, 29 ethmoid, and 4 sphenoid and frontal. Of the maxillary sinus patients, 51 percent received full-course radiation and 41 percent pre- or postoperative therapy. The total overall NED at 3 years was 36 percent: preoperative radiotherapy, 58 percent, and postoperative radiation, 36 percent. Those treated with radiotherapy only, including inoperable cases, had 24-percent NED survival. In terms of T and N stage, T_2 lesions had a 67-percent 3-year NED survival; T_3, 39 percent; and T_4, N_1, or N_2, 0 percent [26]. Lewis and Castro [29] reported on 87 cases of squamous cell carcinoma of the paranasal sinuses. The 3-year survival rate was 30 percent, including 24 patients treated either palliatively or not receiving any therapy at all. The 3-year survival rate in patients treated curatively was 44 percent. Infrastructural maxillary lesions had a 68-percent 3-year survival rate compared to a 29-percent suprastructural survival. Bush and Bagshaw [30] reported results of 38 patients treated at Stanford from 1956 to 1974. Relapse-free survival was 37 percent and absolute survival was 32 percent at 5 years.

SALIVARY GLANDS (Site 3)

The major salivary glands (parotid, submandibular, and sublingual glands) account for 3 to 4 percent of all head and neck tumors (see Chapters 3 through 5).

Treatment

Guidelines

Surgery is the treatment of choice. Low- to moderate-grade malignancies that are excised adequately generally do not require radiotherapy. Postoperative radiotherapy is recommended, however, for close or positive margins, capsular rupture, or recurrent tumors.

Adenoid Cystic Carcinoma

Adenoid cystic tumors are treated aggressively with postoperative radiotherapy, including the perineural pathways and the ipsilateral neck. Preoperative radiotherapy is given to borderline resectable or unresectable lesions.

High-Grade Neoplasms

High-grade neoplasms are given postoperative ratiotherapy to reduce recurrences significantly. Preoperative radiotherapy is given to questionably unresectable tumors. Definitive external beam radiotherapy and brachytherapy are used for unresectable tumors.

Technique

External Beam

The minimum treatment volume includes the tumor bed and regional nodes. In the presence of perineural involvement, the fields also include the neural pathways. The entire neck is irradiated electively for high-grade lesions or for clinically positive nodes in the neck dissection specimen. Microscopic disease requires 5000 to 6000 cGy in 5 to 6 weeks. For gross residual disease or positive margins, higher doses are given. There is no difference in required dose for the various histologies [31,32].

Brachytherapy

Interstitial implants may be used postoperatively for positive margins or in conjunction with external beam radiotherapy.

Recurrence

Recurrences are treated usually by secondary surgery followed by radiation.

Complications
Xerostomia is reduced by sparring the contralateral salivary glands. Trismus, serous otitis media, and localized hair loss are possibilities. Mandibular osteoradionecrosis is rare.

Results
Numerous studies have reported their survival data. The survival is affected by stage, histology, and extent of residual disease after parotidectomy. Thus, depending on the particulars, the reported results vary significantly.

LIP (Site 4)

Squamous cell carcinomas of the lip usually arise on the lower lip and infiltrate the orbicularis early (see Chapters 4 and 5) [33]. Advanced lesions involve the commissures, buccal mucosa, skin of the lip, mandible, and mental nerve. The lower lip drains to the submental, submaxillary, and subdigastric nodes. The upper lip drains to the submaxillary, preauricular, and parotid nodes. Only 5 to 10 percent of the patients present initially with positive necks at diagnosis. However, lymph node involvement is higher (19%) with commissure lesions [34].

Treatment

Guidelines
Early Lesions
Early lesions (0.5–1.5 cm) are treated with surgery. Irradiation is selected for lesions involving the commissure, for lesions greater than 1.5 cm on the lower lip, and for all but the smallest lesions of the upper lip [35].

Moderately Advanced Lesions
Moderately advanced lesions (1.5–5.0 cm) are treated with radiotherapy to preserve function and enhance cosmesis.

Advanced Lesions
Advanced lesions, with bone or nerve invasion, require resection and postoperative irradiation.

Technique
Brachytherapy
Interstitial implants utilize radium, iridium 192, gold, or radon seeds.

External Beam
External beam treatments are given with orthovoltage or electrons over 4 to 6 weeks.

Recurrences
Easily identified, recurrent lip lesions have an increased risk of lymphatic involvement. Therefore, treatment includes the primary site and the neck.

Complications
The late effects of atrophy, telangiectasis, fibrosis, and ulceration are reduced significantly when protracted fractionation is employed [38]. Radiation caries, bone exposure, and osteoradionecrosis are rare and late sequelae of brachytherapy.

Results
McKay and Sellers [36] reviewed 2854 patients with all stages of lip cancer; 92 percent were managed initially by radiation therapy. The primary lesion was controlled in 84 percent of the cases, with an additional 8 percent salvaged by later treatment. They reported a determinate 5-year survival rate of 89 percent and an absolute 5-year survival rate of 65 percent. The M.D. Anderson Hospital reported local control rates for 444 patients. Eighty-three percent initially managed by surgery had 3- and 5-year determinate survival rates of 94 percent [37].

Treatment Guidelines
Irradiation consists of interstitial implants, external beam therapy, or both. Fractionation over 4 to 6 weeks is preferred over shorter regimens to decrease the late effects of atrophy, telangiectasis, fibrosis, and ulceration [38]. The neck is treated for advanced, poorly differentiated, and recurrent lesions.

ORAL CAVITY (Site 5)

Anatomy

The oral cavity, including several subsites, extends from the vermillion border to the hard palate. This area contains the anterior two-thirds of the tongue, buccal mucosa, lower alveolar ridge, upper alveolar ridge, retromolar trigone, floor of the mouth, and hard palate (see Chapter 4).

Pathology

With the exception of verrucous carcinoma, the vast majority of malignant tumors are squamous cell carcinoma and its variants (see Chapter 5). Surgery for verrucous carcinoma is preferable; however, for the remaining lesions, chemotherapy, surgery, and radiotherapy are employed.

Clinical Considerations

The clinical appearance of the tumor is a good predictor of the radioresponsiveness. Well-vascularized exophytic tumors have the best response [41], whereas ulcerative and infiltrative nodular lesions are less responsive [42]. The true extent of an infiltrative lesion is often underestimated.

Results

See Table 9-4 for oral cavity results.

OROPHARYNX (Site 6)

Anatomy

The oropharynx includes several subsites: base of the tongue, tonsils, soft palate, and the posterior and lateral pharyngeal walls (see Chapter 4).

Pathology

The majority of the lesions are of squamous cell origin or one of its variants (see Chapter 5). Lymphoepithelioma occurs in the tonsil and base of the tongue. Lymphomas are reported to occur in this region as well.

Clinical Considerations

See Table 9-5 and Figure 9-5.

Results

See Table 9-5 for oropharynx results.

HYPOPHARYNX (Site 7)

The hypopharynx includes the pharyngeal walls, pyriform sinus, and postcricoid pharynx (see Chapter 4). The majority of lesions originate in the pyriform sinus (see Chapter 5).

Treatment

Technique

Lesions confined to the pyriform sinus with normal mobility (T_1) are controlled locally in 80 percent of the cases by radiation therapy or partial laryngopharyngectomy (Table 9-6) [50–52]. The latter requires careful patient selection (see Chapter 14). More advanced, infiltrative lesions respond poorly to either modality alone. The most radical treatment is total laryngopharyngectomy, neck dissection, unilateral or bilateral, and postoperative radiotherapy.

Field Plan

Due to the tendency for extensive submucosal spread, primary irradiation requires large fields. Bilaterally opposed upper fields to encompass the primary and regional nodes and a single anterior neck field for the lower jugular nodes constitute the standard technique. Appropriately positioned blocks avoid excessive radiation to the spinal cord. Total doses of 6000 to 6500 cGy in 6½ to 7 weeks are recommended for early lesions undergoing definitive radiotherapy.

Postoperative Treatment

Following total laryngopharyngectomy with or without neck dissection, postoperative radiotherapy is recommended for close or positive margins and for multiple or large positive nodes.

Recurrence

The hallmark of local recurrence after radical radiotherapy is persistent edema or poor visualization of the pyriform sinus, odynophagia, and laryngeal fixation. Such suspicious scena-

Table 9-4. Radiotherapy of the oral cavity (site 5)

Subsite	Features	Treatment	Results*	Complications
Anterior tongue	Occurs usually on lateral and undersurfaces Advanced lesions invade floor of mouth, tonsillar pillars, base of tongue, and mandible Subdigastric & submandibular lymph node metastasis 35% occurrence of positive nodes 5% incidence of bilateral nodes	Irradiation is recommended for early tip & dorsal lesions Excisional biopsies with positive margins are treated with interstitial implant (5500–6000 cGy)	Stage I: 90–100% Stage II: 70% Stage III: 35% Stage IV: less than 10%	Xerostomia Dysphagia Mandibular ankylosis Temporomandibular joint syndrome
Floor of mouth	Early involvement of sublingual gland, gingiva, and mandible Frank invasion of the mandible is a late phenomenon 80% present with positive neck nodes; 4% with bilateral disease	Interstitial implant after inadequate excisional biopsies (5000–6500 cGy) Interstitial implant & external therapy for positive margins Surgery for invasive lesions followed by external therapy	Stage I: 75% Stage II: 50% Stage III: 30% Stage IV: 10%	Xerostomia Dysphagia Mandibular ankylosis Temporomandibular joint syndrome
Buccal mucosa	Usually low-grade squamous carcinoma Cervical metastasis 9–31% Frequent site for verrucous carcinoma	Lesions <1 cm are excised Radiotherapy alone for lesions <3 cm Combined therapy for lesions >3 cm	Stage I: 85% Stage II: 50% Stage III: 30% Stage IV: 10%	Xerostomia Dysphagia Mandibular ankylosis Temporomandibular joint syndrome
Hard palate	Most lesions originate on gingiva and spread to hard palate, buccal mucosa, and bone Lymph node metastasis, 13–24%	Surgery is the treatment of choice	Stage I: 70% Stage II: 45% Stage III: 32% Stage IV: 6%	Xerostomia Dysphagia Mandibular ankylosis Temporomandibular joint syndrome
Retromolar trigone	Early spread to adjacent structures Lymph node metastasis, 40%	Radiation therapy is effective in all stages and offers excellent cosmesis Bony invasion may require mandibulectomy	Absolute 5-year survival: 30%	Xerostomia Dysphagia Mandibular ankylosis Temporomandibular joint syndrome

*Radiation initially with surgical salvage.
Source: Adapted from References 39–44.

Table 9-5. Radiotherapy of the oropharynx (site 6)

Subsite	*Features*	*Technique*	*Recurrences*	*Complications*	*Results*
Base of tongue	Frequently asymptomatic & silent Late diagnosis Poor prognosis Bilateral cervical metastasis	Opposing lateral portals to primary and both necks T_1: 6000–6500 cGy in 6½ weeks T_2–T_3: 7500 cGy in 7½ weeks Reduced on shrinking field to protect spinal cord	Usually treated by surgery, i.e., total glossectomy ± total laryngectomy	Tissue necrosis 6–10% Bone necrosis Hemorrhage—uncommon Hypoglossal palsy Dysphagia Trismus	Stage I/II—90% Stage III—45% Stage IV—25%
Tonsil	Usually undifferentiated, exophytic, or ulcerative Posterior tumors to lateral pharynx Anterior tumors to base of tongue 80% have cervical metastases	T_1–T_2: full-course radiation therapy (6000–6500 cGy) T_3: radiation (7000–7500 cGy), but failure rate is 30–50% T_4: combined treatment Opposing lateral portals Dose to spinal cord no greater than 4500 cGy Boosts 1000–1500 cGy with interstitial implants		Tissue necrosis 6–10% Bone necrosis Hemorrhage—uncommon Hypoglossal palsy Dysphagia Trismus	Negative nodes: 70–80% Positive nodes: 40% Local control T_1: 90% $T_2/T_3/T_4$: 50–60%

Source: Adapted from References 45 and 46.

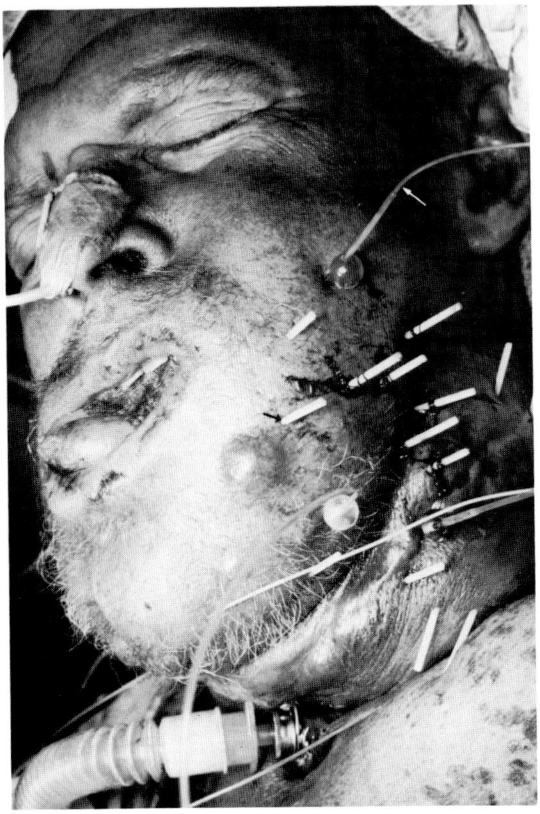

Figure 9-5. Interstitial implantation. This patient with an extensive recurrent cancer has multiple hollow catheters (*black arrow*) inserted for iridium implants (*white arrow*).

rios require direct laryngoscopy and biopsy. However, in the presence of questionable prognosis, salvage surgery may be recommended based on clinical evidence only. In general, salvage results are poor.

LARYNX (Site 8)

Excluding skin cancer, laryngeal cancer is the most common head and neck malignancy (see Chapters 4, 5, and 14). These tumors have little propensity for distant metastases. They affect speech, one of the most important functions in life and the only mode of communication for some patients (see Chapter 26). Therefore, the treatment goal is effective disease ablation while preserving speech and deglutition [53–55].

Treatment

Poor surgical risks and patients who refuse surgery should receive radical irradiation to preserve the voice and for reasonable control of the disease (Table 9-6). Patients with residual and recurrent disease are considered for salvage surgery.

Recurrence

Edema, pain, fixation, and hoarseness are suggestive of recurrent disease or the effects of radical irradiation. Therefore, follow-up must be meticulous and careful. Early laryngoscopy and biopsy are recommended for any patient with new or aggravated old complaints. Salvage after irradiation is total laryngectomy or hemilaryngectomy in carefully selected cases.

Results

Local control correlates directly with the anatomic extent and tumor volume. Recurrence rates generally increase with a greater tumor volume and extension to neighboring anatomic structures. Local control rates for invasive squamous cell carcinomas are in the range of 90 percent for T_1, 70 percent for T_2, and 50 to 60 percent for T_3 and T_4 lesions. The surgical salvage rates for T_1 and T_2 irradiation failures is 90 to 95 percent [54].

THYROID (Site 9)

Carcinomas of the thyroid are rare. The clinical presentation and disease course vary considerably with the particular histology. Therefore, the management of these tumors must be individualized (see Chapters 4, 5, and 15).

Treatment

Surgery

Well-differentiated carcinomas are managed primarily by surgery. They include follicular, papillary, mixed papillary, medullary, and Hürthle cell carcinoma.

Lobectomy and Isthmusectomy

The minimal surgery for a small intraglandular papillary carcinoma or low-grade follicular car-

Table 9-6. Radiotherapy of the hypopharynx and larynx (sites 7 & 8)

Site	*Subsite*	*Features*	*Treatment*	*Complications*
Hypopharynx	Pharyngeal walls Postcricoid pharynx Pyriform sinus	Most lesions are found in the pyriform sinus	T_1 Stage I lesions are controlled locally in 80% of the cases by radiation therapy or partial laryngopharyngectomy Stage III & IV lesions are treated with total laryngopharyngectomy, neck dissections, and postoperative radiotherapy Technique: bilateral opposed upper fields and a single anterior field to the lower neck (6000–6500 cGy in 6½–7 weeks)	Persistent laryngeal edema—usually resolves in one year Laryngeal necrosis, infrequent but potentially fatal
Larynx	Supraglottis Glottis Subglottis	Except for the supraglottic larynx, lesions tend *not* to metastasize	Stage I & II: hemilaryngectomy or 6000–6500 cGy in 6–6½ weeks Verrucous carcinoma is best treated by hemilaryngectomy Stage III & IV: total laryngectomy is the treatment of choice For advanced carcinoma when a neck dissection is not performed For poorly differentiated carcinoma For advanced tumors, higher dosages are given: 7000 cGy with first 4000 cGy given in 200-cGy fractions	Persistent laryngeal edema—usually resolves in one year Laryngeal necrosis, infrequent but potentially fatal

Source: Adapted from Wang CC, Schulz MD: Cancer of the larynx: Its management by radiation therapy. *Radiology* 80:963, 1963.

cinoma is total lobectomy and isthmusectomy. Unsuspected carcinoma found after lobectomy for benign conditions is followed closely; additional surgery or radiotherapy usually is not indicated.

Total Thyroidectomy
The majority of thyroid malignancies require total or near-total thyroidectomy.

Radioactive Iodine
Patients with adequate surgery for well-differentiated thyroid carcinomas do not require postoperative adjuvant radiotherapy. Patients greater than 40 years of age (worse prognosis) require prophylactic postoperative radiotherapy. The residual gland is ablated with radioactive iodine, followed by a diagnostic radioimmunoassay total body scan. If the scan demonstrates residual disease, a therapeutic dose of iodine 131 is administered.

External Radiotherapy
Some patients with an inadequate iodine uptake have a high risk of local recurrence. Approximately 20 percent of patients do not concentrate ^{131}I. In these instances, external beam irradiation is advocated. The indications for external radiation are (1) known gross residual disease in the surgical field, (2) tumor extending beyond the capsule or into the soft tissues, (3) extensive cervical lymph node involvement, and (4) the presence of markedly invasive follicular carcinoma.

Medullary Carcinoma
Medullary and Hürthle cell carcinoma do not concentrate ^{131}I. Therefore, in the presence of poor prognostic variables for local recurrence, external radiation therapy as described is indicated.

Anaplastic Carcinoma
The prognosis for anaplastic carcinomas of the thyroid is poor. These are very aggressive tumors that are usually very advanced and unresectable at diagnosis. Anaplastic tumors do not concentrate ^{131}I and respond poorly to external radiotherapy. However, they often are treated with palliative external radiotherapy.

Portals
The radiation portals should encompass the thyroid gland completely from the mandible to the clavicle and upper mediastinum. Care is taken not to exceed the spinal cord tolerance. Spinal cord shielding in conjunction with an electron beam boost through oblique portals maximizes treatment of the tumor.

Distant Metastasis
Five to 10 percent of patients with distant metastasis from a well-differentiated carcinoma are cured permanently after therapeutic doses of ^{131}I [57,58]. Cure rates for patients with lung metastasis may be as high as 30 percent if the tumor concentrates ^{131}I. Metastatic disease does not concentrate iodine in the presence of normal thyroid tissue. However, not all metastatic lesions that concentrate iodine regress. Iodine concentration can be improved by producing acute thyroid hormone depletion.

The therapeutic doses of iodine are in the range of 150 to 200 mCi, with 6 to 12 months between successive doses to allow for bone marrow recovery.

Complications
Bone marrow depression following radioiodine is usually transient [59]. The risk of developing a second malignancy is small and related to total cumulative dose [60–62]. Patients with lung metastases are at risk of developing radiation-induced pneumonitis or pulmonary fibrosis [63]. There is no apparent increase in infertility or birth defects in female patients treated with radioiodine.

Results
Due to the long natural history of well-differentiated thyroid carcinoma, a 5-year follow-up is insufficient. Tumor recurrence has occurred 25 to 30 years after definitive therapy. Several variables result in decreased survival: large primaries, capsular invasion, soft-tissue involvement, aggressive follicular carcinomas, age

greater than 40 years, sex (males), and diabetes mellitus. Interestingly, the presence or absence of lymph nodes has no prognostic value for well-differentiated carcinomas. However, medullary carcinoma survival correlates with nodal status. Patients with anaplastic carcinoma have a very poor prognosis.

UNKNOWN PRIMARY SITE

A primary tumor site is not identified in 2 to 3 percent of the patients presenting with metastatic cancer in the neck (see Chapter 3) [64]. Approximately 10 percent of these cases represent metastasis from an occult head and neck primary site to the cervical nodes [65]. Aggressive local and regional treatment greatly benefits this group, whose prognosis is good compared to those with tumors at other anatomic sites.

Surgery alone results in the appearance of a head and neck primary tumor in 20 percent of the patients [66]. In comparison, only 6 percent develop a head and neck primary lesion, outside the radiation portals, when definitive radiotherapy is used [66]. The unknown site is infrequently found post mortem [67].

Adenocarcinoma almost always originates from below the clavicles and suggests metastasis from the chest, abdomen, or breast. These tumors usually present as supraclavicular nodes and have a much less favorable prognosis.

Treatment

Guidelines

Prior to 1973, the standard radiation technique for an unknown primary consisted of irradiation of the nasopharynx, oropharynx, and subdigastric and upper posterior cervical nodes through lateral opposed fields [66]. The lower neck was irradiated with 50 cGy fractions through an anterior portal. In those instances when the histology (e.g., lymphoepithelioma) or the location of the nodes (e.g., posterior cervical chain) favored the nasopharynx as the primary site, this standard technique was employed. Today, the modified standard technique includes the hypopharynx when a nasopharyngeal tumor is excluded.

The Upper Neck

Treatment planning in the upper neck is dictated by the location of the node. Upper and midjugular lymph nodes require elective irradiation of the nasopharynx, oropharynx, supraglottic larynx, hypopharynx, and both sides of the neck to the clavicles. A solitary submaxillary lymph node is better treated by neck dissection and observation because of the morbidity induced by irradiation of the entire oral cavity [68]. A preauricular lymph node containing squamous cell carcinoma almost always represents metastasis from a skin cancer and is treated by a combination of parotidectomy and radiation or irradiation therapy alone [68]. Supraclavicular nodes are irradiated through fields that encompass the supraclavicular fossa.

It generally is agreed that 5000 cGy in 25 fractions is adequate to control subclinical disease in a neck that has undergone no surgery [69]. Once the lymphatic channels are disrupted by surgery, a dose greater than 5000 cGy is advised [70]. Additionally, for extranodal disease, boosting the dose at the site of nodal disease to 6300 to 6800 cGy in 180-cGy fractions is advised [71,72].

The Lower Neck

Because of poor prognosis, the goal in the lower neck usually is control of the supraclavicular disease with local irradiation only. These palliative doses may at times be too low to delay massive tumor growth.

Complications

Due to the large volume of mucosa that is irradiated, the main complication is xerostomia. If the mucosal dose is 5000 cGy over 6 weeks to 6000 cGy over 7 weeks, persistent edema of the supraglottic larynx and hypopharynx should not be a problem. Less common complications reported in Carbon and Fletcher's analysis [71] included telangiectasia, skin atrophy, trismus, serous otitis media, external otitis, and hypothyroidism.

NEW HORIZONS

Radiation Modifiers

Tumor hypoxia (low oxygen levels) is one of the most important biologic factors limiting tumor control by irradiation.

The hypoxic portions of a tumor require radiation doses three times higher to achieve a therapeutic effect. To overcome this problem, different modalities and agents have been used. These include chemical sensitizers such as metronidazole (IUdR), 5-bromodeoxyuridine (BruUrd), oxygen, and other modifiers like high linear energy transfer (LET) radiation: neutron, meson, proton, and heat (hyperthermia) [73]. The most common and available radiation modifier is oxygen. The correction of the patient's hemoglobin levels and the use of hyperbaric oxygen are examples of maximizing this radiation sensitizer. The previously mentioned chemical sensitizers and high LET radiations are still investigational. More trials are needed before they are applied routinely to daily patient management.

Hyperthermia

Hyperthermia, the treatment of malignant tumors with heat, is a new addition to radiotherapy. Temperatures of 42.5°C, roughly 5 to 8°C above normal body temperature, destroy tumor cells and enhance radiation sensitivity [74,75]. Laboratory and clinical studies indicate that heat directly destroys cancer cells during specific stages of the mitotic cycle for actively growing mammalian cells. Heat is most effective during the synthesis (S) phase of the cells' mitotic cycle. Radiation, on the other hand, is most effective during the mitosis (M) phase of the cell cycle. Additionally, heat has the capability of preventing repair of sublethally damaged cells.

Theory

The combination of heat with radiation produces radiosensitization as well as a synergistic effect on tumor cell kill. In an experiment done on a transplanted mammary carcinoma, Overguard in 1977 [76] reported no cures with 1600 cGy (rad) delivered in a single fraction, a 22-percent cure rate with heat alone (43°C for 60 minutes), and a cure rate of 77 percent with a combination of both modalities.

Hyperthermia effectiveness is probably due to two distinctly different effects: direct cytotoxicity and cellular sensitization to radiation or drugs. Heat may be more damaging to tumors than to normal tissues for the following reasons [77]: (1) metabolically deprived cells with low pH are more sensitive to heat; (2) the radioresistant phase of the cell cycle, the S phase, is heat sensitive; and (3) hypoxic cells usually have a lower pH than normal cells and therefore are more sensitive to heat. In addition heat itself can reduce blood flow, oxygen tension, and pH.

Techniques

Various methods are utilized to elevate tumor temperature to therapeutic levels: local (external), interstitial, intracavitary, regional, perfusion of specific volumes (e.g., extremities), and whole body. The following physical agents are used most commonly:

1. Electromagnetic radiation at microwave frequencies (50–2450 MHz).
2. Electromagnetic fields with radiofrequency 0.1 to 27 MHz.
3. Ultrasound (0.3–3.0 MHz).

Results

Local or interstitial hyperthermia in combination with radiation therapy produces a 70- to 80-percent complete response rate. This is significantly superior to either modality alone [78,79].

Intraoperative Radiotherapy

Intraoperative radiotherapy, introduced more than 40 years ago [80,81], has the advantage of direct visualization and radiation of a surgically exposed tumor. Intraoperative radiotherapy was first introduced in the United States in 1976 as a result of the collaborative efforts of Henschke and Goldson at Howard University Hospital in Washington, DC (Figure 9-6). A single high dose of radiation, either by particle or photon beam, is delivered to the exposed tumor bed or its local-regional lymph nodes.

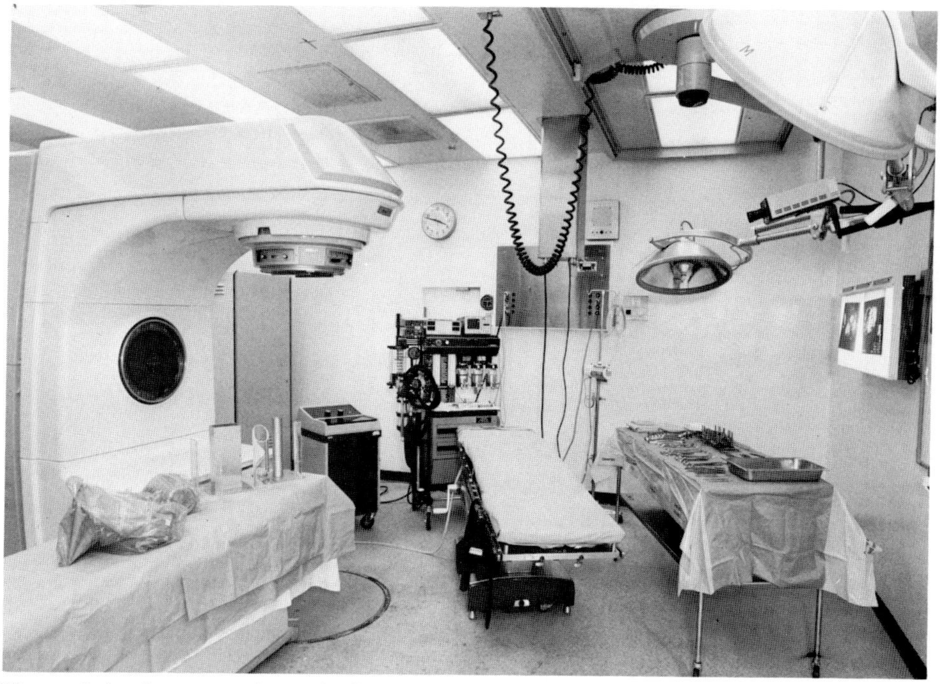

Figure 9-6. Intraoperative radiotherapy suite, Howard University Hospital.

Obviously, close cooperation between the surgeon, anesthesiologist, radiation oncologist, pathologist, operating room nursing staff, and other members of the surgical support team is essential for the success of this procedure [82–84].

Advantages

Intraoperative radiotherapy has several advantages: (1) precise localization of the tumor; (2) accurate beam placement; (3) organ exposure and retraction of normal tissues and sensitive organs (e.g., bowel, lung); (4) protection of sensitive structures (e.g., ureter, nerves) within the irradiation volume by sheets of lead; and (5) precise limitation of irradiation to the tumor volume.

Dose

Doses in the range of 1000 to 2500 rads are delivered in a single fraction. Intraoperative radiotherapy permits delivery of a tumor dose without a concomitant increase in the treatment morbidity or mortality.

Results

It appears that the combination of aggressive surgical resection and intraoperative irradiation to the tumor bed and regional nodal basins may substantially improve local control. The incidence of complications resulting from the addition of intraoperative radiotherapy appears to be no greater than the incidence of complications from extensive surgical treatment alone. With increasing popularity of intraoperative radiotherapy in the medical community in the United States and abroad, additional encouraging clinical trial findings are being reported [85–87].

High Linear Energy Transfer Particle Irradiation

High-LET irradiation offers several potential advantages over low-LET photon or electron irradiation. The higher energy deposition means less dependence on "indirect" free radical–mediated cell killing.

Theory

High-LET radiation is more effective for hypoxic cells than routine irradiation. For fast neutrons, oxygen enhancement ratios are about 1.6, compared with 2.5 to 3.0 for high-energy photons. Also, the damage inflicted by high-LET radiation is repaired less readily by the tumor cells, especially cells in a "resting" or G-phase of the mitotic cycle. Finally, there is less variation in radiosensitivity across the cell cycle with high-LET irradiation than with conventional low-LET irradiation [88].

Results

Hammersmith Hospital and other centers adopting neutron therapy trials have proved the effectiveness of this modality in the treatment role of fast-neutron irradiation in clinical cancer therapy. Uniform clinical trials through multi-institutional collaboration are required prior to routine clinical application of this modality in advanced diseases such as salivary gland tumors, soft-tissue sarcomas, sarcomas of the bone, and cervical lymph node metastases from primary tumors of the head and neck [89–91].

REFERENCES

1. Moss WT, Brand WN, Battifora H (eds): Radiation Oncology, Rationale, Technique, Results. *Introduction to Radiation Oncology* (5th ed). St. Louis: Mosby, 1979. Pp 1–36.
2. Fletcher G: The evolution of the basic concepts underlying the practice of radiotherapy from 1949 to 1977. *Radiology* 127 : 3, 1978.
3. Read J: The effect of ionizing radiation on the broad beam root, part X: The dependence of the x-rays sensitivity on dissolved oxygen. *Br J Radiol* 25 : 89, 1952.
4. Puck TT, Marcus PI: Action of x-rays on mammalian cells. *J Exp Med* 103 : 653, 1956.
5. Hall EJ (ed): *Radiation Biology for the Radiologist* (2nd ed). Hagerstown, MD: Harper and Row, 1982.
6. Casarett AP (ed): *Radiation Biology*. Englewood Cliffs, NJ: Prentice-Hall, 1968.
7. Alper T: Elkind recovery "sublethal damage": A misleading association. *Br J Radiol* 50 : 459, 1977.
8. Moss WT (ed): *Combination of Radiotherapy and Surgery: Radiation Oncology, Rationale, Techniques, Results*. St. Louis: Mosby, 1979. Pp 37–46.
9. Kligerman MM, Urdaneta N, Lafee N: Observations on fifteen inoperable nonresectable cases of rectal cancer given preoperative irradiation. *Am J Roentgenol* 120 : 576, 1975.
10. Inch WR, McCredie JA, Sutherland RM: Effect of x-radiation to tumor bed on local recurrence. In Vaeth JM: *The Interrelationship of Surgery and Radiation Therapy in the Treatment of Cancer*. Baltimore: University Park Press, 1970.
11. Goldson AL: Intraoperative Radiation Therapy. In Devita VT Jr, Hellman S, Rosenbery SA (ed): *Cancer: Principles and Practice of Radiation Oncology*. Philadelphia: Lippincott, 1982. Pp 1922–1935.
12. Ho JHC: An epidemiologic and clinical study of nasopharyngeal carcinoma. *Int J Radiat Oncol Biol Phys* 4 : 183, 1978.
13. Kottaridis SD, et al: Antibodies to Epstein-Barr virus in nasopharyngeal carcinoma and other neoplastic conditions. *J Natl Cancer Inst* 59(1) : 89, 1977.
14. del Regato JA, Spjut HJ (ed): *Cancer, Diagnosis, Treatment and Prognosis* (5th ed). St. Louis: Mosby, 1977. Pp 301–318.
15. Fletcher GH, Million RR: Nasopharynx. In Fletcher GH (ed): *Textbook of Radiotherapy* (3rd ed). Philadelphia: Lea & Febiger, 1980. Pp 364–383.
16. Bedwinek JM, Perez CP, Keys DJ: Analysis of failures after definitive irradiation for epidermoid carcinoma of the nasopharynx. *Cancer* 45 : 2725, 1980.
17. Wang CC, Schulz MD: Management of locally recurrent carcinoma of the nasopharynx. *Radiology* 86 : 900, 1966.
18. Chu AM, et al: Irradiation of nasopharyngeal carcinoma: Correlation with treatment factors and stage. *Int J Radiat Oncol Biol Phys* 10: 2241, 1984.
19. Fu KK, Newman H, Phillips TL: Treatment of locally recurrent carcinoma of the nasopharynx. *Radiology* 117 : 425, 1975.
20. Hilaris BS, Lewis JS, Henschke U: Therapy of recurrent cancer of the nasopharynx: Value of interstitial and intracavitary radiation. *Arch Otolaryngol* 87 : 80, 1968.
21. McNeese MD, Fletcher GH: Retreatment of recurrent nasopharyngeal carcinoma. *Radiology* 138 : 191, 1981.
22. Sooy FA: Experimental treatment of recurrent carcinoma of the nasopharynx with electrodesiccation, radioactive cobalt and x-ray radiation. *Arch Otolaryngol* 65 : 723, 1956.
23. Ashayeri E, et al: Localization technique and afterloading intracavitary irradiation in the treatment of nasopharyngeal carcinoma. *Endocurietherapy/Hyperthermia Oncol* 3 : 115, 1987.
24. Hwang HN: Nasopharyngeal carcinoma in the People's Republic of China: Incidence, treat-

ment, and survival rates. *Radiology* 149 : 305, 1983.
25. Million RR, Cassisi NJ (ed): Nasopharynx. In: *Management of Head and Neck Cancer: A Multidisciplinary Approach*. Philadelphia: Lippincott, 1984. Pp 445–466.
26. Wang CC: *Radiation Therapy for Head and Neck Neoplasms: Indications, Techniques, and Results*. Boston: Wright-PSG, 1983. Pp 213–221.
27. Fletcher GH: *Textbook of Radiotherapy* (3rd ed). Philadelphia: Lea & Febiger, 1980. Pp 408–425.
28. Shukovsky LJ, Fletcher GH: Retinal and optic nerve complications in a high dose irradiation technique of ethmoid sinus and nasal cavity. *Radiology* 104 : 629, 1972.
29. Lewis TS, Castro EB: Cancer of the nasal cavity and paranasal sinuses. *J Laryngol Otol* 86 : 255, 1972.
30. Bush SE, Bagshaw MA: Carcinoma of the paranasal sinuses. *Cancer* 50 : 154, 1982.
31. Katz AD: Unusual lesions of the parotid gland. *J Surg Oncol* 7 : 219, 1975.
32. King JJ, Fletcher GH: Malignant tumors of the major salivary glands. *Radiology* 100 : 381, 1971.
33. Rubin P: *Clinical Oncology: A Multidisciplinary Approach* (6th ed). Rochester, NY: American Cancer Society, 1983. Pp 230–261.
34. Million RR, Cassisi NJ: *Management of Head and Neck Cancer: A Multidisciplinary Approach*. Philadelphia: Lippincott, 1984. P 240.
35. Million RR, Cassisi NJ: *Management of Head and Neck Cancer: A Multidisciplinary Approach*. Philadelphia: Lippincott, 1984. P 241.
36. Mackay EN, Sellers AH: A statistical review of carcinoma of the lip. *Can Med Assoc J* 90 : 670, 1964.
37. MacComb WS, Fletcher GH, Healey JE: Intraoral Cavity. In MacComb WS, Fletcher GH (ed): *Cancer of the Head and Neck*. Baltimore: Williams & Wilkins, 1967. Pp 89–151.
38. Million RR, Cassisi NJ: *Management of Head and Neck Cancer: A Multidisciplinary Approach*. Philadelphia: Lippincott, 1984. P 245.
39. Fletcher GH: *Textbook of Radiotherapy* (3rd ed). Philadelphia: Lea & Febiger, 1980. P 304.
40. Ange DW, Lindbery RD, Guillamondegui OM: Management of squamous cell carcinoma of the oral tongue and floor of the mouth after excisional biopsy. *Radiology* 116 : 143, 1975.
41. Fletcher GH: *Textbook of Radiotherapy* (3rd ed). Philadelphia: Lea & Febiger, 1980. P 287.
42. Gelinas M, Fletcher GH: Incidence and causes of local failures after irradiation in squamous cell carcinoma of the facial arch, tonsillar fossa and base of tongue. *Radiology* 108 : 383, 1973.
43. Million RR, Cassisi NJ: *Management of Head and Neck Cancer: A Multidisciplinary Approach*. Philadelphia: Lippincott, 1984. P 253.
44. Million RR, Cassisi NJ: *Management of Head and Neck Cancer: A Multidisciplinary Approach*. Philadelphia: Lippincott, 1984. P 286.
45. Million RR, Cassisi NJ (ed): Oropharynx. In: *Management of Head and Neck Cancer: A Multidisciplinary Approach*. Philadelphia: Lippincott, 1984. Pp 299–313.
46. Fayos JV: Carcinoma of the oropharynx. *Radiology* 138 : 675, 1981.
47. Hendrickson FR: Cancers of the Oral Cavity and Orothpharynx. Course 518B, Syllabus Head and Neck Cancer, a Categorical Course in Radiation Therapy, 1981, Radiological Society of North America.
48. Perez CA, et al: Nonrandomized comparison of preoperative irradiation and surgery versus irradiation alone in the management of carcinoma of the tonsil. *Am J Roentgenol* 126 : 248, 1976.
49. Fayos JV: The role of radium implants in cancer of the oral cavity and oral pharynx. *Int J Radiat Oncol Biol Phys* 6(4) : 423, 1980.
50. Marks JE, et al: Carcinoma of the pyriform sinus: An analysis of treatment results and patterns of failure. *Cancer* 41 : 1008, 1978.
51. Million RR, Cassisi NJ: Radical irradiation for carcinoma of the pyriform sinus. *Laryngoscope* 91 : 439, 1981.
52. Dubois JB, Guerrier B, Ruggiero JM: Cancer of the pyriform sinus: Treatment by radiation therapy alone and with surgery. *Radiology* 160 : 831, 1986.
53. Moss WT, Brand WN, Battifora H (ed): The Endolarynx and Hypopharynx. In: *Radiation Oncology, Rationale, Technique, Results* (5th ed). St. Louis: Mosby, 1979. Pp 203–232.
54. Million RR, Cassisi NJ (ed): Larynx. In: *Management of Head and Neck Cancer: A Multidisciplinary Approach*. Philadelphia: Lippincott, 1984. Pp 315–363.
55. Nass JM, et al: Radiation therapy of glottic carcinoma. *Int J Radiat Oncol Biol Phys* 1 : 867, 1976.
56. Wang CC, Schulz MD: Cancer of the larynx: Its management by radiation therapy. *Radiology* 80 : 963, 1963.
57. Sedgwick CB, et al: Changing clinical, pathologic, therapeutic and survival patterns in differentiated thyroid carcinoma. *Ann Surg* 1984 : 541, 1976.
58. Tubiana M: External radiotherapy and radioiodine in the treatment of thyroid cancer. *World J Surg* 5 : 75, 1981.
59. Clark RL, et al: Thyroid. In MacComb WS, Fletcher GH: *Cancer of the Head and Neck*. Baltimore: Williams & Wilkins, 1967. Pp 293–328.
60. Rose RG, Kelsey MP: Radioactive iodine in the diagnosis and treatment of thyroid cancer. *Cancer* 16 : 896, 1963.
61. Simpson WJ, Carruthers JS: The role of external radiation in the management of papillary and

follicular thyroid cancer. *Am J Surg* 136 : 457, 1978.
62. Tubiana M, et al: External radiotherapy and radioiodine in the treatment of 359 thyroid cancers. *Br J Radiol* 48 : 894, 1975.
63. Frazell EL, Foote FW Jr: Papillary cancer of the thyroid: A review of 25 years of experience. *Cancer* 11 : 895, 1953.
64. Nordstrom DG, Twefik HH, Latourette HB: Cervical lymph node metastases from an unknown primary. *Int J Radiat Oncol Biol Phys* 5 : 73, 1979.
65. McCunniff AJ, Raben M: Metastatic carcinoma of the neck from an unknown primary. *Int J Radiat Oncol Biol Phys* 12 : 1849, 1986.
66. Jesse RH, Perez CA, Fletcher GH: Cervical lymph node metastasis: Unknown primary cancer. *Cancer* 31 : 854, 1973.
67. Fitzpatrick PJ, Kotalik J: Cervical metastases from an unknown primary tumor. *Radiology* 110 : 659, 1974.
68. Million RR, Cassissi NJ: *Management of Head and Neck Cancer: A Multidisciplinary Approach*. Philadelphia: Lippincott, 1984.
69. Fletcher GH: Elective irradiation of subclinical disease in cancers of the head and neck. *Cancer* 29 : 1450, 1972.
70. Fletcher GH: Letter to the Editor. *Int J Radiat Oncol Biol Phys* 118 : 1060, 1985.
71. Carbon LS, Fletcher GH: Guidelines for radiotherapeutic techniques for cervical metastases from an unknown primary. *Int J Radiat Oncol Biol Phys* 12 : 2101, 1986.
72. Million RR, Cassisi NJ: *Management of Head and Neck Cancer: A Multidisciplinary Approach*. Philadelphia: Lippincott, 1984.
73. Hall EJ (ed): Radiosensitizers . . . "Radioprotectors." In: *Radiobiology for the Radiologist* (3rd ed). Philadelphia, Lippincott, 1988. Pp 179–209.
74. Storm KF: Background Principles and Practice. In: *Hyperthermia in Cancer Therapy*. Boston: Hall, 1983. P 1.
75. Warren JL: Preliminary study of the effects of artificial fever upon hopeless tumor cases. *AJR* 33 : 75, 1935.
76. Overgaard J: Effect of hyperthermia on malignant cells in vivo. *Cancer* 39 : 2637, 1977.
77. Hall EJ (ed): Hyperthermia. In: *Radiobiology for the Radiologist* (3rd ed). Philadelphia, Lippincott, 1988. Pp 293–329.
78. Perez CA, et al: Refresher Course No. 304, Principles and Practice of Localized Hyperthermia (External and Interstitial), American Society for Therapeutic Radiology and Oncology 27th Annual Meeting, 1985.
79. Perez CA, et al: Clinical results of irradiation combined with local hyperthermia. *Cancer* 52 : 1597, 1983.
80. Henschke U, Henschke G: Zur Technik Der Operationsbestrahlung. *Strahlentherapie* 74 : 223, 1944.
81. Goldson A: Past, present and prospects of intraoperative radiotherapy (IOR). *Semin Oncol* 8 : 1, 1981.
82. Goldson A: The outlook for intraoperative radiotherapy. *Int J Radiat Oncol Biol Phys* 7 : 979, 1981.
83. Goldson A, et al: Single high dose intraoperative electrons for advanced stage pancreatic cancer: Phase I study. *Int J Radiat Oncol Biol Phys* P. 869, 1981.
84. Tepper J, Gunderson IL: Progress in intraoperative radiotherapy. *Appl Radiol* 000 : 21, 1983.
85. Abe M, Takahashi M: Intraoperative radiotherapy: The Japanese experience. *Int J Radiat Oncol Biol Phys* 7 : 863, 1971.
86. Abe M, Fukada M, Yamono K: Intraoperative irradiation in abdominal and cerebral tumors. *Acta Radiol* 10 : 408, 1971.
87. Sindelar WF, et al: Experimental and clinical studies with intraoperative radiotherapy. *Surg Gynecol Obstet* 157 : 205, 1983.
88. Hall EJ (ed): LET and RBE. In *Radiobiology for the Radiologist* (3rd ed). Philadelphia: Lippincott, 1988.
89. Laramore GE, Griffin TW: Potential applications of clinical neutron-beam generator in cancer management. *Appl Radiol,* Sept./Oct. 1986, Pp 74–79.
90. Stone RS: Neutron therapy and specific ionization. *AJR* 59 : 771, 1940.
91. Griffin TW: Particle radiotherapy. *Hospital Pract* 91 : 91, 1985.

10

Airway

ERNEST M. MYERS

KEY CONCEPTS

Diagnosis; Management; Intubation; Tracheotomy; Extubation; Percutaneous; Laser Surgery; Ventilation

MILESTONES

124 B.C.	Tracheotomy	Asclepiades
131 A.D.	Anatomy of the Larynx	Galen
1545	Successful Tracheotomy	Brasavola
1733	Double-Lumen Tracheotomy Tube	Martine
1909	Endotracheal Intubation	Meltzer and Auer
1967	Cadaveric Laser Surgery	Jako
1970	Endoscopic Laser Surgery	Bredemeir
1972	Laser Laryngeal Surgery	Strong and Jako
1974	Microscopic Laser Laryngoscopy	Polani, Wallace, and Pejchar
1974	Bronchoscopic Laser Surgery	Strong

Airway management is paramount in all three phases of head and neck oncology. The indications are obstruction, respiratory support, and pulmonary hygiene [1]. Of the three, obstruction is a potential problem in 6 of the 10 sites of head and neck cancer. Upper airway obstruction is associated with site 5, the oral cavity, and site 6, the oropharynx. Lower airway obstruction is associated with site 7, the hypopharynx; site 8, the larynx; site 9, the thyroid/parathyroid; and site 10, the cervical esophagus. This chapter presents a comprehensive system of airway management for the head and neck cancer patient.

RESPIRATORY FAILURE

Although the emphasis is on airway, any discussion is incomplete without a more comprehensive discussion of respiratory failure.

Diagnosis

Respiratory failure is the inability of the respiratory system to sustain effective oxygenation [1]. The four clinical criteria of respiratory failure are (1) acute dyspnea, (2) P_aO_2 less than 50 mm Hg, (3) P_aCO_2 greater than 50 mm Hg, and (4) pH less than 7.30. Most patients with respiratory failure have at least two of these criteria [1].

Symptoms

Unlike patients who exhibit acute respiratory failure, head and neck cancer patients with respiratory problems have chronic symptoms spanning days and weeks (Table 10-1). As the airway gradually compromises, the patients imperceptively and unconsciously decrease their activity. They avoid stairs, running, and other activities requiring exertion. When the airway becomes critically marginal, acute

Table 10-1. Symptoms and signs of airway obstruction

- *Symptoms*
  - Psychological
    - Apprehension
    - Confusion
    - Combativeness
  - Visual
    - Abnormal respirations (tachypnea)
    - Retractions
    - Sweating
    - Anxiety
  - Audible
    - Dysphonia
    - Aphonia
    - Snoring
    - Stridor
    - Gagging
    - Wheezing
    - Grunting
    - Hoarseness
- *Signs*
  - Integumental
    - Cyanosis
    - Sweating
  - Respiratory
    - Glottic edema
    - Glottic obstruction (mass or inflammation)
    - Vocal cord paralysis
    - Rhonchi
  - Cardiovascular
    - Vital signs: tachycardia, hypertension, hypotension
    - Electrocardiogram: ST segment elevation, prolonged QT interval, Q waves
  - Musculoskeletal: use of accessory muscles of respiration

apprehension, confusion, and frank combativeness ensue.

Signs

During the initial patient interview, breathiness, hoarseness, and audible wheezes may be obvious (Table 10-1). Many head and neck cancer patients often appear chronically ill and older than their stated age. In extremis, accessory muscles of respiration may be required to sustain the work of breathing. Imminent danger signs are resting tachycardia, tachypnea, and hypertension.

Physical Examination

As outlined in Chapter 2, the primary step in airway evaluation is indirect or direct laryngoscopy to assess obstruction and/or paralysis. Of secondary importance is cervical palpation and chest auscultation.

X-rays

Soft-Tissue Lateral Neck X-rays

Soft-tissue lateral neck x-rays are incomplete without confirmation by indirect or direct laryngoscopy. However, they do provide valuable information in regard to altered anatomy of the supraglottis, glottis, subglottis, and hypopharynx (Figure 10-1).

Figure 10-1. Airway compromise. Lateral soft-tissue neck film demonstrating hypopharyngeal dilation secondary to lower airway obstruction.

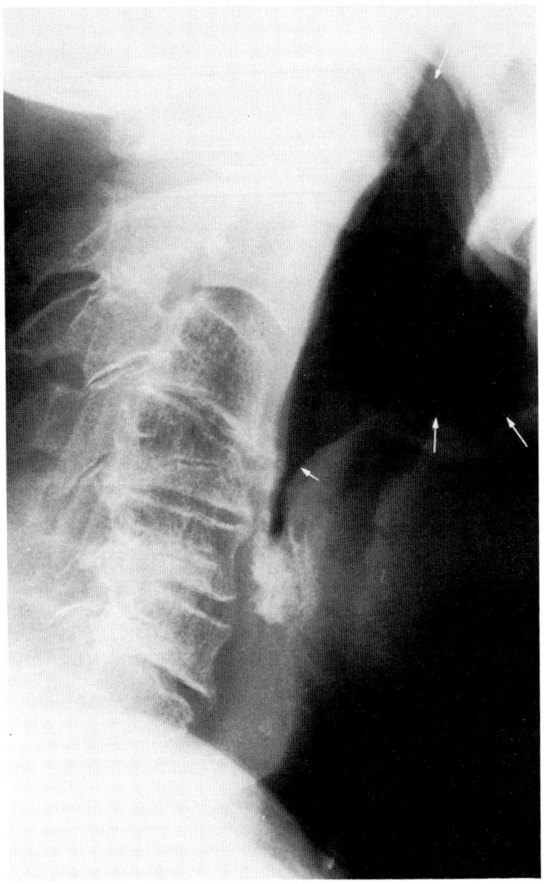

Anteroposterior and Lateral Chest X-rays
A common pattern encountered with some head and neck patients is aspiration pneumonia (right lung field) and/or secondary pleural effusion. Such findings commonly are secondary to large oropharyngeal, hypopharyngeal, laryngeal, and high (cervical) esophageal lesions.

Computed Tomography Scans
Computed tomography (CT) of the neck, mediastinum, and lung, when indicated, is invaluable. CT scan is especially useful in detecting soft-tissue invasion, bony erosion, and regional metastasis (see Chapter 4).

Arterial Blood Gases

Hypoxemia, the hallmark of respiratory failure, is responsible for most of the signs and symptoms. Arterial blood gases are the cornerstone of rapid diagnosis of respiratory failure. They provide pertinent information before initiating therapy—in particular, the adequacy of ventilation and oxygenation [2]. However, although important for clinical management, they are insensitive to overall gas exchange efficiency.

Etiology

The respiratory system consists of a chain of interconnected systems (Table 10-2) [1]. A failure in any one system results in respiratory compromise. Moreover, regardless of the affected system, there are only three mechanisms of abnormal gas exchange: hypoventilation, shunt, and ventilation-perfusion mismatch with secondary diffusion impairment [1].

Table 10-2. Etiology of respiratory failure*

Site	*Examples*	*Mechanism*
Central nervous system	Drugs	Hypoventilation
Brain	Narcotics	
Spinal cord	Barbiturates	
	Closed head injury	
	Spinal shock	
Neuromuscular system	Polio	Hypoventilation
	Guillain-Barré syndrome	
Cardiovascular system	Myocardial infarction	Shunt
	Valve disease	
	Cardiomyopathy	
Upper airway	Head and neck neoplasm	Ventilation-perfusion mismatch
	Trauma	Hypoventilation
	Facial fractures	
	Mandibular fractures	
	Infection	
	Epiglottitis	
	Peritonsillar abscess	
Respiratory system		
Thorax & pleura	Kyphoscoliosis	Ventilation-perfusion mismatch
	Pleural effusion	Shunt
Lower airway & alveoli	Bronchospasm	Ventilation-perfusion mismatch
	Asthma	
	Pulmonary edema	Shunt

*Other factors that impact on respiratory failure are hypovolemia, severe anemia, overwhelming sepsis, and metabolic acidosis.

Phases of Management

Diagnostics

In some patients, even before the initial examination, immediate airway management is required. Depending on the site and stage of the cancer, many patients present with early airway compromise (Table 10-2). Whenever airway compromise is suspected, indirect or direct laryngoscopy is mandatory. Soft-tissue anteroposterior (AP) and lateral neck films may reveal the location and extent of airway compromise. If conditions permit, a CT scan of the neck is even more informative.

Therapeutics

For many patients, the prerequisite for safe therapy is a secure airway. When extensive head and neck surgery or interstitial implantation is planned, an elective tracheotomy may be indicated. Although the carbon dioxide laser is invaluable for airway management, tracheotomy remains the time-honored standard.

Rehabilitation

Even beyond therapy, head and neck cancer patients require eternal vigilance to ensure an airway. For example, after full-course radiation of the larynx or post-hemilaryngectomy, a tenuous airway may demand immediate intervention. Again, in most instances, tracheotomy is the benchmark of airway management. However, intubation followed by carbon dioxide laser is beginning to supplant its usage.

SITE ANALYSIS

A review of laryngeal anatomy and basic flow-volume loop physiology is invaluable in understanding the airway (Figures 10-2, 10-3; Table 10-3).

Table 10-3. Sites of head and neck cancer

Site 1	Nasopharynx
Site 2	Nose and paranasal sinuses
Site 3	Salivary glands
Site 4	Lips
Site 5	Oral cavity
Site 6	Oropharynx
Site 7	Hypopharynx
Site 8	Larynx
Site 9	Thyroid and parathyroids
Site 10	Cervical esophagus

Nasopharynx, Nose, and Paranasal Sinuses, Salivary Glands, and Lips (Sites 1–4)

Sites 1 through 4 rarely are associated with airway compromise, regardless of tumor stage.

Oral Cavity and Oropharynx (Sites 5 and 6)

Malignancies in sites 5 and 6 have the potential for airway compromise, especially in the terminal stages associated with extensive tongue invasion (Figure 10-4).

Hypopharynx (Site 7)

Hypopharyngeal lesions are difficult to manage (Figure 10-5). Establishing an airway under emergency conditions may precipitate acute upper airway obstruction. If urgent intubation is planned, the surgical team should be prepared for an emergency rigid bronchoscopy or tracheotomy. To prevent an open wound and decrease possible stomal recurrence, carbon dioxide laser is the procedure of choice.

Larynx (Site 8)

As indicated, carbon dioxide laser is the first option for laryngeal carcinoma. Again, there are exceptions, such as significant glottic or subglottic involvement. With a patient in extremis, the only choice is tracheotomy (Figures 10-6 to 10-9).

Thyroid/Parathyroid and Cervical Esophagus (Sites 9 and 10)

Sites 9 and 10 have the potential for airway obstruction but usually late in the disease course. The clinical presentation of site 10 may be subtle and treacherous. A patient developing airway obstruction in the cervical esophagus could require laser laryngoscopy, bronchoscopy, or esophagoscopy (Yag laser). The physician must be acutely aware that the obstruction may be distal to the usual tracheotomy location.

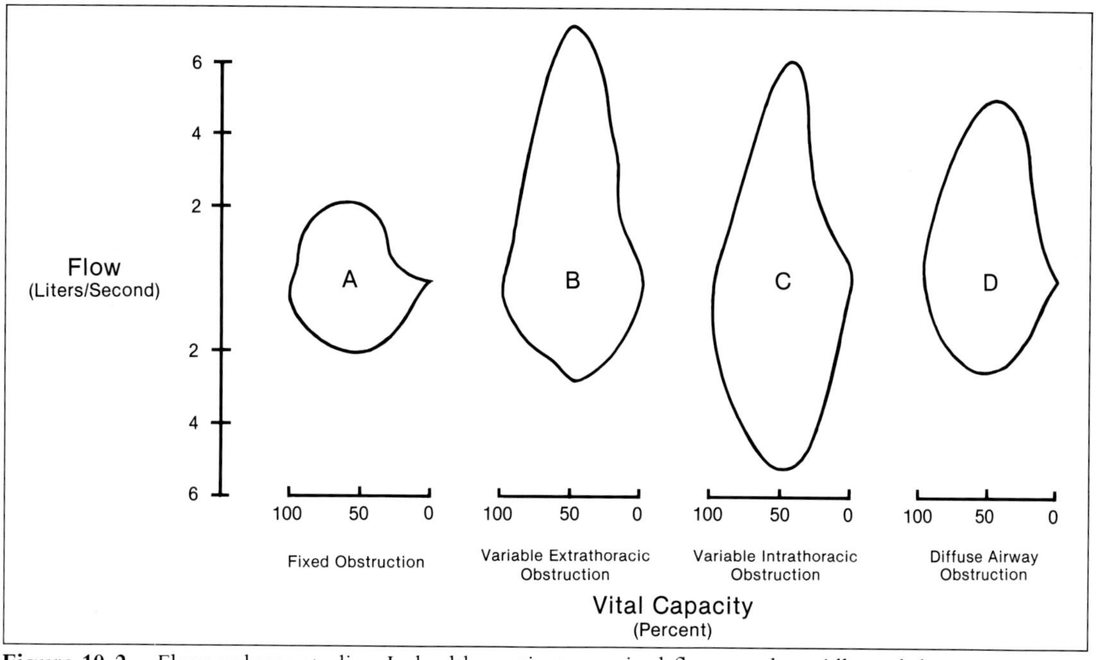

Figure 10-2. Flow-volume studies. In healthy patients, expired flows peak rapidly and decrease linearly with decreasing lung volume. With obstructive lung disease (C, D), flows are low: Flow decreases early during forced exhalation, generating a marked convexity toward the volume axis. In contrast, restrictive lung disease (B) has low absolute flows but normal or slightly high flows when compared to equivalent lung volumes. With fixed upper-airway obstruction (A), a situation most common with head and neck cancer patients, flow-volume curve reaches a plateau at high volumes and decreases with normal configuration at lower volumes.

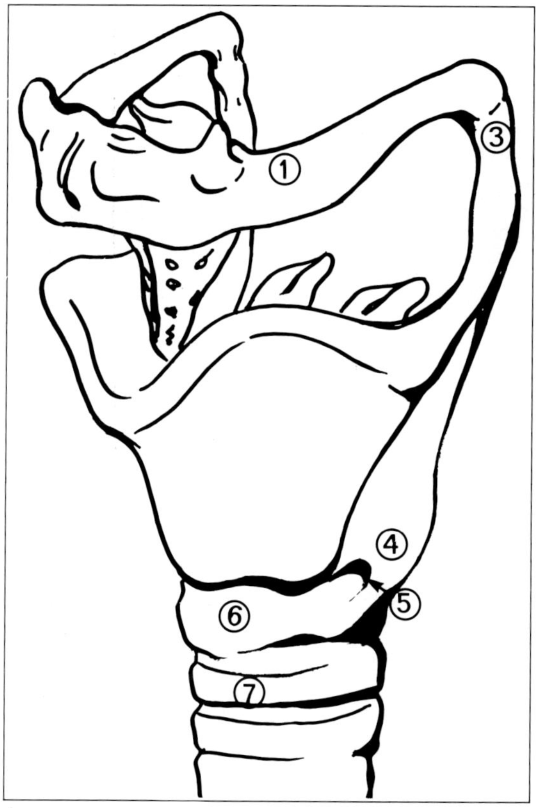

A

Figure 10-3. Laryngeal anatomy. A. Three-quarter view. *1* = hyoid bone; *3* = superior cornu; *4* = inferior cornu; *5* = cricothyroid joint; *6* = cricoid cartilage; *7* = first tracheal ring. B. Direct view. *1* = hyoid bone; *2* = epiglottis; *3* = true vocal cords; *4* = arytenoid cartilages; *5* = cricoid cartilage.

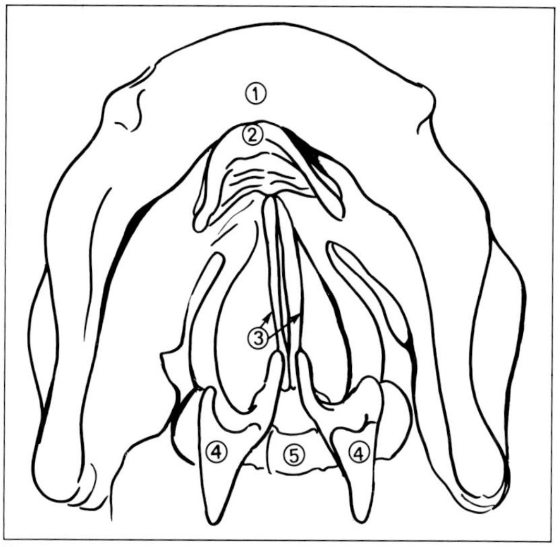

B

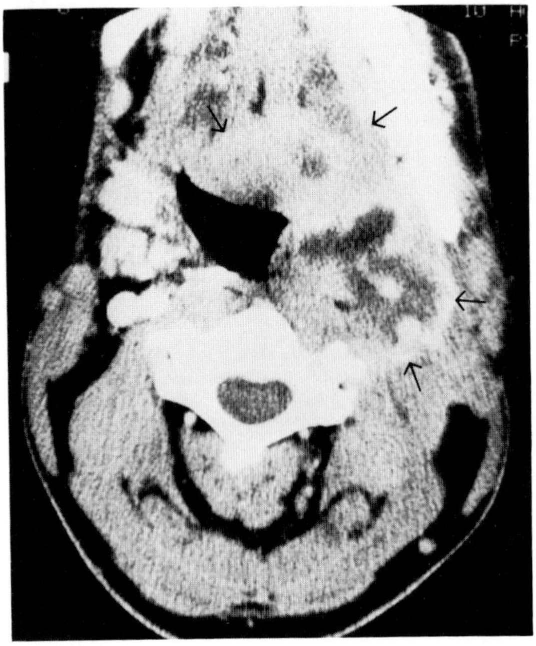

Figure 10-4. CT scan (level of base of tongue) showing upper airway obstruction secondary to a large carcinoma of the left tonsil with base of tongue involvement.

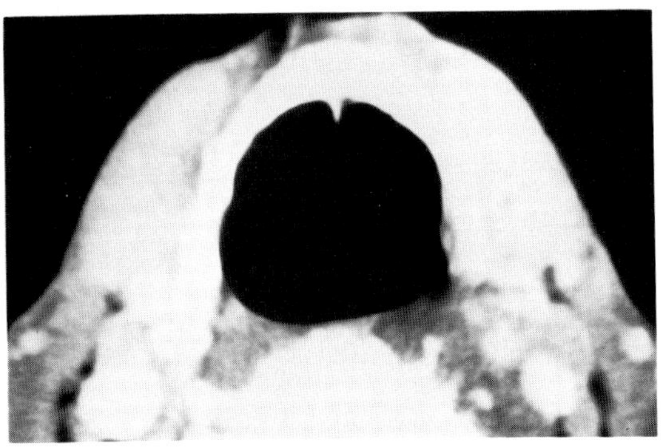

A

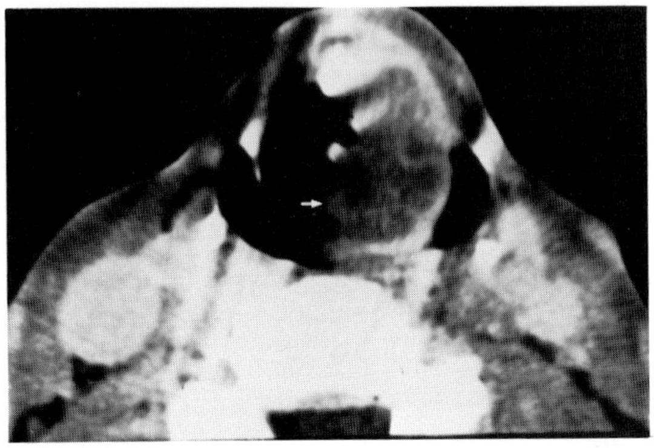

B

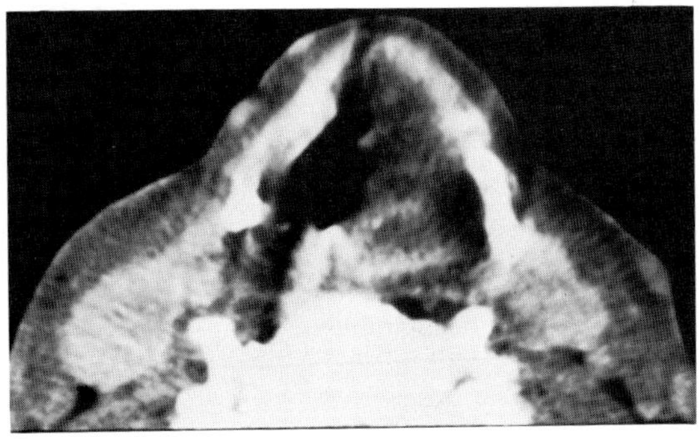

C

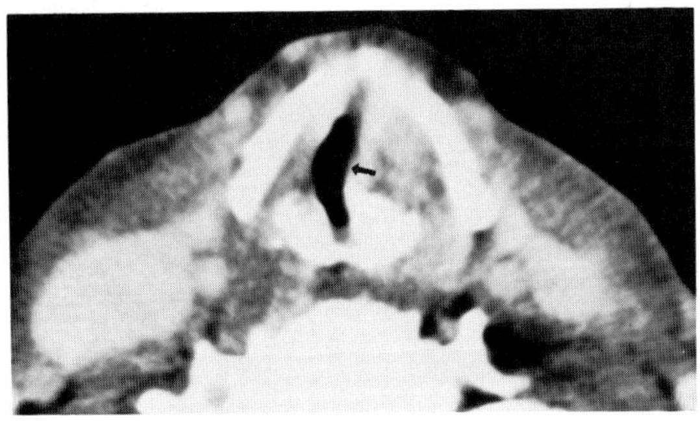

D

Figure 10-5. CT scans at the level of the larynx demonstrating a large hypopharyngeal carcinoma with hypopharyngeal dilatation (A), pyriform obliteration (B), airway compromise (C), and paraglottic space infiltration (D).

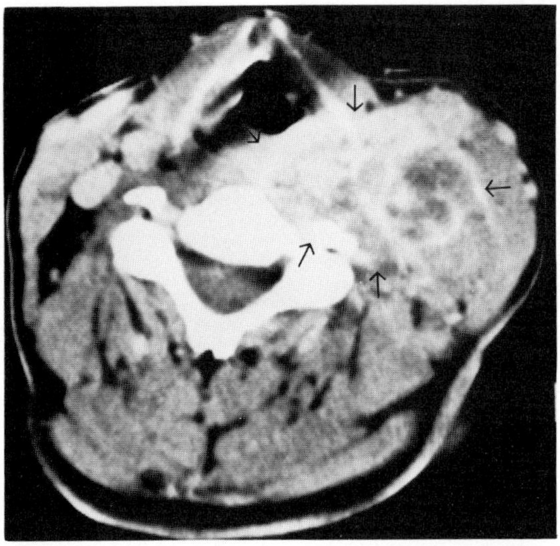

Figure 10-6. CT scan, neck (level of thyroid cartilage). A. Complaining of labored breathing and hoarseness, this 63-year-old man presented with impending airway obstruction and extensive carotid sheath involvement.

Figure 10-7. A horizontal CT scan at the level of the hyoid bone shows a large, fluid-filled, massive metastasis with parapharyngeal space invasion and a compromised lower airway.

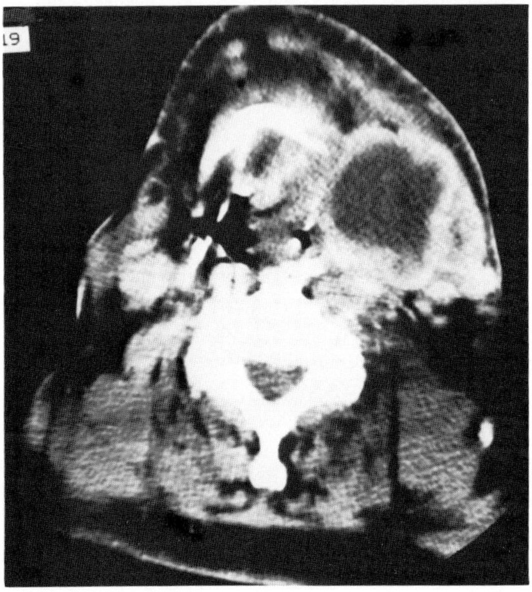

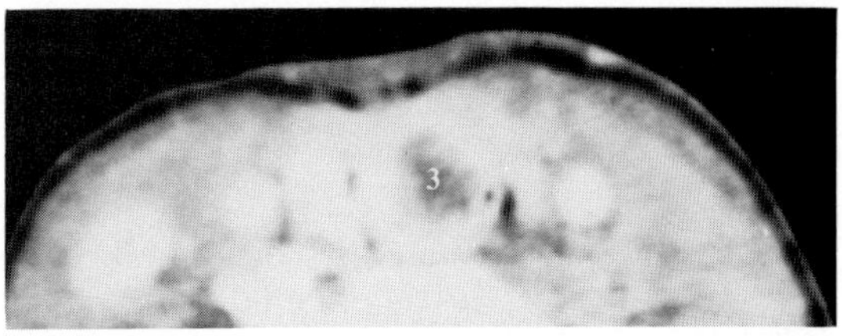

A

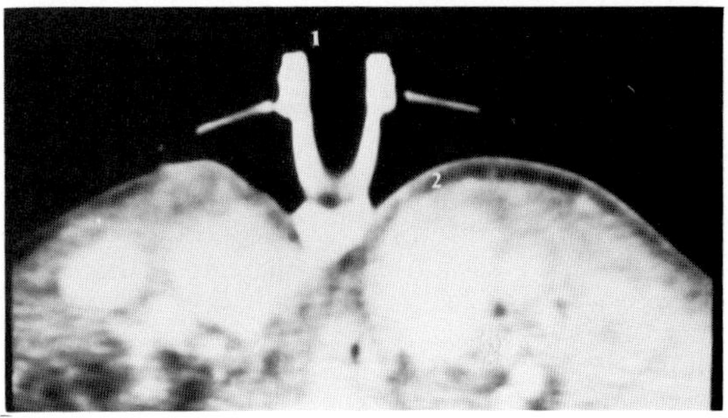

B

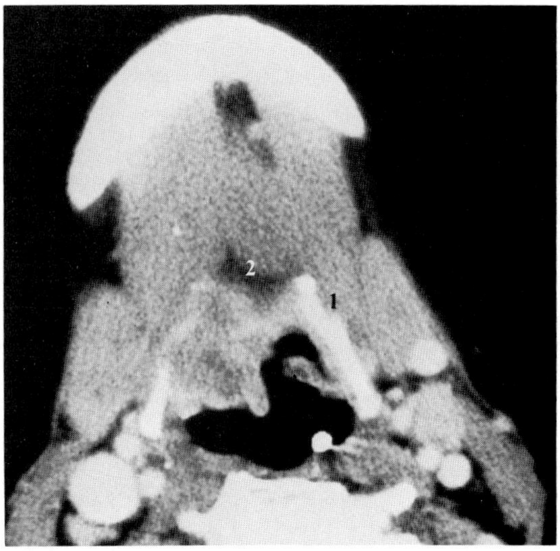

C

Figure 10-8. A and B. Stomal recurrence in a 40-year-old woman after total laryngectomy preceded by an emergency tracheotomy. *1* = tracheotomy tube; *2* = thyroid gland; *3* = stomal recurrence. C. The same patient later developed a recurrence in the base of the tongue (arrow). *1* = hyoid bone; *2* = preepiglottic space. (continued)

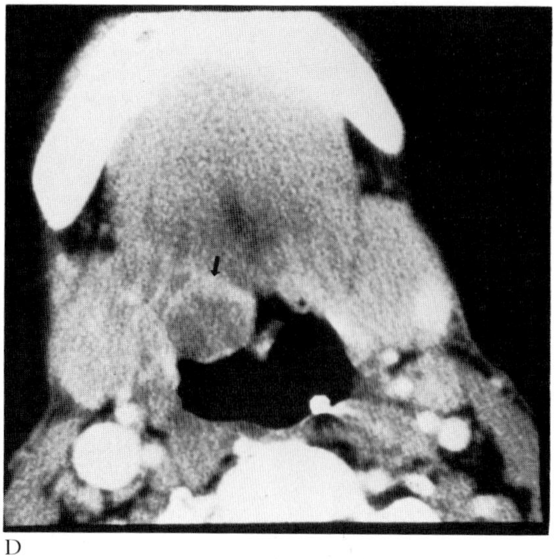

D

Figure 10-8. (continued) D. The same patient later developed a recurrence in the base of the tongue (arrow). *1* = hyoid bone; *2* = preepiglottic space.

Figure 10-9. CT scan, chest (level of upper sternum). This 61-year-old patient had an obstructive laryngeal carcinoma that required an emergency tracheotomy. Following the failure of full-course radiation therapy, a total laryngectomy was performed. Within 8 months of surgery, she developed a peristomal and upper anterior mediastinal recurrence that enveloped the tracheotomy tube.

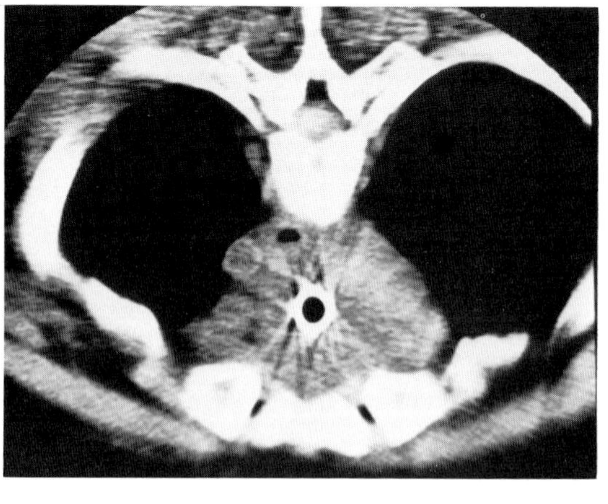

AIRWAY TECHNIQUES

Intubation

Endotracheal intubation is the preferred airway technique for most patients. An adequately inflated endotracheal tube cuff isolates and protect the lower from the upper respiratory system.

Indications

Indications for intubation include significant lower and occasional upper airway obstruction (Tables 10-4 and 10-5) [3].

Table 10-4. The difficult airway: clinical assessment

History
Tracheal stenosis
Maxillofacial trauma
Previous difficult intubation
Preoperative head and neck irradiation
Previous head and neck surgery
Physical examination
Congenital abnormalities
Macroglossia
Micrognathia
Prognathia
Habitus
Obese cervical anatomy
Short, muscular neck
Cervical arthritis or ankylosis
Dental assessment
Loose teeth
Protruding incisors
Long, arched palate
Temporomandibular joint ankylosis
Trismus
Head and neck malignancy
Large oral cavity neoplasm
Large oropharyngeal neoplasm
Marginal airway—associated with large laryngeal, hypopharyngeal, or thyroid malignancy
Anticipated procedure
Panendoscopy
Laser endoscopy
Interstitial implant
Partial laryngectomy
Combined mandibular neck dissection (COMMANDO)

Table 10-5. The difficult airway: objective assessment

Physical examination
Auscultation (neck & chest)
Indirect or direct laryngoscopy
Diagnostic radiology
Soft-tissue films of the neck—AP & lateral
Chest—AP & lateral
CT—neck*
CT—mediastinum*
CT—lungs*
Pulmonary function studies
Arterial blood gases
Flow-volume studies
Spirometry
Fiberoptic laryngoscopy
Laboratory
Complete blood count & differential
Arterial blood gases

*When indicated.

Technique

All head and neck oncologists should be able to intubate, since the potential for emergency airway obstruction exists in all three phases (diagnostics, therapeutics, rehabilitation) of head and neck oncology. Intubation is performed in a controlled environment such as the intensive care unit or operating room (Table 10-6). With the patient placed in the sniffing or neutral anatomic position, a shoulder roll facilitates cervical hyperextension. The straight or Miller blade (battery-operated laryngoscope) is recommended; this blade is invaluable for patients with short, fat, or muscular necks (Figures 10-10 and 10-11). Dentures, mucus, blood, or vomitus is cleared for unobstructed visualization. The operator protects the upper dental arch, holds the laryngoscope with the nondominant hand, and inserts the endotracheal tube with the dominant hand. In an emergency situation, only the most experienced team member intubates. The remainder of the surgical team stands by, if needed, prepared to assist or perform an emergency tracheotomy. With carbon dioxide laser usage, a special fire-resistant endotracheal tube is used.

Table 10-6. The difficult airway: anesthetic technique

Premedication
Mild sedative
Anticholinergic
Induction: awake technique
Nasoendotracheal intubation
Shoulder roll (cervical hyperextension)
Topical nasal & oral anesthesia
Blind versus fiberoptic intubation
Oral-endotracheal intubation
Shoulder roll (cervical hyperextension)
Topical oral anesthesia
Backup
Rigid bronchoscopy
Cricothyrotomy
Tracheotomy

Nasal Intubation

Nasal intubation is the preferred route for unimpeded surgery in the oral cavity. Maxillofacial surgery, mandibulectomy, transoral glossectomy, floor-of-mouth resections, or combined mandibular neck dissection (COMMANDO) procedures are indications for this route.

Oral Intubation

Oral intubation is indicated for patients with anticipated intubation problems, such as those with short, muscular, or fat necks, cervical arthritis, or anteriorly displaced larynges. Nasopharyngoscopy, nasal surgery, and upper maxillofacial surgery are procedures that are indicated for this technique.

Advantage

The advantage of endotracheal intubation is that it requires minimal skill.

Disadvantages

Precipitation of airway obstruction, especially in patients with upper airway lesions, is one disadvantage of intubation (Table 10-7) [4, 5].

Complications

See Table 10-8 for complications of intubation.

Tracheotomy

Tracheotomy is the time-honored standard for a secure, permanent, or semipermanent airway

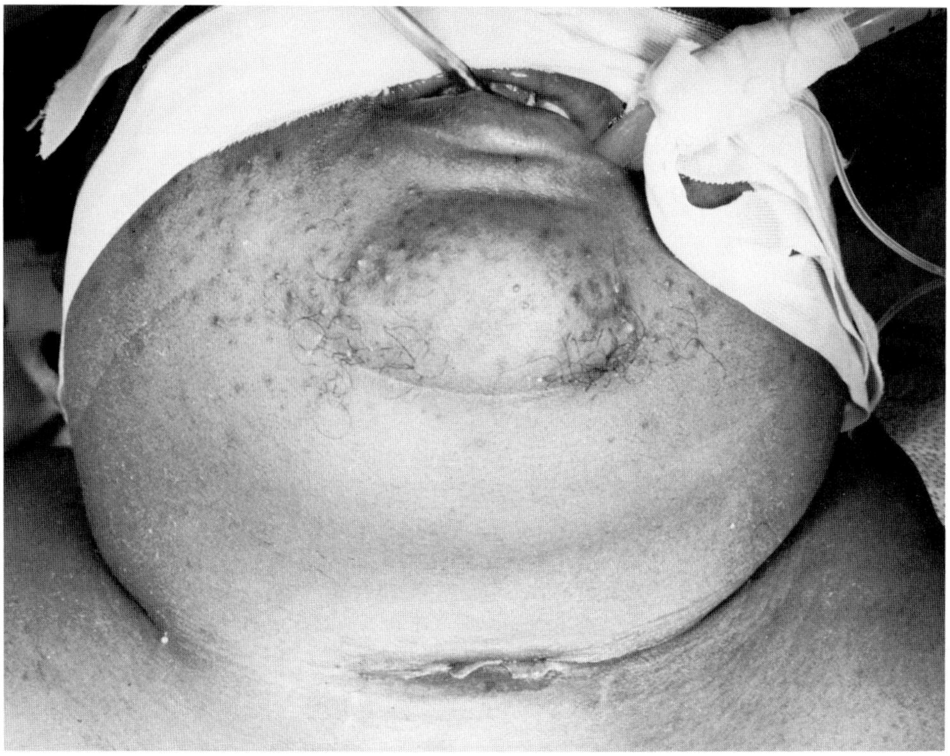

A

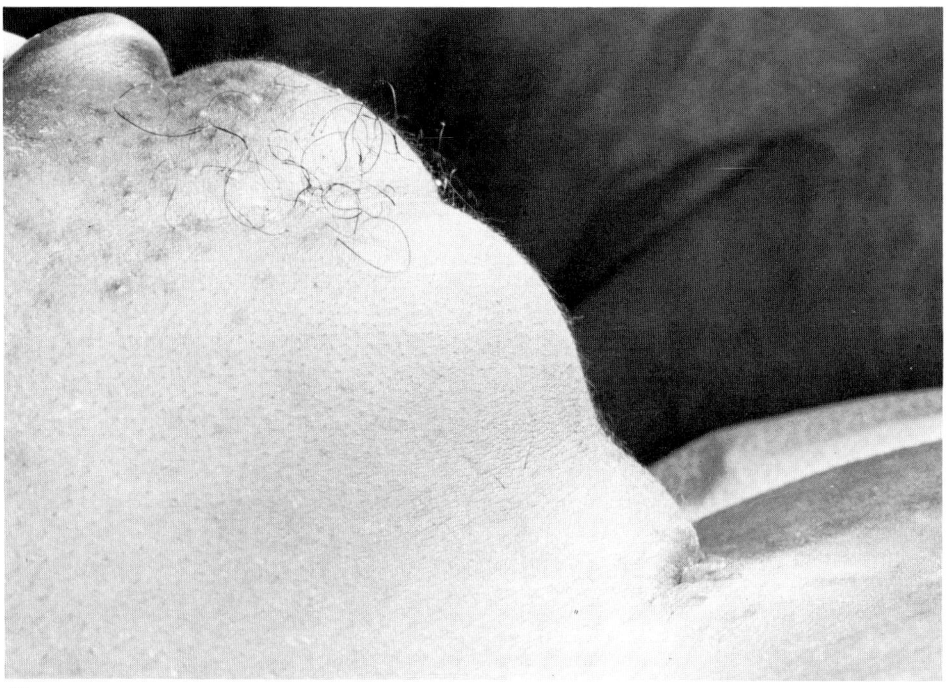

B

Figure 10-10. This patient has two features of a difficult airway: obesity and a short neck. Note the scar from a previous tracheotomy.

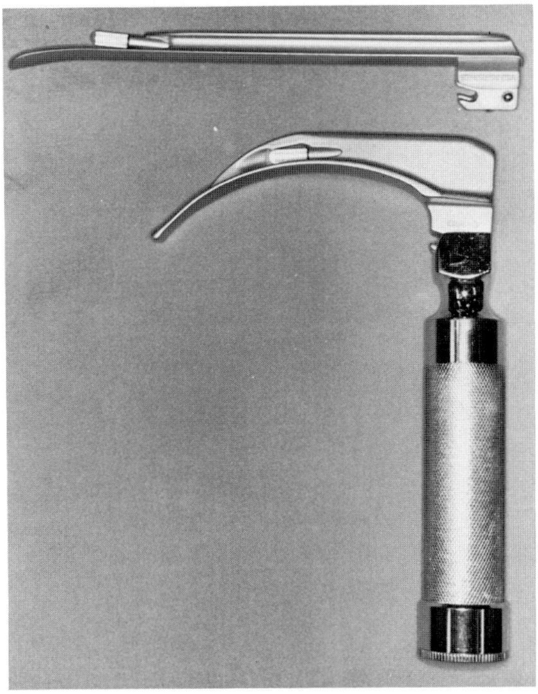

Figure 10-11. The straight (Miller) and curved (MacIntosh) blades for the battery-operated laryngoscope.

Table 10-7. Intubation: disadvantages

Requires constant tube position (assessment above the carina)
- 23 cm from the teeth in men
- 21 cm from the teeth in women

Altered respiratory physiology
- Diminished cough
  - Increased secretions
  - Mucus plugs
- Increased airway resistance (notable with small-diameter tubes)
  - Increases significantly in patients with respiratory insufficiency
  - Increased work of breathing
  - Predisposition for bronchospasm or laryngospasm

[6, 7]. Prior to surgery, a preoperative anesthesiology assessment is invaluable. A chart review may reveal coagulopathy, respiratory compromise, poorly controlled diabetes mellitus, or other potential problems. Ideally, these conditions are stabilized or treated prior to surgery. Tracheotomy is performed, if possible, over an endotracheal tube or rigid bronchoscope, in the operating room. In some emergency situations,

Table 10-8. Intubation: complications

Site	*Acute Complications*	*Chronic Complications*
Oropharynx	Tooth avulsion Tonsil laceration Tongue laceration Palate laceration	Pneumonitis secondary to foreign body Cleft tongue
Hypopharynx	Perforation	Cleft palate Cervical emphysema Pneumothorax Pneumomediastinum Mediastinitis
Supraglottis & glottis	Laceration Cord edema Cord abrasion Arytenoid dislocation	Supraglottic stenosis Polyps Granulomas Cord fusion
Subglottis	Tracheoesophageal perforation Mucosal abrasion	Tracheoesophageal fistula Tracheoesophageal space abscess Mucositis, chondritis, subglottic stenosis Tracheitis Tracheomalacia Tracheal ring necrosis

an endotracheal tube is a luxury, and preoperative intubation may be hazardous. At Howard University Hospital, the overwhelming majority of patients for tracheotomy are evaluated and monitored intraoperatively by the anesthesiologist. Such collaboration has decreased perioperative morbidity.

Indications

Indications for tracheotomy include significant upper and occasional lower airway obstruction.

Technique

Although this procedure usually is performed under local anesthesia, monitoring by the anesthesia service is encouraged, especially for the unstable patient [8]. The patient is placed on a shoulder-roll for hyperextension (Figure 10-12). With the anxious patient, the head is elevated 30 degrees. Oxygen is administered by nasal cannula throughout the procedure. Lidocaine, 1% with or without epinephrine, is infiltrated two fingerbreadths above the suprasternal notch. The surgeon wears an operating headlight to ensure maximum visualization. A horizontal incision is preferred; this incision may be extended for additional exposure and does not compromise future head and neck incisions. In the extreme emergency situation, a slash tracheotomy is performed through a midline incision to prevent transection of the anterior jugular veins. If these veins are injured, troublesome bleeding further aggravates an already grave situation. Regardless of the skin incision, the strap muscles are incised vertically in the midline and retracted laterally to expose the thyroid isthmus. The isthmus is divided or mobilized to uncover the trachea. Lidocaine is injected transtracheally to attenuate the cough reflex. After immobilization with a trachea hook, the trachea is incised vertically between the second and third rings. This location is ideal, since high or low placement is associated with cricoid chondritis or innominate artery hemorrhage respectively. U-shaped incisions or partial ring excisions are discouraged, since these maneuvers predispose stenosis. Next, the opening is widened by an obturator or dilator. Prior to insertion, the tracheotomy cuff is tested. The appropriate size tube is atraumatically inserted, sutured, and tied securely (cervical hyperflexion) to prevent accidental decannulation (Table 10-9).

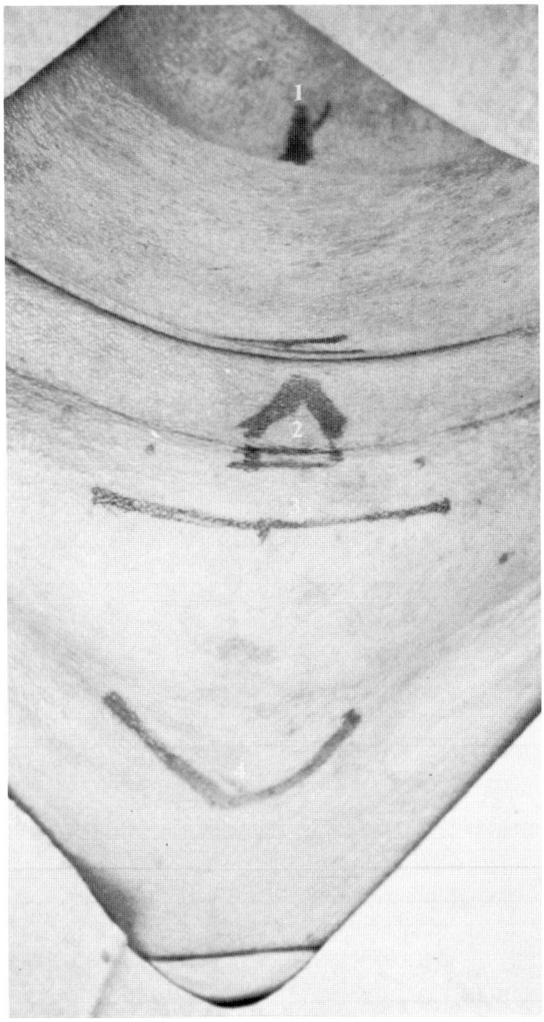

A

High tracheotomy or cricothyroidotomy is encouraged by some authors to establish an emergency airway [9–12]. A horizontal incision is placed in the avascular cricothyroid membrane, avoiding the anterior jugular veins and thyroid gland. In some emergency situations, cricothyroidectomy with a large-bore (14-gauge) venous catheter may suffice; however, in a cardiac arrest, this is inadequate. Some patients with large hypopharyngeal or trans-

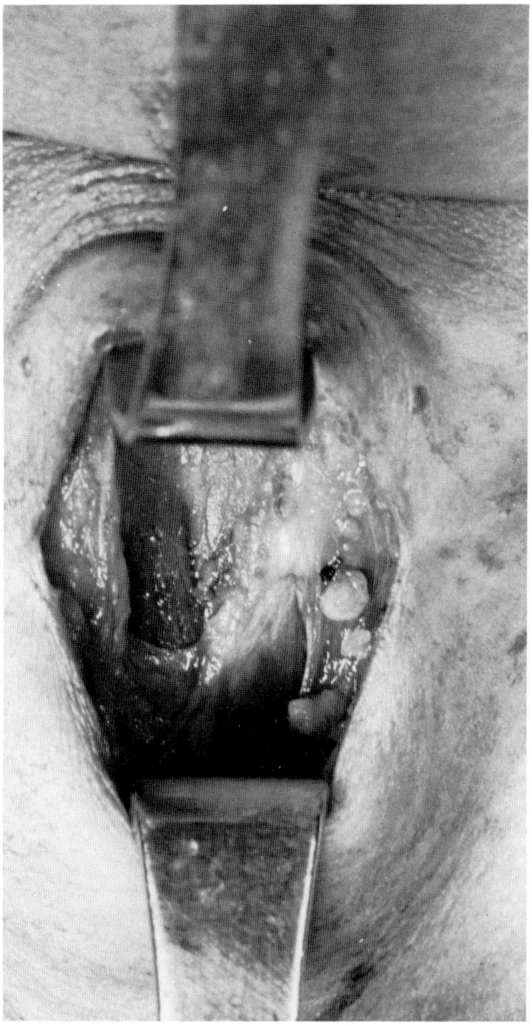

B

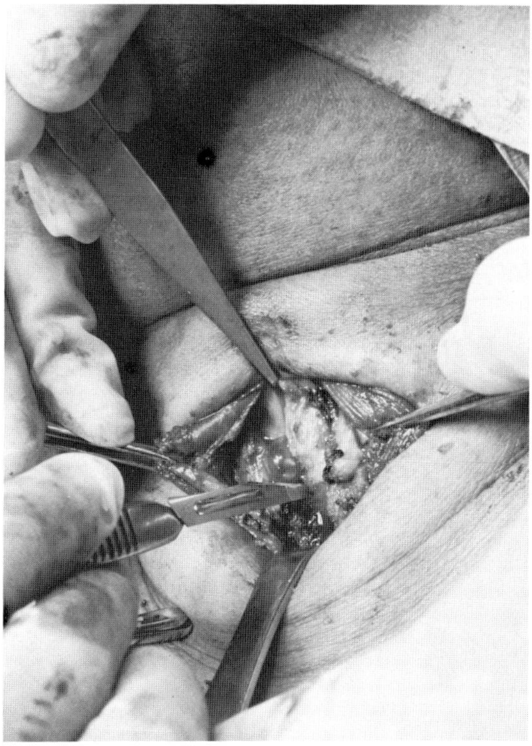

C

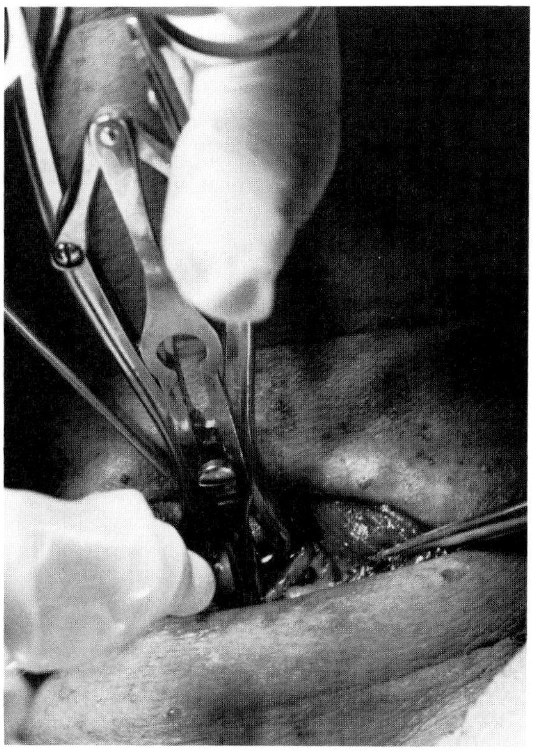

D

Figure 10-12. Tracheotomy. A. The patient is placed in cervical hypertension. *1* = hyoid bone; *2* = thyroid notch; *3* = proposed incision; *4* = suprasternal notch. B. The strap muscles are exposed and divided in the midline. C. The tracheotomy is entered sharply. D. Utilizing a dilator, the trachea is entered gently.

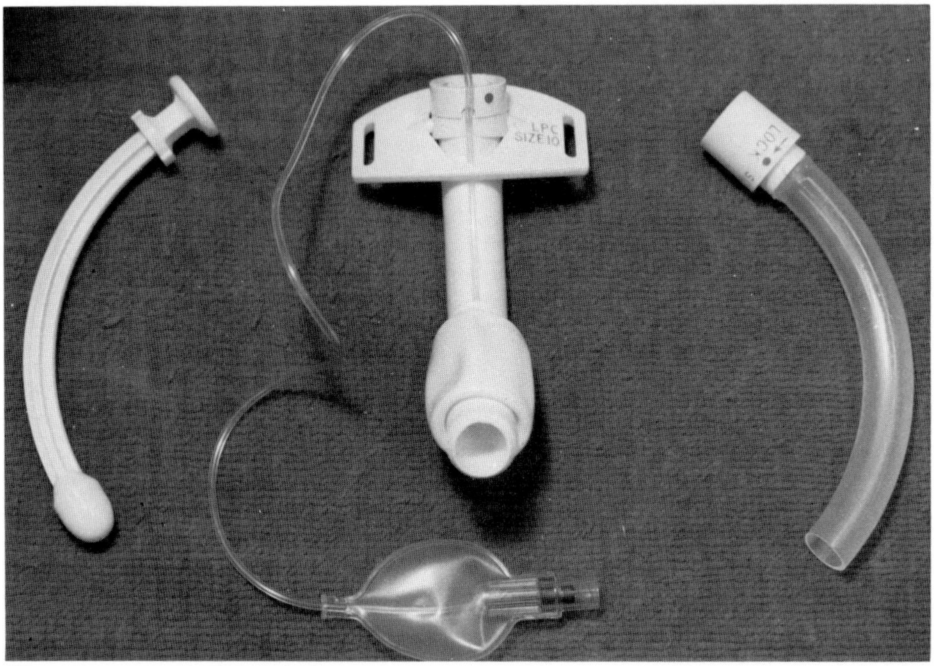

E

Figure 10-12. (continued) E. Typical Silastic tracheotomy tube with (*left to right*) obturator, outer tube with cuff, and inner cannula.

Table 10-9. Tracheotomy general orders

1. 40% oxygen via tracheotomy collar for humidification.
2. Deflate the cuff (if not on a respirator).
3. If the patient is on a respirator, inflate the cuff no greater than 5 cc of air.
4. Deflate the cuff 5 minutes each hour if the patient is on the respirator.
5. Do not change the tracheotomy ties for 72 hours.
6. Daily wound toilet; change the tracheotomy pad as needed.
7. Postoperative chest AP & lateral x-ray (optional).
8. Place the tracheotomy obturator at the bedside.
9. Inspect the tracheotomy site thoroughly if bleeding occurs.
10. Change the tracheotomy tube in 72 hours.

glottic tumors have invasion of the cricothyroid membrane. In general, cricothyroidotomy is discouarged as a definitive airway for the head and neck oncology patient.

Advantage

The advantage of tracheotomy is that it provides a quickly executed, definitive airway after endotracheal intubation and rigid bronchoscopy.

Disadvantage

The disadvantage of tracheotomy is that it requires a moderate degree of surgical skill.

Complications

See Table 10-10 for complications of tracheotomy [4, 8].

Carbon Dioxide Laser

The carbon dioxide laser precisely and bloodlessly vaporizes small lower respiratory lesions. For select patients, it is highly effective in establishing an airway. The primary destructive

Table 10-10. Tracheotomy complications

Immediate
Hemorrhage
Pneumothorax
Pneumomediastinum
Tracheoesophageal fistula
Recurrent largyngeal nerve injury
Immediate (<10 days)
Hemorrhage
Infection
Aspiration
Pneumonia
Late
Hemorrhage
Tracheal stenosis
Stomal recurrence
Tracheoesophageal fistula
Tracheomalacia

effect is thermal energy. The degree of tissue destruction is proportional to tissue absorption and is dependent on power density (watts per square centimeter), exposure (duration), power (watts), and water content. The laser photocoagulates and seals small vessels. With large bulky lesions, a serviceable airway is created, eliminating the need for a tracheotomy [12, 13].

Limitations

The carbon dioxide laser requires direct visualization and a dry field. Vessels greater than 0.5 mm are poorly coagulated.

Technique

Laser therapy is performed following intubation or percutaneous transtracheal ventilation. Endotracheal intubation requires a special fire-resistant tube. The laser, coupled with the microscope, is set in the continuous mode (5–15 watts), depending on tumor size and location (Figures 10-13 and 10-14). The following guidelines are recommended:

WATTS	LESION
5	Nodular lesions
5–10	Polypoid lesions
10–20	Bulky lesions
20–30	Tongue lesions

Precautions

The laser requires diligent precautions to prevent ignition and burns [14]. Although the laser is a precise instrument, it potentially is hazardous. The following protocols are recommended:

Nursing Protocol

1. Check the permit.
2. Make sure all personnel have goggles or glasses.
3. Check the laser for adequate nitrogen, carbon dioxide, and helium levels.
4. The following items must be in the operating room:
   a. Tracheotomy set.
   b. Bronchoscopy set.
   c. Microscope with 400-mm lens.
   d. Cottonoid sponges.
   e. Cold normal saline.
   f. Dexamethasone.
   g. Eye pads.
5. Place moist cloth towels over the entire face.
6. Do not insert the key until the surgeon orders laser activation.

Anesthesiology Protocol

1. The endotracheal tube must be fire-resistant.
2. The cuff is inflated with methylene blue; this alerts the surgeon if the cuff is ruptured.
3. Use only noncombustible anesthetic agents.
4. Dexamethasone (Decadron) always is available to prevent laryngeal edema.

Surgeon's Protocol

1. Check the endotracheal tube flammability with a laser pulse.
2. Check carbon dioxide and helium beam alignment (tongue blade).
3. Check for beam spot size.
4. Check the wattage.
5. Check the duration.
6. Check the foot pedal.

Complications

Ignition is the most dreaded complication of the carbon dioxide laser (Table 10-11) [15–18].

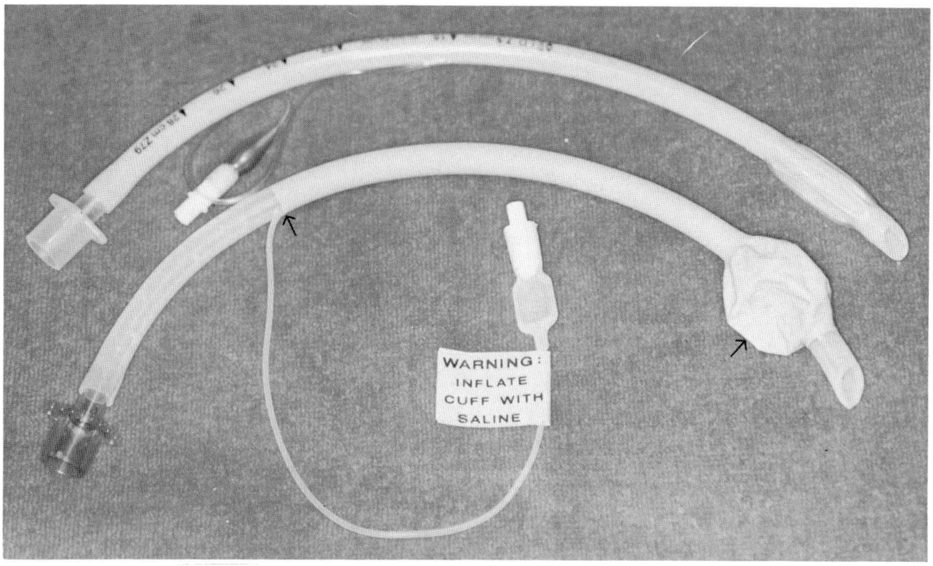

Figure 10-13. Top: Ordinary Silastic endotracheal tube. Bottom: protected, laser-resistant (*arrows*) endotracheal tube.

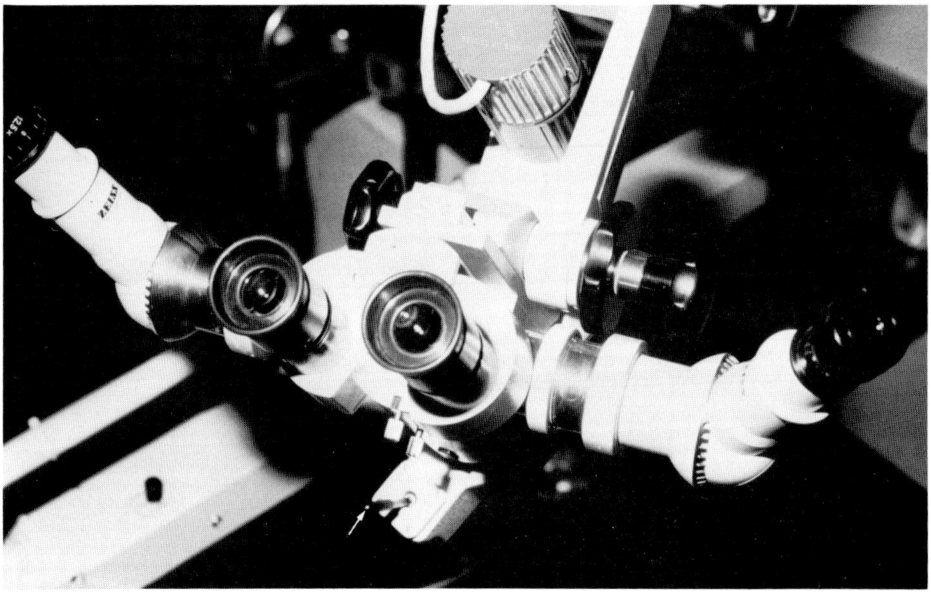

A

Figure 10-14. Carbon dioxide laser with microscope. A. The arrow denotes the joystick that guides the co-axial helium beam on the target.

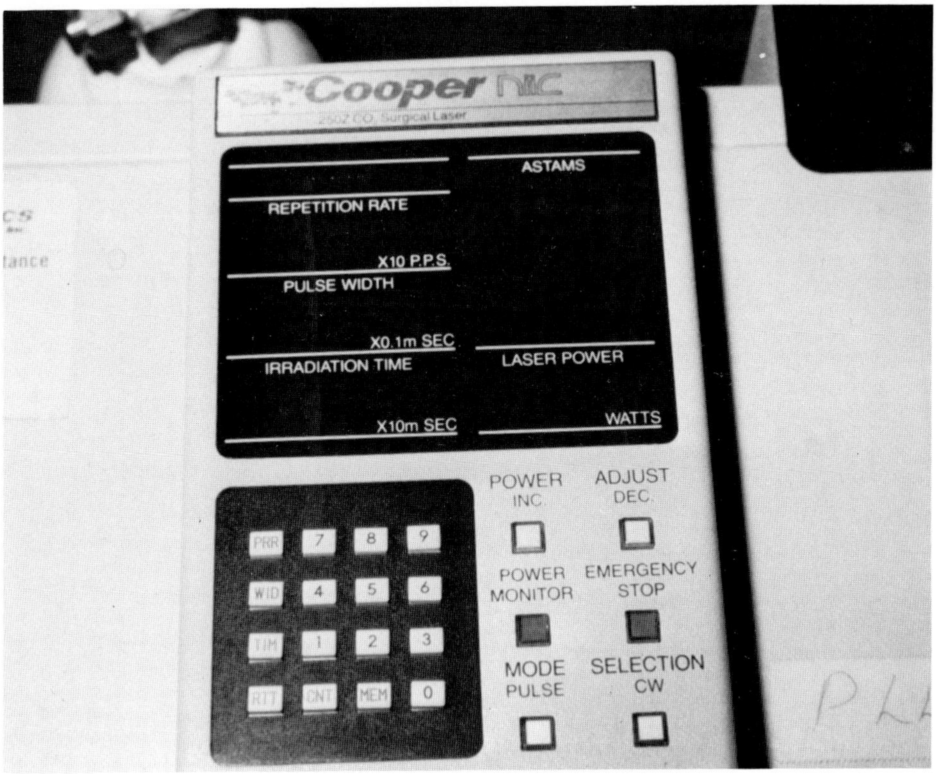

B

Figure 10-14. (continued) B. Laser console with self-monitoring microprocessor.

Table 10-11. Laser complications

Immediate
Facial skin burn(s)
Retinal burn(s)
Mucosal burn(s)
Endotracheal tube cuff laceration
Cottonoid ignition
Endotracheal tube ignition
Pneumothorax
Intermediate
Burns (reflecting surface)
Mucosal char with airway obstruction
Hemorrhage
Edema
Late
Glottic web
Glottic incompetence
Dysphonia

Should a fire ensue, the following emergency measures are recommended:

1. Immediately discontinue the oxygen.
2. Douse the flames.
3. Extubate immediately.
4. Ventilate by mask with 100% room air.
5. Reintubate, carefully.
6. Laryngoscopy and bronchoscopy.
7. Other measures:
   a. Bronchodilators.
   b. Humidification.
   c. Tracheobronchial lavage.
   d. Positive end-expiratory pressure (PEEP).
   e. Steroids.
   f. Antibiotics.

VENTILATION

After the establishment of an airway, some head and neck cancer patients require ventilatory assistance. Ventilation is the movement of ambient air into the body and its distribution throughout the tracheobranchial system for effective alveolar gas exchange [19].

Basic Mechanical Ventilation

Goals

Mechanical ventilation is machine-assisted maintenance of oxygenation and carbon dioxide exchange. Mechanical ventilators prevent lung deterioration by maintaining lung volume and they support alveolar ventilation by various positive pressure techniques (e.g., PEEP) [20]. Finally, ventilators maximize oxygen transport and correct hypoxemia.

Continuous Mandatory Ventilation

Continuous mandatory ventilation (CMV) is positive pressure breathing at fixed intervals. It usually is indicated intraoperatively and immediately postoperatively. CMV may require sedation and muscle relaxation.

Assist-Control Mechanical Ventilation

Assist-control mechanical ventilation (ACMV) is intermittent positive breathing triggered by the patient. ACMV reverts to CMV if the spontaneous respiratory rate is less than the desired preset rate.

Intermittent Mandatory Ventilation

Intermittent mandatory ventilation (IMV) is a predetermined rate of positive pressure breaths interspersed with spontaneous breathing. Its advantages include avoidance of respiratory alkalosis, minimal sedation, and prevention of respiratory muscle atrophy. Its disadvantages are carbon dioxide retention and increased work of breathing.

Pressure Support Ventilation

In pressure support ventilation (PSV), spontaneous breathing effort triggers the ventilator to increase flow to a preselected level above baseline pressure. While it decreases the work of breathing, its disadvantage is air trapping, especially in patients with chronic obstructive pulmonary disease.

Settings

Table 10-12 outlines the basic parameters for mechanical ventilation. The ventilator mode and settings are selected to optimize respiration and minimize complications. With any chosen technique, three basic components are altered: inspiratory phase (flow rate, pause), tidal volume (or frequency), and expiratory phase.

Oxygen Concentration

Oxygen concentration (F_{IO_2}) is 21 to 100 percent; it is usually less than 50 percent to avoid the side effects of oxygen toxicity.

Tidal Volume

Tidal volume is the volume delivered during a normal ventilator breath.

Respiratory Rate

Respiratory rate is the rate or frequency of tidal volume breaths, usually 12 to 14 per minute; it is adjusted according to $PaCO_2$ or pH.

Sensitivity

Sensitivity is the ventilator's response or lack of response to patient effort.

Pressure

CONTINUOUS POSITIVE AIRWAY PRESSURE

Continuous positive airway pressure (CPAP) is maintenance of constant inspiratory and expiratory pressure to overcome air resistance (stiff

Table 10-12. Mechanical ventilation: indications

Mechanical parameters
Respiratory rate > 35/minute
Vital capacity < 15 cc/kg
$FEV_1 < 10$ cc/kg
Inspiratory force < -25 mm Hg
Oxygenation parameters
QS/QT $> 20\%$
PaO_2 (mask) < 70 mm Hg
Ventilation parameters
$PaCO_2 > 55$ mm Hg
$V_D/V_T > .06$

lungs, endotracheal tubes) and maintain functional residual capacity (FRC) *without* mechanical ventilation.

POSITIVE END-EXPIRATORY PRESSURE

Positive end-expiratory pressure (PEEP) is maintenance of constant inspiratory and expiratory positive pressures to maintain FRC *with* mechanical ventilation.

MANIPULATION

By varying the various settings and modes, the arterial PO_2, PCO_2, and ph are adjusted:

DESIRED EFFECT	PARAMETER
↓ PCO_2	↑ Minute ventilation
	↑ Respiratory rate
↑ PCO_2	↓ Minute ventilation sedation
	↑ Ventilator dead space
↑ PO_2	↑ FIO_2
	↑ PEEP

High-Frequency Ventilation

High-frequency ventilation techniques, supervised by the anesthesiologist, are based on high cycling rates (frequency) coupled with low tidal volume [21].

Special Ventilatory Techniques

High-Frequency Positive Pressure Ventilation

In high-frequency positive pressure ventilation (HFPPV), positive pressure is generated greater than 60 breaths/minute in a low compliance circuit.

High-Frequency Jet Ventilation (HFJV)

SANDERS JET

The Sanders jet is a hand-held system that delivers oxygen or anesthesia into the trachea through a small catheter placed just above the carina (110–440 breaths/minute). The primary advantage is its use with laser endoscopy; the main disadvantage is transient or persistent hypercarbia.

PERCUTANEOUS TRANSTRACHEAL JET VENTILATION

Percutaneous transtracheal jet ventilation (PTV) is a hand-held system that delivers oxygen and anesthesia through a needle inserted percutaneously into the cricothyroid membrane [8, 9]. PTV is performed in the operating room by an anesthesiologist familiar with the technique. Special training and equipment are required.

High-Frequency Oscillation

High-frequency oscillation (HFO) is continuous movement of volume by to-and-fro motion as carbon dioxide is removed by either soda lime or a bypass circuit; oxygen flows in at a rate consistent with metabolism.

Indications

High-frequency ventilation techniques are interim means of establishing and maintaining ventilation prior to laser laryngoscopy or tracheotomy. They may also be utilized for repair of bronchopleural cutaneous fistula, tracheal reconstruction, and lung transplantation.

Advantage

High-frequency ventilation techniques are simple lifesaving measures performed prior to the establishment of a long-term airway.

Disadvantage

The disadvantage of high-frequency ventilation is that the necessary equipment and skills are not readily available.

Complications

Complications include subcutaneous emphysema and cervical hematomas.

Weaning

Gradual removal or weaning from mechanical ventilation begins by lowering the IMV and the PEEP (minimum 5 cm H_2O). The minimal support prior to extubation is 5 cm H_2O CPAP or IMV of 2 breaths/minute. The rate of weaning depends on clinical assessment, sequential arterial blood gases, and the duration of mechanical ventilation (Table 10-13).

AIRWAY STRATEGY

Steroids

Powerful steroids such as dexamethasone are invaluable in stabilizing an obstructed patient before establishing a definitive diagnosis. When

Table 10-13. Decannulation or extubation

Clinical assessment
Return to baseline mental status
Elimination of anesthetics and muscle relaxants
Ventilatory assessment
Vital capacity > 15 cc/kg
Peak inspiratory force > −25 cm H_2O
$V_D/V_T < 0.6$
$A\text{-}aDO_2 < 300$ mm Hg with FIO_2 1.0

the patient has acute airway obstruction, steroids and oxygen are given immediately. Utilizing these measures, a marginal airway may be established. This permits unhurried diagnosis to determine whether the obstruction is in the upper or lower airway. Fiberoptic laryngoscopy, soft-tissue lateral films of the neck, and chest x-ray usually locate the site of obstruction.

Upper Versus Lower Airway Obstruction

Once the location, upper versus lower, is identified, airway management is much clearer (Table 10-14; Figure 10-15). Upper airway obstruction is managed usually by tracheotomy, proceeded by intubation, bronchoscopy, or PTV; tracheotomy is safer over an established airway. In patients who have lower airway obstruction, PTV or intubation, followed by laser laryngoscopy, is a possibility. However, these measures may be impractical or even dangerous. Therefore, a tracheotomy is performed forthrightly for the difficult case.

Intubation and Laser Therapy

Intubation is successful for most lower airway obstructions; however, at times it is abandoned for bronchoscopy or emergency tracheotomy. An adjunct to intubation is laser therapy [18]. Successful intubation of a lower airway obstruction followed by laser treatment is ideal and logical management for many patients. Most patients can be extubated within 24 hours after laser surgery.

Tracheotomy

Tracheotomy is performed in a controlled environment, such as the operating room, unless an emergency situation dictates otherwise. If tracheotomy is unsuccessful, especially with lower airway obstruction, bronchoscopy is attempted. When the obstruction is distal to the proposed tracheotomy site (carina or bronchus), laser bronchoscopy is recommended.

Postoperative Care

Chapters 11 and 18 discuss respiratory care in

Table 10-14. Management: site versus technique

Site[a]	*Intubation*	*Laser*	*Tracheotomy*
Upper Airway			
5. Oral cavity	2	3	1
6. Oropharynx	2	3	1
Lower Airway			
7. Hypopharynx	3	2	1
8. Larynx			
Supraglottis	2	1	3
Glottis	2	1	3
Subglottis	2	1	3
9. Thyroids/parathyroids	2	3	1
10. Cervical esophagus	3	2[b]	1

1 First choice.
2 Second choice.
3 Third choice.
[a]Sites 1 through 4 are omitted, since they rarely present with airway obstruction.
[b]May require laser bronchoscopy.

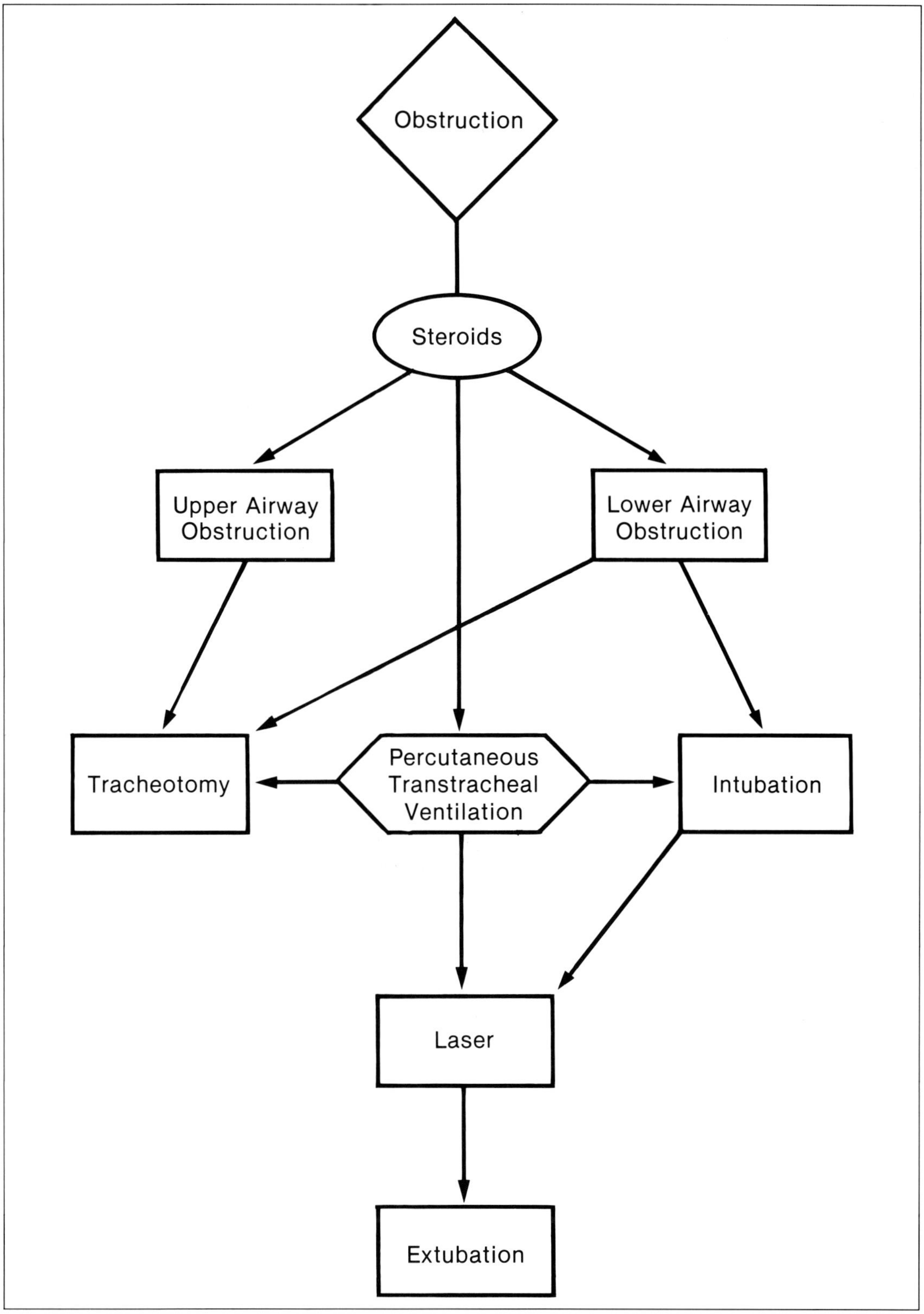

Figure 10-15. Airway strategy.

detail; however, the general guidelines are as follows:

1. Oxygenation and humidification.
2. Sterile suctioning.
3. Intermittent positive pressure breathing or respirator.
4. Sequential arterial blood gases.

Post-Airway Pulmonary Edema

Post-airway pulmonary edema is a phenomenon encountered in a patient with long-standing airway obstruction who is relieved acutely by an artificial airway. The patient with chronic obstruction disease seems especially susceptible. Such a complication is best handled in the intensive care unit by mechanical ventilation, diuretics, and PEEP.

Decannulation

Endotracheal Tube

Once the airway is established (after steroid or laser surgery), the patient is decannulated. Immediately after decannulation, the patient is observed carefully and followed with sequential arterial blood gases. If there is any question of airway compromise, fiberoptic or indirect laryngoscopy is performed.

Tracheotomy Tube

For most patients, tracheotomy is indicated for permanent or long-term airway management. The patient is considered for decannulation for the following reasons: (1) reversal or elimination of the original indication for the tracheotomy, (2) decreased secretions, (3) reversal of coma, and (4) discontinuation of mechanical ventilation.

If the attending or consulting physician is reticent, the patient is decannulated gradually. The usual protocol is to downsize every 24 hours (No. 6 Shiley to No. 4 Shiley) and then decannulate. This conservative approach is preferable to immediate extubation, especially after normal duty hours or over the weekend.

Immediate decannulation is considered if the patient (1) is alert, (2) has an excellent cough, and (3) has fiberoptic or laryngoscopic documentation of clear upper or lower airways. As the tube is removed, the patient is suctioned sterilely. A clean gauze sponge is secured to the tracheotomy site with tape. The patient is instructed not to cough or talk without occluding the tracheotomy site. Tracheotomy site occlusion enhances spontaneous closure by secondary intention. The site is cleansed daily with hydrogen peroxide.

REFERENCES

1. Balk R, Bone RC: Classification of acute respiratory failure. *Med Clin North Am* 67 : 551, 1986.
2. Alonzo GE, Dantzker DR: Respiratory failure, mechanism of abnormal gas exchange and oxygen delivery. *Med Clin North Am* 67 : 517, 1983.
3. Deane RS, Mills EL: Prolonged nasotracheal intubation in adults: A successor and adjunct to tracheotomy. *Anesth Analg* 49 : 89, 1970.
4. Myers EM: Hypopharyngeal perforation: A complication of traumatic intubation. *Laryngoscope* 92 : 5, 1982.
5. Whitted RE: A study of post-intubation laryngeal dysfunction. *Laryngoscope* 95 : 727, 1986.
6. Forst EAM: Tracing the tracheotomy. *Ann Otol Rhinol Laryngol* 85 : 618, 1976.
7. Jackson C: Tracheotomy. *Surg Clin North Am* 15 : 117, 1935.
8. Dayal VS, Masri WE: Tracheostomy in intensive care setting. *Laryngoscope* 96 : 58, 1986.
9. Brantigen CO, Grow JB: Cricothyroidotomy: Elective use in respiratory problems requiring tracheotomy. *J Thorac Cardiovasc Surg* 71 : 72, 1976.
10. Smith RB, et al: Percutaneous transtracheal ventilation for anesthesia and resuscitation: A review and report of complications. *Can Anaesth Soc J* 22 : 607, 1975.
11. Smith RB: Transtracheal ventilation during anesthesia. *Anaesth Analg* 55 : 225, 1974.
12. Strong MS, et al: Transoral resection of cancer of the oral cavity: The role of the CO_2 laser. *Otolaryngol Clin North Am* 12 : 107, 1979.
13. Myers EM, Ogura JH: Stomal recurrences: A clinicopathological analysis. *Laryngoscope* 89 : 112, 1979.
14. Healy GB, et al: Complications of CO_2 laser surgery of the aero-digestive tract: Experience of 4416 cases. *Otolaryngol Head Neck Surg* 93 : 13, 1984.
15. Schramm VL, Mattor DE, Stool SE: Acute management of laser ignited intratracheal explosion. *Laryngoscope* 91 : 1417, 1981.
16. Annyas AA, et al: CO_2 laser in malignant lesions of the larynx. *Laryngoscope* 94 : 836, 1984.

17. Geffin B, et al: Flammability of endotracheal tubes during ND-Yag laser applications in the airway. *Anesthesiology* 65 : 511, 1986.
18. Golden L, Myers EM: CO_2 laser for obstructive laryngeal and hypopharyngeal malignancies. Submitted for publication.
19. Bone RC, Stober G: Mechanical ventilation in respiratory failure. *Med Clin North Am* 67 : 599, 1983.
20. Popvich J: The physiology of mechanical ventilation and the mechanical zoo: IPPB, PEEP, CPAP. *Med Clin North Am* 67 : 621, 1983.
21. Gallagher TJ: High frequency ventilation. *Med Clin North Am* 67 : 633, 1983.

11

Anesthesia

CHERYL R. BURRUSS, SANDRA J. REED, LAWRENCE D. MASON, and ERNEST M. MYERS

KEY CONCEPTS

Respiratory Function, Cardiovascular Function, Thyroid Function, Hepatic Function, Renal Function, Diabetes Mellitus, Fluids, Transfusions

MILESTONES

700 A.D.	"Sweet Vitriol" (Ether)	Lullius
1667	Discovery of Blood Transfusion	Ottenberg
1772	Nitrous Oxide	Priestley
1792	Ether	Frobenius
1798	Nitrous Oxide for Anesthesia	Davy
1806	Morphine	Serturner
1831–32	Chloroform	Guthrie, Soubeiran, Liebig
1846	Ether, First Public Operation	Morton, Wells
1847	Chloroform Obstetrical Anesthesia	Simpson
1860	Cocaine	Nieman
1880	Nitrous Oxide Obstetrical Anesthesia	Klikovicki
1881	Morphine Induction	Crombil
1884	Cocaine Local Anesthesia	Koller
1885	Spinal Anesthesia	Corning
1899	Bier Lumbar Anesthesia	Bier
	Belladonna and Morphine Induction	Korff
1901	Red Blood Cell Typing	Landsteiner
1905	Novocain	Einhorn, Braun
1908	Blood Typing Before Transfusion	Ottenberg
1923	Ethylene	Luckhardt, Carter
1937	American Board of Anesthesia	Dripps, Eichenhoff
1941	Systematic Blood Transfusions	Drew

The anesthetic management of the head and neck cancer patient requires close cooperation between the anesthesiologist and surgeon. Many of these patients are middle-aged or elderly and have multiple medical problems that must be assessed and stabilized carefully prior to general anesthesia. Moreover, most procedures require airway "sharing" by both anesthesiologist and surgeon (see Chapter 10). Major head and neck ablation and reconstruction often are associated with blood loss, fluid replacement, and postoperative mechanical ventilation. Collectively, multiple medical problems, airway management, and fluid resuscitation underscore the necessary cooperation of both disciplines for safe, uneventful patient management of the head and neck (Figures 11-1 and 11-2).

This chapter discusses the anesthesia preoperative evaluation and preparation and perioperative management of the head and neck cancer patient. Discussion of other disease states is beyond the scope of this chapter.

RESPIRATORY FUNCTION

Overview

Many head and neck oncology patients have chronic pulmonary problems stemming from a long history of smoking. These may be compounded by other risks that impact detrimentally on pulmonary function: (1) past thoracic and abdominal surgery, (2) musculoskeletal deformity, (3) morbid obesity, (4) heavy smoking and chronic cough, (5) history of pulmonary disease, or (6) cardiovascular disease.

Figure 11-1. Anesthesia machine.

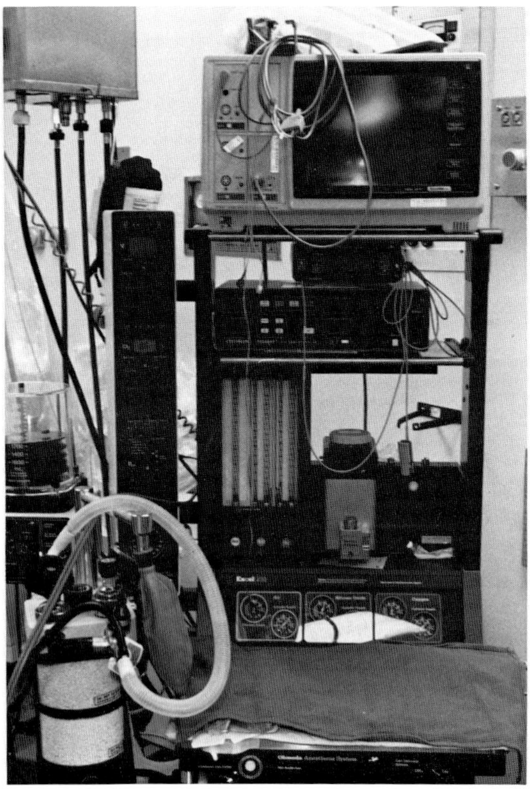

Obstructive Lung Disease

Obstructive lung disease is characterized by decreases in expiratory flow rates (dependent on airway resistance), elastic recoil, and muscular strength. The bedside assessment of expiratory flow includes (1) the ratio of inspiration to expiration (I/E), (2) maximal expiration of forced vital capacity, and (3) adventitial breath sounds (wheezes, rales, rhonchi).

I/E Ratio

The normal I/E ratio is 1 : 2, with expiration including both true expiratory time and apnea. As the patient breathes, the pattern is observed closely. If the ratio decreases (e.g., 1 : 4, 1 : 5), expiration is prolonged clinically, thus implicating obstruction.

Forced Expiratory Time

The volume of air expired either slowly or forcefully from maximal inspiration is the vital capacity (VC). The time to forcibly exhale VC is the forced expiratory time (FET); it is normally less than 3 or 4 seconds. FET greater than 4 seconds indicates increased airway resistance, poor elastic recoil, or abnormal neuromuscular integrity.

Overinflation

On physical examination, many obstructive lung disease patients have increased residual volumes characterized by barrel-chested thoraces and lowered diaphragms. This is indicative of chronic overinflation (air trapping).

Restrictive Lung Disease

The typical restrictive lung disease patient has reduced lung volumes due to an abnormality of the thoracic skeleton, neuromuscular junction, pleura, interstitium, or alveolus. These patients have some combination of the following: diminished skeletal expansion with inspiration, reduced diaphragmatic excursion, and decreased residual volume (Table 11-1).

Vascular Lung Disease

The typical findings of vascular lung disease are right ventricular hypertrophy, palpable pul-

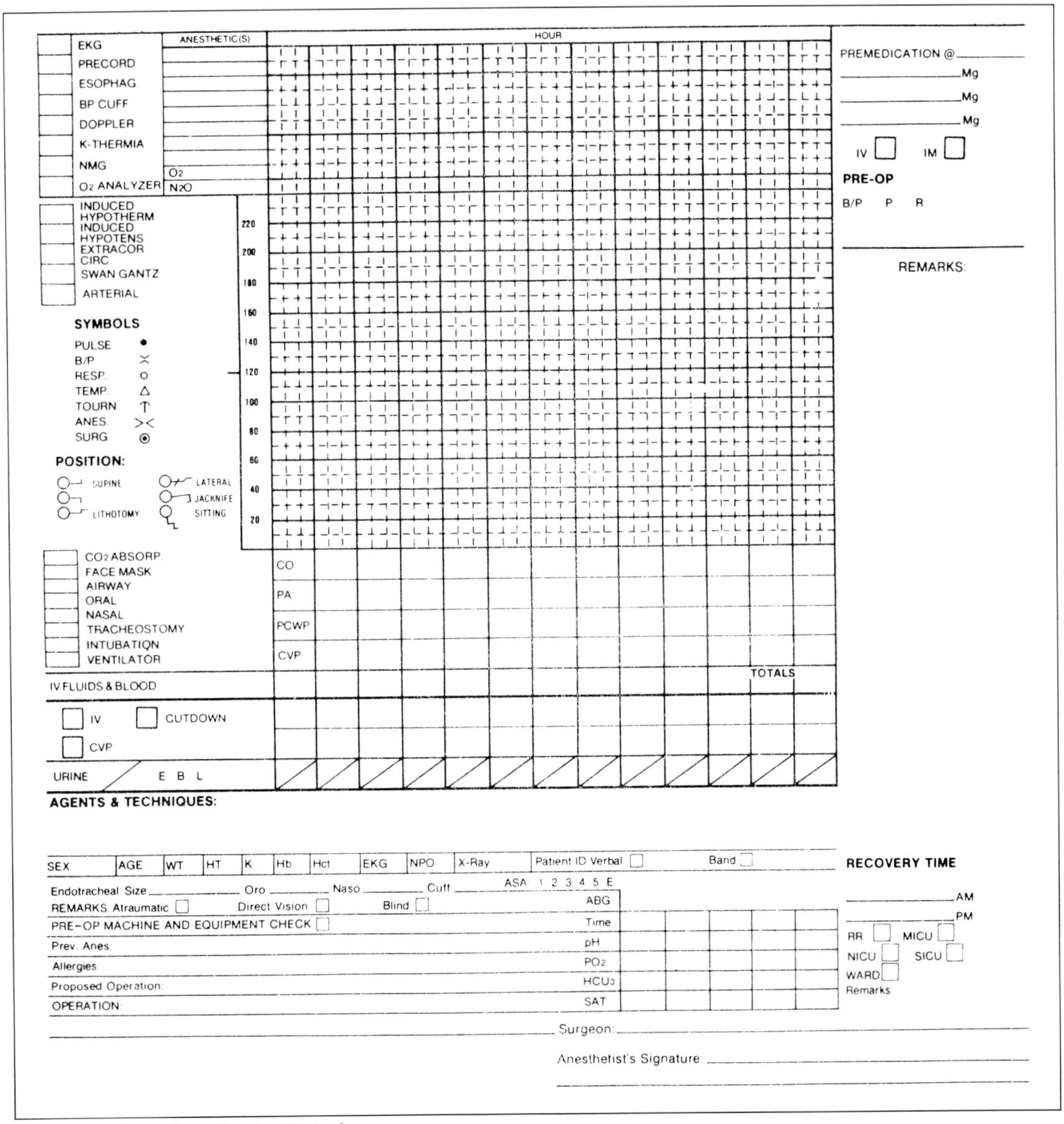

Figure 11-2. Anesthesia clinical report.

Table 11-1. Restrictive lung disease

Component	*Examples*
Thorax (skeletal limitation or restricted expansion)	Kyphoscoliosis, ankylosing spondylitis, rheumatoid arthritis, morbid obesity
Neuromuscular	Diaphragm paralysis, myasthenia gravis, multiple sclerosis, Guillain-Barré syndrome, poliomyelitis
Pleura	Effusion, fibrothorax
Interstitium/alveolus	Pulmonary edema, interstitial fibrosis, diffuse pneumonia, granulomatous disease

monary artery thrill, snappy second heart sound (S_2), prominent pulmonic ejection murmur, and signs of right heart failure. However, in the early asymptomatic patient, the only clue may be dyspnea *without* signs of obstructive or restrictive lung disease. The physical findings of vascular lung disease are corroborated by pulmonary hypertension, primary vascular lung disease (emboli, vasculitis), and cardiac disease (mitral valve disease, left ventricular failure). Pulmonary hypertension may be associated with hypoxemia, hypercapnia, and acidosis.

Assessment

Basically, the preoperative evaluation is an attempt to diagnose and evaluate the three basic lung disease patterns: obstructive, restrictive, and vascular lung disease [1,2]. The evaluation begins with the history and physical examination. Excessive cigarette smoking (> 70 pack years), chronic cough, asthma, and dyspnea are the important historical prognosticators. The physical signs of compromised pulmonary function include rapid (resting) respiratory rate, use of accessory muscles of respiration, forced expiratory time (> 5 seconds), jugular venous distention, and inspiratory paradox.

The preoperative evaluation of patients with potential respiratory compromise has three goals: to define the extent of disease, to assess the degree of anesthetic risk, and to determine reversibility or optimization of pulmonary disease. Arterial blood gas analysis and spirometry are the most cost-effective and informative diagnostic modalities.

Arterial Blood Gases

Although the relationship of abnormal arterial blood gases to perioperative morbidity has been studied extensively, the results are inconclusive. This is a static test that does not measure pulmonary reserve; however, it is performed and interpreted easily. Generally, the values indicative of increased risk are $PaCO_2$ greater than 50 mm Hg and PaO_2 less than 50 mm Hg, with greater emphasis on an abnormal $PaCO_2$ [2].

PaO_2 is not a good prognosticator of postoperative complications. However, patients with resting hypoxemia likely will have further hypoxemia postoperatively because of frequent bed rest with decreased respiratory effort and decreased tidal volume, atelectasis, and decreased ability to clear airway secretions.

$PaCO_2$ identifies those patients with significant obstruction or ventilatory compromise who may develop respiratory failure postoperatively.

Spirometry

Spirometry is indicated when a patient has one of the clinical patterns of lung disease. Utilizing four volumes and four capacities, spirometry objectively measures pulmonary function (Figure 11-3; Tables 11-2 and 11-3). This series of dynamic, simple reliable tests is the best assessment of respiratory reserve. Although it is difficult to assign values that denote risk, the following are generally accepted as poor prognosticators [3]:

Forced vital capacity (FVC) less than 50 percent predicted
Forced expiratory volume ($FEV_{25-75\%}$) less than 50 percent predicted
Forced expiratory volume in 1 second ($FEV_{1.0}$) less than 50 percent predicted or less than 2 liters
Maximum voluntary ventilation (MVV) less than 50 percent predicted or less than 50 liters/minute

Recently, some investigators have emphasized the importance of maximum breathing capacity (MBC = MVV). This is a comprehensive test of ventilatory function that is altered by airway obstruction, elastic properties of the lungs, chest wall compliance, respiratory muscle strength, coordination, and motivation. The normal MBC is 175 liters/minute. An indirect determination of MBC is to multiply FEV (liters/minute) × 35. If the measured MBC is less than this product, patient effort may be suspect. If MBC is less than 50 percent predicted, the patient will not cough effectively postoperatively. If MBC is less than 30 percent, the patient may require intubation to permit suctioning to clear secretions. Still mucus plugging with consequent atelectasis or pneumonia and

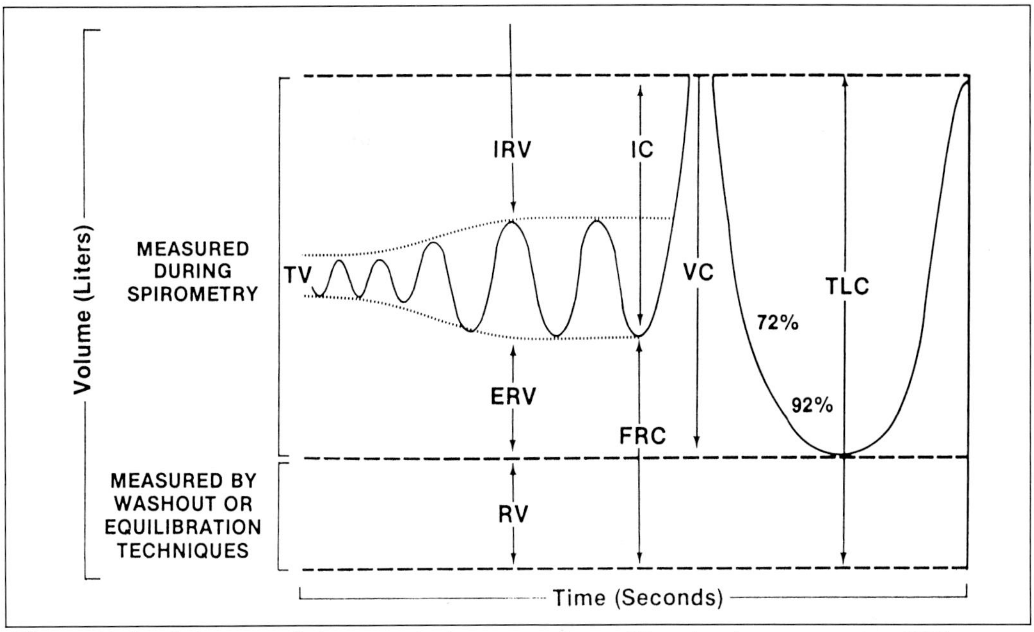

Figure 11-3. Spirogram. Spirometry is the volume measurement of air inhaled and exhaled. IRV = inspiratory reserve volume; ERV = expiratory reserve volume; RV = reserve volume; IC = inspiratory capacity; FRC = functional residual capacity; VC = vital capacity; TLC = total lung capacity.

Table 11-2. Lung volumes in lung disease

Lung disease	*IC*	*ERV*	*IRV*	*RV*	*VC*	*TV*	*FRC*	*TLC*
Obstructive Disease	Nor ↑	Nor ↑	Nor ↓	↑	Nor ↓	Nor ↑	↑	↑
Restrictive Disease	Nor ↓	Nor ↓	Nor ↓	Nor ↓	↓	Nor ↓	Nor ↓	↓

IC = inspiratory capacity: volume of gas inspired from resting end tidal volume to maximal inhalation.
ERV = effective reserve volume: volume of gas exhaled from resting end tidal volume to maximal exhalation.
IRV = inspiratory reserve volume: volume of gas inhaled from end inspiratory tidal volume to maximal inspiration.
RV = residual volume: volume of gas remaining in lungs after maximal exhalation.
VC = vital capacity: volume of gas expired either slowly or forcefully from maximal inspiration.
TV = tidal volume: volume of gas inhaled or exhaled with normal, nonforced breathing.
FRC = functional residual capacity: volume of gas remaining in lungs at end tidal expiration.
TLC = total lung capacity: volume of gas in lungs from maximal expiration to maximal inspiration plus residual volume.
Nor = normal.

Table 11-3. Spirometry of obstructive and restrictive lung disease

Lung disease	*VC*	*FRC*	*TLC*	*FEV_1*	*FEV_3*	*$FEF_{200-1200}$*	*MVV*
Obstructive Disease	Nor ↓	↑	↑	↓	↓	↓	↓
Restrictive Disease	<80%	Nor ↓	↓	Nor ↑	Nor ↑	Nor ↓	Nor ↓

VC = vital capacity.
FRC = functional residual capacity.
TLC = total lung capacity.
FEV_1 = forced expiratory volume: volume of gas forcefully expired from maximal inspiratory level, in 1 second.
FEV_3 = forced expiratory volume achieved in 3 seconds.
$FEF_{200-1200}$ = forced expiratory flow: the difference in air flow measured between 200 ml and 1200 ml of the FVC maneuver. This measurement is useful to evaluate effect of bronchodilator therapy.
MVV = maximum voluntary ventilation (also referred to as maximum breathing capacity): maximum volume a patient can ventilate, deeply and rapidly, over a 15-second period.
Nor = normal.

hypoxemia are risks of perioperative morbidity. The following abnormal values indicate an extreme increased perioperative risk [4,5]:

FVC less than 1.5 liters or less than 20 cc/kg
$FEV_{1.0}$ less than 1.0 liter
MVV less than 50 liters/minute or less than 50 percent predicted
$PaCO_2$ greater than 45 mm Hg

Treatment

Given a patient with marginal pulmonary function and a head and neck malignancy amenable to surgery, the respiratory function must be optimized. The following protocol is suggested [2,3,6,7]:

1. Preoperative cessation of smoking for 12 to 48 hours leads to increased oxygen availability by decreasing the carboxyhemoglobin levels. Cessation for 1 to 2 weeks decreases airway secretions; 4 to 8 weeks improves mucociliary transport, small airway function, and airway vitability [6].
2. Antibiotic treatment of any pulmonary infection.
3. Preoperative bronchodilators for reversible obstructive disease.
4. Good nutrition: minimal carbohydrates (increases both $PaCO_2$ and work of ventilation).
5. Minimal anesthesia time.
6. Judicious use of narcotic anesthesia.
7. Early postoperative mobilization and ambulation.
8. Heparin prophylaxis (in selected patients).
9. Postoperative incentive spirometry.

Risks

Pulmonary complications are likely to occur in patients who (1) have baseline hypoxemia/hypercapnia, (2) have difficulty with clearing airway secretions (may lead to mucus plugging, atelectasis, and pneumonia), (3) require postoperative mechanical ventilation, or (4) experience bronchospasm. Postoperative pulmonary dysfunction varies with the site of surgery (peripheral, upper versus lower abdominal, thoracic, neurologic). Arterial blood gases and pulmonary function tests can identify those patients at risk. The severity of abnormality is directly related to degree of risk, morbidity, and mortality. Pulmonary function tests provide a basis for (1) preoperatively optimizing pulmonary function (e.g., bronchodilators), (2) anticipating postoperative respiratory problems, and (3) an objective assessment of risk-benefit ratio, especially in the patient with severe pulmonary dysfunction. Finally, these tests are only guidelines and somewhat imprecise. The literature does not provide *clear* correlations between pulmonary function and postoperative outcome.

CARDIAC FUNCTION: ATHEROSCLEROSIS

Overview

Every year 1 million people die of cardiovascular disease. Affecting one in four Americans, the morbidity is greater than twice the mortality: myocardial infarctions (1.5 million), cerebrovascular accidents (0.6 million), and congestive heart failure (0.4 millions) [8]. Of approximately 65 million people with cerebrovascular disease, about 59 million have hypertension and 6.7 million have proven or symptomatic coronary artery disease (CAD); a large number of people have "silent" ischemia [8]. In 1988, 25 million people underwent noncardiac surgery: 1 million had diagnosed CAD (angina, Q waves on electrocardiogram [ECG]); 2 to 3 million had two or more risk factors; and 4 to 6 million were older than age 65 (CAD increases with age) [8,9]. Perioperative myocardial infarctions occur in up to 0.7 percent of the general population and 1.1% of patients with CAD. With or without CAD, 1.8% of patients over age 40 have myocardial infarctions. Reinfarction rates are much higher (5–37%) and are dependent on the interval between the infarction and surgery. Of 50,000 patients per year who sustain a perioperative myocardial infarction, 20,000 die [10]. Based on these sobering statistics, the recognition of patients at risk from CAD is crucial.

Assessment

Identifying patients at risk for perioperative cardiac morbidity involves obtaining a careful history, performing a comprehensive physical examination, and interpreting routine and nonroutine diagnostic tests. There are multiple risk factors for CAD as well as historical predictors of outcome. Many predictors are controversial, while recent myocardial infarction and current congestive heart failure are proven [8].

History

Historical data that identify patients at risk from CAD are (1) smoking, (2) positive family history, (3) hypertension, (4) diabetes mellitus, (5) hyperlipidemia, and (6) advanced age [11]. A positive history of angina (Table 11-4), either at rest or exercise induced, decreasing exercise tolerance, paroxysmal nocturnal dyspnea, orthopnea, pedal edema, and palpitations warrant further cardiac evaluation. In addition to symptomatic patients, it is now known that there are approximately 2 to 5 million Americans who have asymptomatic ischemic CAD [11]. Many patients with silent ischemia have diabetes mellitus [11,12]. Since most patients with head and neck cancer are heavy smokers, CAD must be suspected.

Table 11-4. Characteristic Anginal patterns

Angina	*Characteristics*
Stable angina	Substernal chest discomfort (pressure, pain, squeezing sensation) Duration of 5–15 minutes Induced by exercise, emotional stress, cold Relieved by rest or nitroglycerin Pain often radiates to shoulder, jaw, or inner aspect of arm
Unstable angina	New-onset angina occurring within past 2 months or increasing intensity, frequency, or duration of pain Can occur at rest Less responsive to treatment Duration usually greater than 30 minutes Transient ST and T wave changes on ECG
Variant angina	Usually occurs at rest Unrelated to exercise or stress ST changes are seen sometimes Higher incidence of dysrhythmias

Physical Examination

The physical examination may reveal evidence of left ventricular dysfunction, a very high risk of perioperative morbidity. Cardiomegaly as evidenced by a displaced point of maximal impulse indicates an ejection fraction less than 50 percent. A third or fourth heart sound is a sign of increased left ventricular end-diastolic pressure or decreased ventricular compliance, respectively. Extra heart sounds are associated with increased risk of perioperative morbidity. Jugular venous distention, peripheral edema, and rales are classic physical diagnostic signs of congestive heart failure.

Diagnosis

Electrocardiogram

The resting ECG is normal in 25 to 50 percent of patients with CAD [8]. However, some ECG abnormalities portend cardiac compromise: dysrhythmia, injured myocardium, infarction, or ischemia. These abnormal findings may warrant further workup prior to elective surgery.

Chest X-Ray

A routine chest x-ray is a highly specific (68–72%) indicator of abnormal ventricular function in the presence of an increased cardiothoracic ratio, cardiomegaly, enlarged left ventricle, or pulmonary congestion [8]. However, a normal chest x-ray does not rule out abnormal ventricular function.

Exercise Stress Testing

Exercise stress testing is 70-percent sensitive and 90-percent specific in identifying patients with CAD [8]. Each of the different protocols is designed to increase myocardial work progressively while monitoring signs and symptoms of ischemia. The stage at which ST segment changes or symptoms occur and the millimeter change in ST segment position predict the number and locations of CAD [13].

Echocardiography

Echocardiography is a noninvasive ultrasonic assessment of myocardial wall thickness, dyskinesia, valvular function, ejection fraction, and global ventricular function. An ejection fraction less than 40 percent is associated with increased perioperative morbidity and mortality [8].

Thallium Scan

Dipyridamole-thallium perfusion scans are often performed in lieu of treadmill ECG. They can identify areas of potentially ischemic myocardium during stress. Thallium is a radionuclide incorporated into normal myocardial tissue in proportion to regional perfusion. Dipyridamole, a potent coronary vasodilator, vasodilates normal coronaries while being ineffective on atherosclerotic vessels. It causes shunts away from areas of myocardium perfused by diseased coronaries. Thus, myocardium at risk shows an early defect that is reperfused 3 hours later [14].

Coronary Artery Catheterization

Cardiac catheterization is still the most widely used test to identify coronary anatomy and function definitively. However, recent advances in cardiac magnetic resonance imaging may replace catheterization. During catheterization, contrast medium is injected to delineate coronary anatomy and ventricular function. If there is significant coronary stenosis (> 75% luminal narrowing), angioplasty or coronary artery bypass surgery may be indicated before elective head and neck surgery [10].

Treatment

Prior to head and neck cancer surgery, patients with atherosclerosis are evaluated by a cardiologist to ensure optimal cardiac status (i.e., antihypertensives, antianginal agents, antiarrhythmics, diuretics, pacemaker function). Due to the length of surgery and possible blood loss, perioperative management of the patient with ischemic heart disease requires an arterial line to monitor hemoglobin, electrolytes, and arterial blood gases, pulmonary artery catheterization to guide volume management, vasodilator or vasopressor therapy, and inotropic support. With such monitoring, ischemic changes may be diagnosed quickly, and blood pressures are followed closely.

Risks

Multiple studies to assess predictors of cardiac morbidity and mortality in the patient with CAD have produced controversial results. Two of the common risk indices are the New York Heart Association Classification and Goldman's Cardiac Risk Index (Tables 11-5 and 11-6). These indices enumerate physical statistics as well as specific factors: recent myocardial infarction or current congestive heart failure. The time interval between surgery and a previous myocardial infarction can account for a perioperative reinfarction rate between 5 and 36 percent [60].

Table 11-5. New York Heart Association function classification

Class	*Functional classification*
I	Patients with cardiac disease but without resulting limitations of physical activity. Ordinary physical activity does not cause undue fatigue, palpitation, dyspnea, or anginal pain.
II	Patients with cardiac disease resulting in slight limitation of physical activity. They are comfortable at rest. Ordinary physical activity results in fatigue, palpitation, dyspnea, or anginal pain.
III	Patients with cardiac disease resulting in marked limitation of physical activity. They are comfortable at rest. Less than ordinary physical activity causes fatigue, palpitation, dyspnea, or anginal pain.
IV	Patients with cardiac disease resulting in inability to carry on any physical activity without discomfort. Symptoms of cardiac insufficiency or of the anginal syndrome may be present even at rest. If any physical activity is undertaken, discomfort is increased.

Source: From Braunwald E: The History. In Braunwald E (ed): *Heart Disease. A Textbook of Cardiovascular Medicine*. Philadelphia: Saunders, 1984. Pp 1–13.

Table 11-6. Clinical factors independently related to perioperative cardiac complications

Criteria	*Points*
S_3 gallop or jugular venous distention on preoperative physical examination	11
Transmural or subendocardial myocardial infarction in the previous 6 months	10
Premature ventricular beats, more than 5/min documented at any time	7
Rhythm other than sinus or presence of premature atrial contractions on last preoperative ECG	7
Age over 70 years	5
Emergency operations	4
Intrathoracic, intraperitoneal, or aortic site of surgery	3
Evidence for important valvular aortic stenosis	3
Poor general medical condition*	3

*As evidenced by electrolyte abnormalities, renal insufficiency, abnormal blood gases, abnormal liver status, or any condition that has caused the patient to become chronically bedridden. Risks of perioperative morbidity increase with increasing total points.

Source: Adapted from Goldman L, et al: Multifactional index of cardiac risk in non-cardiac procedures. *N Engl J Med* 297 : 843, 1982.

Angina

Angina pectoris is usually associated with significant CAD [15], but it is a controversial predictor of adverse outcome in patients undergoing noncardiac surgery. The impact of vasospasm and the severity and frequency of angina as they relate to increased risk has not been determined [8].

Hypertension

Untreated or poorly controlled and labile blood pressure places the patient at greater risk for myocardial ischemia and stroke [8].

Diabetes Mellitus

Myocardial infarction is the leading cause of death in diabetic patients. Usually the ischemia is "silent," perhaps related to diabetic neuropathy and altered sensory afferent. Altered autonomic tone results in greater blood pressure lability; this increases the risk of adverse cardiac outcome [16].

Dysrhythmias

Patients with CAD and frequent premature ventricular contractions or other dysrhythmia have increased risk for fatal perioperative dysrhythmias.

Peripheral Vascular Disease

There is a very strong correlation between patients with peripheral vascular disease and concurrent CAD.

Cigarette Smoking

Smoking has been associated with accelerated atherosclerosis and increased risk of myocardial infarction.

Summary

The only proven preoperative predictors of adverse cardiac outcome are current congestive heart failure and recent myocardial infarction. Patients should not undergo elective surgery until 6 months after a myocardial infarction or resolution of congestive heart failure. Even though there are multiple studies that support and reflect the same predictors of outcome and risk indices, it is prudent to remember the various population samples, statistical analysis, and research design of these studies. The entire clinical presentation of the patient must be considered if risks are to be identified. Diagnostic testing to objectively assess cardiac functions and pathology should be performed. Appropriate preanesthetic and intraoperative planning decrease the risk of cardiac morbidity and mortality.

CARDIAC FUNCTION: HYPERTENSION

Overview

Hypertension, with associated secondary cardiac, cerebrovascular, and renal complications, has a high risk for perioperative morbidity and mortality. Recent studies suggest that approximately 66 percent of the more than 58 million Americans with hypertension are treated inadequately [17,18]. The severity of preoperative hypertension directly correlates with perioperative morbidity and mortality [19]. There is a definite difference in risk for the controlled versus uncontrolled hypertensive patient [20].

Therefore, it is imperative that hypertension be adequately assessed and treated prior to general anesthesia.

Assessment

The hypertensive patient requires a careful history, physical examination, and objective diagnostic data. The goal is to determine the severity of hypertension, whether it is adequately controlled, and whether systemic complications of hypertension exist that may increase risk.

There are two types of hypertension: essential (primary) and secondary.

Essential Hypertension

Essential hypertension is elevated blood pressure without any known cause. There may be correlations with heredity, diet, renin-angiotensin system alterations, and disturbances in the sympathetic nervous system. It accounts for 80 to 85 percent of the patients with hypertension [21]. Borderline systemic arterial hypertension is a blood pressure between 140/90 and 160/100 mm Hg [22]. Severe hypertension is a diastolic blood pressure greater than 110 mm Hg.

Secondary Hypertension

Secondary hypertension may be due to renal, endocrine, neurogenic, and cardiovascular abnormalities. In addition to adequate therapy for the hypertension, it is necessary to differentiate essential and secondary hypertension. The specific etiology must be corrected or treated to decrease any additional risks of general anesthesia. Hypertension is associated with coronary and systemic atherosclerosis [21,22]. Preoperative studies should include chest radiography (to examine cardiac size and possible signs of failure) and ECG (to assess ventricular hypertrophy, CAD, myocardial ischemia or infarction, and conduction abnormalities). Past medical history and other objective screening data may dictate additional assessments of ventricular function or coronary anatomy. The signs and symptoms of cerebrovascular insufficiency (transient ischemic attacks, syncope, symptomatic carotid bruits) as well as renal function (electrolytes, creatinine, urinalysis) should be investigated [21].

Treatment

Patients with untreated, inadequately treated, or uncontrolled hypertension require adequate therapy. Antihypertensive medications should be continued up to and including the morning of surgery. Postoperatively, the hypertensive patient is still at risk for morbid events, especially if CAD or ventricular dysfunction is present. Therefore, perioperative control of blood pressure and heart rate is very important. Depending on the etiology, there are several classes of antihypertensive agents that can control hypertension. A knowledge of the various pharmacologic agents and their mechanisms of action is important for proper anesthetic management and anticipation of autonomic interactions with anesthesia as well as electrolyte and volume effects. Certain drugs exacerbate the hypertension associated with catecholamine release during intubation, surgical incision, and emergence from anesthesia. Finally, patients on diuretics are usually dehydrated and are at risk from hypotension because of vasodilatation secondary to general anesthesia.

Risks

Patients with well-controlled hypertension have less fluctuation in blood pressures during anesthesia and markedly decreased risk of morbidity and mortality [24,25]. Since hypertensives have an increased incidence of CAD and ventricular hypertrophy, intraoperative labile blood pressure (hypertension and/or hypotension) may cause ischemia or infarction. The mortality from a perioperative myocardial infarction or major cerebrovascular event is 50 percent [26,27].

Adequate antihypertensive therapy decreases the risks of adverse perioperative outcome; therefore elective surgery should be delayed if the diastolic blood pressure is greater than 110 mm Hg. Some authorities advocate additional antihypertensive therapy if the diastolic pressure is greater than 100 mm Hg [22].

Diuretics

Although there are multiple classes of diuretics, the most commonly used, thiazides, produce hypokalemia and hypovolemia. If the patient is not adequately rehydrated, profound hypotension can occur with induction of anesthesia.

Vasodilators

Vasodilators comprise many drugs: alpha blockers (hydralazine), centrally acting inhibitors (alpha-methyldopa), alpha agonists (clonidine), direct smooth-muscle dilators (nitroprusside, nitroglycerin), and ganglionic blockers (trimethaphan).

Calcium Channel Blockers

Four calcium channel blockers are presently available for antihypertensive therapy. Nifedipine vasodilates arteries without a significant effect on heart rate. Verapamil mildly vasodilates but primarily decreases heart rate. Diltiazem is intermediate between these two. Nicardipine is a potent coronary vasodilator.

Angiotensin-Converting Enzyme Inhibitors

Angiotensin-converting enzyme inhibitors are useful to decrease aldosterone by decreasing angiotension levels. Blood pressure is controlled by lowering intravascular volume (less sodium retention). Enalapril and captopril are examples.

Beta Blockers and Combination Drugs

For years propranolol was used to decrease heart rate, especially in patients with CAD. However, beta blockade alone leaves alpha receptors unopposed, and vasoconstriation can occur. Labetalol has a beta-alpha receptor potency ratio of 7:1 intravenously and 3:1 orally to affect heart rate and result in mild vasodilation. Effective plasma concentrations of these medications should be continued up to and including the morning of surgery.

THYROID FUNCTION

Overview

Thyroid disease reflects either the overproduction or underproduction of thyroid hormones. Thyroxine (T_4) and triiodothyroxine (T_3) are the two thyroid hormones. The majority of T_3 is produced by peripheral deiodination of thyroxine. These are the two physiologically active hormones produced by the thyroid gland whose synthesis and secretion are regulated by a positive and negative feedback mechanism (Figure 11-4). Thyroid dysfunction reflects disease involving either the hypothalamus/anterior pituitary or the thyroid gland (primary versus secondary thyroid disease).

Any patient who is hyper- or hypothyroid is not a candidate for an elective surgical procedure (Table 11-7). Until the patient is euthyroid, only emergency surgery is performed.

Assessment

Preoperative screening for patients with suspected or documented thyroid dysfunction includes a history, physical examination, and laboratory evaluations. Laboratory tests are the

Figure 11-4. Pituitary-thyroid axis.

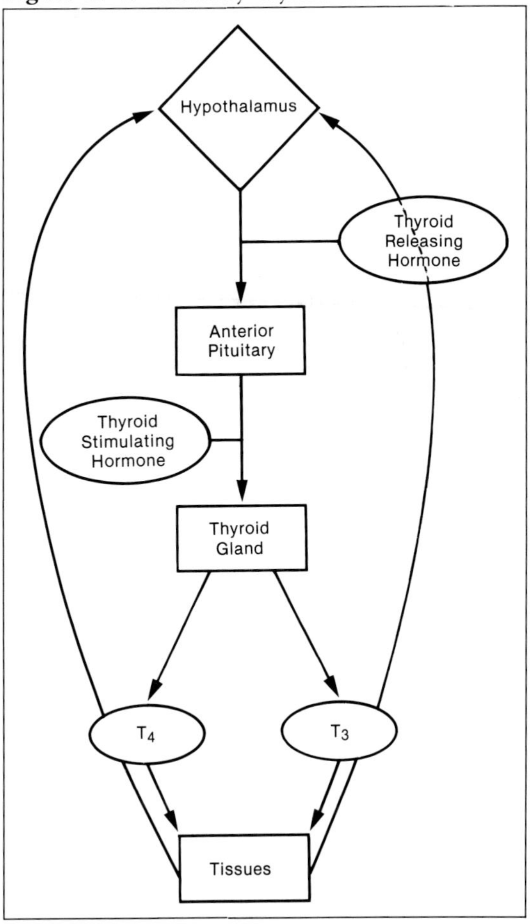

Table 11-7. Signs and symptoms of hyperthyroidism and hypothyroidism

	Hyperthyroidism	*Hypothyroidism*[a]
Habitus	None	Cretinism[b]
Constitution	Weight loss Fatigue Heat intolerance Excitability	Weight gain Lethargy Cold intolerance Somnolence
Skin	Sweating, moist Velvety texture	Dry
Hair	Fine, silky	Coarse, brittle
Eyes	Exophthalmus, widened palpebral fissure	Watery, puffy
Cardiovascular system	Tachycardia, atrial arrhythmias	Bradycardia
Respiratory system	Dyspnea	Pleural effusion
Musculoskeletal system	Muscle weakness Fine tremor (fingers & tongue)	Delayed deep tendon reflexes
Genitourinary system	Oligomenorrhea or amenorrhea	Menorrhagia

[a]Hypothyroidism is insidious and associated with nonspecific complaints.
[b]Neonatal thyroid hormone deficiency resulting in physical and mental retardation.

only way to make a definitive diagnosis of either condition (Tables 11-8 and 11-9) [28,29].

Treatment

Hyperthyroidism

Hyperthyroidism is managed with drugs that inhibit the iodide trapping, oxidation, and iodination of thyroxine, such as propylthiouracil (PTU) and methimazole. This regimen requires weeks for therapeutic effect. Oral iodide solution (Lugol's solution) may be given to reduce glandular vascularity and prevent active hormone release. Propranolol effectively attenuates the sympathetic manifestations of hyperthyroidism and inhibits the peripheral conversion of T_4 to T_3. Subtotal thyroidectomy is an alternative to prolonged medical management. Prior to surgery, the patient should be euthyroid either with PTU, methimazole, or a combination of oral iodide and propranolol. The last combination achieves a euthyroid state in about 7 to 14 days [28].

Table 11-8. Laboratory diagnosis of thyroid function

Test	*Normal value*	*Hyperthyroidism*	*Hypothyroidism*
Thyroxine (total T_4) (screening for thyroid function)	4.4–9.9 ng/dl	Increased	Decreased
Free thyroxine (T_4) (differentiates between altered TBG and thyroid dysfunction)	1–21 ng/dl	Increased	Decreased
Triiodothyronine resin uptake* (differentiates between altered TBG and thyroid dysfunction)	30–40%	High	Low
Total plasma triiodothyronine (detects hyperthyroidism)	150–250 ng/ml	Increased	Decreased
Thyroid-stimulating hormone (detects hypothyroidism)	Up to 7 units ml^{-1}	Decreased	Increased

TBG = thyroxine-binding globulin.
*Total T_4 and T_3 resin uptake must be interpreted together to account for abnormalities in TBG. When total T_4 and T_3 resin uptake move in an opposite direction, an excess or deficiency in TBG is the likely cause, and the patient is euthyroid.

Table 11-9. Factors influencing plasma concentrations of thyroxine-binding globulin

Event	*Thyroxine-binding globulin (TBG)*
Nephrosis	Decreased
Hypoproteinemia	Decreased
Acromegaly	Decreased
Pregnancy	Increased
Oral contraceptives	Increased
Infectious hepatitis	Increased

Hypothyroidism

Hypothyroidism is treated with exogenous thyroid hormone. Rapid intravenous administration of thyroxine is plagued by problems (arrhythmias, angina pectoris, congestive heart failure); therefore, the parenteral route is preferable [28]. Intravenous triiodothyroxine is effective within 6 hours and peaks in 48 to 72 hours [29]. Patients on oral thyroxine are medicated on the day of surgery.

Risks

Thyroid Storm

The major surgical complication of hyperthyroidism, "thyroid storm," occurs in about 10 to 30 percent of patients (Table 11-10). Clinically, the patient experiences hyperpyrexia, tachycardia, and alteration in consciousness. Although it can occur intraoperatively it is most frequent 6 to 18 hours after surgery [30]. The management is both specific and supportive: intravenous fluids to replace losses secondary to hyperthermia, antithyroid drugs to decrease oxidation and release of thyroid hormones, and cortisol for associated acute adrenal insufficiency. Propranolol is given to decrease heart rate and peripheral thyroxine conversion. Patients with thyroid storm may also develop high-output congestive heart failure that requires digitalis. Aspirin displaces thyroxine from its serum protein and should not be given for hyperthermia.

Table 11-10. Management of thyroid storm

Drug	*Dosage*
Propylthiouracil	200–400 mg PO every 8 hours
Sodium iodide	500–1000 mg IV every 8 hours
Cortisol	100–300 mg IV every 8 hours
Propranolol	IV dose adequate to decrease to <100 beats/min

Myxedematous Coma

Myxedematous coma is a severe form of hypothyroidism that is characterized by hypothermia, hypoventilation, altered consciousness, and congestive heart failure [31,32]. Intravenous triiodothyroxine acutely replaces thyroid hormone. Chronic adrenal insufficiency secondary to adrenal atrophy is managed with cortisol. Congestive heart failure, primarily low output failure, is treated with digitalis. Hypoventilation probably is related to myxedematous infiltration of the muscles of respiration. The associated respiratory compromise may require intubation and ventilatory support.

HEPATIC FUNCTION

Overview

Many patients with head and neck malignancies have a history of heavy ethanol abuse. Statistically, heavy alcohol intake is a major contributor to hepatic dysfunction. In the United States, the most common cause of cirrhosis is alcohol (Laennec's) cirrhosis, but hepatitis B may be the most common worldwide etiology [33].

The liver has numerous synthetic and metabolic functions (Table 11-11). A diseased liver

Table 11-11. Hepatic functions

- Glucose homeostasis
- Fat metabolism
- Protein synthesis
  - Albumin
  - Coagulation factors (except factor 8 and platelets)
  - Pseudocholinesterase
- Drug biotransformation
- Bilirubin formation and excretion
- Enzyme production
  - Transaminases
  - Alkaline phosphatase
- Cholesterol synthesis and excretion
- Urea synthesis

can affect many of these functions, thus challenging perioperative and postoperative management. Liver disease can be classified as either acute, chronic, or irreversible (Table 11-12).

Assessment

Important historical information includes fatigue, malaise, jaundice, past history of hepatitis, postoperative jaundice, heavy alcohol use, bleeding varices, and delirium tremens. Physical examination may show little in the absence of significant hepatic dysfunction, except stigmata suggestive of cirrhosis. Preoperative liver function studies may demonstrate hidden hepatic dysfunction (Table 11-13).

Patients with a past history of hepatitis should have an antibody screen preoperatively. Coagulation parameters should also be evaluated; prolonged prothrombin time is the best assessment of acute liver dysfunction. Due to the liver's large functional reserve, most liver function studies are abnormal only when considerable hepatic damage has occurred.

Many surgical procedures, performed under either general or regional anesthesia, are associated with changes in liver function tests [34, 35]. These elevations (transaminases, alkaline phosphatase, and bilirubin) are transient, minor, and of questionable clinical significance. The role of anesthetic agents in causing minor hepatic dysfunction is unclear. However, all anesthetic techniques reduce hepatic blood flow and result in decreased oxygen uptake by the liver and splenic organs and may contribute to dysfunction [34]. The magnitude of postoperative hepatic dysfunction correlates with the

Table 11-12. Causes of hepatic dysfunction

Acute	*Chronic*	*Irreversible Cirrhosis*
Viral hepatitis	Chronic active hepatitis	Hepatitis B
Type A	Chronic persistent hepatitis	Non-A, non-B hepatitis
Type B		Alcoholic (Laennec's)
Non-A, non-B		Chronic active hepatitis
Epstein-Barr virus		Primary biliary
Cytomegalovirus		Hemochromatosis
Drug-induced hepatitis		Schistosomiasis
		Cardiac (chronic right heart failure)

Table 11-13. Liver function tests and differential diagnosis

Hepatic dysfunction	*Bilirubin*	*Transaminase enzymes*	*Alkaline phosphatase*	*Causes*
Prehepatic	Unconjugated (indirect)	Normal	Normal	Hemolysis: Hematoma Resorption: Bilirubin Overload from whole blood
Intrahepatic	Conjugated (direct)	Elevated	Normal to slightly elevated (less than twice normal)	Viral Drugs Sepsis Hypoxemia Cirrhosis
Posthepatic	Conjugated	Normal to slightly elevated	Elevated (more than twice normal)	Stones Sepsis

Source: From Stoelting RK, Dierdorf SF, McCannon RL, *Anesthesia and Co-existing Disease* (2nd ed). New York: Churchill Livingstone, 1988.

nature of the surgery and its proximity to the liver [36,37].

Treatment

Preoperative therapy is directed at correcting or improving the consequences of hepatic disease. Ascites should be controlled. The coagulopathy should be corrected prior to elective surgery. Vitamin K, administered intramuscularly over several days, should result in a normal prothrombin time. For severe hepatic dysfunction, rapid correction is accomplished with fresh frozen plasma. Platelets are given for counts less than 50,000/μl.

Risks

Surgical risk is difficult to estimate. However, the risk is proportionate to the severity of the hepatic dysfunction and the magnitude of the surgery [33]. Current data are mostly from retrospective studies in cirrhotic patients undergoing abdominal procedures and anecdotal surgical experiences [38,39]. Despite these inadequacies, some estimate of surgical risk can be made with recommendations for perioperative management.

Acute Viral Hepatitis

Viral hepatitis is caused by numerous agents, the most common being hepatitis A, B, and non-A, non-B. The usual clinical presentation is low-grade fever malaise, dark urine, light-colored stools, abdominal pain, and jaundice. There are many patients who are anicteric and have subclinical disease. Moderate to marked elevations in transaminase can be seen, with variable increases in bilirubin and minimal to no increases in alkaline phosphatase. The general perception is that patients with viral hepatitis have increased morbidity and mortality, and therefore elective surgery is contraindicated [33,38]. Elective surgery is usually possible about 1 month after liver function studies have returned to normal.

Chronic Hepatitis

Chronic hepatitis is characterized by chronic inflammation of the liver for at least 3 to 6 months. Chronic active hepatitis and chronic persistent hepatitis are the two entities in this category (Table 11-14). A liver biopsy is required to establish the diagnosis.

Chronic Persistent Hepatitis

Chronic persistent hepatitis is a benign nonprogressive disease histologically characterized by a nonnuclear cell infiltrate confined to the portal zone. Patients are usually asymptomatic with only minimal symptoms and elevated transaminases. Progression to cirrhosis does not occur, hepatic function is usually well preserved, and surgery is well tolerated.

Chronic Active Hepatitis

Chronic active hepatitis, a more serious disease, is characterized by widespread inflammation and hepatocyte destruction. Patients with mild disease may be asymptomatic; those with severe disease may experience fatigue, weight loss, fever, and jaundice. Liver function studies are significantly abnormal. Progression to cirrhosis and hepatic failure can occur. In asymptomatic

Table 11-14. Differentiating features in chronic hepatitis

Features	*Chronic active hepatitis*	*Chronic persistent hepatitis*
Jaundice	Common	Rare
Transaminases	Markedly elevated	Mildly elevated
Bilirubin	Elevated	Normal
Gamma globulin	Elevated	Normal
Prothrombin time	Prolonged	Normal
Albumin	Decreased	Normal
HBsAg (incidence)	10–20%	10–20%

Source: From Stoelting RK, Dierdorf SF, McCannon RL, Anesthesia and Co-existing Disease (2nd ed). New York: Churchill Livingstone, 1988.

patients or those with mild disease, the available data suggest that these patients tolerate surgery well [2]. However, in those with severe disease, elective surgery should be avoided [35,39]. Asymptomatic carriers (hepatitis B surface antigen [HB_sAg]–positive) in the absence of elevated transaminases are not at significant risk for postoperative complications [35].

Halothane Hepatitis

Halothane hepatitis is a much discussed entity, whose exact mechanism is unknown. Although some theories postulate direct toxicity or hypersensitivity, it may manifest as a slight elevation in transaminases 4 to 6 weeks after general anesthesia. It is usually a diagnosis made by exclusion.

Alcoholic Liver Disease

Alcoholism is a disease that affects about 10 million persons in the United States [39]. Alcoholic liver disease is a spectrum from fatty liver to alcoholic hepatitis and cirrhosis.

Fatty Liver

Usually occurring after alcoholic binges, a fatty liver produces a mild asymptomatic illness that is associated with hepatomegaly and slight elevations of transaminase and alkaline phosphatase. Fatty liver resolves after abstinence; liver function is preserved, and elective surgery is not contraindicated.

Acute Alcoholic Hepatitis

Alcoholic hepatitis is a major precursor to the development of cirrhosis [33]. It is characterized by fever, nausea, vomiting, tender hepatomegaly, and elevated transaminases. In its severe form, jaundice, prolonged prothrombin time, coagulopathy, ascites, and hepatic encephalopathy can occur. Elective surgery is contraindicated until the illness resolves [40].

Cirrhosis

Cirrhosis due to alcohol ingestion occurs in about 10 percent of those who consume the equivalent of 80 gm of alcohol daily for 10 to 15 years [39]. It is an irreversible disease process with destruction of hepatic parenchyma and replacement by collagen. Surgical risk can be classified using Pugh's modification of Child's classification (Table 11-15). Overall death rates are 20 to 25%; those individuals classified as severe cirrhotics have greater than 35-percent mortality [41,42].

RENAL FUNCTION

Overview

Renal insufficiency is defined as a measurable reduction in renal function with normal serum biochemical values. Renal failure is renal function that has deteriorated to abnormal serum biochemical values and a loss of homeostasis [43]. Today more than 75,000 patients are on dialysis for chronic renal failure in the United States [44]. The need for surgical procedures in patients with chronic renal failure has resulted in a specialized approach to their care. A knowledge of the problems associated with chronic renal failure and appropriate preoperative management are essential to decrease perioperative morbidity and mortality.

Table 11-15. Prediction of surgical risk based on preoperative evaluation

	Minimal	*Modest*	*Marked*
Bilirubin (mg/dl^{-1})	<2	2–3	>3
Albumin (gm/dl^{-1})	>3.5	3.0–3.5	<3
Prothrombin time (seconds prolonged)	1–4	4–6	6
Encephalopathy	None	Moderate	Severe
Nutrition	Excellent	Good	Poor
Ascites	None	Moderate	Marked

Source: From Stoelting RK, Dierdorf SF, McCannon RL, Anesthesia and Co-existing Disease (2nd ed). New York: Churchill Livingstone, 1988.

Assessment

A thorough history and physical examination are necessary. Important historical information includes etiology of renal failure, urine output (anuria, oliguria), and frequency and type of dialysis (hemodialysis versus peritoneal dialysis). Since many medications are metabolized by the kidneys, a complete medication list is required. Chronic renal failure patients have a prolonged and exaggerated effect from many medications. The physical examination should assess the general status (overhydration versus hydration) as well as specific abnormalities associated with chronic renal failure (Table 11-16). The essential laboratory data are listed in Table 11-17.

Table 11-16. Complications of chronic renal failure

Cardiovascular
Hypertension
Pericarditis
Pericardial effusion
Congestive heart failure
Accelerated atherosclerosis
Pulmonary
Infection
Gastrointestinal
Anorexia
Nausea and vomiting
Hiccoughs
Delayed gastric emptying
Peptic ulcer disease
Hepatitis B carrier
Metabolic
Metabolic acidosis
Hyperkalemia
Hypermagnesemia
Hyperphosphatemia
Hypocalcemia
Hematologic
Anemia
Platelet dysfunction
Neuropsychiatric
Uremic encephalopathy
Drowsiness
Asterixis
Myoclonus
Seizures
Peripheral neuropathy
Autonomic neuropathy

Table 11-17. Preoperative laboratory evaluation of renal function

Hematocrit
Complete blood count
Coagulation profile (prothrombin time, partial thromboplastin time, bleeding time, platelet count)
Serum electrolytes
Serum cretinine, blood urea nitrogen
Urinalysis
Electrocardiogram
Chest x-ray

Treatment

Ideally, those chronic renal failure patients on hemodialysis should be dialyzed the day before surgery. Preoperative dialysis optimizes fluid and electrolyte balance, aids in control of hypertension, corrects acidosis, and allows time for heparin metabolism, a medication used in dialysis. It is generally recommended that elective surgery not be performed unless the serum K^+ is less than 5.5 mEg/liter [45]. Platelet dysfunction may be improved by dialysis in some but not all uremic patients [48]. Desmopressin, 0.3 μg/kg IV given slowly, may correct the coagulopathy through the release of von Willebrand factor. This effect is short-lived, and tachyphylaxis can occur with repeated injections [44,46]. Transfusions are given to patients with serum hemacrits less than 25 percent who are having major surgical procedures or who have decreased cardiopulmonary reserve. Transfusions are best given during dialysis to control increased intravascular volume and to eliminate excess serum potassium.

Risks

The uremia, anemia, and malnutrition associated with chronic renal failure appear to suppress leukocytic chemotaxis and immune response. These patients also have decreased resistance to infection [46]; this risk is not decreased with dialysis. Most importantly, healing is impaired in chronic renal failure [46,48]. There are conflicting data as to whether dialysis alters this potential complication [45,46].

DIABETES MELLITUS

Overview

Fifty percent of the 6 million people in the United States who have diabetes mellitus eventually will have surgery. Seventy-five percent of these will be operated on after the age of 50 [47]. Many patients suffer from diabetic complications (cardiovascular disease, renal insufficiency, and peripheral neuropathy) that increase their perioperative risk.

Stress

In normal patients, surgery causes stress hyperglycemia, which is even greater in diabetic patients. This is due to the intraoperative release of insulin antagonists such as catecholamines, cortisol, and glucagon. These insulin antagonists enhance gluconeogenosis and glycogenesis, which further exacerbate hyperglycemia in the diabetic.

Classification

Diabetics usually are classified in one of two groups: type I or type II (Table 11-18). Type I patients, the insulin-dependent group, are prone to ketosis. Type II, non-insulin-dependent patients are not prone to ketosis.

Atherosclerosis

Diabetes is associated with coronary and cerebral atherosclerosis, microneuropathy (penile and retinal), infections, and impaired wound healing. The last two are very important in the immediate perioperative period.

Assessment

Cardiovascular System

The history reviews the presence of recent or past myocardial infarction, congestive failure, and angina. If angina is present, its severity and characteristics must be evaluated preoperatively. Diabetics may present with autonomic nervous system dysfunction manifesting as orthostatic hypotension, resting tachycardia, and decreased or lost beat-to-beat heart rate variability during voluntary deep breathing. Peripheral pulses are examined for deficits suggestive of progressive atherosclerotic disease. A carotid bruit hints of possible cerebrovascular insufficiency.

Electrocardiogram

An ECG is required preoperatively and postoperatively, since diabetics are known to have silent myocardial infarctions. An abnormal ECG in an otherwise asymptomatic patient may be the only evidence of coronary artery disease.

Echocardiogram

Unless the patient has a history of a myocardial infarction or has known left ventricular dysfunction, an echocardiogram is not mandatory. The specific indications for preoperative echocardiogram were discussed earlier in regard to ischemic heart disease.

Electrolytes

Serum Glucose

The serum glucose should be equal to or less than 250 mg/dl for elective surgery. This is con-

Table 11-18. Classification of diabetes mellitus

	Type I—Insulin-Dependent, Juvenile-Onset	*Type II—Non-Insulin-Dependent, Maturity-Onset*
Age of onset	usually ≤16	Usually ≥35
Clinical presentation	Abrupt	Gradual
Symptoms	Polydipsia Polyphagia Polyuria	Can be asymptomatic
Exogenous insulin requirement	Yes	Not always
Ketoacidosis prone	Yes	No
Nutrition	Thin	Obese
Vascular complication	Infrequent	Frequent

trolled by diet, oral hypoglycemics, or insulin. In an emergency, glucose levels are decreased with 5 to 10 units of regular insulin IV, followed by an insulin drip. Intravascular volume is repleted with non-dextrose-containing fluids. When the electrolytes are corrected and the glucose levels are equal to or less than 250 mg/dl, a dextrose infusion is started and the insulin drip is continued.

Sodium and Potassium
Sodium and potassium abnormalities are corrected prior to elective surgery. With ketoacidosis, in addition to the elevated glucose, K^+ moves extracellularly, causing the K^+ to appear normal. However, as the ketoacidosis is corrected, K^+ moves intracellularly to produce significant hypokalemia.

The osmotic diuresis associated with uncontrolled glucose can result in hyponatremia from excessive fluid loss. Thus, many diabetic patients require careful hydration prior to surgery.

Blood Urea Nitrogen and Creatinine
The blood urea nitrogen (BUN) and creatinine are obtained preoperatively to assess renal function.

Treatment
Oral hypoglycemic agents are discontinued the evening before surgery (Table 11-19) [47,48]. Most agents have long half-lives and can cause hypoglycemia during the fasting perioperative period.

Table 11-19. Perioperative insulin regimens

Time	*Classic Regimen*	*Insulin Infusion Regimen*
Day before surgery	NPO past midnight.[a]	1. Determination of preprandial blood glucose. 2. Start 5% D/W infusion (50 ml/gm/70 kg body weight). 3. Start insulin infusion "piggybacked" into dextrose intravenous fluids (50 units of regular insulin in 250 ml of normal saline. $\text{Rate (units/hr)} = \frac{\text{glucose}}{\text{150 plasma}}$ Use 100 as the denominator if patient is on steroids. 4. Frequent glucose checks q2–4h. 5. Adjust insulin infusion to maintain glucose between 100–200 mg/dl. 6. NPO past midnight.[b]
Day of surgery	1. FBS at 6 A.M. 2. Dextrose-containing infusion started at 125 ml/hr/70 kg of body weight. 3. One-half to one-third usual morning dose of insulin SQ.	FBS.
Operative period	1. Continue dextrose-containing fluids. 2. Frequent glucose checks. 3. Treatment with sliding-scale regular insulin.	1. Administration of nondextrose IV fluid through a separate IV. 2. Frequent glucose checks with appropriate adjustment of insulin infusion.
Recovery room	1. Frequent glucose checks. 2. Treatment with sliding-scale insulin.	Frequent glucose check with appropriate adjustment of insulin infusion.

[a] Orange juice at bedside for treatment of hypoglycemia.
[b] One-half ampul of 50% dextrose if blood glucose is less than 50 mg/dl.

Table 11-20. Maintenance fluid guidelines

4 ml/kg/hr for first 10 kg body weight
2 ml/kg/hr for second 10 kg body weight
1 ml/kg/hr for remaining kilograms

Example: 70 kg male	10 kg × 4 ml/kg/hr	= 40 ml/hr	
	10 kg × 2 ml/kg/hr	= 20 ml/hr	
	50 kg × 1 ml/kg/hr	= 50 ml/hr	
	70 kg	= 110 ml/hr	maintenance requirement

Risks

There is a controversy as to whether normal blood sugar levels are a greater benefit than a risk in diabetic patients and how closely blood sugars should be controlled in the perioperative period [49,50]. Those who advocate tight control evoke evidence of decreased wound infections and increased wound healing in the diabetic animal model. In studies involving gallbladder surgery, no increase in wound or systemic infection, perioperative morbidity, or perioperative mortality could be attributed to diabetes. When corrections for age and cardiovascular disease are made, the increased morbidity seems to disappear. The benefit of short-term close control in the perioperative period is in doubt. However, medical evidence indicates that long-term close control reverses neural and renal complications.

FLUIDS

Crystalloids and Colloids

Maintenance fluids replenish the obligate losses from the lungs, skin, urine, and feces (Table 11-20) [37,38]. Since these losses are sodium-free, they are replaced with *hypo*tonic solutions. The losses secondary to tissue trauma, infection,

Table 11-21. Artificial Colloids

Type Colloid	*Effects on coagulation and blood viscosity*	*Uses*	*Complications*
Dextran 70	Decreases platelet adhesiveness due to antithrombin	Volume expansion Microvascular surgery Stroke patients	>20 ml/kg/day can lead to bleeding Problems with cross-matching Anaphylactic or anaphylactoid reactions Volume overload
Dextran 40	Decreases platelet adhesiveness Adsorption onto RBC surface, resulting in prevention of RBC aggregation and decrease in blood viscosity	Volume expansion (controversial) Decrease blood viscosity in patients with burns, trauma, blood loss, endotoxic shock Increases microcirculatory flow	>22 ml/kg/day may lead to renal insufficiency Volume overload Mild allergic reactions
Gelatin		Volume expansion	Allergic reaction
Hetastarch		Volume expansion	Allergic reaction Problems with cross-matching

Table 11-22. Physiologic response to blood loss*

% Blood Loss	*Compensatory Mechanisms*
10–15	Extracellular fluid moves into intravascular space Contraction of great veins
20	Increased heart rate and stroke volume Orthostatic hypotension
30	Further increased heart rate and stroke volume Orthostatic hypotension Blood flow to muscle and skin decreases Arteriolar constriction Glycolysis and lipolysis with consequent metabolic acidosis and compensatory respiratory acidosis Decreased urine output
40	Low resting blood pressure and central venous pressure Markedly symptomatic, air hunger, clammy skin, thready pulse
50	Shock; death is imminent

*Assumes initial normovolemia and normal hemoglobin.

Table 11-23. Estimated calculations for allowable blood loss and guidelines for replacement

ABL = (initial hematocrit − lowest acceptable hematocrit)(EBV)(3)

EBV = (70 − 90 ml/kg)(kg)

If the blood loss is less than one-third of the ABL, it is replaced 3 : 1 with isotonic fluid.

If the blood loss is more than one-third, but less than total ABL, it is replaced with colloid and/or crystalloid.

If the blood loss is more than ABL and the patient is symptomatically anemic, it is replaced with blood.

ABL = allowable blood loss; EBV = estimated blood volume.

Source: Adapted from Lebowitz P, Newberg L, Gillete M (eds): *Clinical Anesthesia Procedures of the Massachusetts General Hospital* (2nd ed). Boston: Little, Brown, 1982. P 340.

burns, gastric drainage, fistulae, weeping and oozing from raw surfaces, pleural effusions or ascites, and interstitial edema are replaced with *iso*tonic solutions. If electrolytes are normal and disease processes limiting specific electrolyte administration (kidney disease, severe liver disease) are not present, maintenance and replacement fluids may be administered liberally (Table 11-21). Blood loss initially is repleted with crystalloids or colloids: 1ml of colloid or 3 to 7ml of crystalloid for each milliliter of blood loss. Crystalloids readily redistribute among the intracellular, interstitial, and intravascular compartments, constituting 30, 15, and 5 percent of body weight respectively, thus explaining the rationale for crystalloid replacement per milliliter blood loss [51].

TRANSFUSIONS

Indications

Blood product transfusions restore and maintain (1) oxygen carrying capacity, (2) volume, (3) hemostasis, and (4) leukocyte function. Red cells are the product of choice for treating most cases of acute anemia [52–54]. However, most patients with chronic anemia adapt to lower hematocrits (often <20 percent) [52]. The anemic patient, whether the anemia is secondary to chronic disease or acute blood loss, compensates by increasing heart rate and stroke volume. In normal patients, data suggest that cardiac output does not significantly increase until the hemoglobin decreases to approximately 7 gm/dl [40]. Anemia also changes the degree of oxygen extraction and hemoglobin affinity for oxygen. When physiologic compensatory mechanisms fail, red cell transfusion is indicated (Tables 11-22 and 11-23) [51,52,55].

Anemia

Good clinical judgment aided by laboratory data (arterial oxygen tension, mixed venous oxygen tension, cardiac output, and/or oxygen extraction ratio) determines the need for perioperative red cell transfusion. Most patients can lose about 30 percent of their estimated blood volume. This assumes that the patient *starts* with a normal hemoglobin level and is being volume repleted with crystalloids and colloids [51,53]; however, each patient must be individualized. There is a minimal hemoglobin level for each individual; below this level, increased morbidity and mortality occur secondary to inadequate tissue oxygenation. In essence, these guidelines are applicable only in the presence of adequate blood volume and cardiac output. The combination of hypovolemia and anemia can result in severe morbidity or mortality [55].

Hemostasis

Perioperative bleeding usually is due to surgical transection of blood vessels (see Chapter 12). Diffuse troublesome bleeding manifests as oozing, hematuria, gingival bleeding, petechiae, bleeding from venopuncture sites, and ecchymoses. This bleeding may be secondary to (1) dilutional thrombocytopenia, (2) low levels of factors V and VIII, (3) disseminated intravascular coagulopathy (DIC), or (4) hemolytic transfusion reaction [51,54]. Astute blood product transfusion is based on an accurate assessment of the etiology of bleeding.

Dilutional Thrombocytopenia

Dilutional thrombocytopenia is the most likely cause of bleeding if multiple units of blood have been transfused [55–56]. Consequently, if multiple units (usually >10) of whole blood (5–10% platelet function after 24 hours of storage) or packed red cells, devoid of platelets are transfused or bleeding continues, resulting in further platelet loss, a dilutional thrombocytopenia develops [55,57,58]. Acute thrombocytopenia is not tolerated as well as chronic thrombocytopenia; the average patient bleeds perioperatively with platelet counts less than 65,000 [58]. Whereas other coagulation factors equilibrate extravascularly and serve as a replenishment pool, platelets, being largely intravascular factors, are diluted easily during volume resuscitation with packed red blood cells or crystalloids and colloids. Usually 1 unit of platelets will increase the platelet count 5000 to 10,000 in adults [55]. If bleeding continues despite adequate platelet transfusion, there is probably a factor deficiency.

Factor Deficiency

Factor deficiency may occur if whole blood devoid of labile factors V and VIII or multiple units of packed red cells are tranfused. Be aware that one deficiency may exacerbate another factor deficiency [51]. If bleeding persists despite adequate platelet and clotting factor replenishment, consider disseminated intravascular coagulation (DIC) or a transfusion reaction.

Disseminated Intravascular Coagulation

DIC results when the coagulation system consumes and depletes clotting factors and platelets. It is activated by the complement system by sepsis, anaphylaxis, transfusion reaction, hypoxia, and acidosis. DIC is confirmed by abnormal prothrombin time (PT) and partial thromboplastin time (PTT), prolonged bleeding time, decreased platelets and fibrinogen, and increased fibrin degradation products [51]. Thromboelastogram (TEG) analysis detects factor deficiency as well as fibrinolysis [54,55]. The results can be obtained in less than 30 minutes. Sonoclot is a similar viscoelastic analysis of coagulopathy [54]. DIC correction requires treatment of the underlying cause as well as fresh frozen plasma, cryoprecipitate, and platelets.

Hemolytic Transfusion Reaction

Hemolytic transfusion reaction may also lead to perioperative bleeding diathesis.

Fresh Frozen Plasma

Factor Deficiency

Hemostasis requires 10 to 40 percent of the normal plasma concentration of coagulation factors [51,52]. Therefore, replacing 15 to 20 percent of the plasma volume with fresh frozen plasma replenishes these factors (2–3 units or 400–600 ml of fresh frozen plasma/plasma volume) (Table 11-24). Massive blood loss may require 3 to 5 units/plasma volume [37]. Some authors recommend 10ml/kg to achieve hemostatic levels of clotting factors [41]; for example, 70 kg × 70 ml/kg = estimated blood volume, or 4900ml. If hematocrit equals 40 percent, then plasma equals 60-percent estimated blood volume, or 3000ml. Therefore, 20% × 3000ml = 600ml of fresh frozen plasma required for hemostasis.

Table 11-24. Hemoglobin level and indications for transfusion

Hb > 10 gm/dl	No transfusion needed.
Hb 7–10 gm/dl	Most healthy patients do not need transfusion. Transfusion of all patients should be based on clinical and physiologic data.
Hb < 7 gm/dl	Most patients will require transfusion.

Assuming normal values of

Hb	15 gm/dl
C.O.	5 l/min
SaO_2	97%
SvO_2	75%

$$CO_2 = (1.37 \times Hb \times \%\ sat) + (0.003 \times PO_2)$$

↑ very small amount dissolved.

$$VO_2 = O_2del - O_2ret$$

$$O_2del = (C.O.)(1.37 \times Hb \times \%_a\ sat)(10)$$
$$O_2ret = (C.O.)(1.37 \times Hb \times \%_v\ sat)(10)$$
$$VO_2 = (C.O.)(1.37 \times Hb)(10)[\%\ art\ sat - \%\ ven\ sat)$$

To meet demands of *consumption,* either
(1) Hb
(2) C.O.
(3) SaO_2
} must ↑

If C.O. ↑ is maximal, then Hb or SaO_2 must ↑. OF COURSE, ideally ↓ consumption requirement is preferable.

Hb = hemoglobin; C.O. = cardiac output; del = delivered; ret = retained; CO_2 = oxygen content.
Source: From *Perioperative Red Cell Transfusion*. Presented at the National Institutes of Health Consensus Development Conference, June 1988.

Coumadin Reversal

Coumadin depletes vitamin K–dependent factors (II, VII, IX, X) [51,53]. After coumadin is stopped, coagulopathy correction may take 2 to 5 days [41]. Vitamin K, 10 to 30 mg IM, corrects the coumadin effect in 6 to 12 hours. However, fresh frozen plasma (usually 2 units) immediately reverses the coumadin effect [59].

Massive Blood Transfusions

Massive blood transfusion is the replacement of greater than 1 calculated blood volume/24 hours [51]. This results in dilutional coagulopathy rarely; the most likely problem is dilutional thrombocytopenia [51]. Extravascular stores of clotting factors can replenish intravascular depletion. The factors present in the plasma of a platelet transfusion can contribute to hemostasis. Rarely do factor levels drop below 25 to 30 percent [45].

Type and Cross Match

Pretransfusion assessment for compatibility between donor and recipient ensures safety in the administration of blood products (Tables 11-25 and 11-26) [51,52,53]. Red cell membranes contain antigens, and serum contains antibodies. The major antigens are A, B, and RH_o (D); the lesser antigens include Kell, Kidd, Duffy, and others. When the hematocrit is reduced acutely to less than 25 percent, it may be necessary to transfuse blood without a complete cross match. Given this emergency situation, the preferred order of transfusion is as follows:

1. Type-specific, partially cross-matched blood: The patient's serum and donor red cells are incubated at room temperature for 5 minutes and observed for macroagglutin-

Table 11-25. Pretransfusion testing

Test	*Procedure*	*Comment*
Blood typing	Patient's red cells incubated with serum containing a known antibody	Naturally occurring antibodies are found in serum. Antibody to $Rh_o(D)$ antigen forms only after exposure. Agglutination confirms presence of A, B, $Rh_o(D)$ antigen. No agglutination denotes type O without A or B antigen.
Cross-matching		
Major	Donor red cells with membrane antigens incubated with recipient serum containing antibodies	Agglutination confirms recipient antibodies against donor red cells.
Minor	Recipient red cells with antigens incubated with donor serum containing antibodies	Agglutination confirms donor antibodies against recipient red cells.
Third phase	Donor and recipient are individually tested for very antigenic red cell antigens and lesser antigenic Duffy and Kidd antigens, as well as others	
Type and screen	Recipient and donor blood individually typed for A, B, $Rh_o(D)$ antigens and screened for antibodies	No cross match for compatibility is performed.

Table 11-26. A summary of ABO/Rh compatibility

Antigens and Antibodies

	Blood group	*Antigens on red blood cells*	*Antibodies in serum*
ABO	A	A	Anti-B
	B	B	Anti-A
	AB	A and B	—
	O	—	Anti-A and anti-B
Rh	Rh-positive	D	—
	Rh-negative	—	Anti-D only if sensitized

Blood Product Compatibility

Whole blood	Must be ABO-identical to patient.
Red blood cells	Must be compatible with patient serum.
Platelets	Should be compatible with patient red cells. Any blood group may be given if need is urgent.
Fresh frozen plasma	Should be compatible with patient red cells.
Cryoprecipitate	Should be compatible with patient red cells. Any blood group may be given if need is urgent.

If the patient is	*Blood group compatible with patient serum*	*Blood group compatible with patient cells*
A	A, O	A, AB
B	B, O	B, AB
AB	AB, A, B, O	AB only
O	O only	O, A, B, AB
Rh-positive	Rh-positive and Rh-negative	Rh not considered
Rh-negative	Rh-negative	Rh not considered

Source: Adapted from *Practical Aspects of Blood Transfusion*. Arlington, VA: American Association of Blood Banks, 1988. P 93.

ation. This quick assessment only eliminates ABO incompatability.

2. Type-specific, uncross-matched blood: The patient's blood type is determined. There is no incubation between patient and donor blood.
3. Uncross-matched, universal donor: When the patient is too hemodynamically unstable for typing, O^- blood (without A, B, or Rh_o [D] antigens) is transfused. Packed cells are safer because some O^- whole blood may have significant plasma titers of IgM, IgG, anti-A, and anti-B against recipient red cells. O^+ transfusion is acceptable when O^- is not available, but it is avoided in patients previously transfused or women of childbearing age because of Rh sensitization. When a patient receives greater than 2 units of uncross-matched O^- blood, the patient should not be switched to type-specific blood; O^- plasma containing antibodies may have produced a significant titer of antibodies against patient red cell antigens [57]. Prior to subsequent type-specific transfusions, antibody titers must be determined.

Complications and Risks

In addition to hemolytic and nonhemolytic transfusion reactions, there are other complications of blood and blood product transfusion (Tables 11-27, 11-28, and 11-29).

Circulatory Overload

Circulatory overload occurs more easily in infants, the elderly, the severely anemic, and cardiac patients. The symptoms include cough, dyspnea, and cyanosis. Under anesthesia, cyanosis, desaturation, difficulty ventilating, and edema may occur. The treatment is reverse Trendelenburg's position and diuretics [57].

Bacterial Contamination

Bacterial contamination leads to gram-negative shock that is manifested by chills, fever, and hypotension. The treatment is transfusion discontinuation, intravenous antibiotics, and supportive measures for treating shock [57].

Table 11-27. Characteristics of viral hepatitis

Characteristic	*Type A*	*Type B*	*Non-A, Non-B*
Transmission	Fecal-oral	Parenteral	Parenteral
Incubation	2–6 weeks	8–20 weeks	3–12 weeks
Prevention	Pooled gamma globulin	Specific hepatitis B immunoglobulin	Pooled gamma globulin
Course	Does not progress to chronic liver disease	10%—chronic liver disease	4–10%—chronic liver disease
Mortality	0–0.2%	0.3–15.0%	Undefined

Table 11-28. Risks: transfusion reactions and disease transmission

Reaction	*Chance/Unit*
Fever, chills, urticaria	1 : 100
Hemolytic transfusion reaction	
Typed and screened	1 : 6000–1 : 10,000
Cross-matched blood	1 : 6000–1 : 10,000
Typed only, uncross-matched	1 : 100
Previous transfusions or pregnancy	1 : 100
Fatal hemolytic transfusion reaction	1 : 100,000
Viral hepatitis	1 : 143–1 : 500
HIV infection	1 : 40,000–1 : 100,000

Source: From *Perioperative Red Cell Transfusion*. Presented at the National Institutes of Health Consensus Development Conference, June 1988.

Table 11-29. Complications of transfusion of blood products

	Etiology	*Signs and symptoms*	*Treatment*
Nonhemolytic			
Allergic[a]	Incompatible plasma proteins in donor blood, especially in atopic patients.	*Awake* patient: pruritus, erythema, and urticaria; increased temperature and eosinophilia often; occasional laryngospasm and bronchospasm. *Anesthetized* patient: erythema along the vein used for infusion; urticaria on face, neck, and chest.	Stop transfusion. Diphenhydramine, 1 mg/kg IV or 50 mg IM. Subsequent transfusions with *washed* packed red blood cells.
Febrile[b]	Recipient antibodies against antigens on donor white cells or platelets. Injured cells release pyrogens.	↑ temperature within 4 hours, which rarely exceeds 38°C Nausea, vomiting, and chest or back pain, chills. Appears like the early signs of acute hemolytic transfusion reaction (AHTR).	Stop transfusion. Aspirin or Tylenol. Rule out AHTR. Subsequent transfusions with leukocyte poor or washed packed red cells, frozen red cells, or type-specific platelets.
Hemolytic			
Acute hemolytic transfusion reaction[c]	Recipient plasma antibodies react with antigens on donor erythrocytes, thus activating the complement system, releasing histamine, increasing capillary permeability and destroying donor red cells. Antigen-antibody complex activates the kinin and coagulation cascade.	Occurs after as little as 20 ml blood. *Awake* patient: immediate chest or back pain, increased temperature, possible shivering, restlessness, nausea, dyspnea, skin flushing, and hypotension. *Anesthetized* patient: immediate hypotension *only*, followed by hemoglobinuria, oliguria or anuria, bleeding diathesis, anemia, jaundice.	Stop transfusion. Maintain urine output (75–100 ml/hr) Alkalinize urine (sodium bicarbonate) Determine plasma and urine hemoglobin concentrations Determine platelet count, PTT, and serum fibrinogen Return unused blood for recross-matching Rescreen patient's blood Maintain adequate renal perfusion
Delayed hemolytic transfusion reaction	Blood transfusion/pregnancy, which triggers undetectable levels of antibodies against Keil, Duffy, Kidd, E, C, D antigens to increase. Once antibody titer is sufficient, donor erythrocytes are destroyed.	4–21 days after transfusion of red cells, fever and anemia. Occasionally jaundice and hemaglobinuria.	Usually subclinical and require no treatment.

[a]Severe anaphylactic reactions are rare but likely to appear after only a few milliliters of blood. This is likely to occur in patients lacking IgA. Rarely an acute pulmonary hypersensitivity response with abrupt fever, cough, and pulmonary edema may occur.

[b]This is the most common transfusion reaction.

[c]Diagnostic tests: serum haptoglobin, plasma hemoglobin from hemolyzed cells, urine hemoglobin, unconjugated bilirubin from heme breakdown (3–6 hours later), direct antiglobulin tests (detects antigen-antibody complexes).

Noncardiac Pulmonary Edema

Noncardiac pulmonary edema is a rare complication that manifests as circulatory overload. The etiology is probably donor leukoagglutinins and recipient leukocytes trapped in the pulmonary circulation. The treatment is transfusion cessation, steroids, and respiratory support [54].

Graft-Versus-Host Disease

Graft-versus-host disease occurs very rarely in transfused patients receiving chemotherapy and irradiation. Fever, skin rash, hepatitis, and diarrhea are its primary manifestations [55].

Metabolic Abnormalities

During storage, red cell metabolism continues, resulting in changes in levels of carbon dioxide, hydrogen ions, 2,3-diphosphoglycerate (2,3-DPG), and potassium. The anticoagulant citrate can also produce metabolic derangement during transfusion [57].

Hydrogen Ions

Hydrogen ions increase after 14 to 21 days due to (1) continued erythrocyte metabolism, (2) glycolysis, (3) the lower pH of stored blood, and (4) carbon dioxide produced by erythrocyte metabolism. Despite the inherent metabolic acidosis from storage, metabolic alkalosis is more frequent because the citrate is converted to bicarbonate by the liver. Patients who have renal dysfunction may experience alkalosis, since they cannot eliminate bicarbonate [57].

Potassium

Potassium increases to about 6 to 8 mEq/300 ml of packed red cells after 21 days of storage. Even after massive transfusions (>10 units of packed red cells), only 70 mEq of potassium in 21-day-old blood would be transfused. Such levels do not increase the serum potassium concentration to a dangerous level. Patients with renal dysfunction are an exception. Furthermore, the relative metabolic alkalosis that accompanies massive transfusion causes intracellular movement of potassium ions [56].

2,3-Diphosphoglycerate

2,3-DPG decreases in stored blood. Although the temperature is lowered, erythrocyte metabolism continues, thereby causing a leftward shift in the oxygen-hemoglobin dissociation curve. This theoretically could result in less effective tissue oxygenation because of the increased affinity of hemoglobin for oxygen. 2,3-DPG levels are maintained after 1 week in citrate phosphate dextrose (CPD)–stored blood, while levels decrease in adenosine citrate dextrose (ACD)–stored blood [56].

Citrate Intoxication

Attributed to citrate chelation of calcium ions, citrate intoxication is usually a problem in the patient with hepatic dysfunction who is unable to metabolize the citrate to bicarbonate. In a healthy patient, hypocalcemia leading to hypotension and a prolonged QT interval does not occur unless blood is transfused at rates greater than 150ml/70 kg/minute (approximately 10 units/hour). The treatment of symptomatic hypocalcemia is calcium chloride, 3 to 6 mg/kg over 5 to 15 minutes with continuous ECG monitoring.

Disease Transmission

Viral Hepatitis

Viral hepatitis is the most common infection related to blood product transfusion. Icteric hepatitis occurs in 1 to 3 percent of all transfused patients, with 3 to 7 percent of those patients progressing to chronic liver disease [58]. The symptoms appear from 90 to 180 days after transfusion. Non-A, non-B hepatitis accounts for 90 percent of cases; there is still no serologic test for this virus. Hepatitis B has decreased dramatically with preoperative testing. Hepatitis A is rare because there is no carrier state viremia. The tests for hepatitis B are hepatitis B surface antigen and core antibody. Volunteer versus commercial or designated-donor blood products, decreased hospitalization, and limited transfusion have decreased the risks of hepatitis transmission [55].

Acquired Immunodeficiency Syndrome (AIDS)

Unquestionably, AIDS is the most feared infection transmitted by blood products. By 1987, only about 2.0 to 2.5 percent of reported AIDS cases were transfusion related [51]. However, this number probably is low because testing for the virus only began in 1985 and the incubation time for HTLV III is more than 2 to 5 years. It is prevented by discouraging donations by high-risk groups, predonation HIV testing, and autologous blood transfusion. Other viral, bacterial, or rickettsial infections have been reported but at much lower incidences [51].

Homologous Transfusion Alternatives

Autotransfusion

In recent years, concern about transfusion-transmitted diseases has led to increased autologous blood donation. There are three types of autologous blood donation: preoperative donation, preoperative phlebotomy with isovolemic hemodilution, and intraoperative "cell-saver" reinfusion. Autotransfusion (1) avoids the risk of disease transmission, (2) avoids autoimmunization of blood components and plasma proteins, (3) ensures the availability of compatible blood, and (4) stimulates red cell production in the preoperative period. The main disadvantage of predonation, as with all banked blood, is clerical error [53].

Predonation

Predonation of blood for perioperative transfusion requires a hemoglobin of 11 gm/dl and the collection of approximately 250 to 300ml of blood at intervals of 7 to 10 days. Presently, up to 4 units may be collected. The last collection is at least 2 days prior to surgery. This technique is contraindicated in some patients with heart disease, aortic stenosis, bacteremia, active infection (requiring antibiotics), and positive HIV or hepatitis antibodies [54].

Acute Phlebotomy with Normovolemic Hemodilution

Acute phlebotomy with normovolemic hemodilution is the collection of blood while concurrently infusing lactated Ringer's solution to maintain normovolemia. Collection is terminated when the targeted hemocrit decreases to 22 to 25 gm/dl. The blood is stored in ACD anticoagulant at room temperature for no more than 6 hours before retransfusion [53].

Intraoperative "Cell-Saver" Technique

Intraoperative cell-saver technique is an excellent intraoperative source of red cells. Blood from patients free of malignancy or a noninfected surgical field is collected, anticoagulated, saline washed, and reinfused. If massive volumes of saline-washed cells are autotransfused, a dilutional coagulopathy requiring plasma or platelets may develop. Intraoperative red cell salvage and infusion is common during thoracic or open heart surgery [53]. This technique is not recommended for most head and neck cancer patients. Predonation and acute phlebotomy are preferred.

Perfluorocarbon Emulsions

Clinically, perfluorocarbon emulsions are ineffective in patients with severe anemia because of the small increase in oxygen content, short half-life of less than 24 hours, and the limited total dose [53].

Recombinant Human Erythropoietin

Recombinant human erythropoietin (r-HuEPO) significantly accelerates endogenous erythropoiesis in uremic patients [59]. It may be a future strategy for decreasing homologous transfusion. Given preoperatively and postoperatively, r-HuEPO may increase hemoglobin levels such that more autologous units may be obtained or that blood loss may not require intraoperative or postoperative transfusion [52].

1-D-Amino-8-D-Arginine Vasopressin (DDAVP)

DDAVP has been shown to decrease blood loss intraoperatively and postoperatively by augmenting platelet adhesiveness, thereby reducing the need for red cell transfusions [52].

Anesthetic Technique

Intraoperative Hypotension

Hypotensive anesthesia may be used to decrease blood loss. Usually, a mean arterial blood pressure of 55 to 60 mm Hg is maintained by a combination of inhalational anesthesia, intravenous vasodilators, or beta blockers in healthy patients. A higher mean blood pressure may be required for patients with medical problems [53].

Oxygen Transporters

Subject of much research, stroma-free hemoglobin is prepared from outdated blood. Hemoglobin is separated from the red cell membrane. A manufactured polystroma-free hemoglobin-P (Poly-SFH-P) has been developed that has a P_{50} of 20 to 22. This is comparable to 2-week-old banked blood. The only problem preventing clinical testing is studies showing renal dysfunction after infusion of Poly-SFH-P [53].

REFERENCES

1. Tisi GM: Pre-operative evaluation of pulmonary function: Validity, indications and benefits. *Am Rev Respir Dis* 119 : 293, 1979.
2. Tisi GM: Pre-operative identification and evaluation of the patient with lung disease. *Med Clin North Am* 71 : 399, 1987.
3. Tantum KR: Respiratory care of the surgical patient with cardiac disease. *Surg Clin North Am* 63 : 1069, 1983.
4. Ayers L, Whipp B, Ziment I: *A Guide to the Interpretation of Pulmonary Function Tests.* New York: Roering Pharmaceuticals, 1978.
5. Gregg R: *Manual of Pulmonary Testing.* St. Louis: Mosby 1986.
6. Benumof J (ed): *Anesthesia for Thoracic Surgery.* Philadelphia: Saunders, 1987.
7. Weitz HH, Goldman L: Noncardiac surgery in the patient with heart disease. *Med Clin North Am* 71(3) : 413, 1987.
8. Mangano D: Perioperative cardiac morbidity. *Anesthesiology* 72 : 153, 1990.
9. Frye RL, et al: Task force III: Major demographic and epidemiologic trends affecting adult cardiology. *J Am Coll Cardiol* 12 : 840, 1988.
10. Mangano D: *Perioperative Cardiac Assessment.* Philadelphia: Lippincott, 1990. P 1.
11. Cohn PF: Silent myocardial ischemia: Dimensions of the problem in patients with and without angina. *Am J Med* 80(suppl 4c) : 1, 1986.
12. Cohn PF: Silent myocardial ischemia as a manifestation of asymptomatic coronary artery disease: What is appropriate therapy? *Am J Cardiol* 56 : 280, 1985.
13. Goldman S, Jpelos S, Cohn K: Marked depth of ST segment depression during treadmill exercise testing: Indicator of coronary artery disease. *Chest* 69 : 729, 1976.
14. London H, Mangano D: Assessment of perioperative cardiac risk. In Thomas S (ed): *Problems in Anesthesia: Cardiovascular Anesthesia.* Philadelphia: Lippincott, 1987. Vol 1, No 3, P 337.
15. Diamond GA, Forrester JS: Analysis of probability as an aid in the clinical diagnosis of coronary artery disease. *N Engl J Med* 300 : 1350, 1979.
16. Burgus LG, et al: Increased intraoperative cardiovascular morbidity in diabetics with autonomic neuropathy. *Anesthesiology* 70 : 591, 1989.
17. The 1988 Report of the Joint National Committee on Determination, Evaluation and Treatment of High Blood Pressure. *Joint Ntl Comm Arch Int Med* 148 : 1023, 1988.
18. Leslie J, Knopes K: *J Cardiother Anesth* 4(5; suppl 2) : 3, 1990.
19. Veterans Administration Cooperative Study Group on Antihypertensive Agents. Effects of treatment on morbidity in hypertension II: Results in patients with diastolic blood pressure averaging 90 through 114 mm Hg. *JAMA* 213 : 1143, 1970.
20. Prys-Roberts C, Meloche R: Management of anesthesia in patients with hypertension or ischemia heart disease. *Int Anesthesiol Clin* 18 : 181, 1980.
21. Estafanous F: Hypertension in the surgical patient: Management of blood pressure and anesthesia. *Clev Clin J Med,* June 1989. p 385.
22. Koplan J: The poorly controlled hypertensive patient. *J Cardiother Anesth* 4(4; suppl) : 19, 1990.
23. Kannel WB, et al: Blood pressure and risk of coronary heart disease: The Framingham study. *Dis Chest* 56 : 43, 1969.
24. Miller E: Mechanisms and treatment of Perioperative Hypertension. *ASA Refresher Course* 224 : 1–6, 1989.
25. Prys-Roberts C, Meloche R, Foex P: Studies of anesthesia in relation to hypertension: I. Cardiovascular response of treated and untreated patients. *Br J Anaesth* 43 : 122, 1971.
26. Leslie J, Knopes K: Pathophysiology of hypertension and tachycardia. *J Cardiother Anesth* 4(5; Suppl 2) : 3, 1990.
27. Goldman L, Colders D: Risks of general anesthesia and elective operation in the hypertensive patient. *Anesthiology* 50 : 285, 1979.
28. Roizen M, et al: Patients with disorders of thyroid function. *Anesth Clin North Am* 5 : 277, 1987.
29. Stoelting RK, Dierdorf SF, McCammon RL: Endocrine Disease. In: *Anesthesia and Co-existing Disease.* New York: Churchill Livingstone, 1988. P 473.
30. Goldman DR: Surgery in patients with endocrine dysfunction. *Med Clin North Am* 71 : 499, 1987.
31. Roizen MF: Endocrine abnormalities and anes-

thesia: Implications for the anesthesiologist. *ASA Refresher Course* 12 : 161, 1984.
32. White VA, Kumagai LF: Preoperative endocrine and metabolic considerations. *Med Clin North Am* 63(6) : 1321, 1979.
33. Freidman L: Surgery in the patient with liver disease. *Med Clin North Am* 71(3) : 453, 1987.
34. Lamont JT: The Liver. In Vandam LD (ed): To Make the Patient Ready for Anesthesia: Medical Care of the Surgical Patient. Reading, MA: Addison-Wesley, 1984. P 47.
35. Strunin L: Anesthetic management of patients with liver disease. *Liver and Biliary Disease*. London: Saunders, 1985. P 1379.
36. Greenwood SM, Leffler CT: The increased mortality rate of open biopsy in alcoholic hepatitis. *Surg Gynecol Obstet* 134 : 600, 1972.
37. Brown B: Anesthetizing the patient with abnormal liver function. *ASA Refresher Course*, 1989. P 532.
38. Hargrove MD: Chronic active hepatitis: Possible adverse effect of exploratory laparotomy. *Surgery* (68)771, 1970.
39. Stoelting RK, Dierdorf SF: Diseases of the Liver and Biliary Tract. In Stoelting RK, Dierdorf SF, McCammon RL (eds): *Anesthesia and Co-existing Disease*. New York: Churchill Livingstone, 1988. P 355.
40. Harville DD, Summerskill WH: Surgery in acute hepatitis. *JAMA* 184 : 257, 163.
41. Garrison RN, et al: Clarification of risk factors for abdominal operations in patients with hepatic cirrhosis. *Ann Surg* 199(6) : 648, 1984.
42. Doberneck RC, Sterling WA, Allison DC: Morbidity and mortality after operation in nonbleeding cirrhotic patients. *Am J Surg* 146 : 306, 1983.
43. Mazze RI: Critical care of the patient with acute renal failure. *Anesthesiology* 47 : 138, 1977.
44. Sladen RN: Perioperative management of the patient with renal failure. *ASA Refresher Course* 1988. P 172.
45. Weir PH, Chung FF: Anaesthesia for patients with chronic renal disease. *Can Anaesth Soc J* 31(4) : 468, 1984.
46. Burke JF, Francos GC: Surgery in the patient with acute or chronic renal failure. *Med Clin North Am* 71(3) : 489, 1987.
47. Goldman DR: Surgery in patients with endocrine dysfunction. *Med Clin North Am* 71(3) : 499, 1987.
48. Stevens A, Roizen MF: Patients with diabetes mellitus and disorders of glucose metabolism. *Anesth Clin North Am* 5 : 339, 1987.
49. Roizen MF: Endocrine abnormalities and anesthesia: Implications for the anesthesiologist. *ASA Refresher Course* 12 : 161, 1984.
50. Moorthy SS: Metabolism and Nutrition. In Stoelting RK, Dierdorf SF, McCammon RL (eds): *Anesthesia and Co-existing Disease*. New York: Churchill Livingstone, 1988. P 485.
51. Miller RD, Brzica SM: Blood, Blood Component, Colloid and Autotransfusion Therapy. In Miller RD (ed): *Anesthesia*. New York: Churchill Livingstone, 1988. P 1329.
52. Calhoun L: The Infusion of Blood and Blood Components. In Reynolds A, Steckler D (eds): *Practical Aspects of Blood Transfusion*. Arlington, VA: American Association of Blood Banks, 1988. P 43.
53. Perioperative Red Cell Transfusion. Presented at the National Institutes of Health Consensus Development Conference, June 1988.
54. McNiece WL: Disorders of Coagulation. In Stoelting RK, Dierdorf SF, McCammon RL (eds): *Anesthesia and Co-existing Disease*. New York: Churchill Livingstone, 1988. P 575.
55. Gravlee G, Hopkins M: Blood Plasma Products. In Enison N, Jobeo D (eds): *Effective Hemostasis in Cardiac Surgery*. Philadelphia: Saunders, 1988. P 69.
56. Peschel M: Adverse Effects of Blood Transfusion. In Reynolds A, Stechler D (eds): *Practical Aspects of Blood Transfusion*. Arlington, VA: American Association of Blood Banks, 1988. P 95.
57. McNiece WL: Transfusion Therapy. In Stoelting RK, Dierdorf SF, McCammon RL (eds): *Anesthesia and Co-existing Disease*. New York: Churchill Livingstone, 1988.
58. Miller RD: Problems Posed by Transfusion. In Orkin F, Cooperman L (eds): *Complications in Anesthesiology*. Philadelphia: Lippincott, 1983.
59. Eschbach JW, et al: Treatment of the anemia of progressive renal failure with recombinant human erythropoietin. *N Engl J Med* 321(3) : 158, 1989.
60. Barash P, Cullen B, Stoelting R (eds): *Clinical Anesthesia*. Philadelphia: JB Lippincott, 1982. p. 422.

12

Wounds

MARK V. ALEXANDER and ERNEST M. MYERS

KEY CONCEPTS

Phases of Healing; Healing Principles; Antibiotics; Surgical Principles; Complications

MILESTONES

60,000 B.C.	Herb Theory	Neanderthal Man (Iran)
1,500 B.C.	Burn Therapy	Elbers Papyrus (Egypt)
700 B.C.	Salves, Ointments, and Fats	Hesiod
300 B.C.	Elements, Qualities, and Humors	*Corpus Hippocraticum*
14–37 A.D.	*Dere Medicina*	Celsus
65 A.D.	*Materia Medica*	Discorides
77 A.D.	*Natural History*	Pliny the Elder
630–640 A.D.	*On Burns*	Paul of Aegina
1628	Circulation of Blood	Harvey
1644	Concept of Disease	Van Helmont
1861	Systematic Asepsis	Semmelweiss
1858	Cell Theory	Virchow
1867	Disinfection	Lister
1870	Practical Clinical Thermometer	Allbut
1905	Koch's Postulates of Contagion	Koch
1908	Chemotherapy for Infection	Ehrlich
1910	Surgeon's Gloves	Halstead
1917	Sulfanilamide Antibiotics	Jacobs
1929	Penicillin	Fleming
1944	Streptomycin	Waksman

An understanding of wounds is essential and germane to head and neck oncology. Modern physiologic principles are utilized in managing these patients from diagnosis through rehabilitation. The following discussion is based on the current medical literature and clinical observations.

PHASES OF HEALING

For most wounds, the primary concern is effective restoration of the skin. The skin consists of three layers: epidermis, dermis, and subcutaneous tissue. The outer layer is a relatively thick layer composed of epithelial cells. Dermis, the thin but tough middle layer, is the collagen sheet responsible for tensile strength. The innermost layer consists of fat and blood vessels interlaced with connective tissue. Altogether these three layers form a pliable, tough organ that wraps, insulates, and protects the entire body [1].

Wound healing is a dynamic process that is divided into four phases: inflammation, destruction, proliferation, and maturation (Table 12-1) [2–4].

Inflammation (0–3 Days): Stage I

The inflammation phase is characterized by vasodilation followed by vasoconstriction. A clot is formed from platelet aggregation; simultaneously fibrin, transudated fluid, mast cells, and polymorphonuclear cells accumulate interstitially. Fibrin, initiated by the inflammatory phase, seals the lymphatics, thus isolating and localizing the reaction. The inflammatory response is mediated by a variety of vasoactive agents: histamines, vasopeptides, prostaglandins, and proteolytic enzymes, and histamines. Early vasodilation and increased permeability are prolonged by prostaglandins.

Destruction (1–6 Days): Stage II

Facilitated by fibrin deposition, the polymorphonuclear cells are gradually replaced by lymphocytes and macrophages. Monocytes, late arrivals in the inflammatory phase, usher in the destructive phase of healing. Acting as scavengers, the monocytes ingest and destroy debris by phagocytosis and autolysis. Excessive necrosis, foreign bodies, and bacterial contamination may prolong this phase. Eventually, some of the monocytes differentiate into fibroblasts.

Table 12-1. Healing phases

Stage	*Phase*	*Cellular response*	*Biochemical response*	*Histophysiology*
I 0–3 days	Inflammation	Mast cells Epithelial migration	Histamine Serotonin	Vasodilation Increased capillary permeability
			Monamine oxidase	Exudation and edema Phagocytosis Chemotaxis
		Red blood cells Platelets	Oxygenation Prostaglandin E_2 Prostaglandin E_1, E_2	Fibrin formation Epithelial maturation and keratinization
II 1–6 days	Destruction	Granulocytes	Norepinephrine Heparin Hydrolytic enzymes	Vasoconstriction Anticoagulation Tissue necrosis and lysis Fibroblastic activation & stimulation
		Macrophages	Chemotactic factors	Phagocytosis
III 3–14 days	Proliferation	Myofibroblasts	Growth factors	Neovascularity
			Mucopolysaccharide formation Collagen formation Glycoprotein formation Fibrinolysis	Capillary proliferation Fibroblast proliferation Granulation tissue Epithelialization
IV 6–12 months	Maturation	Fibroblasts	Collagen reorientation	Decreased capillaries Scarring & wound contraction Decreased wound cellularity

Proliferation (3–14 Days): Stage III

Epithelialization

Within hours of wounding, epithelial migration ensues, beginning with basal cells deeply located in undamaged epithelium, especially hair follicles [1]. This subphase may be prolonged or aborted by excessive local tissue necrosis, foreign bodies, or contamination. When the wound is approximated cleanly and sutured, epithelialization may be completed within 24 hours. Under ideal conditions, little eschar, cellular infiltration, and degeneration occur and healing is excellent.

Granulation

Simultaneously, as the wound is invaded by fibroblasts and capillary buds, granulation tissue is formed. Metabolic activity is high, and the wound contracts centripedally. Fine collagen fibrils appear as the wound rapidly acquires tensile strength.

Angiogenesis

Rapid capillary formation associated with granulation precedes fibroblastic activity. This fibroblastic migration is facilitated by chemotaxis and transudation. The stimulus for angiogenesis is unknown.

Fibroplasia

New fibroblasts, arising from mononuclear cells present in the destructive phase, begin to proliferate. Their movement is enhanced by the fibrin lattice that acts as filamentous highways for cellular migration. Fibroblasts synthesize the collagen, glycoproteins, and mucopolysaccharides that compose the dermis. The key cell in this phase is the myofibroblast, a cell possessing both fibroblastic and smooth muscle characteristics. The introduction of this cell causes the granulating bed to contract rapidly. Collagen deposition and cross-linking further accelerates wound contraction.

Maturation (14 Days–1 Year): Stage IV

The final phase of wound healing is characterized by decreased cellularity and increased tensile strength [4]. Collagen formation seems directly proportional to the decrease in fibroblast and capillary activity. As the cellular component decreases, collagen deposition increases and stabilizes. The wound becomes pale in contrast to the dusky-red, granulation stage. Gradually, the scar matures, softens, and flattens.

COLLAGEN SYNTHESIS

Connective tissue, a continuous fibrous fabric, constitutes 30 percent of the body's weight [1]. It is a family of specialized molecules with common structural features. Connective tissue is composed of collagen, reticulin, and elastin embedded in ground substance (mucopolysaccharides and mucoproteins). Clinging to this weave of connective tissue are fibroblasts, fat cells, histiocytes, mast cells, and plasmacytes.

Fibroblast

The fibroblast is the cell responsible for the manufacture of collagen (Table 12-2) [4]. Trophocollagen, a collagen precursor, is organized into three polypeptide chains that consist of 1050 amino acid residues, each weighing 95,000 molecular weight [3].

Alpha Chains

The triple helix of alpha chains is the definitive structure of all collagen molecules. These chains are manufactured intracellularly in the rough endoplasmic reticulum after RNA transcription. Once formed, they are discharged extracellularly for further modification, cross-linking, and collagen fiber formation [5–7].

Table 12-2. The fibroblast: collagen synthesis

Rough endoplasmic reticulum
1. Amino acid incorporation (proline & lysine)
2. Polypeptide chain assembly
3. Proline & lysine hydroxylation
4. Formation of trophocollagen from polypeptide chains
5. Addition of carbohydrate moiety

Extracelluar space
1. Trophocollagen extrusion
2. Trophocollagen aggregation into collagen fibrils
3. Collagen fibril aggregation into collagen fibers

HEALING

Wound healing is a complex process influenced by a variety of intrinsic and extrinsic conditions. This section analyzes the external and internal milieus that influence healing [8–11]. Table 12-3 outlines general conditions that promote healing.

Environment

Oxygen

Essential for effective wound healing, oxygen consumption increases during active wound healing. The PO_2 in an incised open wound is 30 to 50 mm Hg [7]. Although the minimal PO_2 needed for wound healing is unknown, fibroblast replication is potentiated at a PO_2 of 30 to 40 mm Hg. Collagen synthesis requires increased oxygen partial pressures. Moreover, epithelial cell proliferation is directly proportional to wound arterial oxygen tension. Finally, normal oxygen tensions are needed for hydroxylation of proline and lysine, the amino acids necessary for collagen cross-linking.

Circulation

Blood pressure

Normal blood pressure favors wound healing. Hypotension, acute or chronic, hinders wound healing.

Blood Volume

Normal blood volume and red blood cell counts enhance oxygen carrying capacity and tissue oxygenation.

Microcirculation

Microcirculation may be compromised by low blood volume, hypertension, collagen vascular disease, diabetes mellitus, and widespread atherosclerosis. Certain medications reduce microcirculation temporarily.

Table 12-3. Healing promoters

Infrared
Carbon ruby laser
Electromagnetic fields
Ultrasound

Thyroid Hormone

Thyroid hormone provides DNA and RNA synthesis, increases mitoses, and enhances epithelialization. Hypothyroid patients generally have delayed healing in all phases. Samples of acquired thyroid deficiency are patients who have had post–full course head and neck radiation and those who have had total laryngectomy with thyroid lobectomy. Some authors estimate the incidence to be as high as 20 percent [8].

Vitamins

Vitamins A, C, and E are free radical scavengers along with the amino acid glutathione (Tables 12-4 and 12-5). Vitamin C is essential for collagen synthesis [7]. Wounding or injury leads to reduced vitamin C levels; therefore, vitamin C is recommended after surgery. Vitamin A levels also fall after burns or injury. Restoration of vitamin A reverses the depression of collagen synthesis by steroids. Vitamin E enhances fibroblast growth in vitro and increases collagen formation [7]. It corrects glutathione synthetase deficiency and platelet aggregation deficiency. Finally, it promotes the formation of prostaglandins [9].

Prostaglandins and Thromboxanes

Postaglandins and thromboxanes are potent humoral mediators of inflammation that are capable of inducing the accumulation and regulation of inflammatory cells [9, 10]. Prostaglandins also stimulate smooth muscle contraction.

Synthesis

Prostaglandins and thromboxanes compose a group of polyunsaturated, hydroxylated, long-chain fatty acids. The synthesis of thromboxane and the stable primary prostaglandins (E_2, F, and D_2) is through an endoperoxidase intermediate formed and broken down by a system of enzymes and coenzymes collectively called "prostaglandin synthetase" (Figure 12-1).

Aspirin

The aspirin-like drugs inhibit this multienzyme system acetylation of the active site of cyclooxygenase. This blocks the production of the endoperoxidases and all their derivatives.

Table 12-4. Healing and malnutrition

Deficiency		Healing Phase			
General	*Specific*	*Stage I*	*Stage II*	*Stage III*	*Stage IV*
Hypoxia	Anemia	+	+ +	+ +	+
	Shock	+ +	+ +	+	
	Renal insufficiency	+	+	+ +	+
Glucose			+ +	+ +	
Protein	Hepatic insufficiency			+ +	+
	Kwashiorkor				
Vitamins	A			+ +	+ +
	B			+ +	
	C		+	+ +	+
Trace elements	Zinc			+ +	+
	Copper			+ +	+

+ + Principal effect. + Secondary effect.

Glucocorticoids
Steroids inhibit prostaglandin synthesis, apparently by inhibiting phospholiphase A_2 activity, so that less arachidonic acid is hydrolyzed from intracellular phospholipids. The reduced substrate decreases prostaglandin synthesis.

Inflammation
Blood vessels and many other body tissues can synthesize prostaglandins and thromboxane. These compounds are synthesized and released in tissues in response to a wide variety of stimuli (hormones, enzymes, trauma, inflammation, pyrogens, and immune and allergic reactions).

Chemotaxis
Eicosatetraenoic acid (ETA) is an acetylenic analog of arachidonic acid and an irreversible competitive inhibitor of endoperoxidase production and the products of arachidonic acid lipo-oxygenation called hydoxyeicosatetraenoic acids (HETEs). The HETEs are lipid mediators that elicit potent leukocyte chemotaxis.

Table 12-5. Vitamins: recommended requirements

Vitamin	*Usual*	*Range*	*Maximum (Safe)*
A	5000 IU	5–8000 IU	50,000 IU
C	60 mg	60–5000 mg	5000 mg
E	30 IU	30–1600 IU	56,000 IU

Prostaglandin$_2$ enhances the chemotaxic responsiveness of monocytes. Thromboxane B_2, prostaglandin, and HETE are chemotaxic for polymorphonuclear leukocytes in vitro and may act locally to induce leukocyte migration.

Platelet Aggregation and Inhibition
Although platelets can synthesize arachidonic acid, they lack prostacyclin synthetase; therefore, they cannot convert it into prostacyclin. Instead, they convert arachidonic acid into thromboxane A_2, a potent vasoconstrictor and platelet aggregator [11]. However, adjacent uninjured epithelium inhibits further platelet aggregation and coagulation with protein C, a vitamin K-dependent protein. Platelets also have alpha granules that contain a variety of coagulation proteins (e.g., factor V, fibrinogen). Aggregated platelets plug the wound and release factor X, a factor that initiates the prothrombinase complex for the conversion of prothrombin to thrombin (see Chapter 11). Thus, the first hemostatic plug is platelets interlaced in fibrin strands. Note the interrelationship between wound healing and hemostasis.

Steroids
When present before injury, steroids suppress fibroblast multiplication. This effect is enhanced by starvation or protein deficiency. Steroids also reduce immunologic responses. Single or short-

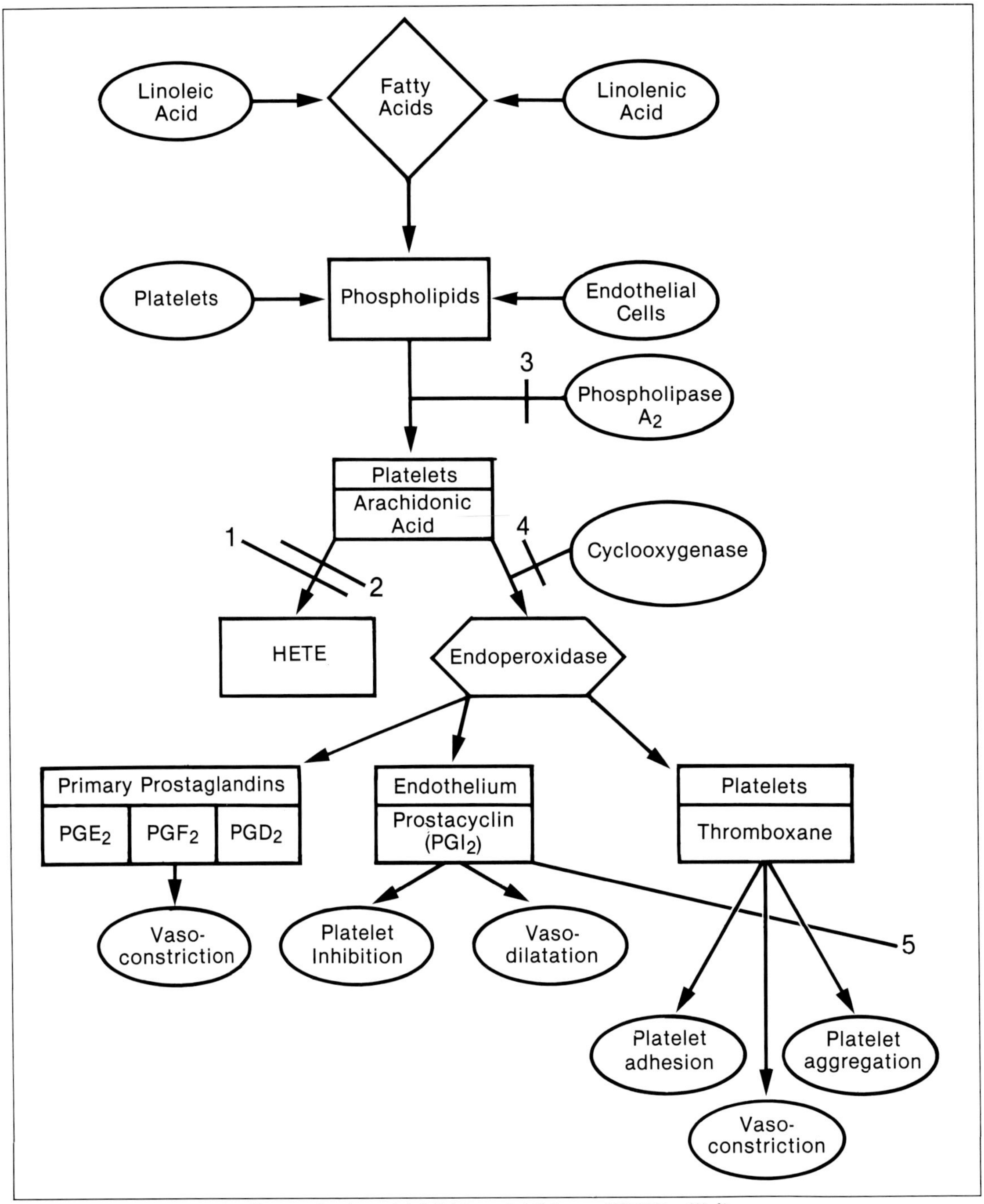

Figure 12-1. Prostaglandin synthesis and inhibition. Inhibitors: (1)ETA, (2) lipooxygenase inhibition, (3) steroids, (4) aspirin, (5) prostacyclin, protein C.

term doses do not impair wound healing, whereas high doses decrease inflammatory cell activity. In the presence of steroids, polymorphonuclear cells have reduced mitosis, phagocytosis, and diapedesis. Steroids also decrease lymphocytes and mast cell activity. Likewise, fibroblasts have decreased mitosis and reduced active transport.

WOUND MANAGEMENT

Infection hinders wound healing by prolonging the inflammatory phase. Epithelialization and secondary collagen production are halted by persistent inflammation or infection.

Preparation

With rare exceptions, aside from shaving the beard, it is unnecessary to remove hair preoperatively for head and neck surgery. A vigorous scrub with an antibacterial solution or detergent is sufficient. Povidone-iodine (Betadine) or Hibiclens commonly are used for the external scrub. Some oral surgeons and dentists rinse the oral cavity with these solutions prior to extractions or extensive oral surgery. Innocuous to the eyes and ears, their use on open incisions is controversial.

Prophylaxis

Preoperative antibiotics, especially with anaerobic agents, effectively reduce the incidence of postoperative infections [12–18]. Prophylaxis usually is recommended for traumatized or contaminated wounds (Tables 12-6 and 12-7), incisions that involve or violate the mucous membranes of the aerodigestive tracts, and surgery in compromised patients (Table 12-8). Finally, it is almost mandatory for the following situations:

1. Preoperative radiation.
2. Chronic steroid usage.
3. Preoperative chemotherapy.

Table 12-6. Surgical wound classification

Class I	Clean; usually a skin incision without entry into an actual or potential space
Class II	Elective entry into gastrointestinal or respiratory tract
Class III	Elective entry into an inflamed area or associated indirect gastrointestinal spillage
Class IV	Dirty wound or gross pus

Table 12-7. Types of healing

Primary intention	Normal healing following a clean incision and tissue approximation
Secondary intention	An open wound that heals by granulation, epithelialization, and contraction.
Tertiary intention	A wound left open for 3–5 days and then approximated (suppurative wounds)

Table 12-8. Past medical history: compromised healing

	Mechanism	*Etiology*
Congenital diseases	Mucopolysaccharidoses (abnormal collagen production & faulty cross-linking)	Rheumatoid arthritis Systemic & discoid lupus Scleroderma Sjögren's syndrome Dermatomyositis Vasculitides Temporal arteritis Giant cell arteritis Wegener's granulomatosis
Endocrinopathy	Decreased inflammation; poor microcirculatory response and delays in all phases of healing	Diabetes mellitus Hypothyroidism
Metabolic dysfunction	Decreased blood volume or protein deficiency	Hepatic insufficiency Renal insufficiency
Previous therapy	Reduced blood supply and scarring; slow collagen production and epithelialization	Chemotherapy Surgery Radiotherapy

Table 12-9. Antibiotics: general considerations

Drug Class	***Features***	***Precautions***
Aminoglycosides	Inhibits protein synthesis Bacteriostatic Often used in combination regimes for life-threatening infections Poor oral absorption Poor crossing of blood-brain barrier	Nephrotoxicity Ototoxicity
Cephalosporins	Inhibits cell wall synthesis Bactericidal Penicillin substitute Surgical prophylaxis	10% cross-reactivity with penicillin-allergic patients
Chloramphenicol	Bacteriostatic Indicated for rickettsial and enteric infections Unsurpassed penetration of blood-brain barrier Effective orally	Bone marrow suppression Aplastic anemia Pregnancy
Clindamycin	Suppresses protein synthesis Bacteriostatic Effective against all gram-positive cocci Poor penetration of blood-brain barrier	Gastroenteritis Pseudomembranous colitis Diarrhea
Erythromycins	Inhibits protein synthesis Bactericidal Inexpensive Pencillin alternative	Gastrointestinal distress
Metronidazole	Bactericidal against *Bacteroides fragilis* Relieves pain of multiple pharyngeal ulcers Favorable effect on painful moniliasis	Wide spectrum of safety
Penicillin	Inhibits cell wall synthesis Bactericidal Widest margin of safety Wide spectrum of activity (see Table 12-10)	Hypersensitivity (5%) Anaphylaxis (1/10,000)
Sulfonamides	Bacteriostatic Synergistic when combined with other antibiotics (bactericidal)	Skin eruptions Poor potential when used alone
Tetracyclines	Inhibits protein synthesis Bacteriostatic Inexpensive	Do not give with antacids Contraindicated for nursing mothers, children (first 8 years) Esophagitis
Vancomycin	Penicillin substitute for serious gram-positive infections Poor gastrointestinal absorption In vitro activity against *Staphylococcus aureus*	Ototoxicity

Source. Adapted from Fairbanks DNF: *Pocket Guide to Antimicrobial Therapy in Otolaryngology Head and Neck Surgery* (4th ed). Washington, DC: AAO-HNS Foundation, 1985. Pp 54–57.

4. Steroid therapy.
5. Cancer chemotherapy.
6. Diabetes mellitus.
7. Renal disease.
8. Exposure of intracranial spaces.
9. Packing or prosthetics.
10. Endocarditis prophylaxis.

At the very least, the antibiotics should be given parenterally 1 to 2 hours prior to surgery. Many surgeons begin the agents 8 to 12 hours preoperatively. Penicillin is a very effective agent. However, if the patient is allergic to penicillin, erythromycin, clindamycin, and chloramphenicol are alternatives (Tables 12-9 through 12-12; Figure 12-2). Suggested guidelines are as follows:

1. Clean cases: First-generation cephalosporin (Ancef, Kefzol): 1 gm IV 1 or 2 hours preoperatively, then 500 mg every 6 hours for four doses or until mucous leakage has stopped or packing has been removed.
2. Contaminated cases: aminoglycoside plus antistaphylococcal penicillin.
3. Anaerobic infection: clindamycin and gentamycin or a third-generation cephalosporin. Johnson and Liu [12] recommend clinidamycin before wound contamination, followed by 600 mg every 6–8 hours for a total of four doses.

Surgical Principles

Surgery may be defined as invasive treatment based on planned improvisation. However, before relying on the latter, sound scientific principles are employed to minimize untoward results (Table 12-13).

Incisions

Unlike surgery in many other areas of the body, access to the head and neck is facilitated by a variety of incisions. Wherever possible, these incisions are placed within skin creases and along natural areas of skin relaxation. Given these basic restrictions, the available surgical approaches are numerous (Table 12-14; Figure 12-3, 12-4).

Table 12-10. Special penicillins

Antistaphylococcal penicillins	Cloxacillin Dicloxacillin* Methacillin Nafcillin Oxacillin
Aminopencillins (gram-negative bacteria)	Ampicillin Amoxicillin* Bacampicillin Cylcacillin Hetacillin
Antipseudomonas pencillins	Azlocillin Carbenicillin Mezlocillin Piperacillin* Ticarcillin

*Drug of choice.
Source. Data from Fairbanks DNF: *Pocket Guide to Antimicrobial Therapy in Otolaryngology Head and Neck Surgery* (4th ed). Washington, DC: AAO-HNS Foundation, 1985. Pp 54–57.

Face

Whenever possible, an incision is placed in a natural skin crease or wrinkle. The nose has multidirectional lines of pull; therefore the direction of incisions in this area is less critical. As a rule, incisions are placed perpendicular to the skin surface; deviation from this dictum compromises coaptation and cosmesis.

Neck

Cervical incisions are planned usually more for utilitarian rather than cosmetic reasons. Wherever possible, however, incisions still are placed within skin creases. Upper neck incisions are placed horizontally at the level of the hyoid bone (usually two fingerbreadths below the mandible). Such an incision can be angled posteriorly to the mastoid tip for additional exposure. Lower neck incisions are made horizontally 2 cm or 2 fingerbreadths above the clavicle.

Technique

In general, the initial incision is performed sharply. However, since the head and neck is divided into a series of interconnected, complex, fascial envelopes, surgery may be facilitated by judicious blunt dissection. A surgeon well versed in the knowledge of cervical planes

Table 12-11. Common infections versus antibiotics

Bacteria	Amino	Cephalo 3	Cephalo 2	Cepha 1	Chloram	Clinda	ERC	Met	Pen	Spec Pen	Sulfa	Tetra	Vanco
Actinomyces				+					+ +	+ +			
Bacteroides fragilis					+	+ +			+ +		+		
Corynebacterium diphtheriae													
Enterobacter					+					+	+		
Escherichia coli	+ +	+ +	+ +							+ +			
Haemophilus influenzae		+	+		+ +		+			+	+	+	
Klebsiella pneumoniae	+ +		+ +		+					+ +	+		
Legionella pneumophila							+ +				+		
Mycoplasma pneumoniae							+ +						
Neisseria gonorrhoeae			+	+					+	+ +	+	+ +	
Peptococcus (anaerobic *Staphylococcus*)		+		+	+	+	+		+				+
Peptostreptococcus (anaerobic *Streptococcus*)					+	+			+ +				
Bordetella pertussis									+	+			
Pneumococcus	+ +	+		+	+		+ +		+ +	+ +			+
Proteus mirabilis	+	+		+	+				+	+ +	+		
Pseudomonas aeruginosa	+	+								+ +			
Staphylococcus aureus					+	+	+		+	+ +			+
Serratia marcescens	+	+ +	+ +							+	+		
Streptococcus pneumoniae					+	+	+		+ +	+			+
Streptococcus pyogenes (beta-hemolytic)		+	+	+		+	+		+ +				+

\+ Effective drug.
\+ + Drug of choice.
Amino = aminoglycoside; Cephalo 1 = first-generation cephalosporin; Cephalo 2 = second-generation cephalosporin; Cephalo 3 = third-generation cephalosportin; Chloram = chloramphenicol; Clinda = clindamycin, ERC = erythromycin; Met = metronidazole; Pen = penicillin; Spec Pen = special pencillins; Sulfa = sulfonamides; Tetra = tetracycline; Vanco = vancomycin.

Table 12-12. Adult dosages of selected drugs

Drug class generic (trade names)	*Oral*	*Parenteral*	*Usual maximum dose/day*	*Usual interval between doses*
Penicillins:				
Penicillin C (1 mg = 1600 U)	250–500 mg q 6 h	1.2 million U IM q 12 h up to 2 million U IV q 2 h	24 million U	4 h
Penicillin V (Pen VK, et al.)	250–500 mg q 6 h	not used	4 gm	6–8 h
Amoxicillin (Amoxil, et al.)	250–500 mg 8 h	not used	3 gm	8 h
Amoxicillin and clavulanate (Augmentin)	250–500 mg q 8 h (based on amoxicillin component)	not used	3 gm	8 h
Ampicillin	250–500 mg q 6 h	0.5–2 gm q 4–6 h	12 gm	4–6 h
Bacampicillin (Spectrobid)	400–800 mg 12 h	not used	1600 mg	12 h
Nafcillin (Unipen, Nafcil)	0.5–1 gm q 6 h	0.5–2 gm q 4–6 h IM, IV	12 gm	6 h
Oxacillin (Prostaphlin, Bactocill)	0.5–1 gm q 6 h	0.5–2 gm q 4–6 h IM, IV	12 gm	6 h
Cloxacillin (Tegopen)	0.5–1 gm q 6 h	not used	4 gm	6 h
Dicloxacillin (Dynapen, Pathocil)	250–500 gm q 6 h	not used	4 gm	6 h
Carbenicillin (Pyopen, Geopen)	not used	5 gm q 4 h IV given over 2 h period	40 gm	4–6 h
Piperacillin (Pipracil)	not used	3 gm q 4 h IV given over 2 h period	24 gm	4–6 h
Ticarcillin (Ticar)	not used	3 gm q 4 h IV given over 2 h period	24–30 gm	4–6 h
Cephalosporins: First Generation				
Cephalothin (Keflin)	not used	0.5–3 gm q 6 h IV	12 gm	4–6 h
Cefazolin (Ancef, Kefzol)	not used	0.25–1 gm q 6 h IM, IV	6 gm	6–8 h
Cephradine (Velosef, Anspor)	250–500 mg q 6 h	0.5–2 gm q 6 h IM, IV	8 gm	6 h
Cephalexin (Keflex)	250–500 mg q 6 h	not used	4 gm	6 h
Cefadroxil (Duricef, Ultracef)	0.5–1 gm q 12 h	not used	4 gm	12 h
Second Generation				
Cefaclor (Ceclor)	500 mg tid to qid	not used	4 gm	8 h
Cefamandole (Mandol)	not used	0.5–2 gm q 4–6 h IM, IV	12 gm	6–8 h
Cefuroxime (Zinacef, IV, Ceftin PO)	not used	1.5 gm q 8 h IM, IV	9 gm	6–8 h
Cefoxitin (Mefoxin)	not used	1 gm q 8 h to 2 gm q 4 h IM, IV	12 gm	6–8 h

Table 12-12. *Continued*

Drug class generic (trade names)	*Oral*	*Parenteral*	*Usual maximum dose/day*	*Usual interval between doses*
Third Generation				
Cefoperazone (Cefobid)	not used	1.5–4 gm q 6–12 h IM, IV	12 gm	
Cefotaxime (Claforan)	not used	1–2 gm q 4–6 h IM, IV	12 gm	6 h
Ceftazidime (Fortaz)	not used	1–2 gm per day IM, IV	6 gm	8–12 h
Moxalactam (Moxam)	not used	1–3 gm q 8 h IM, IV	12 gm	6 h
Erythromycins:				
(E-Mycin, Robimycin, Erythrocin, Ilosone, et al.)	250–500 mg q 6 h	1–4 gm IV q 6 h continuous drip	4 gm	6 h
(EES 400)	400–800 mg q 6 h	not used	4 gm	6–12 h
Chloramphenicol (Chloromycetin)	250–750 mg q 6 h	50 mg/kg/day divided, q 6 h IV only	4 gm	6 h
Clindamycin (Cleocin)	150–450 mg q 6 h	300–900 mg q 6 h IM or IV drip (slow)	4.8 gm	6 h
Tetracyclines:				
(Achromycin, Robitet, Terramycin, Tetrex, et al.)	250–500 mg q 6 h	0.5 gm q 12 h IV; 0.25–0.5 gm q 24 h IM	2 gm	8–12 h
Doxycycline (Vibramycin, Vibra-Tabs)	1st day 100 mg twice subsequent 100 mg daily	1st day 100 mg twice subsequent 100 mg daily		daily
Sulfonamides:				
Sulfisoxazole (Gantrisin)	1–2 gm q 4 h double first dose	not used	8 gm	4–6 h
Sulfamethoxazole (Gantanol)	1–1.5 gm bid double first dose	not used	8 gm	12 h
Trimethoprim-sulfa (Bactrim, Septra)	2 tabs bid	not used	4 tabs	12 h
Vancomycin (Vancocin)	500 mg q 6 h	0.5 gm q 6 h IV (slowly)	2 gm	6 h
Metronidazole (Flagyl)	500 mg qid	30 mg/kg/day IV	4 gm	6–8 h
Aminoglycosides:				
Amikacin (Amikin)	not used	15 mg/kg/day IM, IV divided, q 8–12 h	1.5 gm	8 h
Gentamicin (Garamycin) Tobramycin (Nebcin)	not used	3–5 mg/kg/day IM, IV divided, q 8 h (usually 80 mg tid)	5 mg/kg 8 h	8 h

Source. Condensed and reprinted from Fairbanks DNF: *Pocket Guide to Antimicrobial Therapy in Otolaryngology—Head and Neck Surgery* (4th ed). Washington, DC: AAO-HNS Foundation, 1985.

All antibiotics must be ordered on this sheet and include an indication for use

ALLERGIES: ______________________________

____

Patient's weight ______________ CHECK ONE: ☐ New Order ☐ Renewed Order

DATE ORDERED	TIME ORDERED	ANTIBIOTIC	DOSE	ROUTE	FREQUENCY
					☐ q 4 hours ☐ q 6 hours ☐ q 8 hours ☐ other ______
					☐ q 4 hours ☐ q 6 hours ☐ q 8 hours ☐ other ______
					☐ q 4 hours ☐ q 6 hours ☐ q 8 hours ☐ other ______
					☐ q 4 hours ☐ q 6 hours ☐ q 8 hours ☐ other ______
					☐ q 4 hours ☐ q 6 hours ☐ q 8 hours ☐ other ______

SELECT ONE:

Surgical Prophylaxis Operation: ______________	Automatic stop order after 48 hours
Empiric Therapy – Site or Pathogen Unknown Suspected Site: ______________ Suspected Pathogen: ______________ (Cultures must be obtained) **Documented Infection** (Refer to culture report) Site: ______________ Pathogen: ______________ **Non Surgical Prophylaxis** For: ______________ **Other** ______________	Automatic stop order after 7 days

PATIENT IDENTIFICATION PLATE

NURSING: Please indicate time first dose scheduled

____

____
Signature M.D.

____
Signature Nurse Time

HUH 104

Figure 12-2. Antibiotic order sheet.

Table 12-13. Basic principles of head and neck surgery

1. Prophylactic antibiotics
2. Appropriate incision
3. Gentle traction & countertraction
4. Blunt fascial plane dissection
5. Sharp tumor ablation
6. Vigilant hemostasis
7. Dead-space obliteration
8. Preplanned reconstruction with options
9. Meticulous closure
10. Adequate wound drainage

Table 12-14. Common incisions

Site		*Incision*	*Indications*	*Pitfalls*
Face	Upper	Coronal	Temporal fossa, frontal sinus	Male pattern baldness
		Brow	Frontal sinus, orbit	Loss of eyebrows, frontalis hypesthesia
		Lynch	Orbit, lacrimal fossa	Medial palpebral synechia
		Supraciliary	Orbit, infraorbital rim	Ectropion
	Middle	Weber-Ferguson	Orbit, maxilla, palate	Lip scar
		Midfacial (sublabial)	Anterior ethmoids	Midfacial hypesthesia
		Deglovement	Nose, Maxilla	
	Lower	Blair	Parotidectomy	Lobule deformity
		Lip-splitting	Median & lateral osteotomy, anterior floor of mouth, mandibulectomy	Noticeable lip scar
		Visor flap	See above	Lower facial hypesthesia
Neck	Simple	Submandibular	Submandibular triangle	Marginal mandibularis denervation
		Submental	Submental triangle	
		Suprasternal	Tracheotomy, thyroidectomy	Hemorrhage
		Anterior sternocleidomastoid	Common, internal and external carotid arteries	Noticeable scar
	Intermediate	Hockey stick	Neck dissection, larynx, thyroid	Limited access to submandibular & submental triangles
		Cervical degloving	Bilateral neck dissections, total thyroidectomy	Patients with long necks or upper neck disease
	Complex	Schrobinger	Jaw-neck dissection	Carotid artery exposure
		Conley	Neck dissection	
		McFee		Flap slough
Chest		"T" incision	Inferior neck, upper chest	Keloid formation
		Median sternotomy	Anterior—mediastinum	Osteomyelitis—sternum/ clavicle

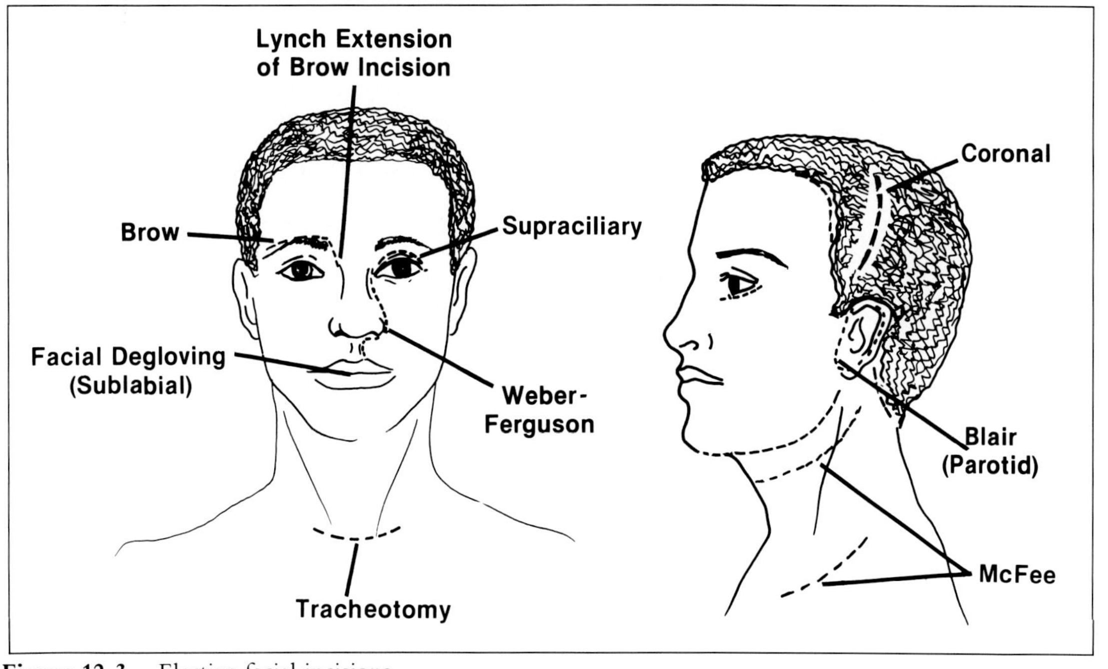

Figure 12-3. Elective facial incisions.

Figure 12-4. Common head and neck incisions.
A. Submandibular triangle incision.
B. Submandibular/submental triangle(s) incision. (continued)

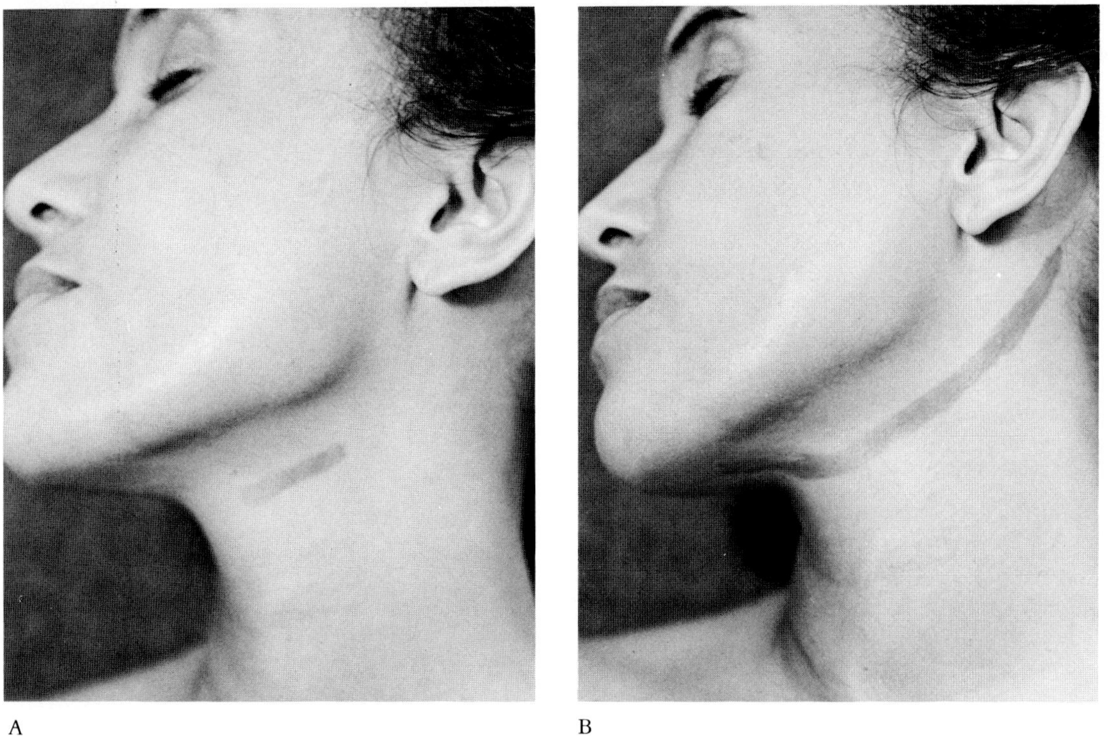

A

B

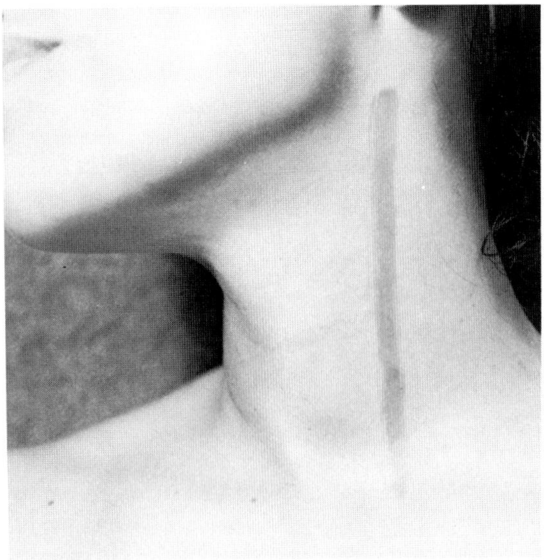

C

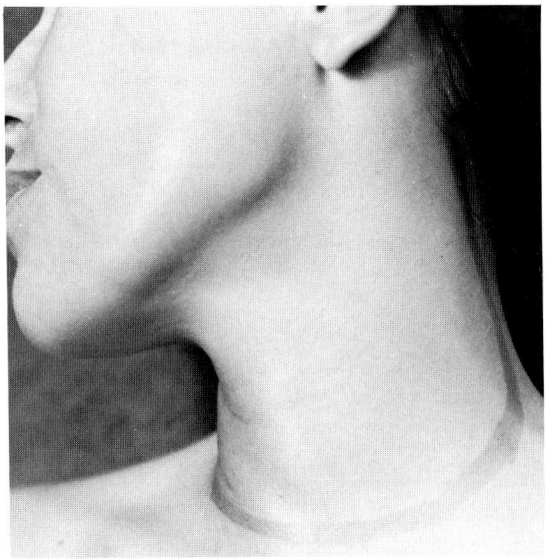

D

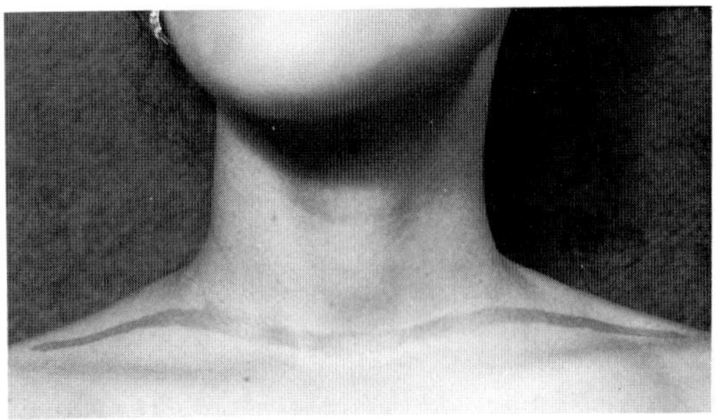

E

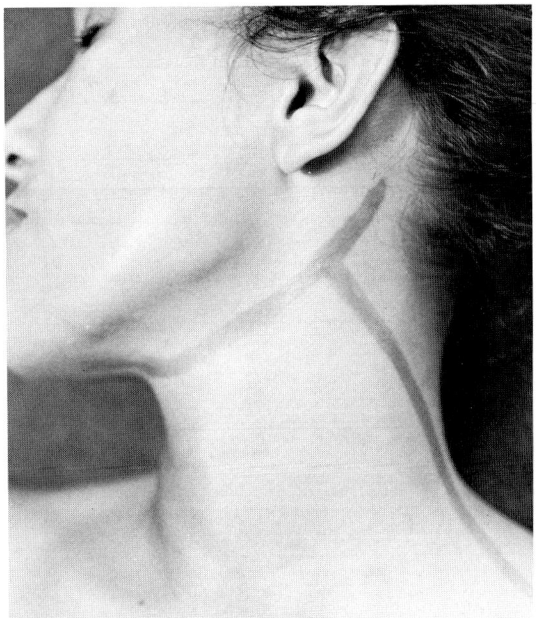

F

Figure 12-4. (continued)
C. Anterior sternocleidomastoid incision. D. Hockeystick incision. E. Cervical deglovement incision. F. Schrobinger incision. G. McFee (modified) incision. H. "T" incision.

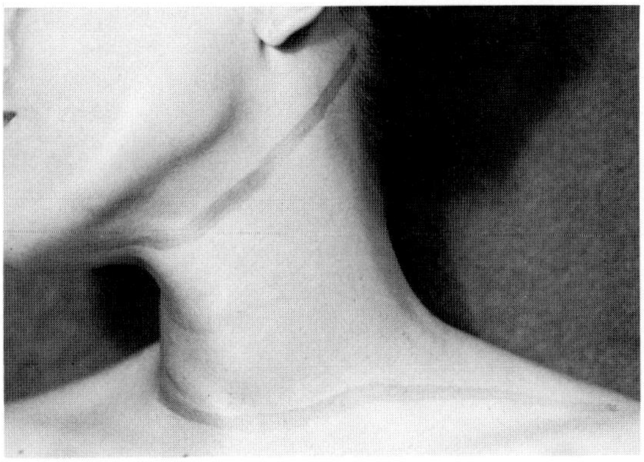

G

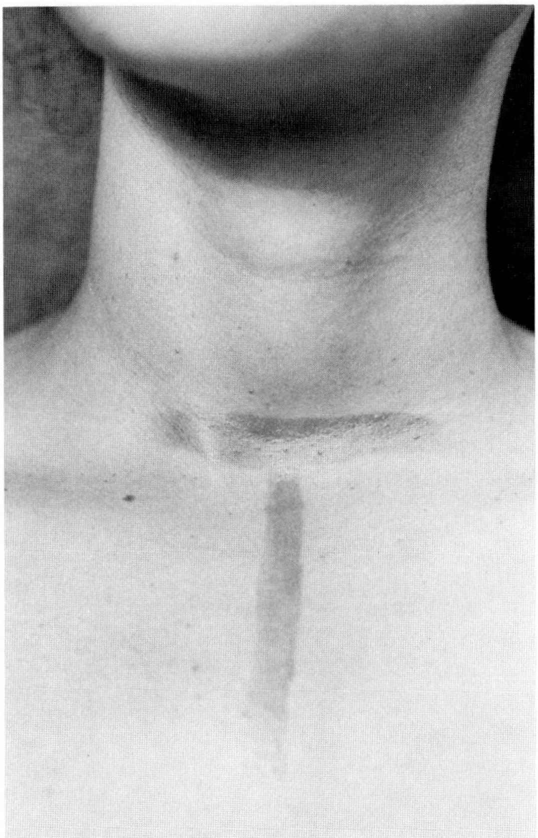

H

and the location of various anatomic landmarks and vital structures can proceed expeditiously. A prime example of surgical technique combining both blunt and sharp dissection is the neck dissection (see Chapter 16). Finally, regardless of the procedure, good surgical technique always is clean, gentle, and precise.

Hemostasis

Once any incision is made the surgeon must assiduously maintain steadfast control of bleeding (see Chapter 11). The basic hemostatic techniques are pressure, packing, precise clamping, ligatures, and electrocautery. More sophisticated measures include heated or laser scapels that seal and weld small blood vessels and lymphatics as they incise. Occasionally, topical agents are applied to wide areas of diffuse bleeding. They are especially useful for diffuse bleeding or if the patient has local or systemic coagulopathy. Of all the hemostatic techniques, they are the most unreliable.

Ligatures and Suture Ligatures

A ligature is a freehand tie facilitated by a hemostat, whereas a suture ligature is tissue immobilization and coaptation with a needle-carried material (Table 12-15) [13]. In the head and neck, most surgeons use silk for midsize and large vessels and chromic or plain catgut for small vessels. Silk, being permanent and natural, may initiate a local inflammatory reaction. Catgut, also natural and somewhat inflammatory, eventually dissolves after a brief time period. Dissolvable synthetics that incite little tissue reaction also are available.

Clips

In small or inaccessible areas, stainless steel or synthetic hemostatic clips are utilized for hemostasis. They are precise, fast, and produce little inflammatory reaction. Metal clips may also be used as landmarks for the radiologist and radiotherapist.

Drains

Most head and neck wounds are drained (Table 12-16). Drains serve two purposes: wound decompression and fluid egression. Serum,

Table 12-15. Sutures

	Natural	*Synthetic*	*Tissue reaction*	*Knot stability*	*Surgeon's comfort*	*Tensile strength*
Absorbable	Catgut		+ + +	+ +	+ + +	+
	Collagen		+ + +	+ +	+ + +	+
		[Polymers]				
		Glycolide (Dexon)	+	+	+ +	+ +
		Polydioxane (PDS)	+	+	+ +	+ +
		Polylactide (Vicryl)	+	+	+ +	+ +
Nonabsorbable	Silk		+ + +	+ +	+ + +	+
	Linen		+ + +	+ +	+ + +	+
	Cotton		+ + +	+ +	+ + +	+
		Polyester (Dacron)	+	+	+ +	+ +
		Polyamide (nylon)	+	+	+ +	+ +
		Stainless steel	+ +	+ + +	+	+ + +

\+ Weak/worse.
\+ + Intermediate.
\+ + + Strongest/best.

Table 12-16. Drains

Open
- Penrose
- Rubber band
- Ribbon gauze
  - Selvage
  - Iodoform

Closed: self-contained
- Soft
  - Silastic
  - Silicone (Jackson-Pratt)
- Hard
  - Silastic (Hemovac)

blood, or pus that accumulates in dead spaces retards healing, harbors infection, predisposes to dehiscence, and encourages fistulization. Suture lines, especially in the early phases of wound healing, undoubtedly benefit from local decompression. Finally, although very useful, drains are not substitutes or saviors for poor surgical technique.

Open Drains

Flat, tubular open drains (rubber bands, Penrose) are the simplest drains. They are sutured for security. Usually after 48 hours they are removed. If they remain longer than 72 hours, they are potential sources of retrograde wound contamination and possible infection.

Closed Drains

Self-contained Silastic or silicone drains are manufactured in a variety of configurations. Designed for long term placement, they may remain days without the threat of retrograde contamination.

MAINTENANCE

Self-contained drains are checked every shift and declotted manually every day (see Chapter 18). Drains are connected to wall suction at 60 cm of H_20 negative pressure. When the patient ambulates, the drains are connected to a self-contained suction reservoir or bellows.

SUCTION

The drain is connected to the suction reservoir and then to the wall suction. This arrangement confirms whether the wall suction is working properly. Self-contained drains are removed when the drainage is less than 20 ml/day. With thoracic duct injury they may remain in place for longer periods of time.

Closure

Careful wound approximation in layers helps all phases of healing. Sloppy closures encourage hematomas, seromas, and infection. Like many phases of surgery, closure is subject to personal preference. The following are provided as general suggestions.

Skin

The skin is closed in layers with interrupted, buried absorbable sutures beginning with the platysma and followed by the dermis. The epithelium may be approximated in an interrupted or running fashion with synthetic sutures. Some surgeons prefer stainless steel staples for skin closure.

Skin Grafts

Hemostasis must be meticulous. Grafts are immobilized with bolsters over a sheet of antibiotic-impregnated gauze. They are generally covered by a bulky dressing for strict immobilization for 3 to 5 days.

Flaps

The blood supply to both cervical and regional flaps must be preserved at all times (see Chapter 22). The closure should be secure with well-placed sutures that do not compromise vitality. When in doubt, intravenous fluorescein dye and a Wood's lamp confirm viability.

Dressings

Self-contained drains, meticulous closure, and prophylactic antibiotics have lessened the need for dressings (Tables 12-17 and 12-18). However, a good dressing remains invaluable for promoting sterility, insulation, immobility, and security.

COMPLICATIONS

Wound complications clinically are divided into early, intermediate, and late phases (Figure 12-5). Usually, the early complications are related to surgical technique. The intermediate and late complications are an interplay of patient factors and possibly technique (Tables 12-19 to 12-23). Unforeseen events that impact on wound complications are discussed in detail in Chapter 16. The following are the major wound-related complications.

Table 12-17. Qualities of the ideal dressing

Sterility
Porosity
Aeration
Humidification
Drainage
Insulation
Immobility
Security

Table 12-18. Comprehensive dressings*

First layer: seal
Dry
Fine mesh gauze (FMG)
Telfa
Wet
Saline FMG
Petroleum FMG
Bismuth tribronopherate (Iodoform) FMG
Second layer: absorption
Fluff gauze
Combined dressing
ABD
Surgipad
Gauze sponge layers
Third layer: security
Gauze wrap
Kling
Fluff wrap
Kerlex
Soft band
Elastic wrap
Elastoplast

*A comprehensive dressing is composed of *one* component from each layer.

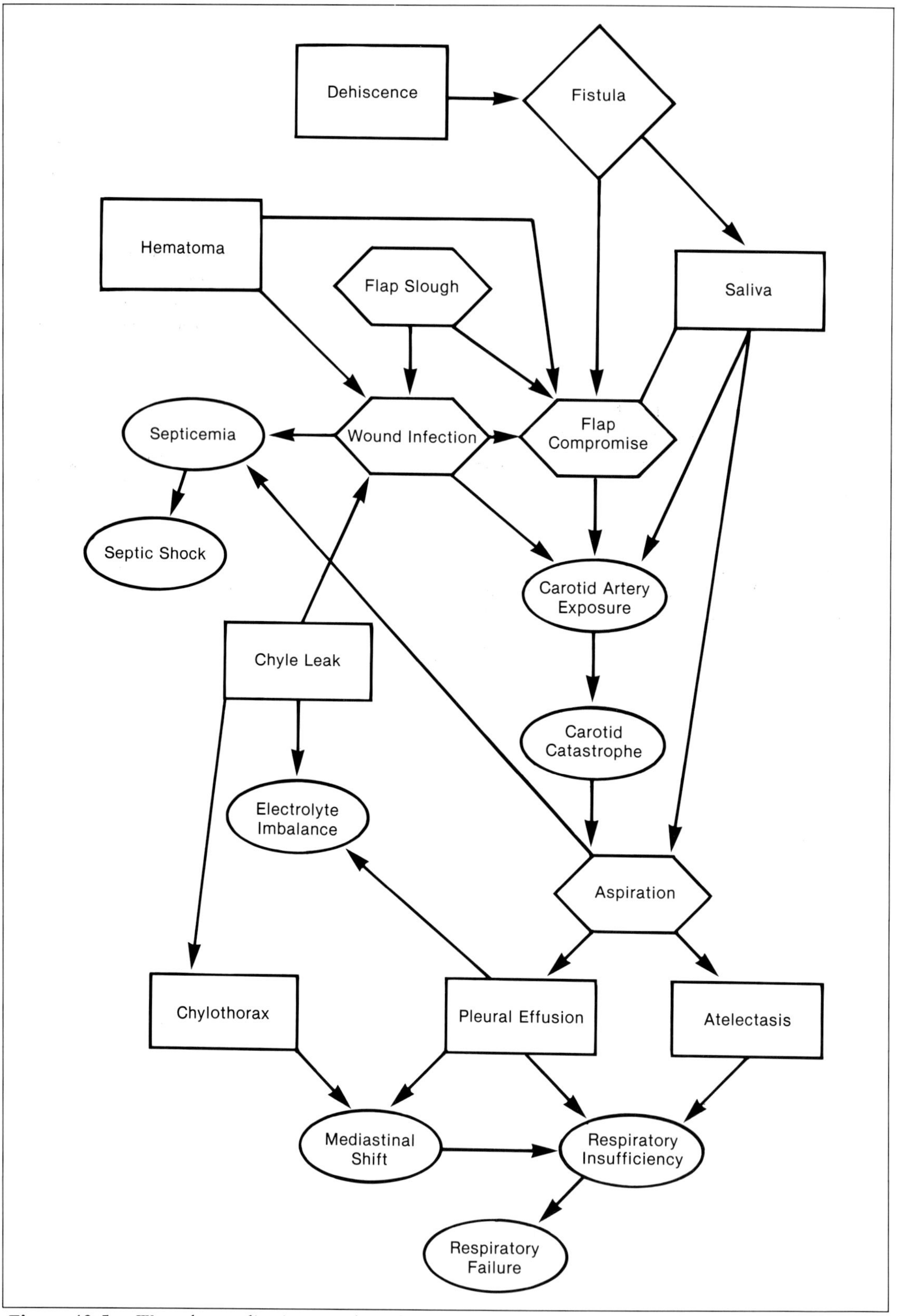

Figure 12-5. Wound complications. (Adapted from Myers EM: Complications in surgery for stomal recurrences. *Laryngoscope* 93(3) : 285, 1983.)

Table 12-19. Complications: acute

Wound infection
Skin slough
Fistula
Carotid artery exposure
Carotid castastrophe
Chyle fistula
Air embolism
Cerebrovascular accident
Myocardial infarction

Table 12-20. Complications: chronic

Drooling
Altered phonation
Dysphagia
Aspiration
Pneumonia
Lung abscess
Pleural effusion
Tracheotomy
Gastrostomy
Osteomyelitis
Altered body image
Depression
Impotence

Hemorrhage (Immediate or within 10 Days of Surgery)

Immediate

In the overwhelming majority of cases, immediate hemorrhage is secondary to improper hemostasis of minor, secondary blood vessels (Figure 12-6). However, occasionally a major blood vessel is transected partially or completely. Arteries notoriously contract, retract, and vasoconstrict when transected. Later, after delayed vasodilation, active bleeding ensues. The search for a retracted, bleeding artery requires proper lighting, a keen eye, and patience. Veins tend to tear longitudinally and present a different and more perplexing problem. A scenario combining brisk hemorrhage from both an artery and vein is a prodrome to potential hemorrhagic shock.

Delayed

Unchecked hemorrhage results in a hematoma and potential cervical flap compromise. In rare instances this is controlled at the bedside. Ideally, the patient is returned to the operating room, reanesthetized, and the wound is explored. Attempts at bedside control may

Table 12-21. Complications versus surgical procedure: I

		Deglutition				*Speech*	
Procedure	***Vision/ hearing***	***Drooling***	***Malocclusion***	***Mastication***	***Swallowing***	***Articulation***	***Phonation***
Floor of mouth resection		+ +	+	+		+	
Glossectomy							
Partial		+ +		+ +	+ +	+ +	
Total				+ + +	+	+ + +	+ + +
Mandibulectomy							
Partial		+ +	+	+ +	+		
Subtotal		+ + +	+ + +	+ + +	+ + +	+ + +	+ + +
Palatectomy	+ +			+ +	+	+ +	
Laryngectomy							
Partial					+ +		+ +
Total							+ + +
Neck dissection		+					
Maxillectomy	+ +	+	+	+ + +	+ +	+ +	
Tracheotomy					+ +		+ + +

\+ Possible.
\+ + Probable.
\+ + + Likely.

Table 12-22. Complication versus surgical procedure: II

	Respiratory system			*Cardiovascular system*			*Nervous system*			
Procedure	***Breathing***	***Cough***	***Aspiration***	***Myocardial infarction***	***CVA***	***Air embolism***	***Facial N.***	***Hypoglossal N.***	***Sympathetics N.***	***Spinal acc. N.***
Floor of mouth resection				+	+		+	+ +		
Glossectomy										
Partial		+	+ +	+	+		+	+ +		
Total				+	+					
Mandibulectomy										
Partial			+	+	+		+			
Total	+	+ +	+ +	+	+					
Palatectomy				+	+					
Laryngectomy										
Partial	+	+ + +	+ + +	+	+					
Total	+			+	+					
Neck dissection			+	+	+ +	+ +	+	+	+	+ + +
Maxillectomy				+	+					
Tracheotomy	+	+ +	+ + +	+						

\+ Possible.
\+ + Probable.
\+ + + Likely.
MI = myocardial infarction; CVA = cerebrospinal accident; N. = nerve; Acc. = accessory.

Table 12-23. Complications versus surgical procedures: III

	Psyche			*Infection*			
Procedure	***Facial asymmetry***	***Depression***	***Impotence***	***Flap necrosis***	***Wound infection***	***Oseomyelitis***	***Fistula***
Floor of Mouth resection		+			+		+
Glossectomy							
Partial		+			+		
Total		+ + +			+		+ +
Mandibulectomy							
Partial	+ +	+			+	+ +	+
Total	+ + +	+ +			+	+ +	+
Palatectomy		+			+	+ +	
Laryngectomy					+		+ +
Partial							
Total		+ + +	+ + +		+		+
Neck dissection	+			+	+		+
Maxillectomy	+ +	+ +			+	+ +	
Tracheotomy		+ +	+		+		

\+ Possible.
\+ + Probable.
\+ + + Likely.

result in injury to other vital structures. Only under controlled conditions is the skin opened in the presence of a major hematoma. The cervical flaps may tamponade and control major bleeding; once the suture lines are incised, major hemorrhage may occur. Of course adequate plasma products and blood should be available (see Chapter 11).

The most dreaded delayed hemorrhage is a carotid blow or rupture. Heralded by the so-called sentinel bleed, impending blows must be diagnosed early. Vigorous and timely aggressive treatment will avoid uniformly fatal hemorrhagic shock (see Chapter 16).

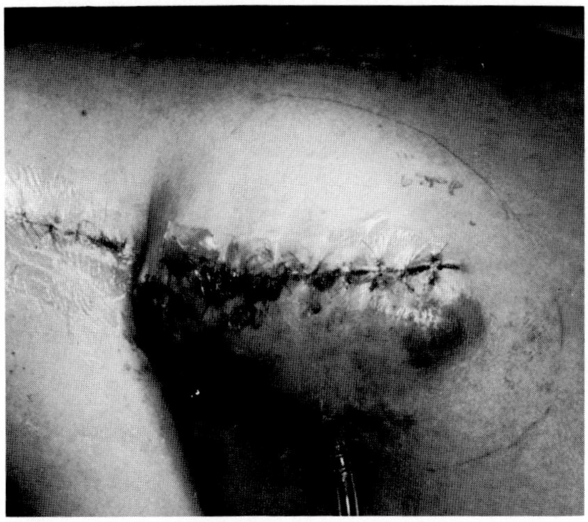

Figure 12-6. Hematoma. A tense chest hematoma that developed within 24 hours after surgery (first-stage deltopectoral or Bakamjian flap).

Infection (36–48 Hours After Surgery)

A cervical wound infection fortunately is rare, particularly if prophylactic antibiotics have been used.

Cellulitis

When the flaps become gradually erythematous and the patient has a low-grade fever, impending infection is likely. Cephalosporins are notorious for producing indolent, smouldering infections. When a cellulitis is suspected, the initial antibiotic (e.g., cephalosporin, penicillin) is discontinued and another is started empirically, such as clindamycin or chloramphenicol.

Abcess

Localized pockets of purulence are evacuated at the bedside after limited removal of interrupted sutures. Subsequently, the wound is irrigated daily with half-strength peroxide. The exteriorized pocket is paced with fine-mesh gauze, impregnated with iodinated ointment or acetic acid ($^1/_4$% or $^1/_2$%).

Recurrence

Some persistent tumors masquerade as cellulitis (Figure 12-7).

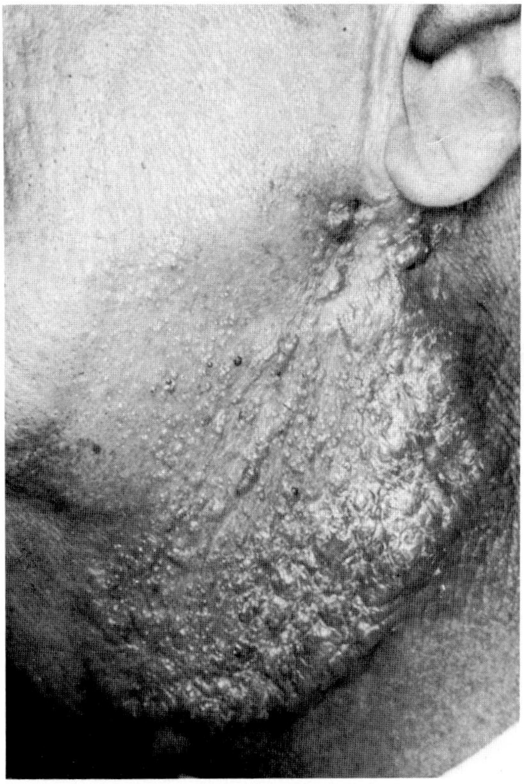

A

Figure 12-7. Skin metastasis. A. An erythematous, confluent intradermal eruption over the neck and angle of the mandible. (continued)

Flap Necrosis (<5–10 Days After Surgery)

Flap devitalization may arise in either the cervical or regional flaps. The earliest signs are pallor and coldness (<24 hours). A late sign is

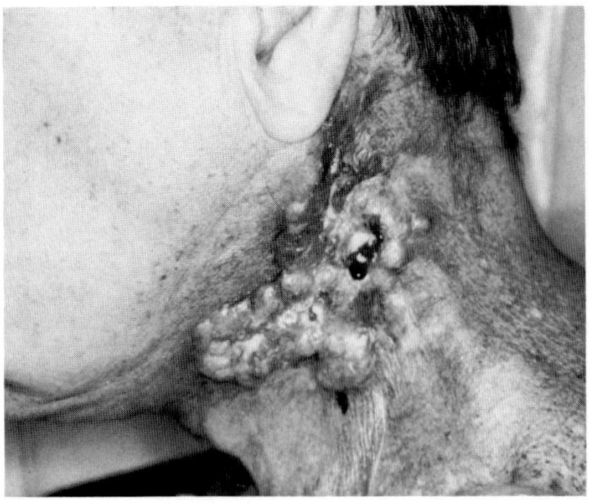

B

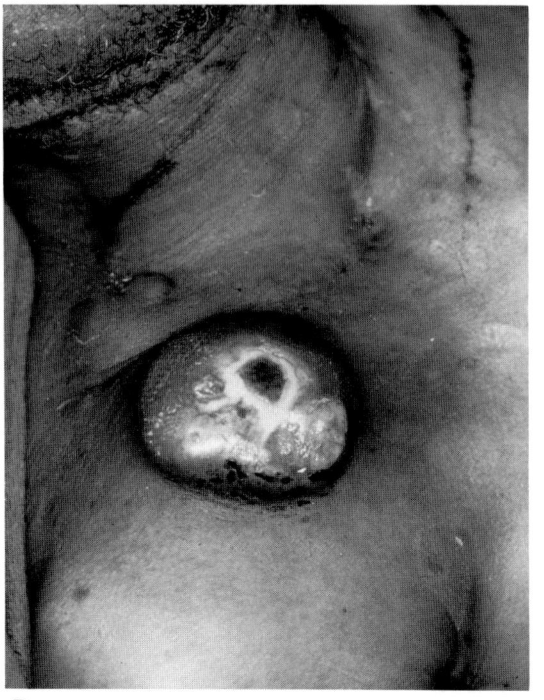

D

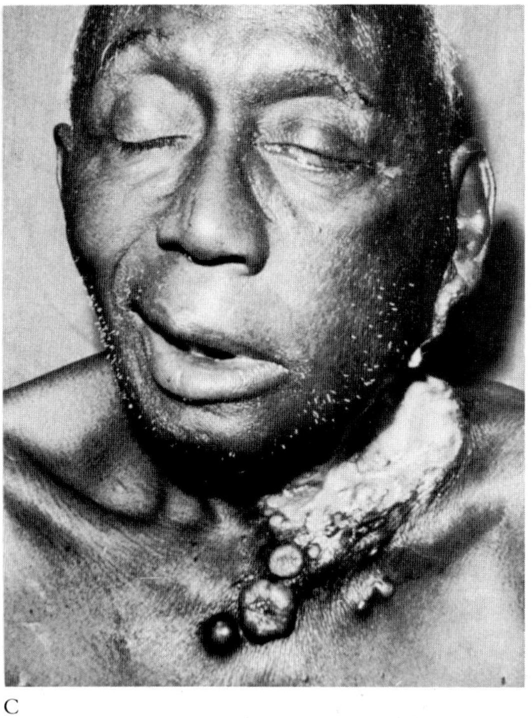

C

Figure 12-7. (continued) B. A large, weeping, exophytic squamous cell carcinoma over the left upper neck. This luxuriant metastasis deeply surrounds the carotid sheath, a situation that portends of carotid catastrophe. C. Massive left cervical metastasis with carotid sheath, skull base involvement, and left peripheral facial paralysis. D. A right shoulder metastasis in a patient who had an advanced floor-of-mouth cancer treated previously with chemotherapy, surgery, and radiotherapy.

suture-line contraction or retraction (Figures 12-8 and 12-9). Prophylactic antibiotics may mask systemic responses such as fever and leukocytosis. When in doubt, intravenous fluorescein dye and a Wood's lamp usually confirm or deny the worse clinical suspicions.

Etiology

Ultimately, necrosis is the result of vascular compromise. Some predispositions are complex skin incisions, hematoma, seroma, abscess, chyle leak, and fistula.

Treatment

When confirmed, the surgeon either allows demarcation or debrides the area. Passive flap demarcation is a form of biologic bandage. Some surgeons may elect to debride aggressively to encourage secondary healing by granulation.

Table 12-24. Fistula: the high price

Extended hospitalization
Nursing care
  Intravenous fluids
  Tube feeding
  Dressings
  Trach care
Carotid artery precautions
Reconstructive surgery
Psychological support

Fistula (5–21 Days After Surgery)

A fistula is defined as a wound breakdown and communication between the aerodigestive tract and the skin (Table 12-24); Figures 12-10 and 12-11). Any complication prolongs hospitalization, but fistulization is perhaps the most dreaded complication (see Chapter 16). A serosanguineous discharge 3 to 4 days after surgical incision suggests impending wound dehiscence or fistula. The presence of edema, fever, odor, and saliva in the wound confirms the diagnosis.

Etiology

As presented in Figure 12-11, the causes of a fistula are a dynamic interplay of events. The overall incidence of fistualization is 5 to 14 percent. With combined surgery and radiation, it increases dramatically. Early recognition allows the surgeon to short-circuit the dynamics and reduce to manageable proportions the potential late and morbid sequelae.

Figure 12-8. Flap slough, McFee incision. The wound is granulated and clean. Two weeks of meticulous debridement and dressing changes were necessary to prepare the wound for closure.

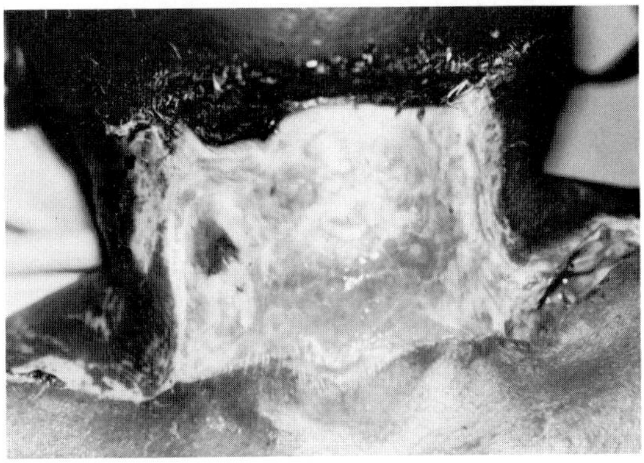

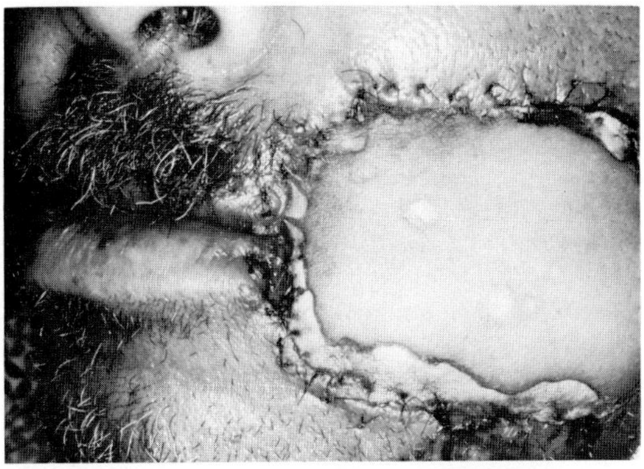

Figure 12-9. Flap necrosis. This pectoralis myocutaneous flap was mobilized and placed 1 week previously for a massive buccal mucosal squamous cell carcinoma. The skin is pale, and the suture line is beginning to retract.

Figure 12-10. A. Centralized, direct pharyngocutaneous fistula (*arrow*) that occurred 1 week after total laryngectomy for full-course radiation failure. The endotracheal tube is in the tracheostoma. (continued)

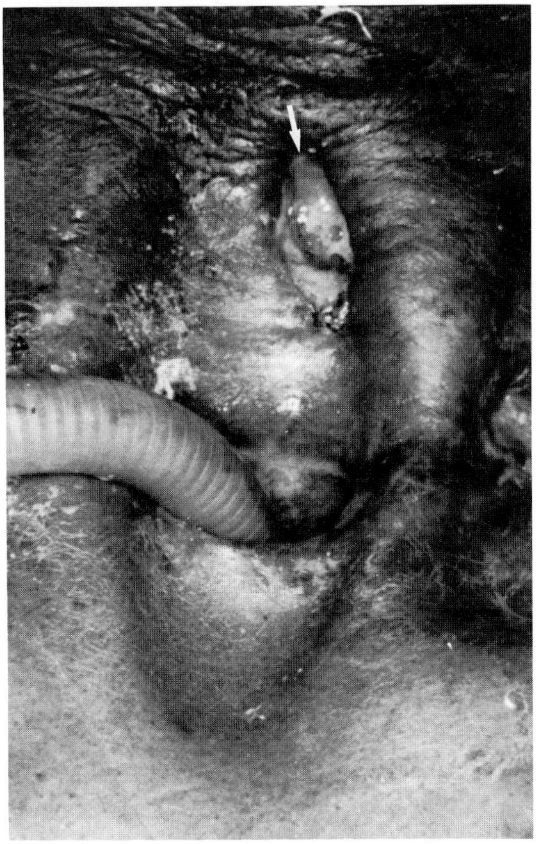

A

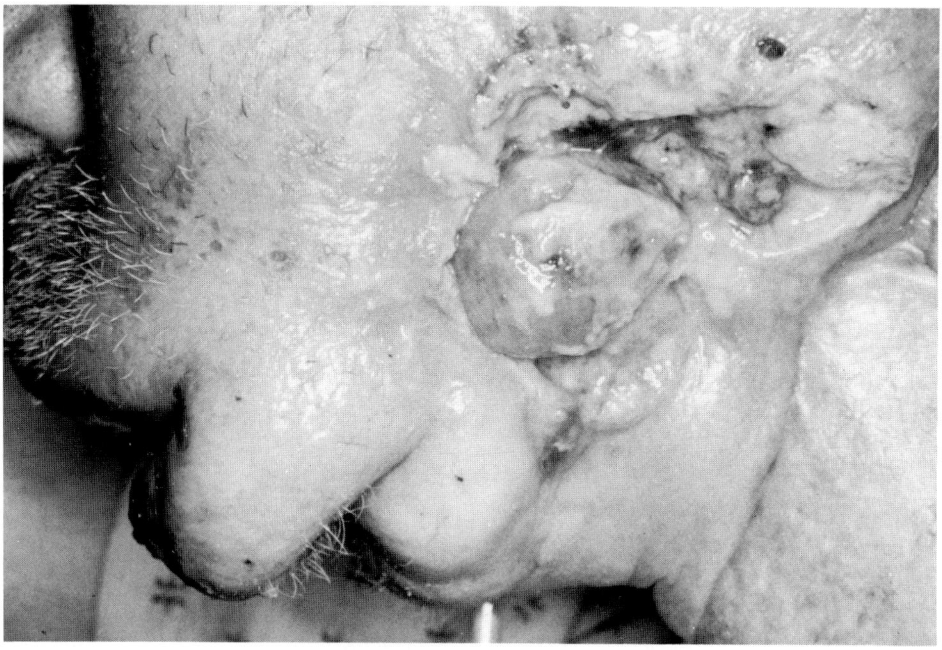

B

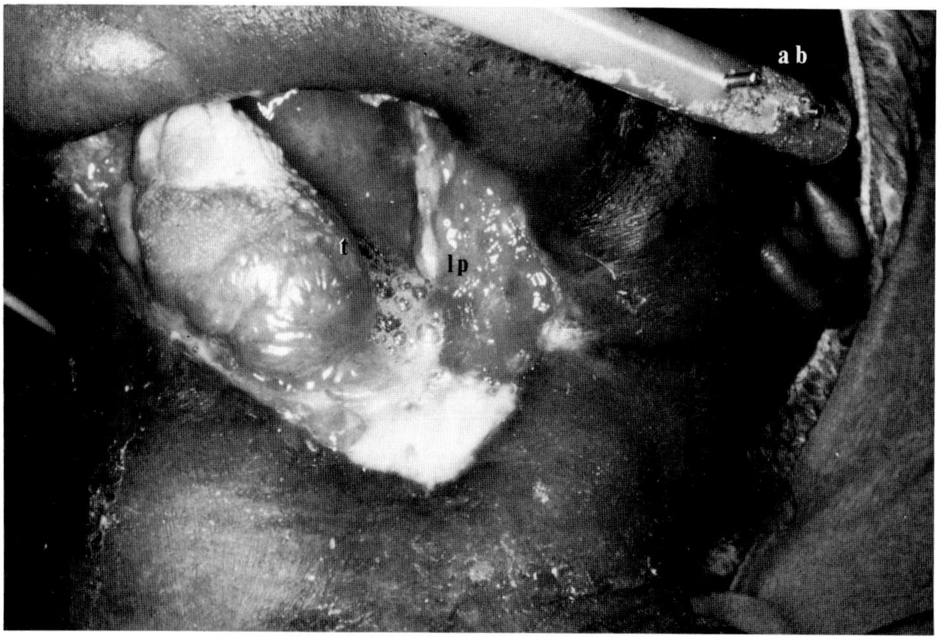

C

Figure 12-10. (continued) B. Left buccal, direct, orocutaneous fistula associated with a superficially infected recurrence. Note the upper and lower lip edema. C. A massive left, direct, orocutaneous fistula. Originally, an indirect fistula, opening the suture line and pressure dressings, diverted saliva away from the carotid artery. ab = acrylic bar for external mandibular fixation; t = tongue; lp = lateral pharyngeal wall.

Diagnosis

Since healing and infection are intimately interrelated, problems that affect one can affect the other. Quite often, fistulae are associated with wound infections. Fistulae are suggested by erythema, incision-line fluctuance, drainage, or fluid accumulation under skin flaps. They are confirmed by oral ingestion of methylene blue or intravenous radioactive tracers [19,20,21].

Classification

Direct Fistula

A direct fistula is a straightforward communication between the aerodigestive tract and the cervical flaps without flap compromise or carotid exposure.

Indirect Fistula

The most dangerous form, indirect fistula, is a circuitous communication between the aerodigestive tract and the skin, complicated by flap elevation or compromise and carotid exposure. Saliva and purulence bathing the carotid artery are a prodrome for a potential cascade of complications and ultimately carotid catastrophe.

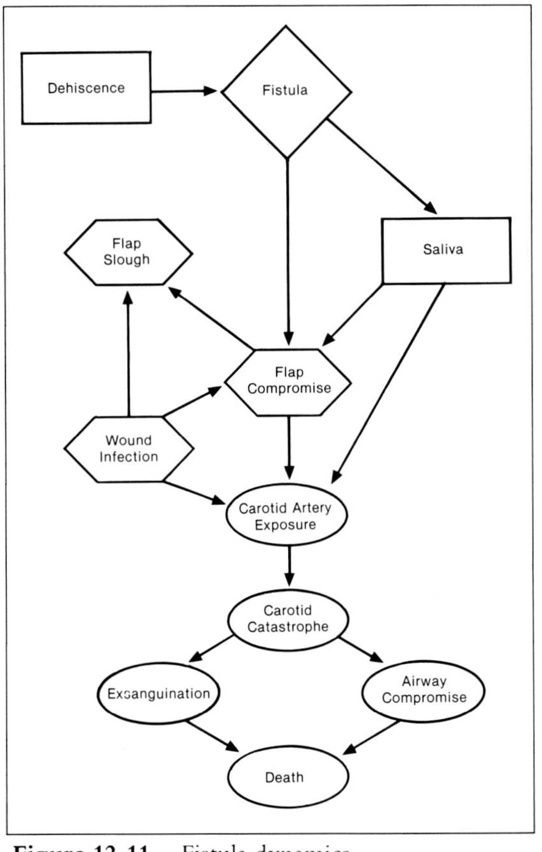

Figure 12-11. Fistula dynamics.

Treatment

The first step in treatment is the conversion of an indirect fistula to a direct fistula. The purulence and saliva must be directed away from the carotid artery. The cervical flaps are protected from devascularity. This is accomplished by exteriorization. Similar to the treatment of an abscess, the wound is opened partially and drained. This is followed by careful debridement, irrigation, and packing. Pressure dressings are invaluable; they discourage cervical flap elevation and isolate the carotid artery from the infected drainage. Laborous daily dressing changes may encourage spontaneous closure of small fistulae. However, large fistulae require major reconstruction to reestablish aerodigestive continuity and cervical skin resurfacing.

REFERENCES

1. Baur PS, Parks DH, Larson DL: The healing of burn wounds. *Clin Plast Surg* 4(3) : 389, 1977.
2. Boucek RJ: Factors affecting wound healing. *Otolaryngol Clin North Am* 17 : 2, 1984.
3. Carrico TJ, Mehrhoff AI, Kelman C: Normal and Pathological Wound Healing. In Georgiade NG, et al (eds): *Essentials of Plastic, Maxillofacial, and Reconstruction Surgery*. Baltimore: Williams & Wilkins, 1987. Pp. 11–17.
4. Hunt TK: Wound Healing. In Paperella MM, Shumrick DA (eds): *Otolaryngology*. Philadelphia: Saunders, 1973.
5. Sasaki GH, Krizek TH: Biology of Tissue Injury and Repair. In Georgiade NG, et al (eds): *Essentials of Plastic, Maxillofacial, and Reconstruction Surgery*: Baltimore: Williams & Wilkins, 1987. Pp 3–10.
6. Eyre DR: Collagen molecular diversity in the body's protein scaffold. *Science* 207 : 1315, 1980.
7. Rojkind M: Chemistry and biosynthesis of collagen *Bull Rheum Dis* 30 : 1006, 1979.
8. Alexander MV, Zajtchuk JT, Henderson RL: Hypothyroidism and wound healing, occurrence after head and neck radiation and surgery. *Arch Otolaryngol* 108 : 289, 1982.

9. McGrath M: The effect of prostaglandin inhibitors on wound contraction and the myofibroblast. *Plast Reconstr Surg* 69(1) : 74, 1982.
10. Sasaki GH, Pang CY: Experimental evidence for involvement of prostaglandins in viability of acute skin flaps. *Plast Reconstr Surg* 67(3): 335, 1981.
11. Collen D: On the regulation and control of fibrinolysis. *Thromb Haemost* 43 : 77, 1980.
12. Johnson, J, Liu UL: Role of aerobic gram-negative rods, anaerobes, and fungi in wound infection after head and neck surgery: Implications for antibiotic prophylaxis. *Head Neck,* Jan/Feb, 1989. Pp 27–29.
13. Johnson JT, et al: Efficiacy of two third-generation cephalosporins in prophylaxis for head and neck surgery. *Arch Otol Head Neck Surg* 110 : 224, 1984.
14. Goode, RL, et al: Effect of prophylactic antibiotics in radical head and neck surgery. *Laryngoscope* 89 : 601, 1979.
15. Johnson JT, et al: Antimicrobial prophylaxis for contaminated head and neck surgery. *Laryngoscope* 94 : 46, 1984.
16. Becher GD, Parell GJ: Cefaxolin prophylaxis in head and neck cancer surgery. *Ann Otol Rhinol Laryngol* 88 : 183, 1979.
17. Fairbanks, DNF: *Pocket Guide to Antimicrobial Therapy in Otolaryngology Head and Neck Surgery* (4th ed). Washington, DC: AAO-HNS Foundation, 1985. Pp 54–57.
18. Westaby SA: *Fundamentals of Wound Healing: Wound Care.* St. Louis: Mosby, 1985. Pp 11–21.
19. Larsen LR, Schuller DE: Wound amylase as an early indicator of orocutaneous fistulae. *Laryngoscope* 94 : 1302, 1984.
20. Weiland FL, et al: Salivary scan after major ablative head and neck surgery with prediction of postoperative fistulization. *Ann Otol Rhinol Laryngol* 92 : 366, 1983.
21. Beahrs OH: Complications of surgery of the head and neck. *Surg Clin* North Am 57(4) : 823, 1977.

13

Skull Base

GARY C. DENNIS

KEY CONCEPTS

Anterior Skull Base; Middle Skull Base; Posterior Skull Base; Complications

MILESTONES

1906	Transcranial Hypophysectomy	Horsley
1910	Intranasal Hypophysectomy	Hirsch
1910	Combined Approach to Acoustic Nerve	West
1912	Sublabial Transseptal Hypophysectomy	Cushing
1917	Acoustic Surgery Monograph	Cushing
1923	Operating Microscope	Holmgren
1925	Complete Excision of Acoustic Tumor	Dandy
1957	Transsphenoidal Hypophysectomy with Image Intensifier	Guiot
1962	Extradural Excision of Acoustic Tumor	Kurze et al.
1963	Microsurgical Acoustic Tumor Resection	House
1965	Microsurgical Facial Nerve Preservation	Rand, Kurze
1968	Acoustic Tumor Excision with Cochlear Nerve Preservation	Rand, Kurze
1969	Microsurgical Transsphenoidotomy	Hardy

LOCATION

In contrast to other head and neck neoplasms, skull base tumors are rarely visualized or palpated. Largely inaccessible, these tumors historically have been difficult to diagnose and treat (Table 13-1; Figure 13-1). Moreover, with either an intracranial, osseous, or extracranial location, their clinical presentation is varied and confusing. Today their diagnosis and treatment are more feasible [1–4].

TREATMENT

Skull base tumors require sophisticated and multidisciplinary management [5]. Frequently, due to lower cranial nerve involvement, a neurologist, neurosurgeon, or otolaryngologist first encounters these patients. When the visual pathways or cranial nerves that affect extraocular movements are involved, the ophthalmologist is first consulted. The neuroradiologist performs complex diagnostics and preoperative embolization. The otolaryngologist or plastic surgeon reconstructs the extensive skull base defects. The neuroanesthesiologist monitors and manages intraoperative complications, including cerebral ischemia, air embolism, hypothalamic or pituitary dysfunction, and brain stem and cranial nerve dysfunction [6]. Working as a well-coordinated team, these var-

Table 13-1. Skull base tumors and cranioneuropathies

Cranial Nerve	*Location*	*Tumor*
II (or optic chiasm)	Sella Parasella	Pituitary, optic schwannoma or glioma, sella meningioma, esthesioneuroblastoma, craniopharyngioma
III, IV, VI, V_1 (60% V_2)	Cavernous sinus	Nasopharyngeal carcinoma, schwannoma
III, IV, VI, V_1 (no V_2)	Superior orbital fissure	Meningioma of medial sphenoid wing, orbital carcinoma
V_1, VI	Petrous apex	Dermoids, epidermoids, cholesteatomas, meningiomas
VII, VIII	Internal auditory meatus	Acoustic neuroma, epidermoid
V, VII, VIII (sometimes IX)	Cerebellopontine angle	Meningioma, acoustic neuroma, epidermoids, sarcoma of local origin
IX, X, XI (sometimes XII, VII, VIII, V)	Jugular foramen	Glomus tumors, schwannoma, meningioma

Figure 13-1. Intracranial locations of skull base lesions. *1* = nasal olfactory groove meningioma; *2* = medial sphenoid wing meningioma; *3* = lateral sphenoid wing meningioma; *4* = tuberculum sella meningioma, pituitary tumor craniopharyngioma, esthesioneuroblastoma teratoma; *5* = clivus meningioma, chordoma; *6* = tentorial meningioma, trigeminal neuroma; *7* = acoustic neuroma, meningioma, epidermoid; *8* = glomus tumor, meningioma, schwannoma.

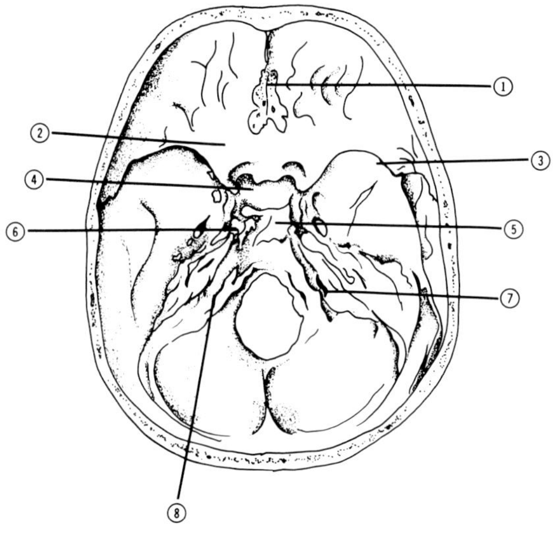

ious specialists diagnose, excise, and reconstruct complex skull base neoplasms.

In addition, sophisticated equipment and instrumentation are necessary. Digital subtraction angiography is a must for the neuroradiologist (see Chapter 4). The anesthesiologist requires intraoperative brain-stem evoked response audiometry and electroencephalography (see Chapter 11). The operating microscope, carbon dioxide laser, ultrasonic aspirator, and microsurgical drill are necessities for the neurosurgeon and neuro-otologist. Without sophisticated diagnostics and instrumentation, these tumors cannot be ablated safely while preserving vital structures.

ANTERIOR SKULL BASE TUMORS

Pathology

Anterior intracranial tumors include meningioma, sarcoma, pituitary adenoma, craniopharyngioma, dysgerminoma, esthesioneuroblastoma, optic nerve schwannomas and gliomas. Other tumors which may affect the anterior skull base that are extradural include chondrosarcomas, chordomas and nasopharyngeal carcinomas.

Clinical Presentation

Benign skull base tumors usually grow very slowly, with few symptoms, until they are quite large. The nasal olfactory groove meningioma is a good example of a tumor presenting with late anosmia and optic atrophy.

Visual Complaints

Due to the proximity of the optic nerves and chiasm, pituitary adenomas, dysgerminomas, esthesioneuroblastomas, and craniopharyngiomas present with unilateral or bitemporal visual disturbances and signs of optic nerve or chiasmal compression. Ultimately, they may produce optic atrophy, decreased visual acuity, blind spots, bitemporal hemianopsia, or blindness.

Hormonal Dysfunction

Anterior skull base tumors typically alter hypothalamic-pituitary function and are associated with acromegaly (enlargement of hands and feet and coarse features). Cushing's disease (moonlike faces, buffalo hump, truncal obesity, and cutaneous striae), or hyperprolactinemia (impotence, infertility, amenorrhea, and galactorrhea) (Tables 13-2, 13-3) [7].

Hypothalamic-Pituitary Dysfunction

Nonfunctional pituitary tumors and other parasellar tumors cause hypopituitarism with decreased libido, a decrease in pubic and axillary hair, cold intolerance, generalized weakness, and stress intolerance. Involvement of the pituitary stalk or hypothalamus causes polydipsia, polyuria, loss of thirst, and poor appetite.

Diagnosis

Laboratory

Functional pituitary tumors are diagnosed by high levels of growth hormone, thyroid-stimulating hormone (TSH), prolactin, and adrenocorticotropic hormone (ACTH). Nonfunctional pituitary tumors have low serum and urinary cortisol, ACTH, follicle-stimulating hormone (FSH), luteinizing hormone (LH), growth hormone, and TSH levels. A high prolactin assay is a good tumor marker.

Table 13-2. Pituitary hormones

Site	*Hormone*	*Target Organ(s)*	*Action*
Anterior pituitary	Thyroid-stimulating hormone (TSH)	Thyroid gland	Thyroid—growth & secretion
	Adrenocorticotropic hormone (ACTH)	Adrenal glands	Adrenocortical secretion
	Growth hormone (GH)	Bony epiphysis	Bone growth
	Follicle-stimulating hormone (FSH)	Women—ovaries Men—testicles	Ovarian follicle growth Spermatogenesis
	Luteinizing hormone (LH)	Women—ovaries Men—testicles	Ovulation Testosterone production
	Prolactin	Breasts	Milk production
Posterior pituitary	Antidiuretic hormone	Kidneys	Water retention
	Oxytocin	Breasts	Lactation

Table 13-3. Anterior skull base tumors: hormonal dysfunction syndromes

Site	*Affected Hormone*	*Syndrome*	*Clinical Presentation*
Anterior hypophysis	Growth (increased)	Acromegaly	Enlargement of jaw, hands, and feet; coarse facial features
	Adrenocorticotropic hormone (ACTH) (increased)	Cushing's disease	Moon-like facies, buffalo hump, truncal obesity, cutaneous striae
	Prolactin (increased)	Hyperprolactinemia	Impotence, infertility, amenorrhea, galactorrhea
	Luteinizing hormone (decreased)	Hypogonadism	Decreased libido, pubic and axillary hair
	Follicle-stimulating hormone (decreased)	Hypogonadism	
	Thyroid-stimulating hormone (decreased)	Hypothyroidism	Cold intolerance, change in hair texture, weakness
	ACTH, cortisol (decreased)	Hypocortisolism	Stress intolerance, Hypertension
Posterior hypophysis	Antidiuretic hormone (ADH) (decreased)	Inappropriate ADH	Water intolerance, polydipsia, polyuria, loss of thirst

Diagnostic Radiology

Plain skull films show sellar enlargement (intrasellar tumors), optic foramen expansion (optic nerve glioma), hyperostosis, or erosion (meningioma) (see Chapter 4).

Although computed tomography (CT) scan is the diagnostic modality of choice, magnetic resonance imaging (MRI) is coming to the forefront. Both ascertain vascularity, proximity to adjacent vascular structures (carotid artery, cavernous sinus), and the presence or absence of bony landmarks. Coronal views are very helpful for planning surgery—that is, transsphenoidal, transethmoidal, or transbasal approaches.

Treatment

Preoperative Preparation

Hormonal Replacement

The endocrine status of the patient is evaluated to include prolactin, serum cortisol, and thyroid function. For suspected hypocortisolism, hydrocortisone is administered prior, during, and after surgery as a continuous infusion (300 mg/day) or intramuscular injections. Hypothyroid patients are treated prior to surgery.

Prophylactic Antibiotics

Antibiotics are obligatory. Ampicillin is the drug of choice unless nasal or oral cultures suggest otherwise.

Surgery

Surgery is indicated for increased intracranial pressure, cranial nerve compression, hypothalamic/pituitary dysfunction, or tissue diagnosis. The patient must be able to tolerate general anesthesia and the stress of surgery (Figures 13-2, 13-3, 13-4).

Transsphenoidotomy and Transethmoidectomy

Transsphenoidotomy and transethmoidectomy are used to approach pituitary tumors. Intrasellar lesions that enlarge the sella and have small parasellar or suprasellar extensions usually are amenable to transsphenoidotomy [8,9]. Other tumors that occur in this area are intrasellar teratomas, esthesioneuroblastomas, lymphomas, craniopharyngiomas, and dysgerminomas (Figure 13-5). The transethmoidal approach, requiring a facial incision, is hampered by limited field of vision.

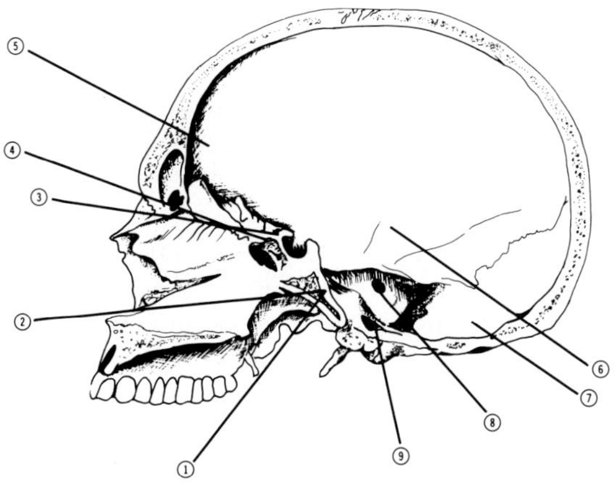

Figure 13-2. Approaches to skull base tumors. *1* = transoral; *2* = transseptal; *3* = transethmoidal; *4* = transbasal; *5* = craniotomy; *6* = subtemporal; *7* = suboccipital craniectomy; *8* = translabyrinthine; *9* = infratemporal.

Craniotomy
Craniotomy is indicated for lesions affecting the anterior skull base with suprasellar extension (Figure 13-2). Large pituitary tumors with significant anterior or middle fossa involvement are approached by formal craniotomy. To achieve wider exposure, a meningioma that invades the anterior skull base (tuberculum, medial or lateral sphenoid wing, planum sphenoidale, and nasal olfactory groove) usually is resected through craniotomy [10].

Transbasal Approach
The transbasal approach, alone or augmented by the transpalatal approach, is indicated for clivus meningiomas (Figure 13-2) [11,12]. Often, the transsphenoidal and transethmoidal approaches are combined with the transbasal approach (in a staged fashion) for large tumors.

Reconstruction
Regardless of the approach, the anterior fossa and skull base between the paranasal sinuses and

Figure 13-3. Management of skull base tumors.

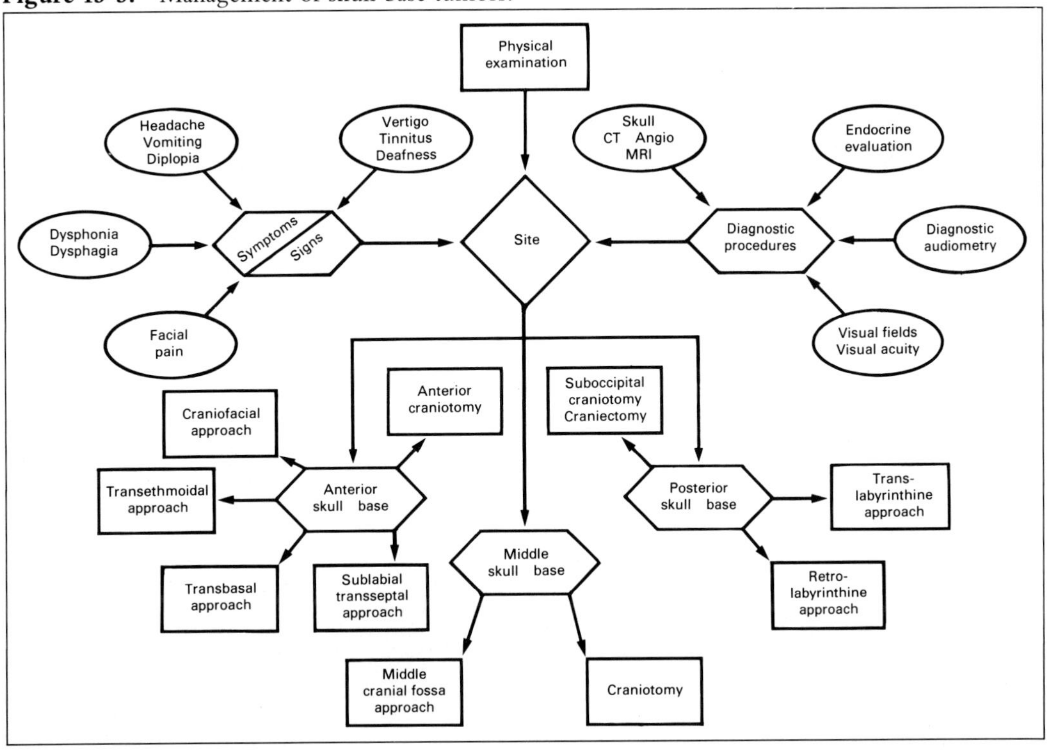

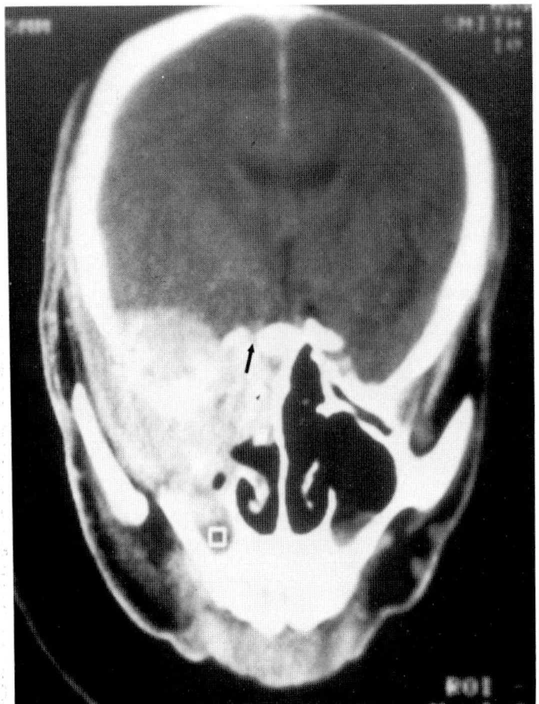

Figure 13-4. CT scan, paranasal sinuses (coronal view). Extensive (anterior skull base) squamous cell carcinoma of the ethmoid sinuses with invasion of the supratemporal space, cribriform plate (*arrow*), and maxillary sinus.

intracranial cavity require reconstruction. With a craniotomy, the anterior floor is covered with temporalis fascia, fascia lata, fat, muscle, or pericranium. This may be reinforced with wire mesh, methyl methacrylate, and Gelfoam. After transbasal surgery, similar techniques ensure a barrier between the subarachnoid space and the contaminated paranasal sinuses [13].

When radical resections of the cavernous sinus are undertaken reconstruction of the carotid artery with a vein graft or extracranial/intracranial bypass may be required.

MIDDLE SKULL BASE TUMORS

Pathology

Middle tumors include meningiomas, neuromas, and epidermoids.

Clinical Presentation

Cranial Nerve Dysfunction

Middle fossa tumors frequently are diagnosed after cranial nerve deficits or brain compression. Medial middle fossa tumors, such as tentorial edge meningioma, are associated with cranial III and IV palsies; anterior extension along the

Figure 13-5. CT scan, paranasal sinuses (coronal view). An unusually aggressive malignant lymphoma of the sphenoid sinus in a 33-year-old man. The presenting complaint was bilateral sudden blindness and a dull, retro-orbital headache. Decompression and biopsy were accomplished by sublabial transnasal sphenoidotomy.

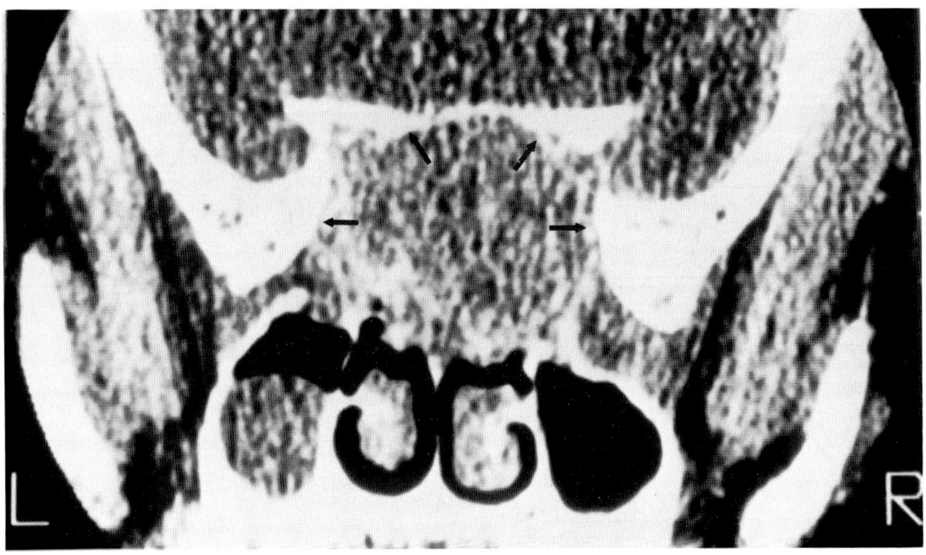

superior orbital fissure or cavernous sinus invasion affects cranial nerves III, IV, VI, and V_1 [4]. Lesions extending to the cavernous sinus usually envelop V_2. Involvement of Meckel's cave, lateral tentorial edge, and the motor branch of V_2 produces temporalis, masseter, and pterygoid dysfunction. Trigeminal neuromas frequently involve one or all three divisions V_{1-3}, resulting in facial pain, numbness, or difficulty chewing.

Intracranial Complaints

When the dominant temporal lobe is compressed, receptive speech may become impaired, thus prompting earlier diagnosis. However, tumors unassociated with cranial neuropathies, especially with involvement of the nondominant temporal lobe, may become quite large before detection. Temporal lobe seizures, associated with visual or auditory hallucinations and behavioral changes, occur in addition to grand mal seizures.

Diagnosis

Diagnostic studies include computed tomography (CT) scan, magnetic resonance imaging, (MRI) and cerebral angiography. Neuroforaminal enlargements are common plain skull film and CT scan findings. A unique vascular pattern (angiography) distinguishes the meningioma from other tumors. Usually benign, the occasional sarcomatous epidermoid or meningioma is diagnosed more readily by CT scan.

Treatment

Surgical indications are an expanding intracranial mass, focal neurologic deficit, cranioneuropathy, and brain stem compression. These tumors, due to the paucity of early symptoms, may grow very large and cause brain stem compression before being diagnosed.

Tumors involving the middle skull base are excised by craniotomy or craniectomy (Table 13-4). The patient usually is positioned laterally, especially for the medial tumors. A subtemporal approach with elevation of the temporal lobe exposes these tumors. They are approached, anteriorly, through the sylvian fissure [14]. The operating microscope, carbon dioxide laser, and the microsurgical drill are essential for resection.

Table 13-4. Treatment of middle skull base tumors

Tumor	*Preparation*	*Surgical Approach*	*Post-op Follow-up*
Meningiomas	Dexamethasone	Microsurgery	Taper steroids
Neuromas	Embolization if possible Spinal drainage	Craniotomy with or without CUSA, laser	Consider radiotherapy
Epidermoids	Dexamethasone Spinal drainage	Craniotomy or craniectomy, laser	Taper steroids

CUSA = cavitron ultrasonic surgical aspirator.

These tumors often are difficult to resect totally and recur when incompletely excised. Therefore, both skull base resections and craniotomy are often necessary (Figures 13-6, 13-7) [15,16]. Reconstruction of the anterior skull base or cranial nerves, carotid artery bypass, or angioplasty may be required.

POSTERIOR SKULL BASE TUMORS

Pathology

The common neoplasms are meningiomas, neuromas, epidermoids, sarcomas, and glomus jugulare tumors.

Clinical Presentation

Cranial Nerve Dysfunction

Posterior skull base neoplasms typically present with lower cranial nerve dysfunction. The precise location within the posterior fossa is determined usually by the cranial nerve deficits. Patients who have tumors within the cerebellopontine angle classically complain of hearing disturbances, tinnitus, vertigo, facial weakness, and sometimes facial numbness due to involvement of cranial nerves V, VII, VIII, and IX (Figure 13-8). Those with internal auditory canal neoplasms have hearing disturbances and facial weakness due to the involvement of cranial nerves VII and VIII.

Extracranial and Intracranial Complaints

Some patients with a glomus tumor, meningioma, or schwannoma at the jugular foramen complain of dysphagia, a change in voice, and weak cervical range of motion (compression of cranial nerves IX, X, and XI). Large tumors compress the cerebellum, causing ataxia and incoordination.

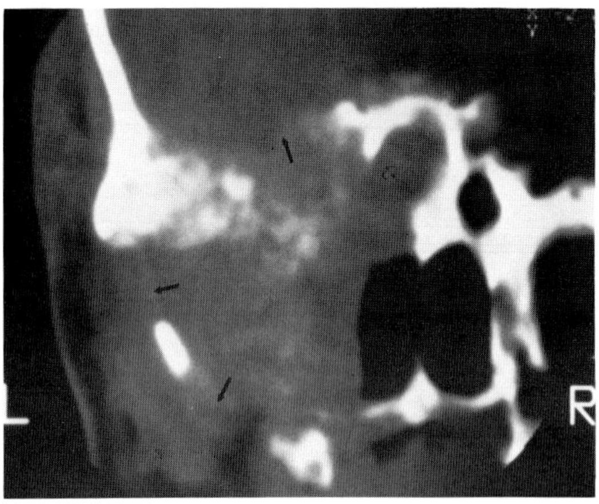

A

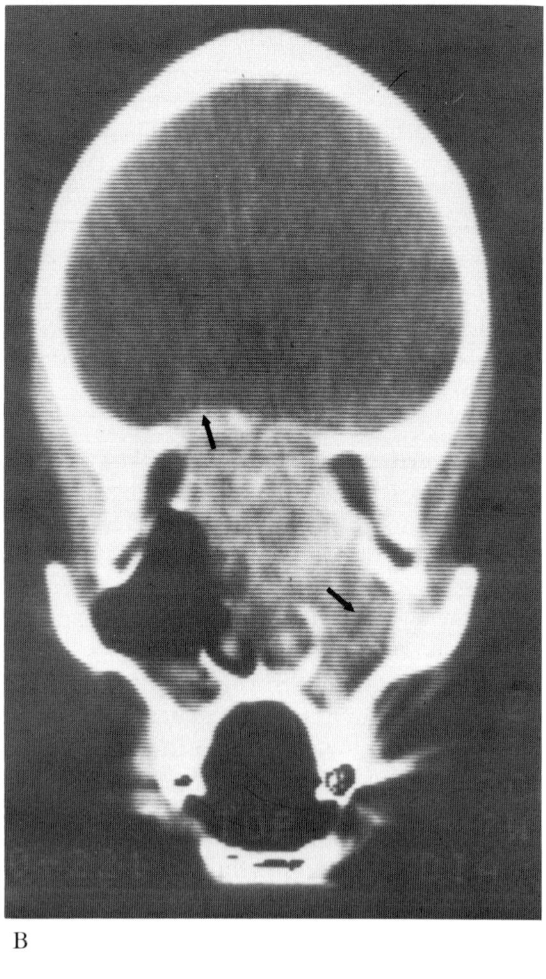

B

Figure 13-6. CT scan, skull base (coronal view). A. Squamous cell carcinoma of the middle skull base with pterygomaxillary space, cavernous sinus, and sphenoid sinus (*open arrow*) invasion. B. A different patient with extension from the middle cranial fossa to the left pterygomaxillary space. The initial complaint was a dull headache with numbness in the distribution of the left infraorbital nerve.

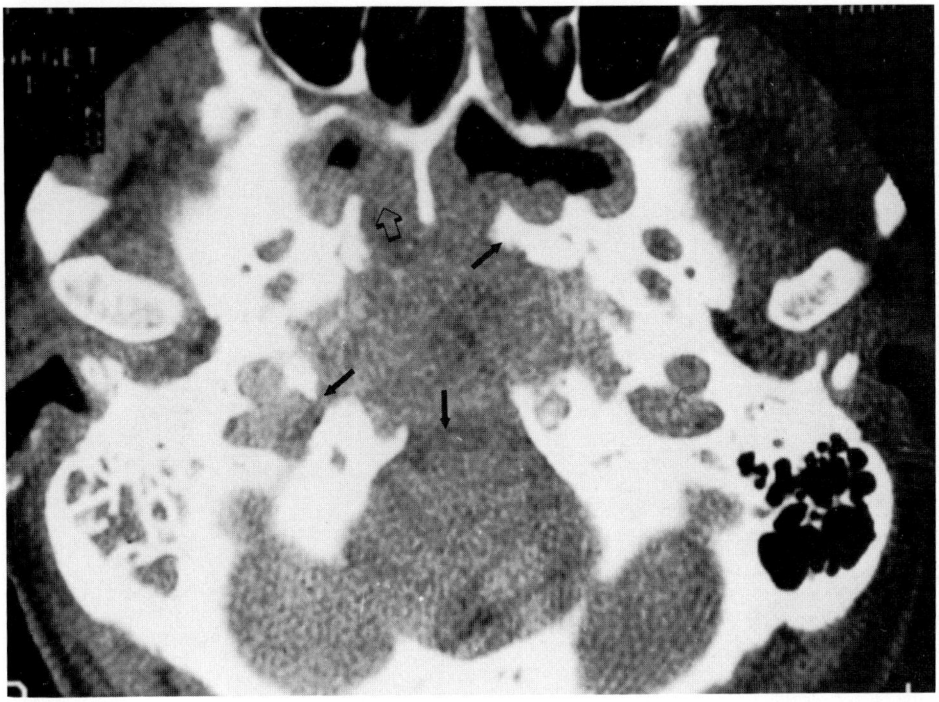

Figure 13-7. CT scan, skull base. Squamous cell carcinoma of the nasopharynx in a 73-year-old man. Tumor has invaded the clivus and the sphenoid sinus (*open arrow*). The complaints were occipital headache and neck pain aggravated by cervical hyperextension.

Diagnosis

Preoperative evaluation includes skull series, CT scan, air contrast CT scan, MRI, and cerebral angiography. Internal auditory canal enlargement is diagnostic of acoustic neuromas. Audiograms, electronystagmography, and brain stem–evoked response audiometry help localize the lesion to the auditory nerve or the brain stem (see Chapter 27) [17]. Mass compression and shift of the fourth ventricle necessitate timely surgical decompression. As a temporizing measure, these patients often require emergency ventriculostomy to reduce or prevent hydrocephalus prior to formal posterior fossa decompression.

Treatment

Posterior skull base tumors continue to grow intracranially if they are not resected. Recurrences after partial resection cause certain neurological dysfunction and possibly death. Therefore, these tumors are removed unless there are medical contraindications (see Table 13-5).

Preoperative Embolization

Posterior skull base tumors usually have a significant extracranial blood supply. Such highly vascular tumors, especially the glomus jugulare, are embolized preoperatively with silastic beads, Gelfoam, bucrylate, or Ivalon. Embolization causes infarction and significantly reduces intraoperative blood loss. These patients should have surgery within 24 hours of embolization to avoid the rapid increase in collateral circulation. Unlike bucrylate and Ivalon, Gelfoam (resorbable) is used only when surgery is performed within days of embolization [18].

Preoperative Preparation

Posterior skull base surgery requires coordination between the neuroanesthesiologist and surgeon (see Chapter 11). Patients are positioned either sitting, prone, or lateral [19,20]. If the

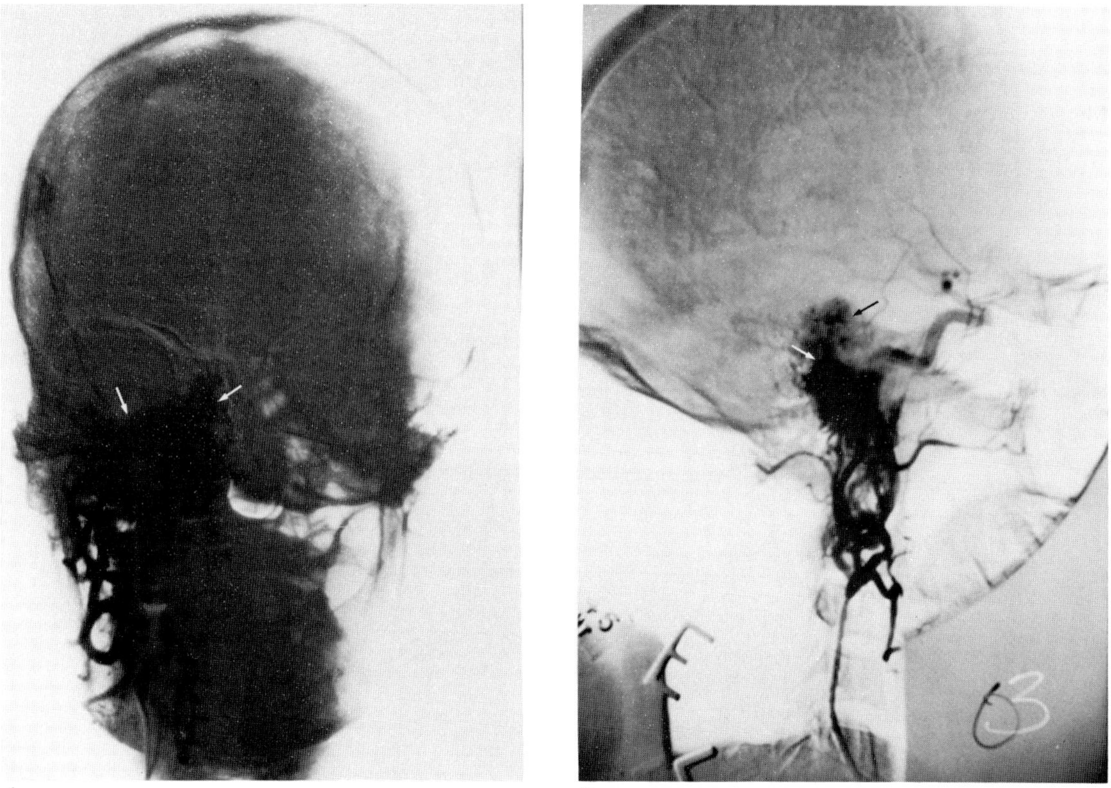

A

B

Figure 13-8. Cerebral angiogram. A. Anteroposterior view of an intensely vascular glomus jugular tumor. B. Lateral view shows extension into the otic capsule. The patient complained of gradual unilateral hearing loss.

sitting position is used, a central venous catheter, Doppler monitor, or end tidal carbon dioxide monitor (for early detection of air embolism) is used. Brain stem–evoked responses are recorded intraoperatively to monitor brain stem function during surgical manipulation. Intraoperative facial nerve stimulation in the cerebellopontine angle and facial electromyography are helpful; large tumors may displace and distort the facial nerve. Long-acting muscle relaxants are contraindicated when intraoperative facial nerve stimulation is likely.

Surgical Approaches

Translabyrinthine and Middle Cranial Approaches

The acoustic neuroma and epidermoid (cholesteatoma) tumors are removed by both the neurosurgeon and otolaryngologist. Such teamwork ensures excision with preservation of vital structures, especially the facial nerve. Intracanalicular acoustic and facial neuromas are removed through the middle fossa or translabyrinthine approach alone or in combination with a suboccipital craniectomy. This affords facial nerve preservation at the expense of the labyrinth. Labyrinthectomy is indicated when ipsilateral hearing is poor or absent [15,21,22].

Suboccipital Craniectomy

Suboccipital craniectomy is the standard neurosurgical approach to the cerebellopontine angle [2]. This procedure decompresses both the brain stem and cranial nerves. The residual tumor is removed through a transmeatal resection within the internal auditory meatus. This best preserves facial, labyrinthine, and cochlear function. Tumors, originating in the posterior skull base, may extend into the petrous portion

Table 13-5. Treatment of posterior skull base tumors

Tumor	*Preparation*	*Surgical Approach*	*Post-op Follow-up*
Meningioma	Dexamethasone	Microsurgery	Taper steroids
Sarcomas, epidermoids	Embolization if possible	Suboccipital craniectomy Laser, CUSA	Observe for hydrocephalus and cerebrospinal fluid (CSF) leak
Schwannomas	Dexamethasone Angiogram Electronystagmography Brain stem–evoked response audiometry (BSER)	Translabyrinthine Middle fossa Suboccipital craniectomy Laser, CUSA Facial nerve stimulation	Taper steroids Facial nerve stimulation Lateral tarsorrhaphy
Glomus jugulare	Embolization BSER Dexamethasone	Ligation of external carotid Infratemporal, suboccipital excision of sigmoid sinus Cricopharyngeal myotomy	Taper steroids Observe for hydrocephalus and CSF leak Consider radiotherapy for residual tumor

CUSA = cavitron ultrasonic surgical aspirator

of the temporal bone and necessitate petrous apicotomy.

Infratemporal Approach

The infratemporal approach, alone or in combination with the suboccipital craniectomy, is a good technique for complete exposure of large glomus tumors in the jugular foramen, intrapetrous carotid, sigmoid sinus, and internal jugular vein [23].

COMPLICATIONS

Anterior Skull Base

Table 13-6 summarizes the complications of skull base surgery.

Frontal Lobe Injury

Contusion

Anterior skull base surgery is associated with frontal lobe contusion and edema. Usually due to excessive retraction, these complications are prevented by intraoperative mannitol and cerebrospinal fluid drainage as well as frequent release of retractor pressure (Figure 13-9). Adequate cerebral perfusion, head elevation, reduced carbon dioxide, and steroid therapy are other prophylactic measures.

Hematoma

Subdural and epidural hematomas are associated with sweeping hemispheric deficits, alteration in sensorium, and eventual compression and death. Any significant deterioration in neurologic function is considered a neurosurgical emergency that requires immediate CT scan, hematoma evacuation, and cerebral decompression [24].

Cerebrospinal Fluid Rhinorrhea

Cerebrospinal fluid (CSF) rhinorrhea may occur following anterior skull base surgery. After craniectomy, meticulous dural closure and sealing with pericranium, fascia, muscle, or fat help prevent this complication.

Cerebrospinal Fluid Fistula

CSF fistula following transethmoidal, transsphenoidal, or basal surgery is due to ineffective fascial and fat packing. When a CSF fistula is suspected, the fluid is analyzed for glucose; it should be low in nasal secretions but high (60 percent of the serum glucose) in CSF.

When the leak is immediate and copious, the patient is returned to the operating room for closure [25]. If the leak is delayed or minor, the patient is placed on bed rest (10 degrees head result in CSF fistulization. This is prevented by watertight closure, soft-tissue coverage of dural defects, and fat obliteration of the mastoid cavity.

Due to dysphagia and aspiration following suboccipital and subtemporal surgery, cricopharyngeal myotomy frequently is performed in anticipation of lower cranial nerve palsies [27].

Cranial nerve transection is repaired by nerve grafts or primary suture; good results are possible.

Facial to hypoglossal anastomosis restores tone to the face in patients with permanent facial nerve paralysis [28–30].

Vascular Injury

Following posterior skull base surgery (suboccipital craniectomy through the middle fossa or the translabyrinthine approaches), small brain stem arterial injury (especially of the anterior inferior cerebellar artery) may result in stroke and death. To avoid this tragedy, maintenance of cerebral blood flow, reduction in posterior fossa mass, and prevention of hydrocephalus, collectively, are the keys.

REFERENCES

1. Kennedy DW, et al: Transsphenoidal approach to the sella: The Johns Hopkins experience. *Laryngoscope* 94 : 1066, 1984.
2. Kazan R: The neurosurgeon in skull base operations. *Otolaryngol Clin North Am* 15 : 925, 1982.
3. Sami M, Draf W: The Diagnosis and Operative Strategy of Large Glomus Tumors. In Scheunemann H, Schurmann K, Helms J (eds): *Tumors of the Skull Base*. New York: Walter de Gruyter, 1986. Pp 237–244.
4. Adams RD, Victor M: *Principles of Neurology*. New York: McGraw-Hill, 1977. Pp 455–456.
5. Helms J, Schurmann K: Interdisciplinary Approach to Benign Tumors of the Lateral Skull Base. In Scheunemann H, Schurmann K, Helms J (eds): *Tumors of the Skull Base*. New York: Walter de Gruyter, 1986. Pp 227–229.
6. Rafferty TD: Neuroanesthetic Management in Surgery of the Skull Base. In Sasaki CT, McCabe BF, Kirchner JA (eds): *Surgery of the Skull Base*. Philadelphia: Lippincott, 1984. Pp 9–14.
7. Weiss MH: Neuroendocrine Evaluation of Pituitary Disorders. In Brackmann DE (ed): *Neurological Surgery of the Ear and Skull Base*. New York: Raven, 1982. Pp 119–122.
8. Laws ER Jr.: Transsphenoidal Approach to Lesions In and About the Sella Turcica—Operative Technique. In Schmidek HH, Sweet WH (eds): *Current Techniques in Operative Neurosurgery*. New York: Grune & Stratton, 1977. Pp 161–172.
9. Kirchner JA: Transethmoidal Approach to the Sella. In Sasaki CT, McCabe BF, Kirshner JA (eds): *Surgery of the Skull Base*. Philadelphia: JB Lippincott, 1984. Pp 63–78.
10. Koning W, Frowein RA, Wilcke O: Bifrontal Meningioma of the Skull Base. In Scheunemann H, Schurmann K, Helms J (eds): *Tumors of the Skull Base*. New York: Walter de Gruyter, 1986. Pp 131–137.
11. Derome PJ: The Transbasal Approach to Tumors Invading the Base of the Skull. In Schmidek HH, Sweet WH (eds): *Current Techniques in Operative Neurosurgery*. New York: Grune & Stratton, 1977. Pp 223–246.
12. Jenkins HA, Canalis RF: Transpalatal Approach to the Skull Base. In Sasaki CT, McCabe BF, Kirchner JA (eds): *Surgery of the Skull Base*. Philadelphia: Lippincott, 1984. Pp 113–124.
13. Baker SR: Surgical reconstruction after extensive skull base surgery. *Otolaryngol Clin North Am* 17 : 591, 1984.
14. Harker, LA, McCabe BF: Middle Cranial Fossa Approach to Skull Base. In Sasaki CT, McCabe BF, Kirchner JA (eds): *Surgery of the Skull Base*. Philadelphia: Lippincott, 1984. Pp 161–176.
15. Brackmann DE: The Translabyrinthine Approach. In Sasaki CT, McCabe BF, Kirchner JA (eds): *Surgery of the Skull Base*. Philadelphia: Lippincott, 1984, Pp 177–192.
16. Glasscock, III ME, Kveton JF, Jackson CG, Levine SC, McKennan, KX: A Systematic Approach to the Surgical Management of Acoustic Neuroma. Laryngoscope, 96 : 1088–1094.
17. Brackmann DE, Selter SA: Auditory Brainstem Response Audiometry in Acoustic Tumor Detection. In Brackmann DE (ed): *Neurological Surgery of the Ear and Skull Base*. New York: Raven, 1982. Pp 109–117.
18. Hieshima GB, et al: Embolization for tumors of the skull base. In Brackmann DE (ed): *Neurological Surgery of the Ear and Skull Base*. New York: Raven, 1982. Pp 391–394.
19. Norrell H: The Sitting Position for Surgery: Techniques and Pitfalls. In Brackmann DE (ed): *Neurological Surgery of the Ear and Skull Base*. New York: Raven, 1982. Pp 213–218.
20. Hitselberger WE: The Supine Lateral Position for Removal of Ear and Skull Cerebellopontine Angle Tumors. In Brackmann DE (ed): *Neurological Surgery of the Ear and Skull Base*. New York: Raven, 1982. Pp 219–221.

21. Sekhar LN, Estonillo R: Transtemporal-Infratemporal Approach to the Skull Base. In Scheunemann H, Schurmann K, Helms J (eds): *Tumors of the Skull Base.* New York: Walter de Gruyter, 1986. Pp 199–207.
22. Fisch U, Pillsbury III HC, Sasaki CT: Infratemporal Approach to the Skull Base. In Sasaki CT, McCabe BF, Kirchner JA (eds): *Surgery of the Skull Base.* Philadelphia: Lippincott, 1984. Pp 141–160.
23. Shaheen OH: *Surgical Concepts in Malignant Tumors of the Lateral Skull Base.* New York: Walter de Gruyter, 1986. Pp 141–158.
24. Myers DL, Sataloff RT: Spinal fluid leakage after skull base surgical procedures. *Otolaryngol Clin North Am* 17 : 601, 1984.
25. Sasaki CT: Transseptal-Transsphenoidal Approach to the Sella. In Sasaki CT, McCabe BF, Kirchner JA (eds): *Surgery of the Skull Base.* Philadelphia: Lippincott, 1984. Pp 79–94.
26. Levine RE: Protection of the Exposed Eye in Facial Paralysis. In Brackmann DE (ed): *Neurological Surgery of the Ear and Skull Base.* New York: Raven, 1982. Pp 81–87.
27. Ey W, Denecke HJ: Rehabilitation of Swallowing Following Paresis of the Caudal Cranial Nerves. In Scheunemann H, Schurmann K, Helms J (eds): *Tumors of the Skull Base.* New York: Walter de Gruyter, 1986. Pp 245–247.
28. Conley J: Hypoglossal-Facial Nerve Anatomosis. In Brackmann DE (ed): *Neurological Surgery of the Ear and Skull Base.* New York: Raven, 1982. Pp 93–98.
29. May M: Late Facial Nerve Rehabilitation. In Brackmann DE (ed): *Neurological Surgery of the Ear and Skull Base.* New York: Raven, 1982. Pp 89–92.
30. Arnold H, Herrmann HD: Skull Base Chordoma-Neurosurgical Problems. In Scheunemann H, Shurmann K, Helms J (ed): *Tumors of the Skull Base.* New York: Walter de Gruyter, 1986. Pp 209–216.
31. Austin MB, Mills SE: Neoplasms and neoplasm-like lesions involving the skull base. *Ear Nose Throat J* 65 : 57, 1986.
32. Bosley JH, Martinez DM: Practical surgical anatomy of the skull base. *Ear Nose Throat J* 65 : 52, 1986.
33. Cece JA, et al: Complications in the management of large glomus jugulare tumors. *Laryngoscope* 97 : 152, 1987.
34. Horwitz NH, Rizzoli HV: *Postoperative Complications of Intracranial Neurological Surgery.* Baltimore: Williams & Wilkins, 1982.

Table 14-1. Laryngeal spaces

Space	*Subsite*	*Boundaries*						*Natural dehiscences*	*Lymphatics*	*Pathologic considerations*
		Anterior	*Posterior*	*Superior*	*Inferior*	*Medial*	*Lateral*			
Preepiglottic space	Supraglottis	Thyroid cartilage Thyrohyoid membrane	Epiglottis Quadrangular membrane	Valleculae Hyoepiglottic ligament	Petiole	Airway	Paraglottic space	Petiole of epiglottis	Superior bilateral via thyrohyoid membrane	Easy access to the base of tongue Egress into paraglottic space Potential for bilateral lymphatic metastasis
Paraglottic space	Glottis & subglottis	Thyroid cartilage	Pyriform fossa mucosa	Vocalis muscle Conus elasticus	Conus elasticus	Ventricle Quadrangular membrane	Thyroid cartilage	Cricothyroid membrane	Inferior: ipsilateral via inferior constrictor muscle	Associated with early vocal cord paralysis Direct extension via cricothyroid membrane may invade thyroid gland Easy egress into prelaryngeal soft tissues and pyriform sinus

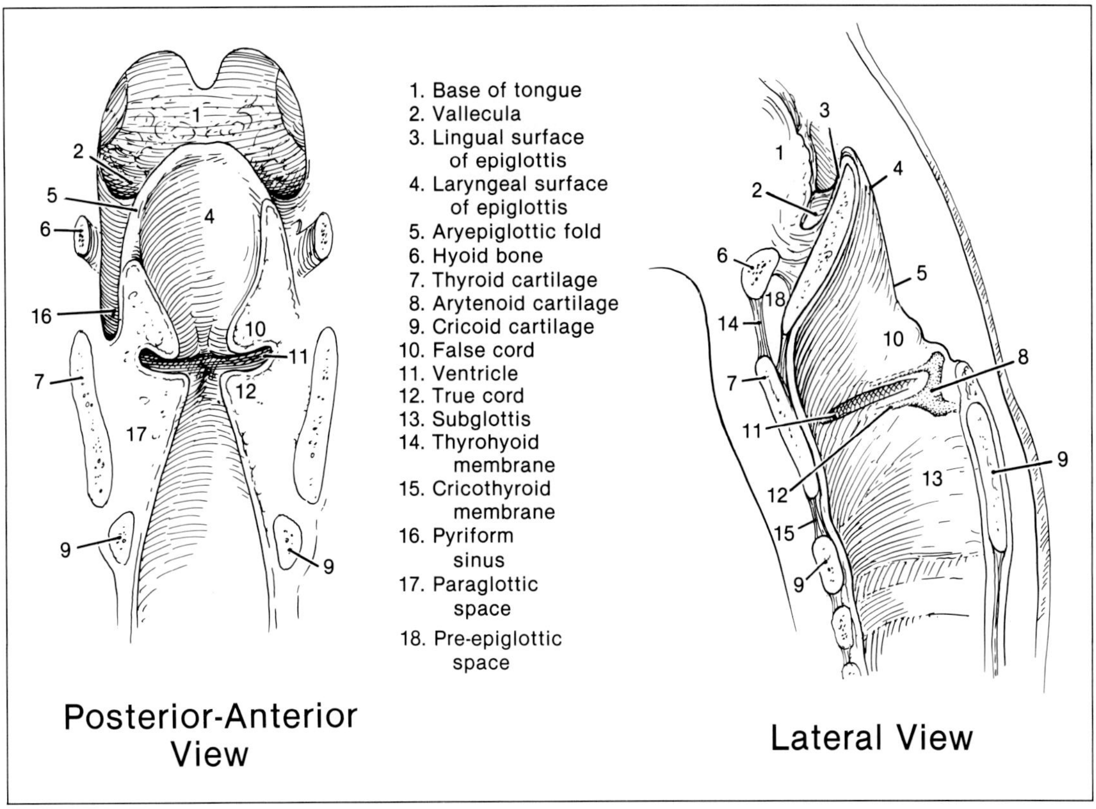

Figure 14-1. Basic laryngeal anatomy.

Cartilages

Thyroid

The alae or wings of the thyroid converge anteriorly in the midline to form the keel-like thyroid prominence or Adam's apple. Posteriorly and laterally, each ala projects into the superior and inferior cornua. The superior cornua are attached to the hyoid bone by the tough thyrohyoid membrane. The inferior cornua articulate with the cricoid cartilage at two synovial (cricoid) joints.

Epiglottis

The epiglottis is a leaf-shaped cartilage attached posteriorly and superiorly to the thyroid cartilage at the inferior border or petiole. The free border of its anterior surface is attached to the posterior aspect of the horseshoe-shaped hyoid bone by soft-tissue attachments.

Cricoid

The cricoid is a signet-ring shaped cartilage. Its anterosuperior border is attached to the inferior border of the thyroid cartilage by the cricothyroid membrane.

Arytenoids

The arytenoids are paired pyramidal-shaped cartilages superior to the posterior surface of the cricoid cartilage. The bases allow medial to lateral movement and rotation; the remaining two sides are the vocal and muscular processes. Extending anteriorly from each vocal process and inserting into the posterior surface of the thyroid cartilage are the thyroarytenoid ligaments or vocal cords.

Muscles

Suspended from the complex cartilaginous framework are the intrinsic laryngeal muscles,

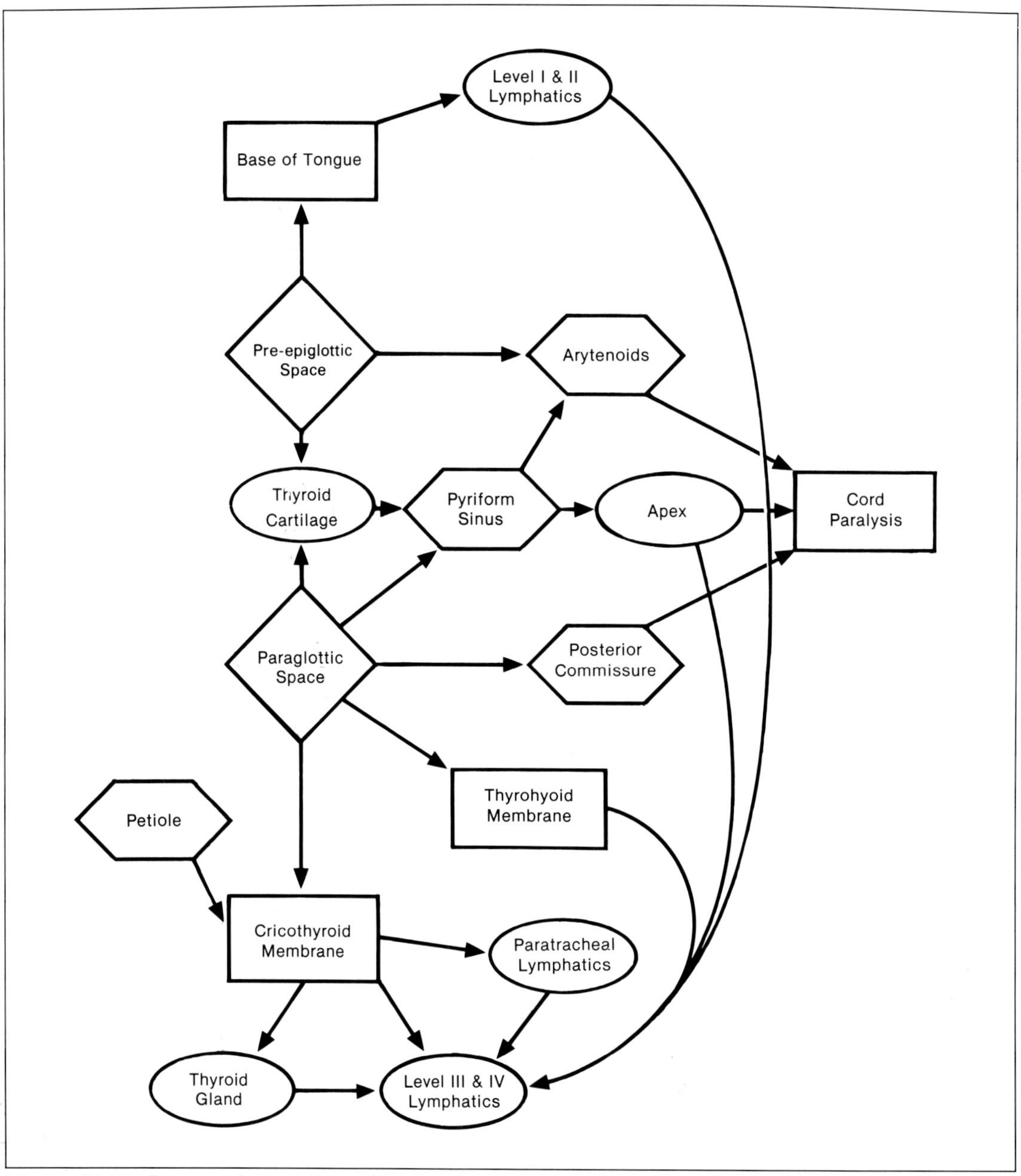

Figure 14-2. Laryngeal space dynamics.

covered intraluminally by respiratory epithelium.

Nerves

The right and left vagus nerves bilaterally innervate the larynx. The superior laryngeal branch of the vagus supplies supraglottic sensory innervation and cricothyroid motor innervation. The recurrent laryngeal nerve supplies glottic and subglottic sensory innervation and motor innervation to the remaining intrinsic laryngeal muscles.

Blood Vessels and Lymphatics

Both blood vessels and lymphatics are divided into superior and inferior divisions by the glottis. The vocal cords and their subepithelial spaces are largely devoid of blood vessels and lymphatics. The superior laryngeal lymphatics traverse the thyrohyoid membrane via the superior thyroid vascular pedicle. The inferior laryngeal lymphatics enter and exit beneath the inferior constrictor muscle via the inferior thyroid vascular pedicle.

CLINICAL PRESENTATION

History

There is no substitute for an accurately analyzed chief complaint and a well-formulated history. The minimal requirements are onset, duration, and associated problems. In addition, social and past medical history, habits, occupation, and medications also are pertinent (see Chapter 2). Initially, the patient is encouraged to describe the problem after open-ended questions. Later, if the discussion digresses, more direct questions are posed.

The following biographic data should be included:

1. Age. Cancer of the larynx is primarily an adult disease; it is seen most frequently in patients over the age of 40.
2. Sex. Men are more frequently afflicted than women.
3. Race. There is a higher incidence among blacks than whites [3].
4. Life-style. Patients exposed to chronic irritation (cigarette smoke, alcohol, infection) have a higher incidence of laryngeal malignancy [4–7].

Symptoms

The larynx, unlike some head and neck sites, presents with early complaints (see Chapter 2).

Chronic Hoarseness

Chronic hoarseness is the most frequent early symptom; the vast majority of laryngeal lesions originate from the free vocal cord edges. All patients with hoarseness for more than 2 weeks should be laryngoscoped.

Odynophagia

Odynophagia is associated with ulcerative and inflammatory lesions of the epiglottis, postcricoid area, and hypopharynx.

Dyspnea

Dyspnea is a late symptom, found with large obstructive lesions of the supraglottis or subglottis. It is also caused by vocal cord fixation secondary to invasion of the intrinsic laryngeal muscles or intraluminal obstruction.

Dysphagia

Although most frequently associated with upper alimentary tract disease, dysphagia occurs with invasive laryngeal lesions involving the hypopharynx.

Pain

Pain is a late symptom that implies an ulcerative or invasive lesion. An unusual variant is referred pain or pain originating from another site that shares a common sensory innervation, such as otalgia, related to supraglottic and hypopharyngeal lesions.

Hemoptysis

Hemoptysis is a late symptom associated with ulcerative or invasive lesions.

Cough

Possibly caused by laryngeal cancer, cough is also associated with pneumonia, chronic bronchitis, mediastinal involvement, or lung metastasis.

Signs

Commensurate with laryngeal symptoms, the significant signs usually reflect early disease.

Endolaryngeal Lesion

An endolaryngeal lesion is the earliest sign of a laryngeal carcinoma [3]. It presents as an exophytic mass, leukoplakia, erythroplasia, or ulcer. Most lesions are located in the glottis.

Cord Paralysis

Cord paralysis is an intermediate sign that is secondary to invasion of the endolaryngeal musculature or recurrent laryngeal nerve involvement.

Airway Obstruction

Airway obstruction is a late sign associated with either cord paralysis or an extensive endolaryngeal lesion in the supraglottis, glottis, or subglottis. If another subsite adjacent to the glottis is involved, supraglottis or subglottis, the lesion is designated as transglottic.

Neck Mass

Neck mass is a late sign (see Chapters 3 and 6). Depending on the subsite and its propensity for metastasis, a neck mass is either ipsilateral, contralateral, or bilateral.

DIAGNOSIS

Physical Examination

In reality, the physical examination begins with careful observation as the patient elaborates the chief complaint (see Chapter 2). Posture, respirations, and voice reveal valuable clues. The neck is scrutinized for asymmetry. Regardless of seemingly innocent complaints and symptoms, a complete physical examination is performed, with emphasis on the neck and indirect laryngoscopy.

Palpation

Palpation is a valuable but underutilized procedure that detects laryngeal mobility, fixation, abnormal position, or pain. Although rare in glottic carcinoma, direct extension and fixation are found with advanced lesions.

Indirect Laryngoscopy (Mirror Laryngoscopy)

A time-honored procedure, indirect laryngoscopy is a simple technique that exposes the larynx and hypopharynx using a mirror and an external light source. It is usually performed in the office under topical anesthesia with the patient in the sitting position.

Direct Laryngoscopy

Direct laryngoscopy, a component of panendoscopy, is the keystone of laryngeal diagnosis.

Rigid Laryngoscopy

Rigid laryngoscopy is direct laryngeal visualization through an open, rigid endoscope. The procedure is performed under topical or general anesthesia in the recumbent position. The operating microscope and carbon dioxide laser are useful adjuncts to laryngoscopy (see Chapter 10).

Fiberoptic Laryngoscope

After topical anesthesia, the flexible fiberoptic laryngoscope is passed transnasally with the patient in the sitting position. This procedure is performed easily in the office and is invaluable for anxious patients with a hyperactive gag reflex. Special video and still camera attachments are available for recording the findings.

Diagnostic Radiology

Fortunately, there are a variety of cost-effective and extremely accurate diagnostic modalities for laryngeal cancer (Table 14-2). Their easy availability and interpretation usually results in quick diagnostic assessments (see Chapter 4). Many times, a precise diagnosis is determined during the initial visit.

Plain X-ray Films

Lateral x-ray films are of greatest diagnostic value. The proper interpretation of these films requires only a basic knowledge of laryngeal anatomy.

Xeroradiography

Xeroradiography produces great soft-tissue detail, especially of the anterior commissure and subglottis. However, it exposes the patient to high radiation levels. It has largely been replaced by computer tomography.

Tomography

Tomography offers sequential visualization of the laryngeal structures at various levels. It detects tumor invasion in the horizontal and coronal planes.

Contrast Laryngography

Contrast laryngography consists of instilling radiopaque material into the larynx and imaging

Table 14-2. Imaging modalities: larynx

Modalities	*Advantages*	*Disadvantages*	*Indications*
Soft-tissue films	Availability Inexpensive	Soft-tissue detail	Airway assessment Nasopharngeal soft-tissue assessment Retropharyngeal assessment
Xeroradiography	Good soft-tissue visualization	Radiation Availability	Airway assessment Foreign bodies
Tomography	Mucosal detail	Radiation Patient cooperation Anteroposterior projection only	Pyriform sinus assessment Paraglottic space assessment Ventricle Subglottis
Laryngography	Mucosal detail	Aspiration Contrast allergy Topical anesthesia Availability	Preepiglottic space Epiglottis Subglottis
Computed tomography	Soft-tissue detail	Cartilage invasion Mucosal detail Contrast allergy Expensive Availability	Preepiglottic space Paraglottic space Subglottis Postcricoid area Lymphadenopathy
Magnetic resonance imaging	Soft-tissue detail Multidimensional views Allergic (contrast) patients Cartilage invasion	Availability Equipment expense Procedure cost Pacemaker malfunction	Base of tongue Preepiglottic space Paraglottic space Pyriform sinus

its distribution over the laryngeal surface. Today, it is supplanted largely by computed tomography.

Computed Tomography (CT Scan)

An advanced radiographic technique, CT scan is invaluable for evaluating the supraglottis and subglottis, and for detecting soft-tissue involvement.

Magnetic Resonance Imaging

Considered the state of the art, magnetic resonance imaging (MRI) is excellent for soft-tissue detail. Presently, its routine use is limited by availability and cost.

Precancerous Lesions

Early recognition of precancerous lesions is important (see Chapter 5). Once confirmed, the patient is urged to change his life-style immediately. Such pathologic changes imply prior or current exposure to carcinogens, principally tobacco.

Leukoplakia

Hyperkeratotic lesions, appearing clinically as white plaques, are referred to as leukoplakia.

Hyperkeratosis

Hyperkeratosis is thickening of the superficial laryngeal epithelium. It presents as irregular gray patches or papillomas.

Pachydermia Laryngitis

Pachydermia laryngitis is a diffuse hyperkeratotic lesion of the posterior commissure that typically involves the interarytenoid area. It characteristically interferes with complete glottic closure, resulting in chronic hoarseness.

Malignant Lesions

Once the subsite is ascertained, a tissue diagnosis is required. Biopsies are obtained under local or general anesthesia. Most pathologists can diagnose the common laryngeal malignancies with certainty.

Carcinoma In Situ

The earliest stage of laryngeal cancer is a carcinoma in situ. It is characterized by atypical cells, bizzare mitosis, large nucleoli, and irregular cell alignment. The absence of any basement membrane invasion or penetration is the distinguishing feature.

Squamous Cell Carcinoma

Squamous cell carcinoma is the most common laryngeal malignancy. It typically arises from the free edges of the anterior two-thirds of the vocal cords.

Adenocarcinoma

Although there is a paucity of endolaryngeal glands, adenocarcinoma arises from the ventricle where these glands are most abundant. Adenocarcinoma constitutes a small percentage of laryngeal malignancy.

Verrucous Cancer

Verrucous cancer is an unusual malignancy that appears benign on physical examination. Pathologically, it is characterized by luxuriant hyperkeratosis with deep rete pegs. Actual cartilage destruction, although rare, does occur. Usually conservation surgery suffices and radiotherapy is contraindicated [8,9].

Sarcoma

Only a small percentage of laryngeal cancers are sarcomas. Histologically, they are classified as fibrosarcoma, chondrosarcoma, leiomyosarcoma, hemangiosarcoma, or neurosarcoma.

Metastatic Carcinoma

Although infrequent, tumors originating from the kidneys, breasts, or prostate metastasize to the larynx. Melanoma is another rare metastatic source.

TREATMENT

Radiation Therapy

Megavoltage radiation is delivered precisely to a limited area without damaging the adjacent soft tissue or skin (see Chapter 9). Dosages range from 6000 to 7000 cGy [10].

Supraglottic Cancers

The size of the treatment portals vary with the size and location of the lesion. Since supraglottic cancer has a high incidence of metastasis, the portals must include both the neck bilaterally. Survival rates for patients treated with radiation range from 30 to 70 percent. However, the prognosis greatly depends on the size, the location, and the presence or absence of lymph node metastasis.

Glottic Cancer

Radiotherapy is the treatment of choice for early glottic tumors and some supraglottic cancers. With radiotherapy, morbidity is minimal and function is preserved. As the primary treatment modality, radiotherapy is recommended for reliable patients who have small unilateral lesions and no cervical metastasis.

Subglottic Cancers

Unlike most laryngeal cancers, subglottic tumors present late. The usual complaints are hoarseness and dyspnea. Due to their late presentation, total laryngectomy and upper mediastinal dissection are the treatments of choice. These are followed by postoperative irradiation.

Surgery

The current surgical philosophy is summarized in Tables 14-3, 14-4, and 14-5.

Table 14-3. Subsites of the larynx (site 8)

Supraglottis
Epiglottis
False cords
Glottis
Ventricle
True vocal cords
Subglottis

Table 14-4. Supraglottic carcinoma: treatment options

	Stage I			Stage III*		
Treatment	***A***	***B***	***Stage II***	***A***	***B***	***Stage IV****
Treatment of choice	Laser Subtotal supraglottic laryngectomy	Radiotherapy (full-course)	1. Subtotal supraglottic laryngectomy 2. Radiotherapy (postoperative)	1. Chemotherapy 2. ¾ laryngectomy or total laryngectomy 3. Radiotherapy	1. Chemotherapy 2. Total laryngectomy 3. Radiotherapy	1. Chemotherapy 2. Total laryngectomy 3. Radiotherapy
Modality available after 1st treatment failure	Radiotherapy	Total laryngectomy	Completion laryngectomy	Chemotherapy	Chemotherapy	Chemotherapy
Modality available after 2nd treatment failure	Completion laryngectomy	Chemotherapy	Chemotherapy	Chemotherapy	Chemotherapy	Chemotherapy

A. Best option.
B. Second best option.
*Neck dissections(s).

Table 14-5. Glottic carcinoma: treatment options

		Stage II		Stage III*		
Treatment	***Stage I***	***A***	***B***	***A***	***B***	***Stage IV****
Treatment of choice	Laser or radiotherapy	Hemilaryngectomy	Radiotherapy (full-course)	1. Chemotherapy 2. Extended hemilaryngectomy or total laryngectomy 3. Radiotherapy	Radiotherapy (full-course)	1. Chemotherapy 2. Total laryngectomy 3. Radiotherapy
Modality available after 1st treatment failure	1. Hemilaryngectomy 2. Radiotherapy (postoperative)	Radiotherapy (postoperative)	Total laryngectomy	Completion laryngectomy	Total laryngectomy	Chemotherapy
Modality available after 2nd treatment failure	Completion laryngectomy	Completion laryngectomy	Chemotherapy	Chemotherapy	Chemotherapy	Chemotherapy

A. Best option.
B. Second best option.
*Neck dissection(s) (±).

Laryngoscopy

Endoscopy is indicated for carcinoma in situ or small stage I carcinomas, especially located on the true vocal cords. Radiotherapy may also be employed, but the endoscopic techniques are more simple and cost-effective. The common endoscopic procedures are endoscopic cordectomy, microlaryngoscopy and cord stripping, and laser microlaryngoscopy. Today, laser laryngoscopy, which is precise and has a low morbidity, is advocated for in situ or small stage I lesions [11,12].

Partial Laryngectomy

Many of the great names in otolaryngology have contributed to the development of conservation or partial laryngeal surgery. These techniques are based on intimate knowledge of laryngeal embryology, physiology, and lymphatics [13–16]. Patient selection depends on the extent of disease, age, habits, physical and mental condition, economics, and occupation. In properly selected cases, acceptable cure rates are obtained and function is preserved. Whenever possible, conservation surgery is employed for laryngeal malignancies [13–18]. These techniques ablate the disease but preserve respiration, phonation, and deglutition (Tables 14-6, 14-7, and 14-8).

Table 14-6. Indications for partial laryngectomy

- Subtotal supraglottic laryngectomy (SSL)
  - Epiglottis & false cords
  - Valleculae & base of tongue (limited)
- Partial laryngopharyngectomy (PLP)
  - Aryepiglottic fold
  - Anterior and medial wall of pyriform sinus
- Hemilaryngectomy (HEMI)
  - Anterior commissure
  - Arytenoid (ipsilateral)
  - Verrucous carcinoma
  - Highly selected lesions
    - Transglottic carcinomas
    - Cord fixation
    - Postradiation failures
    - Subglottis (<1 cm)

Table 14-7. Partial laryngectomy or conservation surgery

- Supraglottic larynx
  - Subtotal supraglottic laryngectomy
  - Partial laryngopharyngectomy
  - Three-quarter laryngectomy
- Glottic larynx
  - Hemilaryngectomy
  - Extended hemilaryngectomy
    - ± Stent
    - ± Muscle flap (free or pedicle)
  - Anterior commissure resection
  - Subtotal vertical laryngectomy with epiglottic reconstruction

Table 14-8. Partial laryngectomy pitfalls

- Subtotal supraglottic laryngectomy (SSL)
  - Any post full-course radiotherapy recurrence
  - Cryptic preepiglottic space involvement
    - Base of tongue
    - Thyrohyoid membrane
    - Petiole
    - Pyriform sinus apex
  - Cryptic paraglottic space involvement
    - Thyroid cartilage
    - Cricothyroid membrane
    - Cricoid cartilage
    - Pyriform sinus
    - Subglottis (>1 cm)
- Partial laryngopharyngectomy (PLP)
  - Post full-course radiotherapy involvement
    - Apex
    - Thyroid cartilage
    - Paraglottic space
    - Petiole
    - Posterior commissure
- Hemilaryngectomy (HEMI)
  - Post full-course radiotherapy
    - Cord fixation
    - Skip lesions
    - Bilateral arytenoid involvement
    - Posterior commissure
  - Cryptic preepiglottic space involvement
    - Thyrohyoid membrane
    - Petiole
    - Thyroid cartilage
  - Cryptic paraglottic space involvement
    - Thyroid perichondrium
    - Cricoid cartilage
    - Cricothyroid membrane
  - Transglottic lesions
  - Paratracheal metastasis

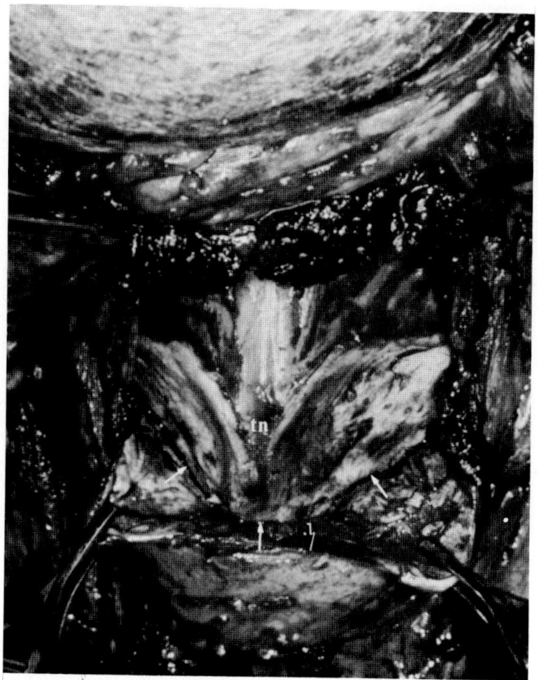

A

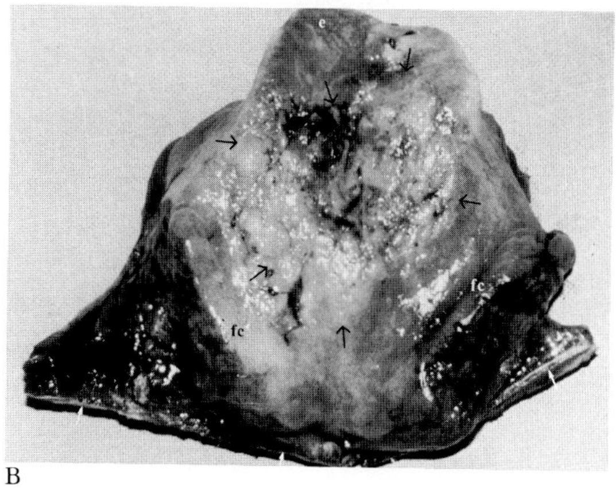

B

Figure 14-3. Subtotal supraglottic laryngectomy (SSL). A. The cartilage cuts required to remove the upper two-thirds of the larynx. *tn* = thyroid notch; *white arrows* = cartilage cuts; *black arrow* = thyroid perichondrium. B. SSL specimen with a large central ulceration on the laryngeal surface. *e* = epiglottis; *white arrows* = cartilage cuts; *fc* = false cords.

Subtotal Supraglottic Laryngectomy

Horizontal partial laryngectomy or subtotal supraglottic laryngectomy is indicated for tumor involvement of the epiglottis or false cords [14]. Invasion of the ventricles or cord paralysis is a contraindication. This procedure is recommended for stage II lesions (Figure 14-3).

Partial Laryngopharyngectomy

Partial laryngopharyngectomy is indicated for lesions involving the epiglottic fold and pyriform sinus unassociated with vocal cord paralysis or apex obliteration (stage II—hypopharynx) (Figures 14-4 and 14-5) [19].

Hemilaryngectomy

Hemilaryngectomy vertically removes one-half of the larynx (Figure 14-6). It is limited to cases without subglottic or posterior commissure involvement [19–24]. For selected lesions involving the ipsilateral arytenoid and contralateral cord (anterior two-thirds), this approach may be extended. Such an extended hemilaryngectomy requires a stent, muscle flap (free or

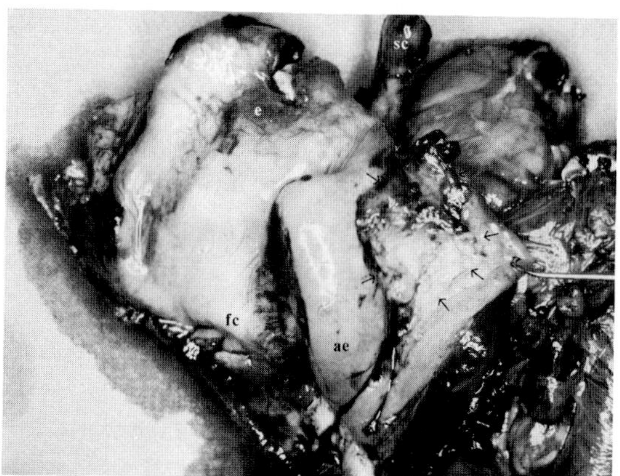

Figure 14-4. Right partial laryngopharyngectomy specimen. *e* = epiglottis, *fc* = false cord; *ae* = aryepiglottic fold; *sc* = superior cornu.

pedicled), or mobilized epiglottis to ensure posterior commissure competence (Figures 14-7 and 14-8).

Three-Quarter Laryngectomy

Three-quarter laryngectomy is a horizontal supraglottic laryngectomy with arytenoidec-

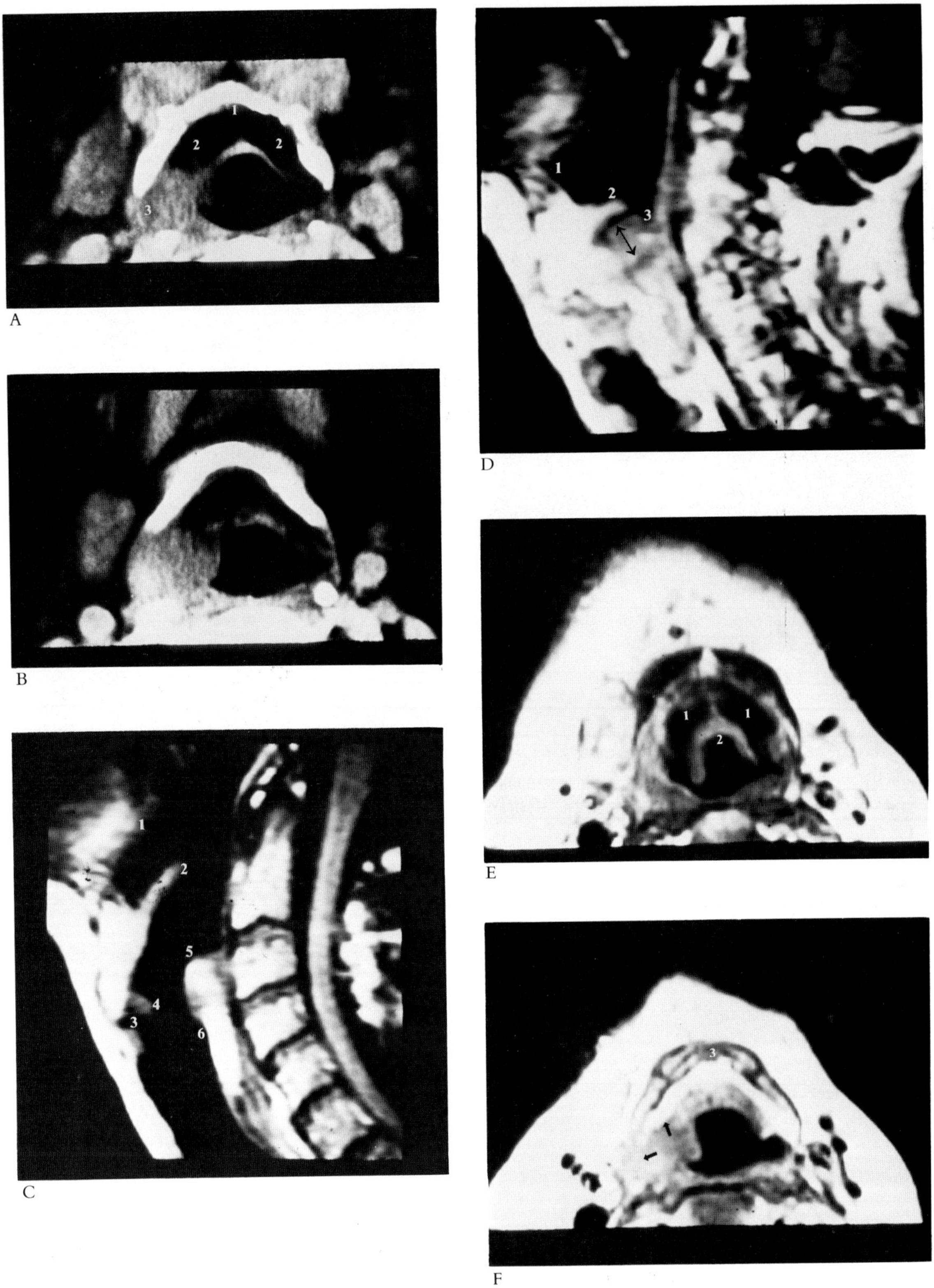
A
B
C
D
E
F

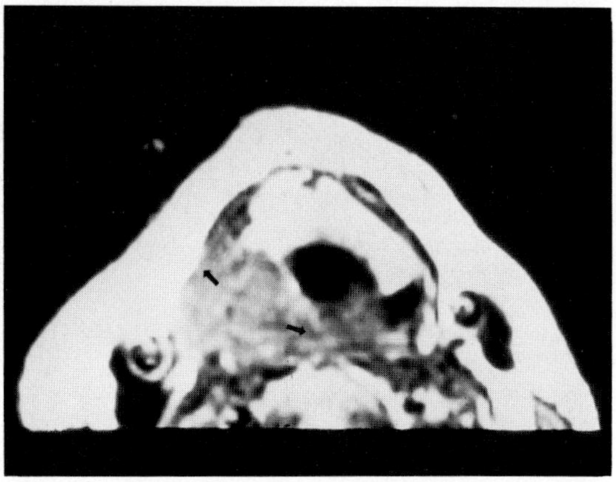

G

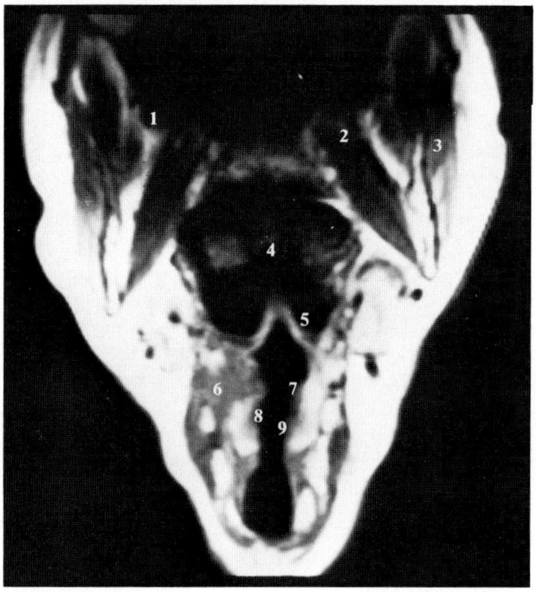

H

Figure 14-5. Hemoptysis and persistent right-sided sore throat were the complaints of this 75-year-old heavy drinker and smoker. Although CT scans were helpful, the multiple views of the MRI were invaluable in determining the feasibility of partial surgery. A and B. CT axial views of the larynx and hypopharynx. *1* = hyoid bone; *2* = valleculae; *3* = pyriform lesion. C. MRI midline sagittal views. *1* = base of tongue; *2* = epiglottis; *3* = ventricle; *4* = true cord; *5* = arytenoid; *6* = cricoid cartilage. D. MRI pyriform sagittal view. *1* = vallecula; *2* = thyroid cartilage; *3* = arytenoid. E–G. MRI axial views. *1* = valleculae; *2* = epiglottis; *3* = thyroid cartilage. H. MRI coronal view: *1* = pterygoid plate; *2* = pterygoid muscle; *3* = masseter; *4* = base of tongue; *5* = aryepiglottic fold; *6* = tumor in the right pyriform sinus; 7 = false cord; *8* = ventricle; *9* = true cord. The patient had a successful partial laryngopharyngectomy and modified neck dissection.

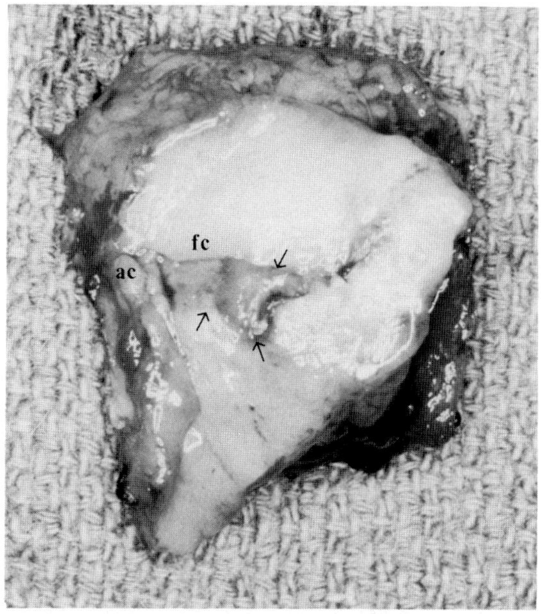

Figure 14-6. Right hemilaryngectomy specimen. *ac* = anterior commissure; *fc* = false cord.

tomy and glottic reconstruction. A sophisticated procedure, it is associated with postoperative aspiration and prolonged tracheal decannulation [19]. Preoperative evaluation excludes those patients with severe chronic obstructive pulmonary disease or emphysema. For patients with severe pulmonary disease, full-course radiotherapy or total laryngectomy is recommended.

Completion Laryngectomy

Completion laryngectomy is the removal of the entire remaining portion of the larynx after partial laryngectomy. It is indicated for tumor recurrence or persistence after an antecedent hemilaryngectomy, supraglottic laryngectomy, or partial laryngopharyngectomy [25].

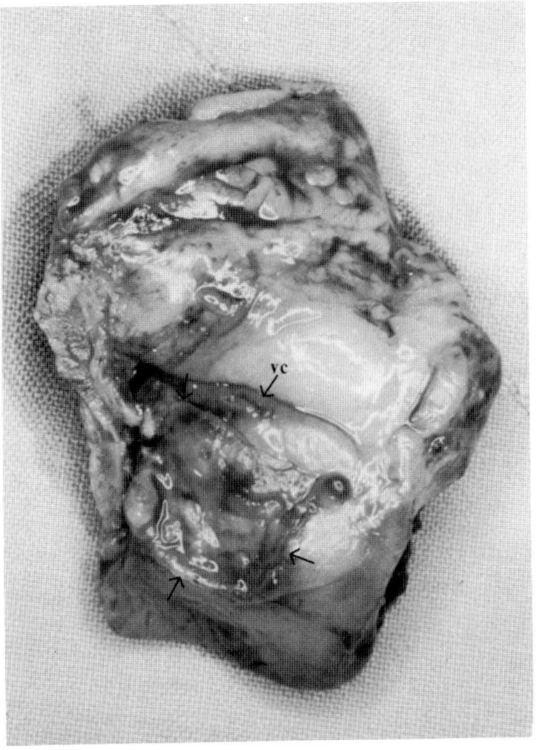

Figure 14-7. Right hemilaryngectomy specimen with a large (anterior two-thirds) lesion; *vc* = vocal cord.

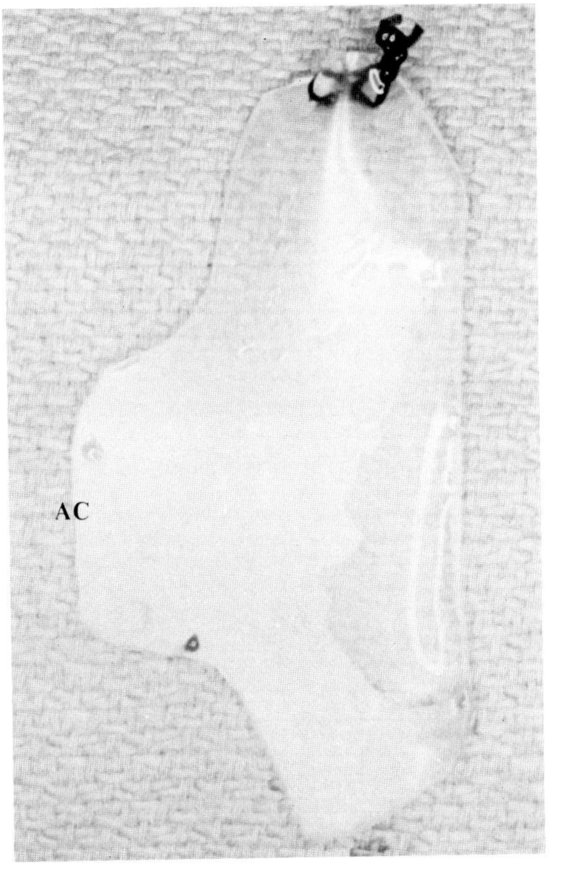

Figure 14-8. Silastic stent. A stent aids reconstruction after an extended hemilaryngectomy: silk suture, proximal (superior) aspect. *AC* = tapered portion for insertion in the anterior commissure.

Table 14-9. Indications for total laryngectomy

Full-course radiation failures
Partial laryngectomy failures
Extensive preepiglottic space involvement
Base of tongue
Thyrohyoid membrane
Petiole
Pyriform sinus apex
Extensive paraglottic space involvement
Thyroid cartilage
Posterior commissure
Cord fixation
Cricothyroid membrane
Cricoid cartilage
Subglottis (1 cm)
Extensive hypopharyngeal involvement
Soft-tissue involvement
Strap muscle
Skin
Thyroid gland
Paratracheal metastasis

Total Laryngectomy

The most widely accepted single procedure for stage III or IV cancer is total laryngectomy (Tables 14-9 and 14-10) [26–31]. However, this operation greatly affects the quality of life. The principal morbidity is aphonia and permanent tracheostomy. For advanced cancers, with cervical metastasis, treatment consists of wide-field total laryngectomy and neck dissection (ipsilateral or bilateral). For advanced laryngeal cancers, most radiotherapists advise postoperative radiation. Therefore, advanced cancers with or without cervical metastasis require surgery as well as radiotherapy (Figures 14-9 through 14-12). The chance of cure with radiotherapy alone is dismal.

Combined Therapy

Surgery and radiotherapy are the primary treatment modalities for cancer of the larynx. Either may be used alone or conjointly in appropriately selected cases [32]. For advanced lesions, there is a definite role for chemotherapy.

Surgery and Radiation

Surgery and radiation are indicated for stage II or III supraglottic, glottic, and subglottic tumors.

Chemotherapy

In the past, chemotherapy was reserved for treatment failures or terminal disease. Today, it is administered inductively, for stage III or IV car-

Table 14-10. Adjuncts to total laryngectomy

Glossectomy
Partial
Total
Pharyngectomy[a]
Partial
Complete
Cervical esophagectomy
Thyroidectomy
Partial
Total
Neck dissection[b]
Unilateral
Bilateral
Mediastinal dissection[c]

[a]See Chapter 24.
[b]See Chapter 16.
[c]See Chapter 17.

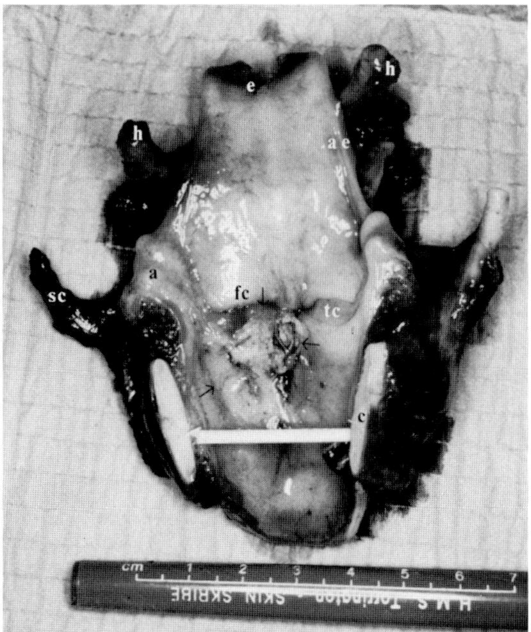

A

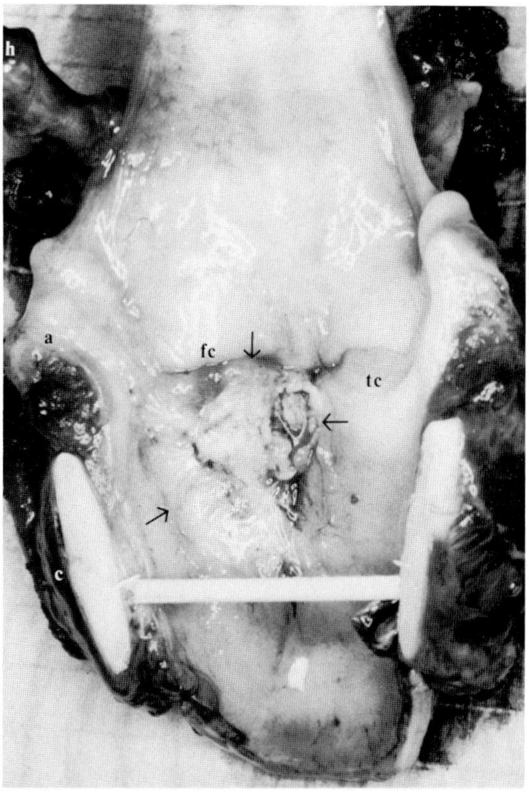

B

Figure 14-9. Total laryngectomy specimen of a moderate size lesion. *e* = epiglottis; *ae* = aryepiglottic fold; *fc* = false cord; *vn* = ventricle; *tc* = true cord; *c* = cricoid cartilage; *h* = hyoid bone; *sc* = superior cornu; *a* = arytenoid.

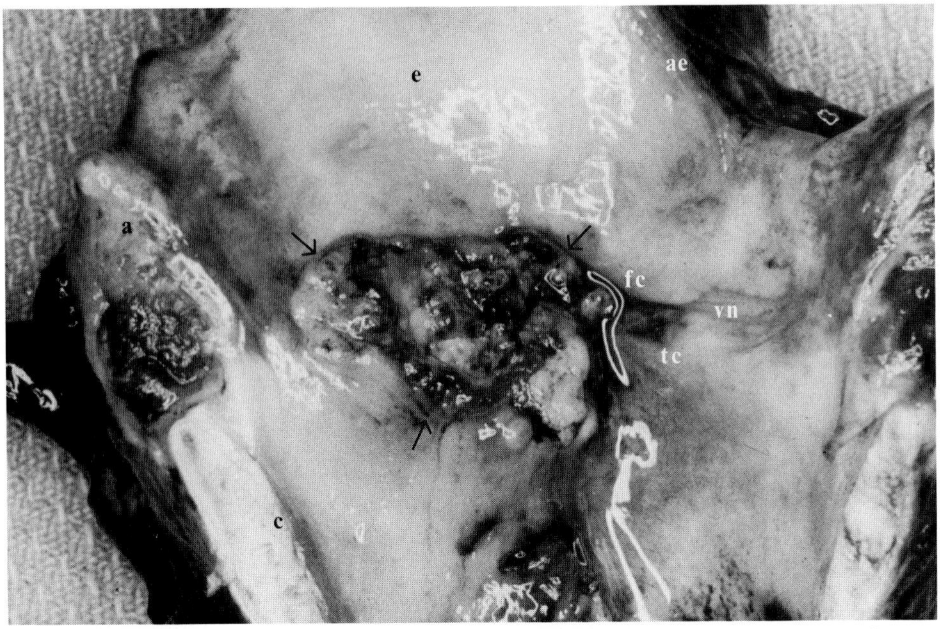

Figure 14-10. Total laryngectomy for obstructive glottic carcinoma. *a* = arytenoid; *e* = epiglottis; *ae* = aryepiglottic fold; *fc* = false cord; *vn* = ventricle; *tc* = true cord; *c* = cricoid cartilage.

Figure 14-11. Total laryngectomy specimen of an extensive lesion involving the left pyriform sinus and postcricoid area. *h* = hyoid bone; *black arrow* = subtotal glottic obstruction.

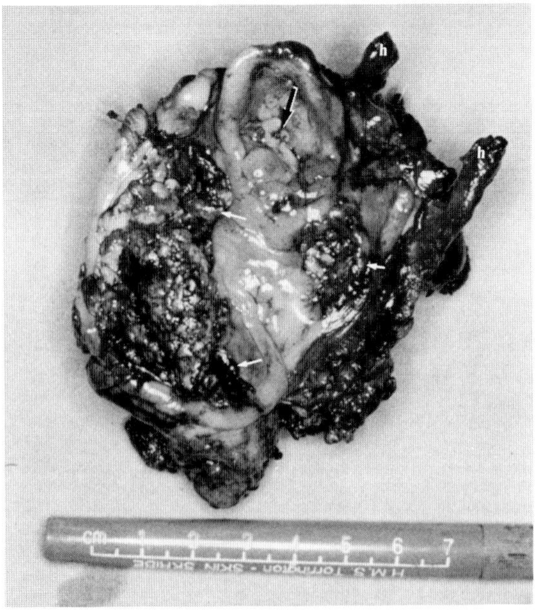

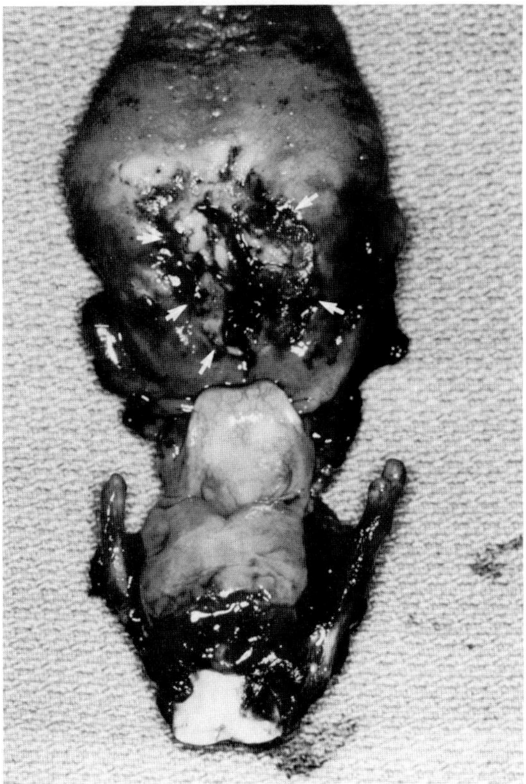

Figure 14-12. Carcinoma of the base of the tongue. The extensive nature of the disease required both total glossectomy and total laryngectomy.

cinomas, followed by surgery and radiotherapy (see Chapter 8). Chemotherapy is invaluable palliation for tertiary treatment failures.

REFERENCES

1. Young JL, Perry CL, Asize AJ (eds): *Surveillance, Epidemiology and End Results: Incidence and Mortality Data, 1973–77*. National Cancer Institute 57 (NIH) 81-2330. Washington, DC: Government Printing Office, 1981.
2. Silverberg E, Lubera E: Cancer statistics, 1988. *CA* 38 : 5, 1988.
3. National Institutes of Health, Public Health Service: *Third National Cancer Survey: Incidence Data*. National Cancer Institute Monograph DHEW Publication (NIH) 75-757. Washington, DC: Government Printing Office, 1975.
4. Jussawalla DJ, et al: Cancer incidence in Greater Bombay: Assessment of the cancer risk by age. *Br J Cancer* 22 : 623, 1968.
5. Watherhouse J, et al (eds): *Cancer Incidence in the Continent*. Lyon, IRC Scientific Publications, 1976. Vol 3, No 15.
6. Doll R: The geographical distribution of cancer. *Br J Cancer* 23 : 1, 1969.
7. Eiband JD, et al: Prognostic factors in squamous cell carcinoma of the larynx. *Am J Surg* 158 : 314, 1989.
8. Myers EM, Sobol S, Ogura JH: Hemilaryngectomy for verrucous carcinoma of the larynx. *Laryngoscope* 90(4) : 693, 1980.
9. Edstrom S, et al: Verrucous squamous cell carcinoma of the larynx: Evidence for increased metastatic potential after irradiation. *Otolaryngol Head Neck Surg* 97 : 381, 1987.
10. Constable WC, Marks RD, Robbins JP: High dose preoperative radiotherapy and surgery for cancer of the larynx. *Laryngoscope* 82 : 1861, 1972.
11. Strong, MS: Laser excision of carcinoma of the larynx. *Laryngoscope* 85 : 1286, 1975.
12. Wetmore SJ, Key JM, Suen JY: Laser therapy for T_1 glottic carcinoma of the larynx. *Arch Otolaryngol Head Neck Surg* 112 : 853, 1986.
13. Robbins KT, et al: Conservation surgery for T_2 and T_3 carcinomas of the supraglottic larynx. *Arch Otolaryngol Head Neck Surg* 114 : 421, 1988.
14. Bocca E: Supraglottic cancer. *Laryngoscope* 85 : 1318, 1975.
15. Alonso JM: Conservation of function in surgery of larynx: Basics, technics, and results. *Trans Am Acad Ophth* 56 : 722, 1952.
16. Ogura JH: Surgical pathology of cancer of larynx. *Laryngoscope* 65 : 867, 1955.
17. Ogura JH, Sessions DG, Spector GJ: Conservation surgery for epidermoid carcinoma of the supraglottic larynx. *Laryngoscope* 85: 1808, 1975.
18. Brandenburg JH, Condon KG, Frank TW: Coronal sections of larynges from radiation therapy failures: A clinical-pathologic study. *Otolaryngol Head Neck Surg* 95 : 213, 1986.
19. Ogura JH, Sessions DD, Ciralsky RH: Supraglottic carcinoma with extension to the arytenoid. *Laryngoscope* 85 : 1327, 1975.
20. Biller HG, Ogura JH, Pratt LL: Hemilaryngectomy for T_2 glottic cancers. *Arch Otolaryngol* 93 : 238, 1971.
21. Sessions DG, Ogura JH, Fried MP: The anterior commissure in glottic carcinoma. *Laryngoscope* 85 : 1627, 1975.
22. Rothfield RE, et al: The role of hemilaryngectomy in the management of T_1 local cord cancer. *Arch Otolaryngol Head Neck Surg* 115 : 677, 1989.
23. Laccourreye H, et al: Supracricoid hemilaryngopharyngectomy. *Ann Otolaryngol Rhino* 96 : 217, 1987.
24. Tucker HM, et al: Near-total laryngectomy with epiglottic reconstruction. *Arch Otolaryngol Head Neck Surg* 115 : 1341, 1989.

25. Myers EM, Ogura JH: Completion laryngectomy. *Ann Oto* 88 : 172, 1979.
26. Razack MS, et al: Management of advanced glottic carcinomas. *Am J Surg* 158 : 318, 1989.
27. Griebie MS, Adams GL: Emergency laryngectomy and stomal recurrence. *Laryngoscope* 97 : 1020, 1987.
28. Sultan MR, Coleman JJ. Oncologic and functional consideration of total glossectomy. *Am J Surg* 158 : 297, 1989.
29. Kirchner JA, Som ML: Clinical significance of fixed cord. *Laryngoscope* 81 : 1029, 1971.
30. Kirchner JA: One hundred laryngeal cancers studied by serial section. *Ann of Oto* 78 : 680, 1969.
31. Sessions DG, Ogura JH, Fried MP: Carinoma of the subglottic area. *Laryngoscope* 85 : 1417, 1975.
32. Nichols RD et al: Partial laryngectomy after radiation failure. *Laryngoscope* 90 : 571, 1980.

15

Thyroid

ROBERT M. WHITE, JR.

KEY CONCEPTS

Thyroid Nodule; Fine Needle Biopsy; Multiple Endocrine Neoplasia Syndrome (MEN II); Thyroidectomy; Radioiodine Therapy; Thyroid Suppression

MILESTONES

1938	Thyroid Lymphatics	Rouviere
1949	Cervical Metastasis and Thyroid Carcinoma	Warren and Feldman
1951	Retrospective Analysis of Thyroid Carcinoma	Lahey and Hare
1952	Solitary Nodule and Thyroid Carcinoma	Cause et al.
1955	Microscopic Cervical Metastasis	Frazell and Foote
1959	Cold Nodule and Malignancy	Groesbeck
1962	Childhood Radiation and Thyroid Carcinoma	Nishiyama
	Classification of Thyroid Lesions	Shimaoka et al.
	Frozen Section Diagnoses of Thyroid Carcinoma	Jones et al.
1963	Thyroid Carcinoma and the Atomic Bomb	Socolow et al.
1966	Surgical Indications for the Thyroid Nodule	Welch
1970	Thyroglossal Duct Cysts and Thyroid Carcinoma	Jacque et al.
1972	Thyroid Sonography	Blum et al.
1973	Fine Needle Aspiration	Crile and Hawk
1975	Familial Medullary Thyroid Carcinoma	Wells et al.
1976	Thyroid Angiography and Carcinoma	Ghosh

In 1990, approximately 12,000 new cases of thyroid malignancy will be diagnosed in the United States. Of these new cases, 3200 will be men and 8900 will be women. There will be 1100 disease-related deaths, of which 400 will be men and 700 will be women [1]. The female to male ratio in papillary and follicular carcinoma is 3 : 1; the female to male ratio in medullary and anaplastic carcinoma is 1 : 1 [2,3].

The risk for developing papillary carcinoma and benign nodular disease is related to low-dose head and neck (<2000 cGy) external radiation [4] (Table 15-1). Higher doses of radiation

Table 15-1. Risk factors for thyroid neoplasia

Benign adenoma and papillary carcinoma
- External radiation to head and neck (latency period 15–25 yr) for
  - Enlarged thymus gland
  - Enlarged tonsils
  - Acne
  - Tinea capitis

C-cell hyperplasia and medullary carcinoma
- Family history (autosomal dominant transmission)
- Multiple endocrine neoplasia II

usually do not cause neoplastic transformation because the gland is ablated by the radiation [5]. Radioactive iodine 131 (^{131}I) therapy is not associated with neoplasia [6]. Medullary carcinoma is associated with a family history of multiple endocrine neoplasia syndrome II (MEN II), that is, medullary carcinoma, pheochromocytoma, and parathyroid adenoma or hyperplasia [2,7].

MANAGEMENT OF THE THYROID NODULE

In order of descending frequency, solitary thyroid nodules are nontoxic nodular goiter, adenoma, thyroiditis, toxic adenoma, cyst, and carcinoma. A thyroid malignancy is suspected when a nodule is hard, solitary, enlarging, or fixed (Figures 15-1 and 15-2). Malignancy is strongly suspected if the patient is young, has cervical adenopathy, and is male. Less frequently, thyroid malignancy is associated with dysphagia, hoarseness, hemoptysis, and dyspnea. Papillary carcinoma is suspected with a history of low-dose external radiation to the head and neck region. Medullary carcinoma is suggested with a familial history of thyroid tumors or MEN II [2,5,8].

Thyroid Function Tests

Thyroid function tests are nondiagnostic for thyroid carcinoma. However, calcitonin assay is useful in the diagnosis of medullary carcinoma [2]. This assay is especially valuable in conjunction with the calcium or pentagastrin provocative tests to detect c-cell neoplasia (a premalignant lesion of medullary carcinoma) in asymptomatic individuals with a family history of MEN II [7].

Thyroid Scans

A technetium 99m thyroid scan detects hyperactive versus hypoactive nodules; hypoactive nodules usually are benign. Cold nodules are benign 80 percent of the time; about one-third of the cold nodules in patients with a history of external radiation are cancerous. Normal thyroid tissue accumulates ^{131}I more efficiently than papillary and follicular carcinomas, thus the association of cold nodules and thyroid carcinoma.

Sonography

Ultrasound distinguishes cysts from solid lesions. Although rarely malignant, cystic lesions should be aspirated for cytology [2].

Computed Tomography Scan

Computed tomography (CT) scan best outlines the regional extent, infiltration, and destruction by a suspected malignant lesion. It is invaluable for presurgical planning (see Chapter 4) [2].

Thyroglobulins

Thyroglobulin elevations detect metastatic disease in patients with documented well-differentiated papillary carcinoma. Since thyroglobulin can be elevated in other thyroid diseases, it is a poor screening test for thyroid cancer [4].

Plain Films

Plain roentgenographs of the neck might detect thyroidal calcifications in the patient suspected of medullary carcinoma.

Fine-Needle Aspiration

Fine-needle biopsy is an accurate alternative to open biopsy of solid or cold thyroid nodules (see Chapters 3 and 5). Patients diagnosed with malignancy, adenoma, follicular cells, or suspicious cells for malignancy are clear candidates for open biopsy and definitive surgery. The majority of patients diagnosed with a non-neoplastic disease are followed and placed on thyroid suppression. Fine-needle biopsy is repeated in 6 months if the nodule increases in size. Urgent surgery is not as crucial in well-differentiated thyroid malignancy because of its low virulence. However, good clinical judgment with regard to other characteristics of the nodule suggesting malignancy outweighs a negative fine-needle aspiration [8–12].

STAGING AND NATURAL HISTORY

Table 15-2 illustrates a staging classification for malignant thyroid neoplasms.

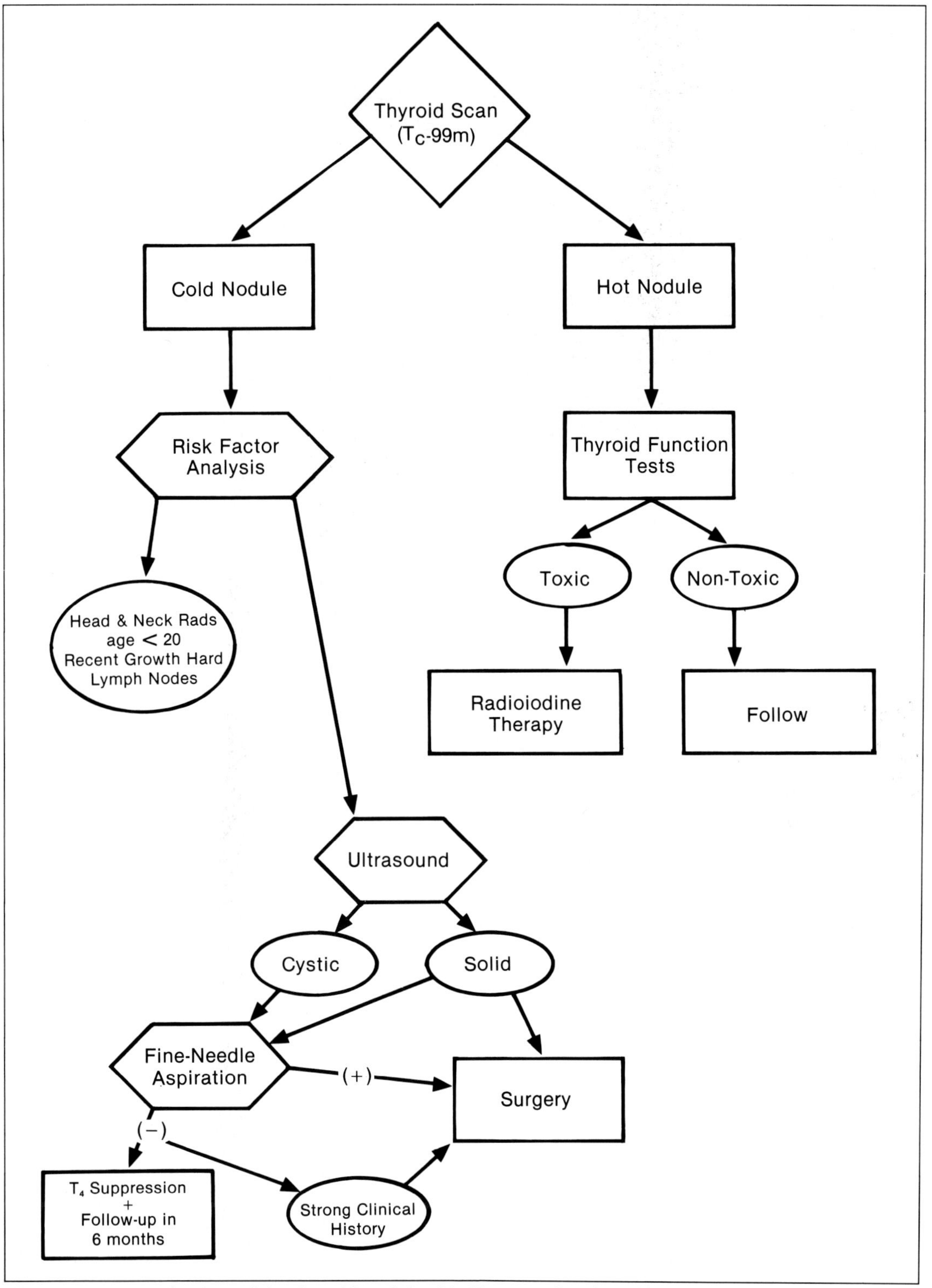

Figure 15-1. Evaluation of the thyroid nodule. *Tc-99m* = technetium 99m.

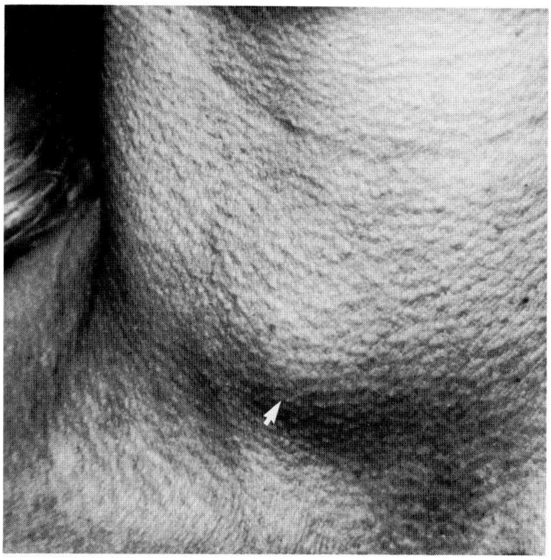

A

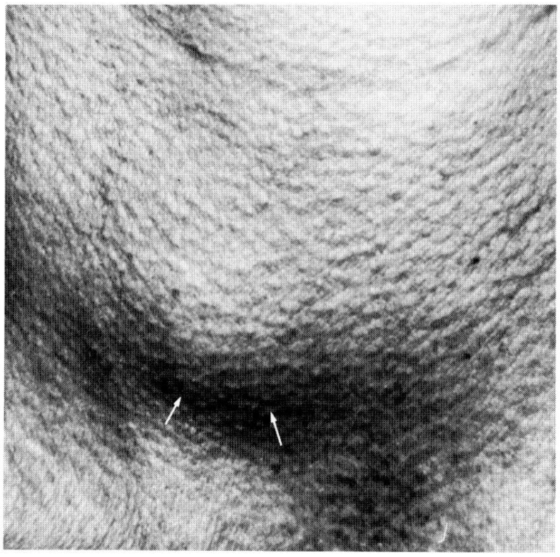

B

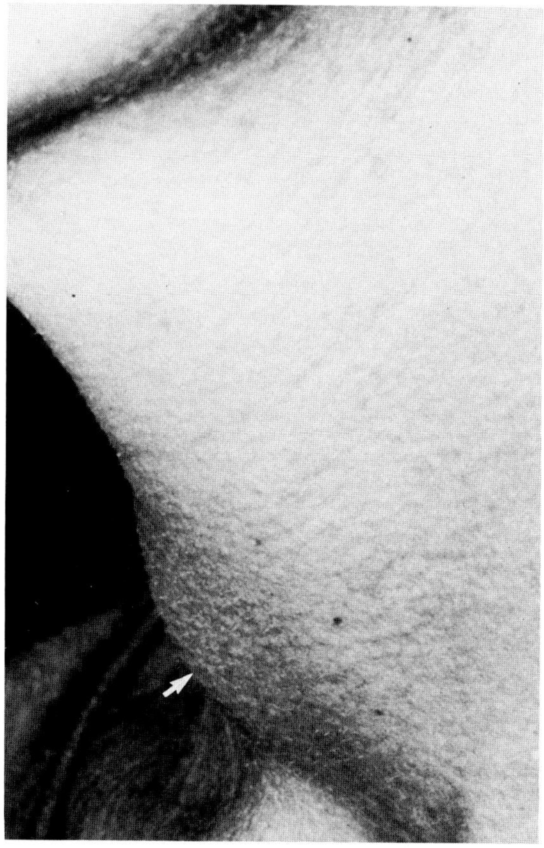

C

Figure 15-2. A 34-year-old woman with an asymptomatic, slowly enlarging right thyroid mass. Fine needle aspirate revealed findings consistent with follicular carcinoma.

Table 15-2. Staging malignancies of thyroid

Stage I	Tumor confined to thyroid gland
Stage II	Metastatic disease to cervical nodes
Stage III	Locally advanced disease, i.e., local invasion and/or fixation to cervical structures
Stage IV	Distant metastasis

Eighty percent of the thyroid malignancies are papillary and follicular carcinomas [13]. Most of the papillary tumors have follicular elements, but these mixed tumors behave biologically as pure papillary tumors. Moreover, radiation-induced papillary tumors behave biologically as sporadic papillary tumors. In contrast to malignancy in other anatomic sites, lymph node metastasis by a well-differentiated tumor has a good prognosis; that is, positive lymph node patients have a better prognosis than patients with negative lymph nodes [13,14]. Finally, the determinants of biologic behavior within any given histology correlate with tumor size, degree of invasion, extracapsular spread, angioinvasion, and metastasis. Women and patients under the age of 40 fare better than men [13].

Tables 15-3 and 15-4 summarize the natural history of thyroid malignancy.

THERAPY VERSUS PATHOLOGY

Seventy to eighty percent of malignant neoplasms in the thyroid gland are well-differentiated carcinomas (see Chapter 5) [13]. Therapy includes surgery (Fig. 15-3), thyroid hormone suppression, and ^{131}I therapy [2,5,9,10,14–16]. Table 15-5 summarizes this concept by stage of disease.

Papillary Carcinoma

Papillary carcinoma has an overall mortality of 11 percent. Surgical indications are multicen-

Table 15-3. Thyroid cancer pathogenesis

Pathology	*Incidence*	*Vascular invasion*	*Extension through capsule*	*Cervical nodes*	*Distant metastasis*
Papillary (includes mixed papillary-follicular)	62%	–	5–10%[a]	50%[b]	–[c]
Follicular	17%	+	–	–[d]	–[d]
Medullary	8–10%	+	+[e]	50%[e]	+
Anaplastic (spindle cell, large cell, & small cell)	10–15%	+	+	+	+

+ Present.
– Absent.
[a]Patients over age 40 at risk.
[b]Children under 15 yr. 90%.
[c]10% develop lung metastasis at some time in course.
[d]Frequent in patients with capsular and vascular invasion.
[e]Early detection by provocative testing.

Table 15-4. Natural history of thyroid cancer

Pathology	*Growth rate*	*Recurrence rate*	*Endocrine abnormalities*	*Median years*	*Survival range*[b]	*Prognosis*
Papillary[a]	Slow	18%	–	8.8	21 mo–17 yr	Good
Follicular	Slow	19%	–	2.9	1 wk–8 yr	Good
Medullary	Variable		+[c]	6.0	3 mo–18 yr	Poor[d]
Anaplastic	Rapid		+	0.8	2 days–39 yr	Poor
Metastasis and lethality: occult < papillary < follicular < medullary < anaplastic						

+ Present.
– Absent.
[a]10% are pure papillary; 70% are mixed papillary and follicular; no survival difference.
[b]Data from Silverberg SG, et al: Fatal carcinoma of the thyroid: Histology, metastases, and causes of death. *Cancer* 25 : 792, 1970.
[c]In familial variant: pheochromocytoma and parathyroid hyperplasia/adenoma.
[d]Early detection by provocative testing improves prognosis when c-cell hyperplasia diagnosed.

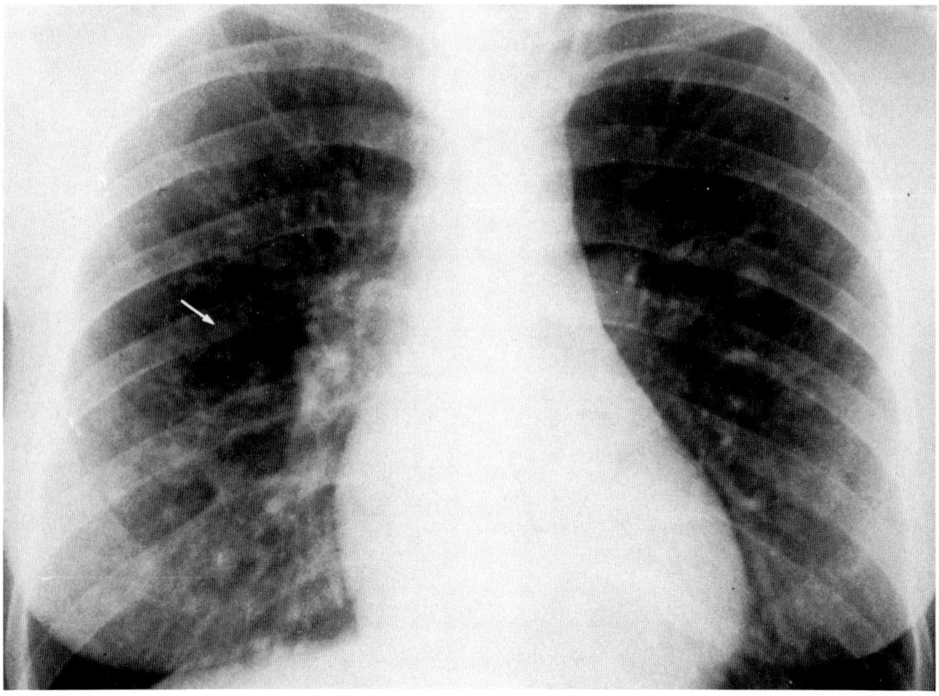

A

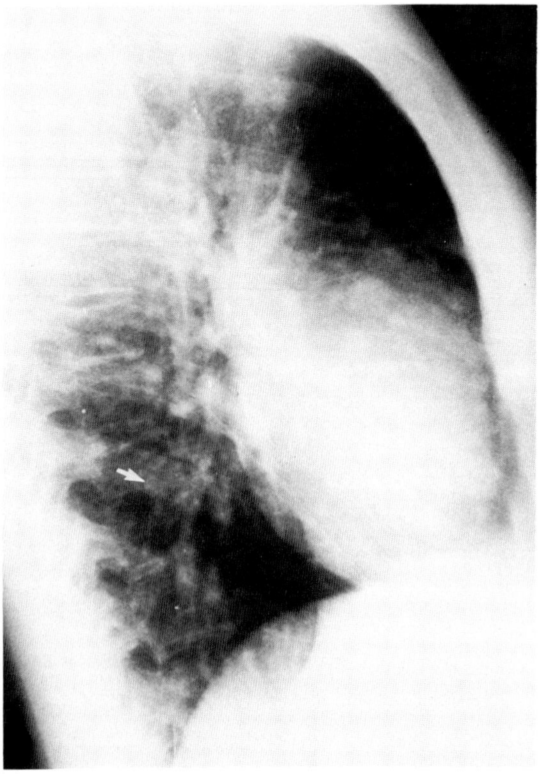

B

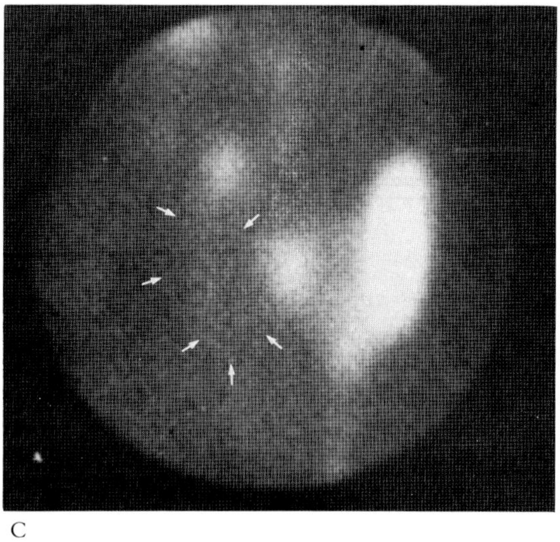

C

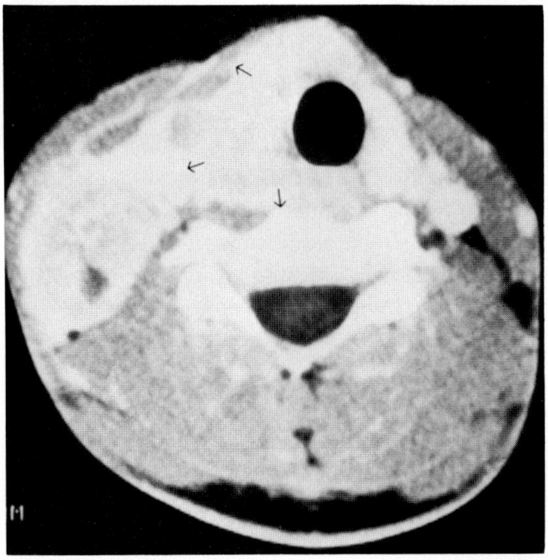

D

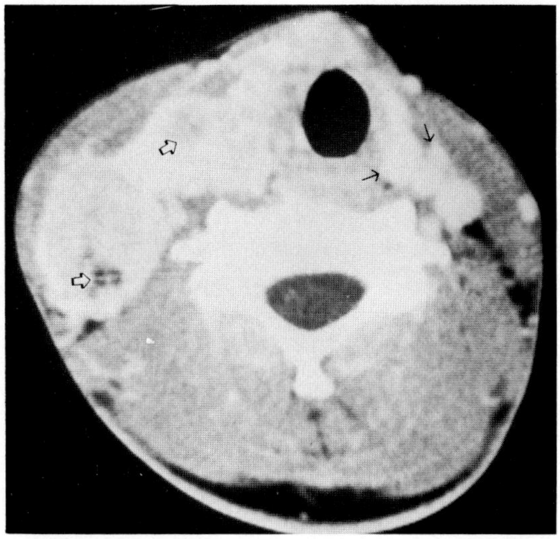

F

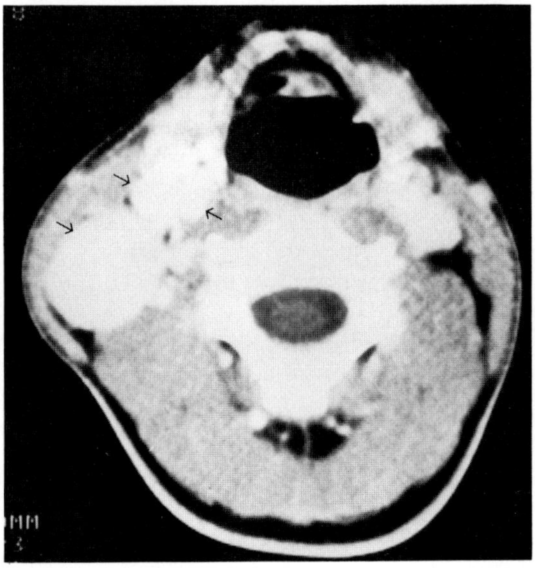

E

Figure 15-3. Metastatic papillary thyroid carcinoma in a 19-year-old woman presenting with a large right neck mass. Eventually, the patient required total thyroidectomy and bilateral functional neck dissections, followed by radioactive iodine therapy. A. Anteroposterior chest x-ray demonstrating multiple metastatic nodules in both lung fields. B. Lateral chest x-ray. C. ^{131}I thyroid scan. The right lobe is replaced by a "cold mass." D. CT scan of the subglottis. The arrows denote the expanding mass involving the thyroid lobe. There is a large metastasis in the right carotid sheath. E. A view at the level of the hyoid bone shows the multinodular nature of the cervical metastases. F. Several necrotic areas (*open arrows*) and suspicious nodes (*black arrows*) in the right carotid sheath are present.

Table 15-5. Treatment of papillary and follicular carcinoma

Stage	*Treatment*
0	Partial thyroidectomy
I	Subtotal or total thyroidectomy; ^{131}I
II	Total thyroidectomy + neck dissection, modified or functional; ^{131}I
III	Total thyroidectomy + appropriate cytoreduction; ^{131}I
IV	Total thyroidectomy or ^{131}I ablation

tricity (especially with previous radiation) and the aggressive nature of recurrent disease. Subtotal thyroidectomy best treats this disease, reducing the need for ablative doses of ^{131}I and protecting the recurrent laryngeal nerve and parathyroid glands. Occult papillary carcinoma, that is, a lesion less than 1 cm, is managed adequately with a partial thyroidectomy. Since mixed papillary and follicular carcinomas biologically mimic papillary carcinoma, they are managed similarly.

Follicular Carcinoma

The surgical management of follicular carcinoma is essentially the same as for papillary carcinoma. Cervical lymph node metastasis is unusual; therefore, neck dissections seldom are indicated. Surgical intervention or open biopsy is often necessary prior to definitive diagnosis, since fine-needle aspirates are difficult to interpret.

Medullary Carcinoma

Medullary carcinoma, a multicentric disease, requires total thyroidectomy with unilateral or bilateral (modified) neck dissection as needed. Surgery limited to thyroidectomy is adequate in familial cases diagnosed by screening provocative tests. The parathyroids are identified and autografted; in cases of parathyroid hyperplasia, a portion of a hyperplastic gland is autografted. Patients with mediastinal involvement are approached by sternotomy and mediastinal node dissection. About two-thirds of the patients risk recurrence due to positive lymph nodes (cervical mediastinal) or a persistent elevation of calcitonin. Postoperative radiation to the neck and mediastinum is an option.

Postoperatively, patients are monitored in 1 to 2 weeks and then every 6 to 12 months with a pentagastrin or calcium infusion provocative test [2,7]. The pentagastrin provocative test is performed as follows: pentagastrin (0.5 μg/kg) is given by IV bolus, and calcitonin levels are measured at 0, 2, 5, 10, and 15 mintues. Except for chest tightness and rare allergic reactions, side effects are minimal. The calcium infusion provocative test is performed as follows: calcium gluconate (15 mg of elemental calcium/kg) is infused over 4 hours, and calcitonin levels are measured at 0, 3, and 4 hours. Severe nausea and vomiting are the side effects associated with this test. Since the pentagastrin test can be done rapidly in the outpatient setting and the toxicities are of shorter duration, it is preferred. A positive test is a stimulated calcitonin greater than 0.58 μg/ml; basal calcitonin is less than 0.4 μg/ml.

Familial Follow-up

Individuals with familial histories of medullary carcinoma are recommended for thyroidectomy if they have two positive calcitonin provocative tests [7]. In patients with familial medullary carcinoma or a history suggestive of MEN II, it is of utmost importance to **rule out pheochromocytoma** prior to surgery. This will prevent a hypertensive catastrophe during induction of general anesthesia. The diagnosis of pheochromocytoma is made by measuring urine levels of catecholamines and the metabolic products of catecholamines (vanillylmandelic acid or metanephrines). Pheochromocytoma is best treated prior to surgery for medullary carcinoma. Patients who postoperatively have persistent elevations of basal or stimulated calcitonins and clinically have no evidence of disease are a diagnostic problem. Selective venous catheterization in conjunction with a pentagastrin provocative test localizes neck or mediastinal disease. Surgery has a limited role; the best option for disease control is radiation [2].

Anaplastic Carcinoma

Surgery is only of diagnostic and palliative value in anaplastic carcinoma. Debulking is questionably beneficial; tracheotomy is an important palliative procedure. For the few resectable tumors, postoperative radiation is indicated.

Caution is exercised for suspected small-cell anaplastic carcinoma. On pathologic review, some of these patients may have a primary lymphoma of the thyroid [3]. This is a potentially curable lesion. Therefore, special stains, immunochemistry, and electron microscopy are strongly encouraged.

THERAPY

Complications of Surgery

Table 15-6 outlines the postoperative complications of thyroid surgery [2].

Hypocalcemia

Ten to 25 percent of patients develop hypocalcemia postoperatively. The nadir calcium occurs 48 to 72 hours after surgery. Patients who develop symptomatic hypocalcemia improve with intravenous or oral elemental calcium therapy. Patients who have permanent hypoparathyroidism are managed with oral calcium supplements and vitamin D therapy. 1,25-Dihydroxycholecalciferol is rapid acting (1–2 days) and expensive. Chronically, patients can be controlled with the slower acting derivatives, vitamin D and 25-hydroxycholecalciferol. The patient who excretes greater than 300 mg/day of calcium in the urine benefits from hydrochlorothiazide, a drug that increases renal absorption and serum calcium levels. Caution should be exercised in administering furosemide (Lasix); it increases calcium and steroid excretion in the urine. Hydrochlorothiazide also blocks the vitamin D effect of calcium absorption in the gastrointestinal tract of hypoparathyroid patients.

Table 15-6. Complications of thyroid surgery

Bleeding
Acute—arterial
Delayed—venous
Airway obstruction
Wound hematoma
Vocal cord paralysis—bilateral
Laryngeal edema
Tracheomalacia
Hoarseness
Unilateral recurrent laryngeal nerve damage
Superior laryngeal nerve damage (aspiration)
Traumatic mucositis of vocal cords
Wound problems
Cosmesis
Skin flap necrosis
Infection—superficial and deep
Seroma
Endocrine
Hypothyroidism
Hypoparathyroidism
Miscellaneous
Chylous fistula
Pneumothorax
Air embolism
Horner's syndrome
Esophageal/tracheal laceration

Recurrent Laryngeal Nerve Injury

One to 7 percent of postoperative patients experience recurrent laryngeal nerve injury. Bilateral recurrent laryngeal nerve section rarely occurs. Transient injury usually recovers in less than a year. The risk of the complication increases in patients with previous neck surgery. Edema, inflammation (acute), or fibrosis (chronic) obscure nerve identification. Patients with bilateral recurrent nerve injury require permanent tracheostomy or unilateral arytenoidectomy.

Hypothyroidism

Essentially all patients become hypothyroid after near total thyroidectomy or ablative radioiodine therapy. Patients who were chronically hypothyroid are given slow thyroid hormone replacement. Those with a history of angina or coronary artery disease are replaced cautiously with beta-blockade assistance (propranolol, 20 mg PO every 8 hours), which is withdrawn slowly after full thyroid replacement.

Postoperative thyroid replacement has two roles. First, hypothyroidism is treated. Second, thyroid-stimulating hormone (TSH) suppression reduces the hormone effect on well-differentiated carcinomas. Thyroid suppression is a surgical adjunct, not an alternative. Thyroxine (T_4) is the preferred hormone preparation, since the body deiodinates T_4 to active liothyronine (T_3) hormone, as needed. The dosage range for TSH suppression is 100 to 200 μg/day of T_4. Euthyroidism is best monitored by T_3 radioimmunoassay, and hypothyroidism is documented by TSH.

Radioiodine Therapy

Normal thyroid tissue competes better for ^{131}I than does well-differentiated carcinoma. Ablative ^{131}I therapy destroys residual thyroid tissue after near total thyroidectomy; thereafter, ^{131}I detects metastatic diseases. Also, these malignancies are multicentric and recur in residual tissue. Ablative therapy is of questionable value in small thyroid lesions and in patients less than age 40 who have a normal life expectancy despite a cancer diagnosis [2,5,13,15,17].

Ablative Radioactive Iodine

Four to 6 weeks post-surgery, an ^{131}I scan (2–5 mCi) is performed. If residual thyroid tissue is detected, an ablative dose of ^{131}I (30–60 mCi) is administered. After thyroid ablation, the ^{131}I scan is repeated to detect metastatic disease. Follicular carcinoma accumulates and responds to radioiodine better than does papillary carcinoma; follicular variants of papillary carcinoma are intermediate in their response. Lung metastases accumulate radioactivity better than do bone metastases. About 5 to 10 percent of well-differentiated metastatic carcinomas are cured with ^{131}I; only 30 percent of patients with pulmonary metastases are cured.

Metastatic Therapy

After the patient is made hypothyroid, 100 to 150 mCi of ^{131}I is administered for metastatic therapy. Up to 200 mCi of ^{131}I is administered for bone metastases. Patients are scanned yearly with ^{131}I until there is no further uptake; afterward they are scanned every 3 to 5 years. Another follow-up study is serum thyroglobulin in patients with well-differentiated papillary carcinoma.

Hormone Replacement

To enhance radioiodine uptake into metastases, T_4 is discontinued for 4 to 6 weeks, or liothyronine T_3 is discontinued for 2 to 3 weeks. A patient on T_4 who is switched to liothyronine T_3 for 2 weeks usually will be hypothyroid (elevated TSH) 2 weeks after cessation of T_3. Elderly patients who tolerate hypothyroidism poorly are controlled symptomatically with 5 μg of T_3 without interfering with the TSH elevation. Also a low iodine diet 3 to 4 weeks prior to radioiodine therapy and hydrochlorothiazide plus potassium chloride supplementation further enhance uptake [2].

Complications

The complications of radioiodine therapy include sialadenitis, myelosuppression, impaired spermatogenesis, pulmonary fibrosis, leukemia, and bladder cancer [5].

Chemotherapy

The role of cytotoxic agents in thyroid cancer is not defined. However, patients with the following are candidates for investigational chemotherapy: (1) well-differentiated carcinoma, refractory to thyroid suppression and radioactive iodine; (2) metastatic medullary carcinoma; and (3) metastatic anaplastic carcinoma [2,9,18]. These patients should be symptomatic, be in good medical condition, and have measurable disease that can be palliated with doxorubicin and cisplatin, combined or as single agents.

REFERENCES

1. Boring CC, Squires TS, Silverberg E: Cancer Statistics, 1990. *CA* 40 : 9–26, 1990.
2. Parsons JT, Pfaff WW: Carcinoma of the Thyroid. In Million RR, Cassis HJ (eds): *Management of Head and Neck Cancer: A Multidisciplinary Approach.* Philadelphia: Lippincott, 1984. Pp 579–596.
3. Barney PL: Pathology of thyroid cancer: Summary and update. *Laryngoscope* 9 : 525, 1983.
4. Favus MJ, et al: Thyroid cancer occurring as a late consequence of head-and-neck irradiation: Evaluation of 1056 patients. *N Engl J Med* 294 : 1019, 1976.
5. Powell BL, Craig JB, Muss HB: Thyroid cancer. *Am Fam Physician* 30 : 185, 1984.
6. Holm L, et al: Malignant thyroid tumors after iodine-131 therapy: A retrospective cohort study. *N Engl J Med* 303 : 188, 1980.
7. Graze K, et al: Natural history of familial medullary thyroid carcinoma: Effect of a program for early diagnosis. *N Engl J Med* 299 : 980, 1978.
8. Van Herle AJ, et al: The thyroid nodule. *Ann Intern Med* 96 : 221, 1982.
9. Frable WJ: The treatment of thyroid cancer: The role of fine-needle aspiration cytology. *Arch Otolaryngol Head Neck Surg* 112 : 1200, 1986.
10. Thompson NW: The resection therapy of carcinoma of the thyroid. *Surg Rounds,* pp. 100–111, Jan 1984.
11. Miller JM, Hamburger JI: Needle biopsy of the thyroid: An update. *Surg Rounds,* pp. 72–81, Jan 1984.
12. Blum M, Rothschild M: Improved non-opera-

tive diagnosis of the solitary "cold" thyroid nodule: Surgical selection based on risk factors and three months of suppression. *JAMA* 243 : 242, 1980.
13. Dunn JT: Thyroid suppression and medical ablation for differentiated thyroid cancer. *Arch Otolaryngol Head Neck Surg* 112 : 1207, 1986.
14. Ward PH: The surgical treatment of thyroid cancer: The primary disease. *Arch Otolaryngol Head Neck Surg* 112 : 1204, 1986.
15. Maxon HR, et al: Relation between effective radiation dose and outcome of radioidine therapy for thyroid cancer. *N Engl J Med* 309 : 937, 1983.
16. Mazzaferri EL, Young RL: Papillary thyroid carcinoma: A 10-year follow-up report of the impact of therapy in 576 patients. *Am J Med* 70 : 511, 1981.
17. DeGroot LJ, et al: Retrospective and prospective study of radiation-induced thyroid disease. *Am J Med* 74 : 852, 1983.
18. Shimaoka K: Adjunctive management of thyroid cancer: Chemotherapy. *J Surg Oncol* 15 : 283, 1980.

16

Neck Dissection

ERNEST M. MYERS

KEY CONCEPTS

Anatomy, Radical Neck Dissection, Modified Neck Dissection, Functional Neck Dissection, Bilateral Neck Dissection, Complications, Prognosis

MILESTONES

1902	Head and Neck Lymphatics	Polya
1906	Radical Neck Dissection	Crile
1932	Composite Resection	Ward
1944	Combined Mandibular Neck Dissection (COMMANDO)	Martin
1960	Transverse Neck Incision	McFee
1967	Functional Neck Dissection	Bocca
1969	Spinal Accessory Nerve Preservation	Roy and Beahrs
1975	Opthalmoplethysmography	Nolph et al.
1980	Posterolateral Neck Dissection	Goepfert and Jesse

The neck dissection is the en bloc excision of overt or occult cervical lymph node metastasis. The goal is tumor ablation with preservation of all vital and uninvolved neck structures [1]. A neck dissection is either a component of a primary resection or a procedure unto itself. Ideally, radiation controls the primary disease, while the neck dissection is reserved for unresponsive cervical disease. Depending on the extent and location of the disease, the appropriate procedure is chosen: radical, modified, functional, or bilateral neck dissection.

INDICATIONS

Neck dissection is indicated for metastatic disease in the superfical or deep cervical fascia [2–4]. Indications for neck dissection follow:

1. Cervical metastasis whose primary has responded to treatment.
2. Cervical metastasis unresponsive to radiotherapy and/or chemotherapy.
3. Anticipated primary resection contiguous with occult or overt cervical metastasis.

CONTRAINDICATIONS

Neck dissection is contraindicated in disease beyond the superficial or deep cervical fascia. The six contraindications are:

1. Poor surgical candidate.
2. Rampant distant metastases.
3. Base of skull disease.
4. Mediastinal or infraclavicular disease.
5. Unresectable or uncontrollable primary disease.
6. Extension into deep or vital structures of the neck.

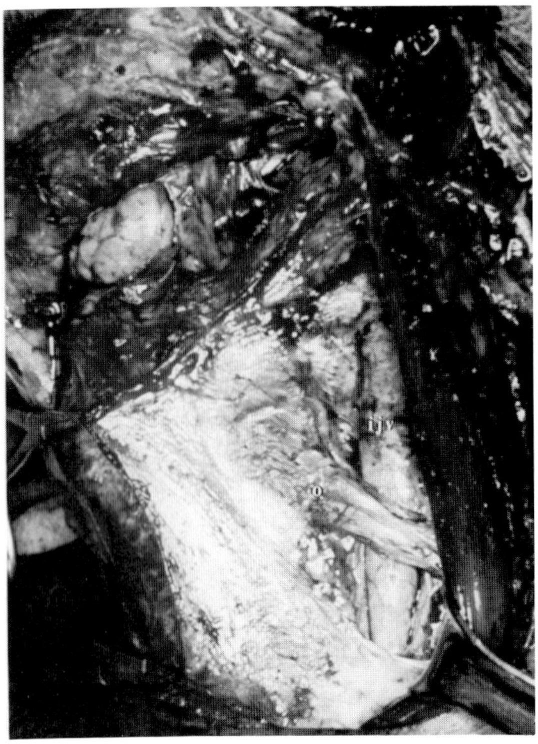

E

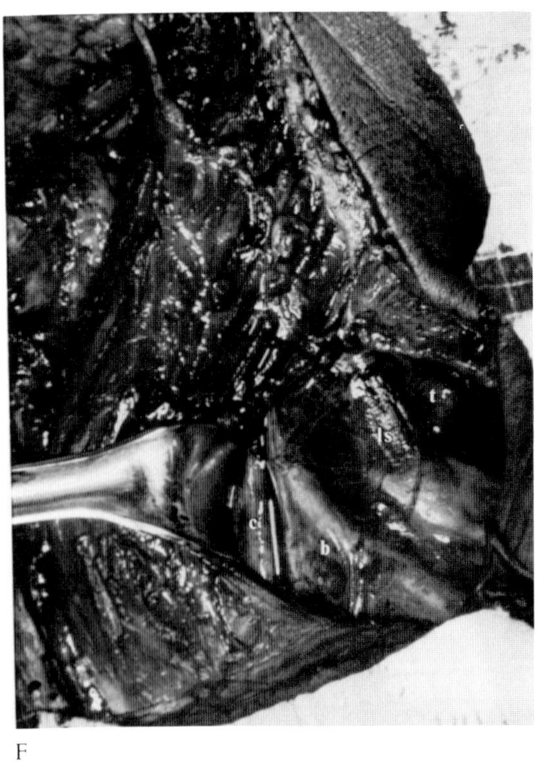

F

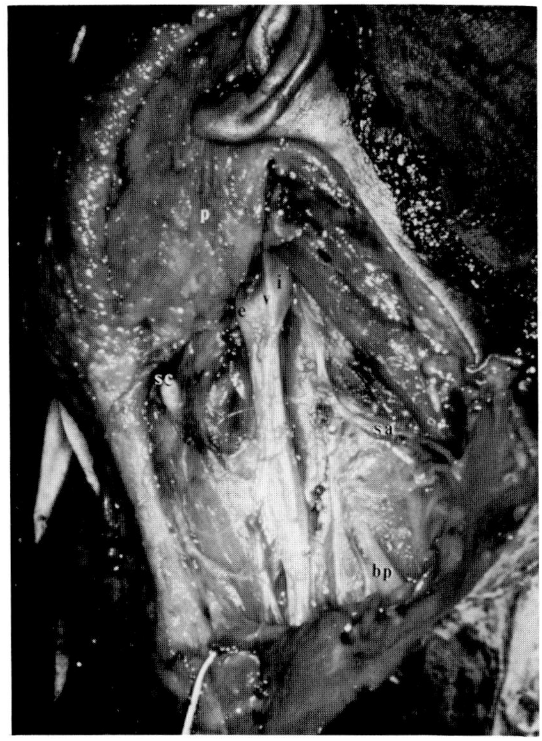

G

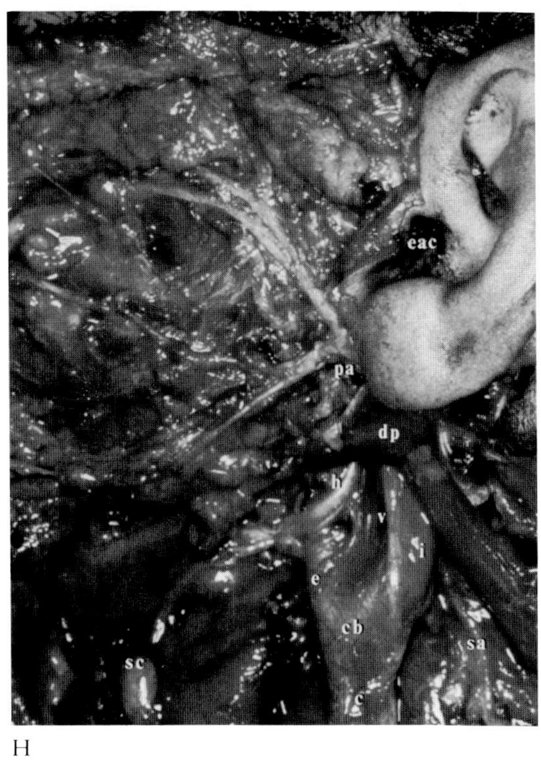

H

Figure 16-3. (continued) C. Submandibular triangle. *smg* = submandibular gland; *f* = facial artery and vein; *dp* = posterior belly of the digastric muscle; *s* = sternohyoid muscle; *double arrow* = carotid sheath. D. Deep submandibular triangle. *n* = metastasis in submandibular lymph node; *tp* = tail of parotid gland; *smg* = submandibular gland; *f* = facial artery and vein; *scm* = sternocleidomastoid muscle; *l* = larynx. E. Anterior carotid triangle. *o* = omohyoid muscle; *ijv* = internal jugular vein. F. Posterior cervical triangle. *c* = carotid artery; *b* = brachial plexus; *ls* = levator scapular muscle; *t* = trapezius muscle. G. Deep neck anatomy (after removal of radical neck dissection specimen). *sc* = superior cornu (thyroid cartilage); *p* = parotid gland; *e* = external carotid artery; *v* = vagus; *i* = internal carotid artery with nearby vagus nerve; *sa* = spinal accessory nerve; *bp* = brachial plexus. H. Deep parotid dissection. *pa* = pes anserinus; *eac* = external auditory canal; *dp* = posterior belly of the digastric; *h* = hypoglossal nerve; *e* = external carotid artery; *cb* = carotid bulb; *c* = common carotid artery; *v* = vagus nerve; *i* = internal carotid artery; *sa* = spinal accessory nerve; *sc* = superior cornu (thyroid cartilage).

Modified Neck Dissection

Also indicated for N_2 or N_3 neck disease, modified neck dissection is a series of operations or variations of the original procedure. Several reports confirm the low risk of recurrent disease associated with modified procedures [5, 6]. Today, most neck dissections are modified neck dissections.

The variations are preservation of (1) the sternocleidomastoid, (2) the spinal accessory nerve, (3) either the submental or submandibular triangles, (4) the internal jugular vein, or (5) any combination of 1 through 4. Common to all variations is the removal of the deep cervical fat pad and usually the internal jugular vein.

The advantage of modified neck dissection is selectivity according to patient pathology. The disadvantages are the longer operative time and the more sophisticated surgical expertise required.

Functional Neck Dissection

Teleologically, for functional neck dissection is indicated for N_0 or N_1 disease [7–9]. It is the meticulous dissection of deep cervical lymphatics and the fatty, lymph node–bearing tissue intimately associated with the vital structures. Basically, it is ablation with preservation of all uninvolved neck structures. It usually does not include the submental and submandibular triangles or internal jugular vein. For some pri-

Table 16-4. Procedure versus primary site

Site	*Radical neck dissection*	*Modified neck dissection*	*Functional neck dissection*	*Bilateral neck dissection*
1. Nasopharynx	+	+	–	+/–
2. Sinus/nose	+	+	–	–
3. Salivary gland	–	+	+	–
4. Lips	–	+	–	+
5. Oral cavity	+	+	–	+/–
6. Oropharynx	+	+	–	+/–
7. Hypopharynx	+	+	+	+/–
8. Larynx	+/–	+	+	+/–
9. Thyroid	–	+	+	+
10. Esophagus	+/–	+/–	–	+/–

+ Indicated.
+/– Equivocal.
– Contraindicated.

pharynx implicates a fistula until proved otherwise.

5. If a tracheotomy has been performed, note the character of the drainage near the tracheotomy site.
6. The following factors predispose to fistulization:
   a. Chemotherapy.
   b. Radiotherapy.
   c. Diabetes mellitus.
   d. Marginal renal function.
   e. Steroids.
   f. Marginal hepatic function.
   g. Complex neck incisions.
   h. Combined procedures.
   i. Prolonged anesthesia and wound exposure.
   j. Tumor adherent to the carotid artery.
   k. Flaps.

Unfortunately, many head and neck patients frequently have more than one predisposition.

Treatment

Diversion

Early recognition leads to safe management. When a fistula is suspected, the site is opened, usually within one of the neck incisions; anesthesia is not necessary. Early drainage releases the purulence and converts the fistula from an indirect to direct fistula. Timely intervention prevents skin flap disruption and devascularity. When a skin flap is elevated by fluid collection, vascular compromise and subsequent slough may develop. More importantly, proper drainage diverts the saliva away from the carotid artery. Inadequate diversion pools saliva and purulence around the carotid artery—predispositions for impending carotid catastrophe. Parenteral nutrition is maintained, since contamination by food and liquids further aggravates the situation and thwarts conservative management.

Closure

Conservative management (diversion, parenteral nutrition, antibiotics, and daily wound care) closes most fistulae. With massive or dangerous fistulae, however, there is no other recourse but prolonged hospitalization (4–6 additional weeks). During this time period, the fistula is cleaned meticulously and closed by a variety of sophisticated reconstructive techniques (see Chapter 22).

PROGNOSIS

A comprehensive retrospective analysis of neck dissections from Roswell Park is very revealing [25]. The size of the primary tumor, extent of nodal involvement, and recurrence in the neck were the important factors identified in the survival of patients with oral cavity, pharyngeal, and laryngeal cancer. Over a 30-year period, 457 dissections were performed. Of the 390 procedures analyzed, 315 (81 percent) were classic radical neck dissections, and 75 (19%) were not radical neck dissections. Of those 75, 55 were functional neck dissections. Some of the conclusions are as follows:

1. Survival was affected by the size of the primary tumor (T_1/T_2, 50%; T_3/T_4, 44%) and the failure to control the neck disease (N_0, 68%; N_1/N_2, 50%; N_3, 29%).
2. Survival was not affected by the type or timing of the neck dissection (elective versus therapeutic) or the addition of radiation therapy.
3. Supraomohyoid neck dissection was not an effective therapeutic procedure.
4. Only 16% (65 patients) developed neck failure when the primary tumor remained controlled; 20 (5%) of the failures developed on the ipsilateral side; 40 recurred contralaterally.

REFERENCES

1. Crile G: Excision of cancer of the head and neck: With special reference to the plan of dissection based on one hundred and thirty-two operations. *JAMA* 47 : 1780, 1906.
2. Drinker CK: *The Lymphatic System.* Stanford, CA: Stanford University Press, 1942.
3. Fakih AR, et al: Elective versus therapeutic neck dissection in early carcinoma of the oral tongue. *Am J Surg* 158 : 309, 1989.
4. Weissler MC, et al: Treatment of the clinically negative neck in advanced cancer of the head and neck. *Arch Otol Head Neck Surg* 115 · 691, 1989.
5. Lingeman RE, et al: Neck dissection: Radical or conservative. *Ann Otol Rhinol Laryngol* 86 : 737, 1977.

6. Deutsch EC, et al: The conservative neck dissection. *Laryngoscope* 95 : 561, 1978.
7. Jesse RH, Ballantyne AJ, Larson D: Radical or modified neck dissection: A therapeutic dilemma. *Am J Surg* 136 : 516, 1978.
8. Bocca E, Pignataro O: A conservation technique in radical neck dissection. *Ann Otol Rhinol Laryngol* 76 : 975, 1967.
9. Bocca E, et al: Functional neck dissection: An evaluation & review of 843 cases. *Laryngoscope* 94 : 942, 1984.
10. Razack MS, Baff R, Sako K: Bilateral radical neck dissection. *Cancer* 47 : 197, 1981.
11. Reed GF, Harrington PC: Dermal grafts: Clinical experience in head and neck surgery. *NY J Med* 69 : 2563, 1969.
12. Schweitzer RJ: Use of muscle flaps for protection of carotid artery after radical neck dissection. *Ann Surg* 156 : 811, 1962.
13. Nolph MB, et al: Ophthalmophlethysmography in head and neck surgery. *Arch Otolaryngol* 105 : 492, 1979.
14. Kennedy JT, Krause C, Lowy S: The importance of tumor attachment to the carotid artery. *Arch Otolaryngol* 103 : 70, 1977.
15. Ogura JH, Thawley SE: Complications of Laryngeal Surgery. In Conley JJ (ed): *Complications of Head and Neck Surgery*. Philadelphia: Saunders, 1979. Pp 246–273.
16. Cummings CE, et al: Complications of laryngectomy and neck dissection following planned pre-operative radiotherapy. *Ann Otolaryngol* 88 : 745, 1977.
17. Ketcham AS, Hoge RC: Spontaneous carotid artery hemorrhage after head and neck surgery. 110 : 649, 1965.
18. Sobel SM, et al: Management of inadvertent injury to the carotid artery during head and neck surgery. *Head Neck Surg* 4 : 475, 1982.
19. Short SO, et al: Shoulder pain & function after neck dissection with or without preservation of the spinal accessory nerve. *Am J Surg* 148 : 478, 1984.
20. Nahum AM, Mullally W, Marmor L: A syndrome resulting from radical neck dissection. *Arch Otolaryngol* 74 : 82, 1961.
21. Ewing MR, Martin H: Disability following neck dissection. *Cancer* 5 : 873, 1952.
22. Cantrell RW: Pharyngocutaneous fistula: Prevention and treatment. *Laryngoscope* 88 : 1204, 1978.
23. Shumrick DA: Carotid artery rupture. *Laryngoscope* 83 : 1051, 1975.
24. Dedo DD, Alonso WA, Ogura JH: Incidence, predisposing factors and outcome of pharyngocutaneous fistulas complicating head and neck cancer. *Ann Otolaryngol* 84 : 833, 1975.
25. Whafif RH, et al: Thirty year experience with 457 radical neck dissections in cancer of the mouth, pharynx, and larynx. *Am J Surg* 158 : 303, 1989.

17

Chest

ROBERT C. LOWERY, JR.

KEY CONCEPTS

Closed Tube Thoracostomy; Mediastinoscopy; Median Sternotomy; Mediastinal Tracheostomy; Jejunal Interposition; Colonic Interposition, Thoracic Drainage

MILESTONES

124–40 B.C.	First Tracheotomy	Asclepiades
1545	Successful Tracheotomy	Brasavola
1854	Practical Laryngoscopy	Garcia
1871	Cuffed Tracheostomy Tube	Trendelenburg
1875	Closed Tube Drainage of Empyema; Physiology of Pneumothorax	Bulau
1904	Avoidance of Pneumothorax During Intrathoracic Surgery	Sauerbruch
1909	Endotracheal Anesthesia	Meltzer and Auer
1913	Transpleural Esophagectomy	Torek
1920	Gastric Transposition	Kirschner
1960	Cervical Esophagogastrostomy	Ong and Lee

Progress in otolaryngology and thoracic surgery has been made possible by the development of new procedures and technology. Fortunately, in many cases, the two specialties have drawn on the advances of the other. This chapter explores the thoracic and abdominal surgical procedures that pertain to head and neck oncology.

THORACIC PROCEDURES

Thoracic Catheterization

Usually performed with local anesthesia, needle or catheter aspiration of intrathoracic fluid collections is a valuable diagnostic and therapeutic procedure.

Indications and Contraindications

1. Indications: diagnosis of pleural effusions; drainage of small, uncomplicated pneumothoraces and pleural effusions.
2. Contraindications: hemothoraces, empyemas.

Technique

The insertion of intravenous access-type catheters entails the aspiration of air or fluid through the needle and leaving the silastic catheter within the chest activity. This minimizes the risk of lung laceration by an indwelling needle.

Table 17-1. Selected mediastinal contents

Mediastinal lymph nodes
Trachea
Esophagus
Thyroid gland
Thymus
Recurrent laryngeal nerves
Phrenic nerves
Aortic arch
Innominate artery and vein

Complications

Complications include pneumothorax; hemorrhage due to intercostal vessel injury; and inadvertent catheterization of the heart, aorta, spleen, or liver.

Closed Thoracic Tube Thoracostomy

Chest tube insertion is one of the most basic and useful of all thoracic surgical procedures. Not uncommonly, an extrathoracic procedure is complicated by a hemothorax or pneumothorax. Opacification of a hemithorax can be caused by increased pleural fluid, intrapleural space hemorrhage, or ipsilateral bronchial obstruction. Bronchoscopy is required for suspected bronchial obstruction whereas diagnostic thoracentesis is indicated for intrapleural fluid collections. Bloody aspiration after thoracentesis necessitates tube thoracostomy for evacuation and monitoring of blood loss.

Indications and Contraindications

1. Indications: large fluid collections, malignant effusions, empyemas, hemothorax, chylothorax, pneumothorax.
2. Contraindications: empyema necessitatis, tuberculous effusions.

Technique

Chest tube insertion requires some experience. It is not inordinately dangerous as long as basic surgical principles are followed. A 2- to 3-cm incision, over an appropriate intercostal space, is carried to the fascia. With a clamp, the intercostal muscles are dissected bluntly and the pleura is entered. Importantly, a finger palpates the smooth pleura to avoid lung parenchymal injury. Once the intrapleural location is assured by digital examination, the tube is passed and directed apically for pneumothoraces and basally for effusions. The drain size ranges from small (16-gauge) venous access-type catheters to the more traditional (28–40F) chest tubes. Minor or small pneumothoraces (10% or less) are treated with aspiration and followed by serial x-rays. However, those associated with significant air leaks or hemothoraces require large-bore tube drainage for adequate resolution.

Complications

Injury to the lung, intercostal vessels, heart, liver, and spleen can occur if the operator is not careful. Significant hemorrhage can result from blunt dissection of lung adhesions to the chest wall.

Mediastinoscopy

Mediastinoscopy is indicated for staging and diagnosis of various neoplastic and benign thoracic processes. Recently, the technique has largely been supplanted by less invasive procedures such as fine-needle biopsy. However, it remains a reliable diagnostic modality.

Indications and Contraindications

1. Indications: undiagnosed mediastinal, paratracheal, and right hilar masses; staging for carcinoma of the lung.
2. Contraindications: previous mediastinoscopy (relative); superior vena caval syndrome; bleeding diathesis; anterior mediastinal masses.

Technique

A small transverse incision is made just above the sternal notch. This incision is carried to the pretracheal fascia where a plane is developed along the anterior tracheal wall. After the pathology is palpated (if possible), the mediastinoscope is passed along the dissected plane. Biopsies are obtained under direct vision.

Complications

The most feared, but rare, complication is hemorrhage from inadvertent biopsy of a major vessel. This may be immediately life-threatening and is avoided by careful aspiration prior to biopsy. Small pneumothoraces that may occur are managed by serial chest x-rays. Phrenic nerve and recurrent laryngeal nerve injuries, also rare, have been reported.

Median Sternotomy

As a result of open heart surgery, median sternotomy is a common approach (Table 17-1, Figures 17-1 and 17-2). When extended superiorly along either sternocleidomastoid, it provides excellent exposure to the root of the neck.

Indications and Contraindications

1. Indications: exploration of anterior mediastinal masses; most common approach for thymectomy; great-vessel exposure; cardiac exposure.
2. Contraindications: sternal osteomyelitis, skin or subcutaneous infection, heavy regional irradiation (relative).

Figure 17-1. Basic chest anatomy. *R.* = right; *L.* = left.

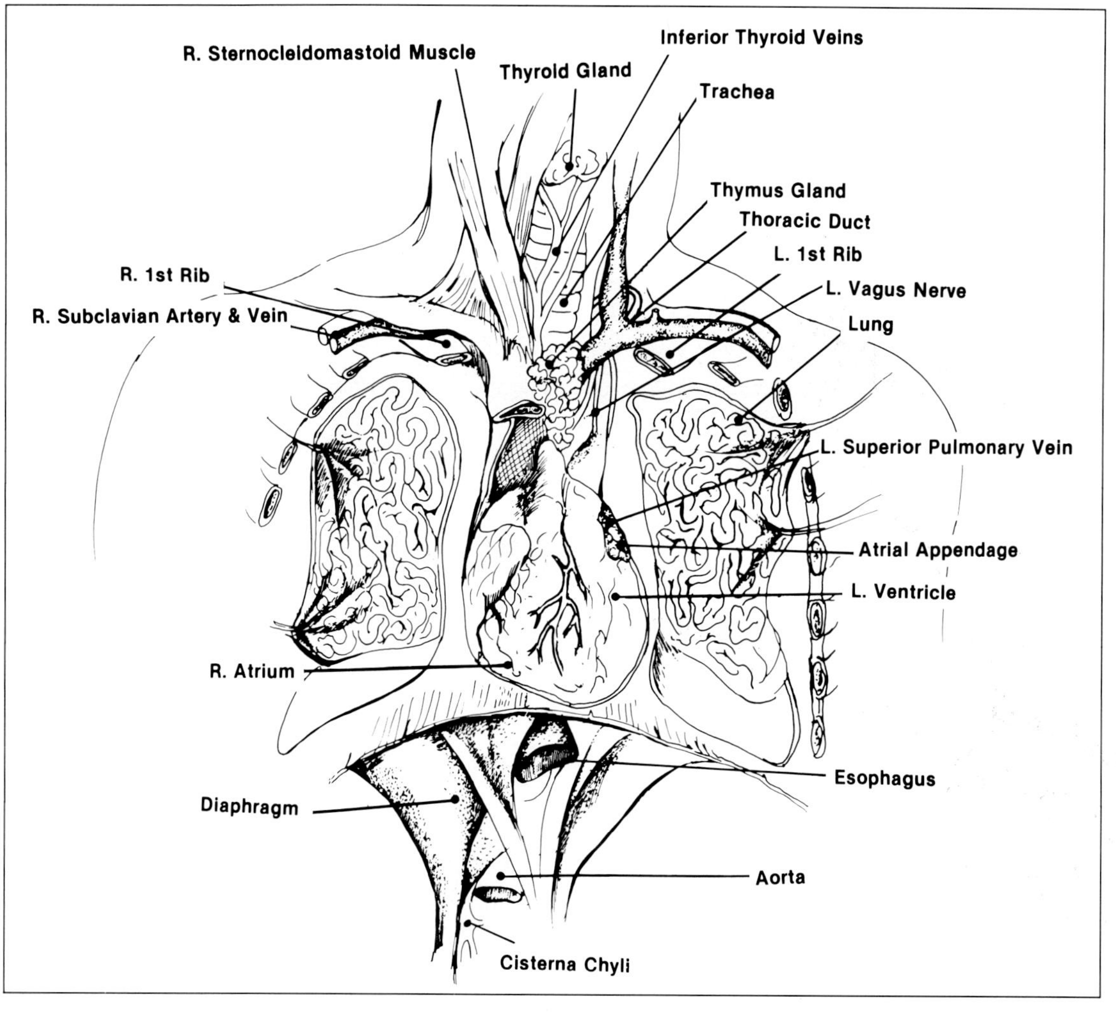

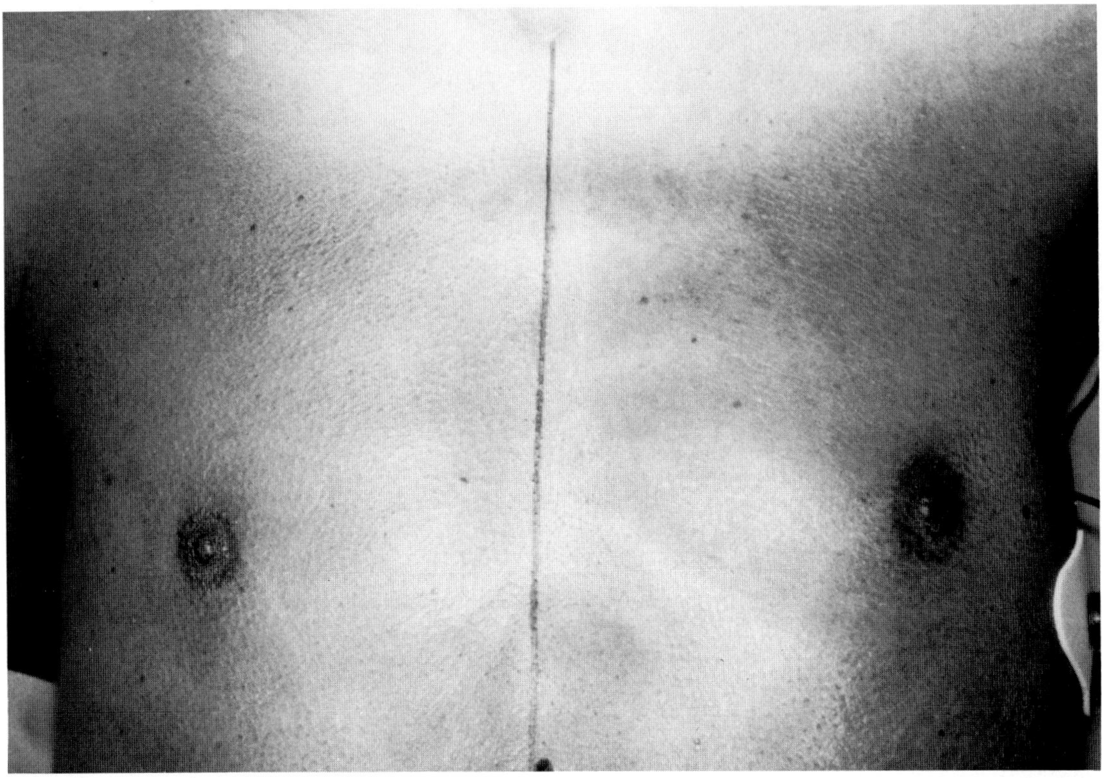

A

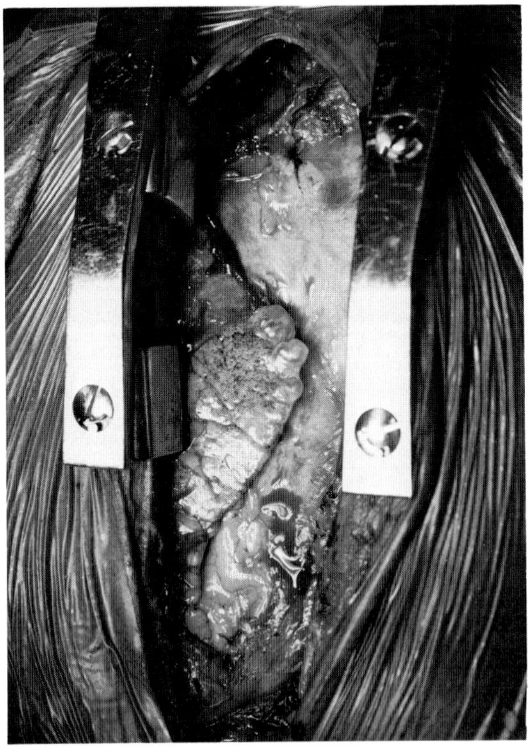

B

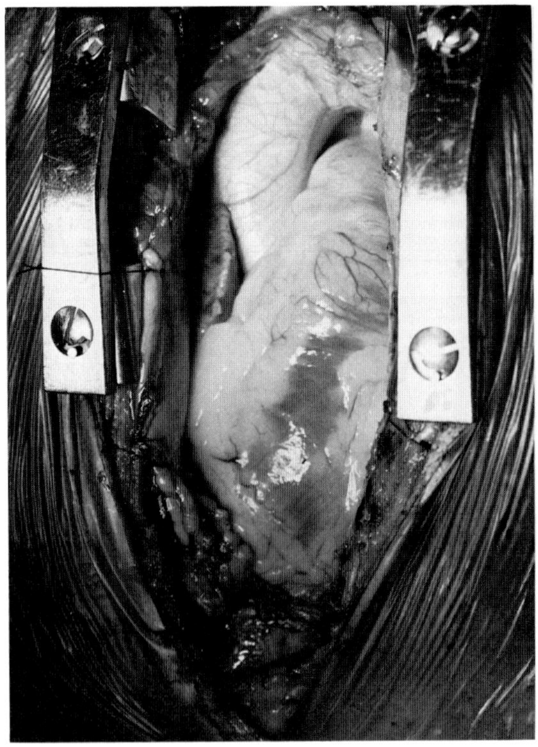

C

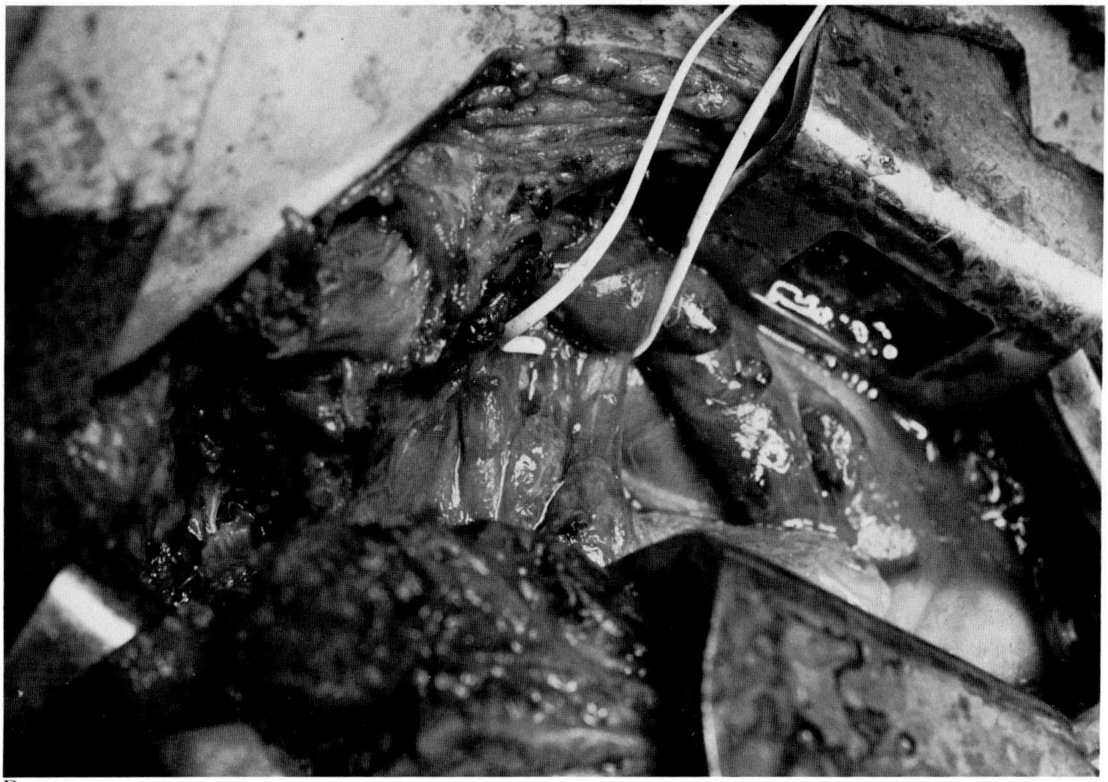

D

Figure 17-2. A. Median sternotomy: proposed incision. B. Lung overlying the percardium. C. Mobilizing the lung and entering the pericardium expose the heart and aorta. D. A vascular tape isolates the innominate artery and vein.

Technique

The vertical skin incision is initially made with a scalpel but is carried to the sternal periosteum with electrocautery. In descending order of safety, the methods of dividing the sternum are air-driven reciprocating saws, power-driven oscillating saws, and the Lebsche knife with mallet. All methods require experience for consistent, safe performance. Once the sternum is divided, marrow and periosteal bleeding is controlled with bone wax and electrocautery. The split sternum is separated by one of a variety of retractors. After the procedure, the sternum is closed with stainless steel wires. The pectoralis fascia is reapproximated with sturdy absorbable suture; the skin and subcutaneous tissues are closed in layers using absorbable sutures.

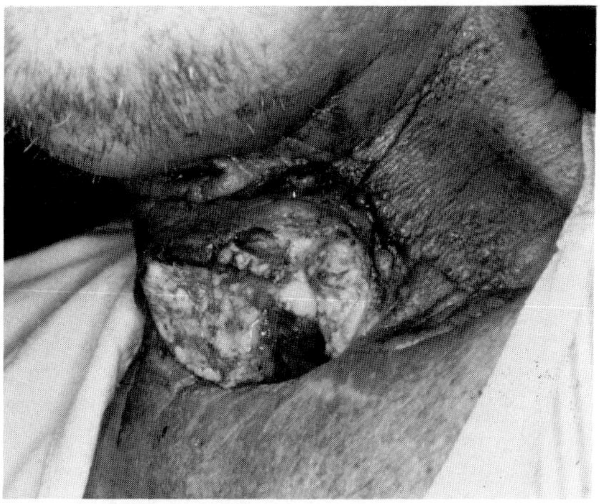

Figure 17-3. A large stomal occurrence with an associated fistula.

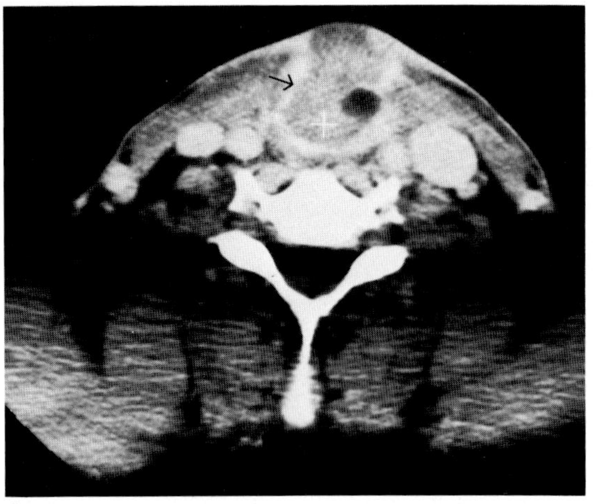

A

Figure 17-4. A. An axial CT scan demonstrates a large stomal occurrence. B. A large left pectoralis myocutaneous flap reconstructs the defect remaining from resection of a stomal occurrence. C. A close-up view of pectoralis myocutaneous flap and tracheostoma.

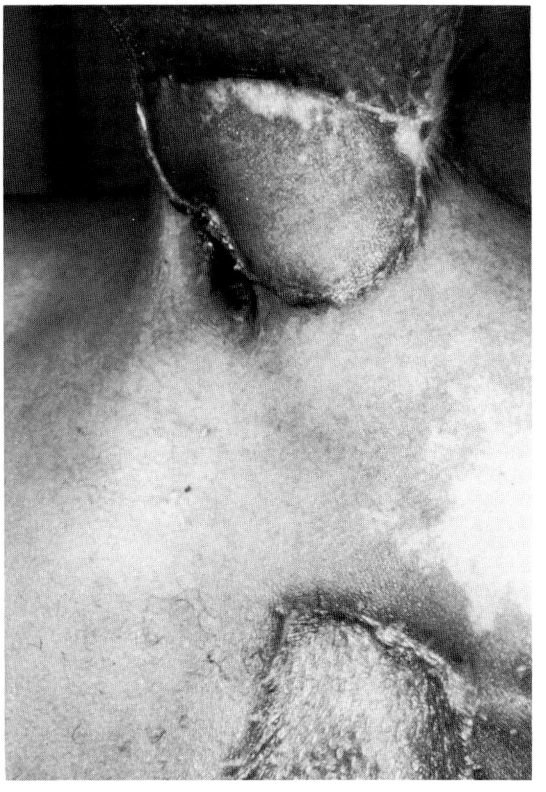

B

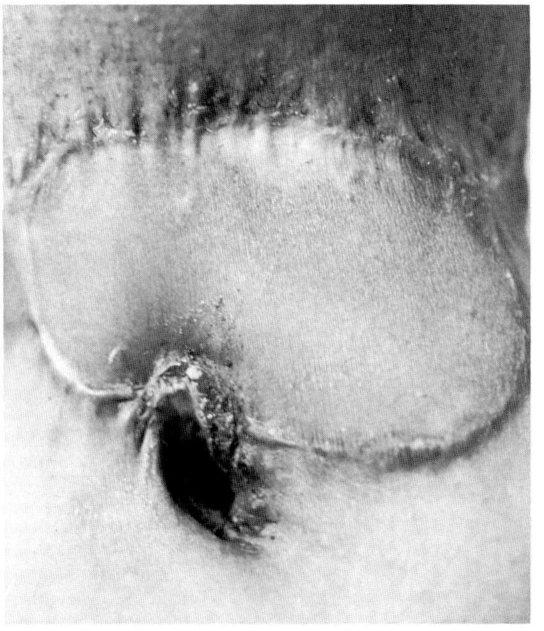

C

Complications

Complications include eccentric sternal division, malunion, wound infection, mediastinitis, and dehiscence.

Mediastinal Tracheostomy and Stomal Resection

Originally described by Watson [9] and advanced by Sisson, mediastinal tracheostomy is indicated for patients with cervical esophageal carcinoma or stomal recurrence after total laryngectomy (Figure 17-3) [2–5]. Although this formidable undertaking may be attended by mediastinitis and great-vessel hemorrhage, deltopectoral and pectoralis myocutaneous flap closure has enhanced its safety (Figure 17-4).

Indications and Contraindications

1. Indications: total pharyngolaryngoesophagectomy, tracheostomal recurrences, postcricoid or proximal tracheal resections.
2. Contraindications: premorbid patients, extensive tumor, great-vessel invasion.

Technique:

For tracheostomal recurrence, an elliptical incision encompassing the stoma is extended over the manubrium to either side of the neck. The carotid arteries and the mobilized esophagus are examined carefully. If the tumor does not involve the great vessels, it is resectable. Following mobilization of the inferior skin flaps, the sternocleidomastoids are transected. A saw removes the upper manubrium and clavicular heads, thus exposing the trachea in the anterior mediastinum. An adequate amount of tumor-free trachea is isolated (usually two to three rings) and separated from the esophagus.

Following these preliminary procedures to determine resectability, the abdomen is explored. The stomach is mobilized, preserving the blood supply from the right gastric and gastroepiploic vessels. The spleen is carefully preserved. The distal esophagus is encircled, and the diaphragmatic hiatus is enlarged manually. A Kocher maneuver allows for adequate mediastinal excursion; a standard Heineke-Mikulicz pyloroplasty is performed. Gently, the stomach is guided through the posterior mediastinum into the neck. The gastroesophageal junction is divided (by a stapler), and the fundus is anastomosed to the remaining pharynx. Prior to abdominal closure, a feeding jejunostomy is performed. Although a nasogastric tube is passed, the jejunostomy ensures adequate postoperative nutrition.

The skin defect is measured, and a corresponding pectoralis myocutaneous flap is fashioned. The stump of the trachea is centered bluntly in the flap and secured. With this technique, some groups have reported encouraging early survival rates [2]. Long-term survival awaits further follow-up.

Complications

Complications include hemorrhage, flap necrosis, mediastinitis, esophageal perforation, pneumothorax, chylothorax, and air embolism (Figure 17-5).

ALIMENTARY CONTINUITY

There are numerous methods for reestablishing alimentary tract continuity following extirpative procedures of the upper esophagus or esophageal bypass for caustic injuries or malignant tracheoesophageal fistulae (see Chapter 24) [5]. Each has its proponents, but substernal gastric bypass, colonic interposition, and free jejunal grafts are the most reliable.

Substernal Gastric Bypass

Originally described by Kirschner and recently popularized by Orringer, substernal gastric bypass procedure is invaluable for the management of malignant aerodigestive fistulae [6,8].

Indications and Contraindications

1. Indications: tracheoesophageal fistulae; esophagobronchial fistulae; unresectable esophageal carcinomas; iatrogenic esophageal perforation associated with unresectable carcinomas.
2. Contraindications: extremely poor operative risk; caustic injury to stomach; previous gastrectomy; inadequate gastric blood supply; existing peptic ulcer disease; tumor infiltration of the fundus.

Technique

It is expedient to perform this procedure using two teams. Abdominal exploration determines whether the stomach is suitable; the lesser sac is entered by dividing the gastrocolic omentum. The incision, continued on the greater curvature, divides the short gastric vessels and preserves the spleen. Care is taken to preserve the right gastroepiploic vessels. The posterior stomach wall is inspected for fundal tumor involvement. If free, the esophagus is encircled with a Penrose drain and the dissection is carried along the lesser curvature, dividing the gastrohepatic ligament. The left gastric artery is suture-ligated near the stomach. A generous Kocher maneuver is executed carefully to avoid right gastric artery injury. Finally, a pyloroplasty is performed.

Simultaneously, the second team explores the neck. A right or left anterior sternocleidomastoid incision is performed. This incision is placed ipsilateral to a nonfunctioning vocal cord. Usually, the middle thyroid vein is

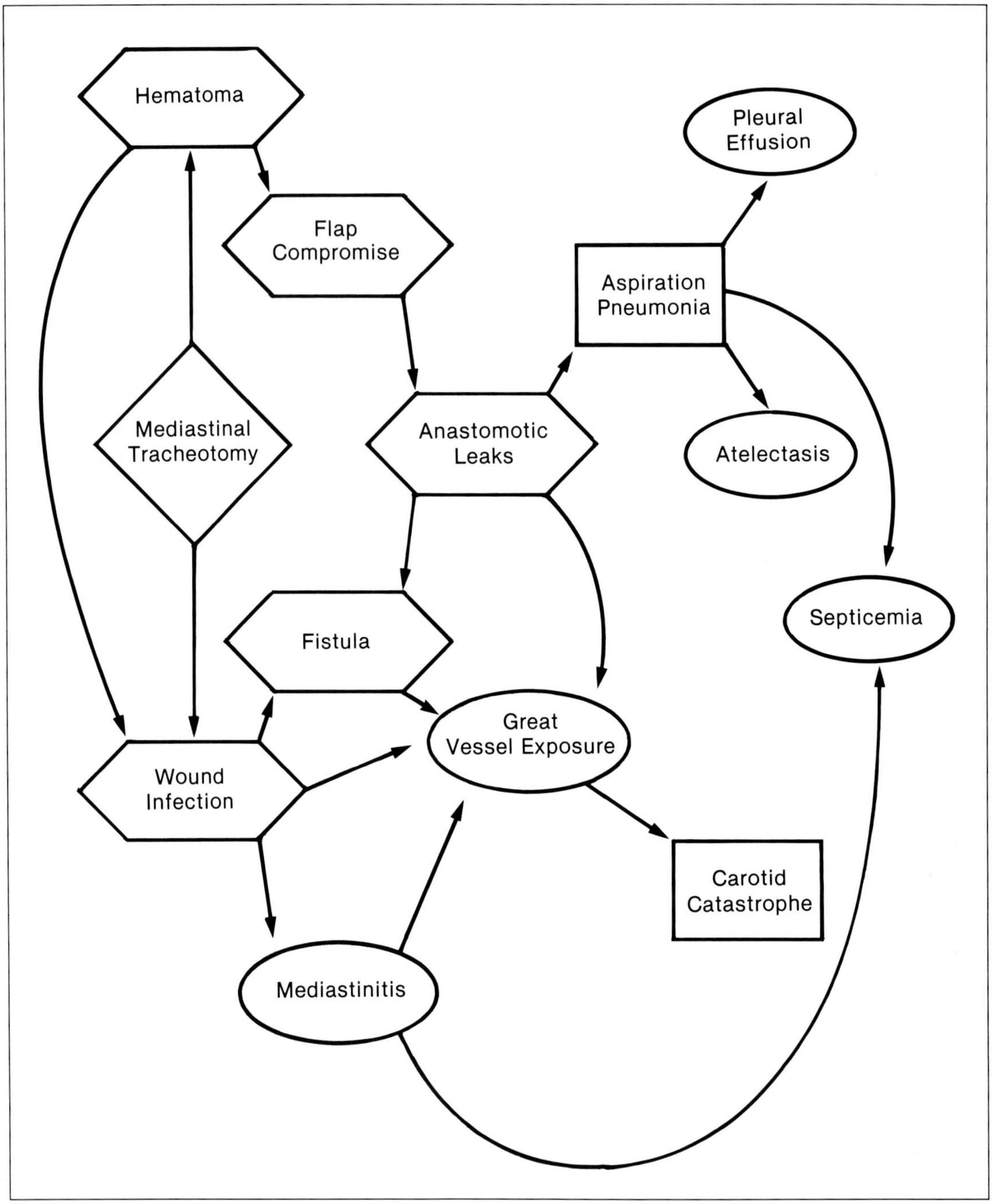

Figure 17-5. Complications of mediastinal tracheotomy.

divided. The carotid sheath is exposed and retracted laterally. The esophagus is encircled with a Penrose drain while the recurrent laryngeal nerves are protected. The esophagus is palpated well into the mediastinum to ensure that distal disease does not preclude anastomosis.

A stapler is then passed across the gastroesophageal junction. The stomach is measured on the anterior chest wall to determine adequate length. A substernal tunnel is created bluntly, by passing a hand into the neck incision. Pressure on the heart is avoided. The esophagus is divided with a GIA stapler as far distally as possible. The stomach is brought up through the widened tunnel without twisting the organ. Occasionally, sternal and clavicular resection is necessary for adequate mobilization.

Complications

Complications include anastomotic leaks and strictures, recurrent nerve injury, esophageal pouch mucocele, mediastinitis and gastric stasis.

Colonic Interposition

The colon is still a useful conduit for upper alimentary continuity. Although perhaps not quite as reliable as the stomach, it is available for situations when the stomach cannot be used. Anastomotic leaks, stricture formation, avascular colon necrosis, and pneumothorax are the common complications. Operative mortality has been reported to be as high as 25 percent [10].

Indications and Contraindications

1. Indications: inadequate stomach for pull-up, surgeon's experience or preference.
2. Contraindications: colonic carcinoma, carcinomatosis, poor operative risk, inadequate colonic blood supply.

Technique

A preoperative barium enema excludes any intrinsic colonic abnormalities. Angiography is advocated by some to detect significant vascular lesions, especially in patients over age 60.

During surgery, the vascular pattern is noted carefully as the blood supply to the proposed conduit segment is temporarily occluded with atraumatic "bulldog" clips. Following colonic moblization and after vascular occlusion, the bowel is inspected for ischemia. As the colon is transected appropriately, spillage is avoided and the vessels are protected gingerly from kinking, tension, or torsion. The bowel is passed into the neck substernally, subcutaneously, or through the posterior mediastinum. The cologastric anastomosis, placed anteriorly on the lesser curvature (via the substernal route) is simplified with the EEA stapler. The substernal tunnel is developed and the conduit passed into the neck, maintaining axial alignment. A pyloroplasty or pyloromyotomy is always performed.

The cervical anastomosis is performed either end-to-end or end-to-side using interrupted absorbable sutures. A nasogastric tube is placed and secured. Intestinal continuity is reestablished by a colocolonic or ileocolonic anastomosis. Prior to abdominal closure, a feeding jejunostomy is performed. Colonic transposition may be accomplished with either right or left transverse segments, although more length is available with the left colon.

Complications

Complications include redundancy, anastomotic leaks, colon necrosis, and stricture formation.

Jejunal Interposition

Free jejunal transposition was performed first experimentally by Carrel [11]. With the development of reliable microvascular techniques, this procedure has become a viable alternative for hypopharyngeal and cervical esophagus reconstruction [7]. Although the jejunum is not as useful as the stomach or colon for the thoracic esophagus, the relative freedom from stricture formation and its generous diameter make the jejunum an attractive conduit.

Indications and Contraindications

1. Indications: short benign esophageal strictures; trauma; bridging gaps; salvage of failed colon interposition.

2. Contraindications: inexperience; too long a gap to bridge; diseased recipient vessels.

Technique

A standard laparotomy is performed, and a jejunal segment is isolated 30 to 40 cm distal to the ligament of Treitz. Grafts greater than 18 to 20 cm require more than one vascular arcade. While small-bowel continuity is restored by enteroenterostomy, the isolated segment perfuses on its vascular pedicle. Following exposure of the cervical anastomotic site, the jejunal segment is transferred to the neck. The proximal pharyngoesophagojejunal anastomosis is performed first with absorbable suture.

The vascular anastomoses are accomplished with standard microvascular techniques using 9-0 or 1-0 monofilament suture. Recipient vessels include the transverse cervical thyroid and the external carotid or common carotid artery. The venous anastomosis is to the internal jugular or thyroid vein. A return of color and peristaltic activity should be observed on reperfusion. Finally, the distal anastomosis is completed. The abdomen is closed after placement of a feeding jejunostomy.

When the neck is closed, a small segment of the free graft, protruding through a "window" in the closure, permits postoperative monitoring of graft viability. The basic limitation is imposed by the length of jejunum that can safely be transplanted.

Complications

Complications include graft necrosis, mediastinitis, peritonitis, fistula formation, stenosis, and dysphagia.

REFERENCES

1. Fishman NH: *Thoracic Drainage: A Manual of Procedures.* Chicago: Year Book, 1983.
2. Sisson GA, Bytell DE, Becker SP: Mediastinal dissection—1976: Indications and newer techniques. *Laryngoscope* 87 : 751, 1976.
3. Myers EM: Complications in surgery for stomal recurrences. *Laryngoscope* 93 : 285, 1983.
4. Krespi YP, Wurster CF, Sisson GA: Immediate reconstruction after total laryngopharyngoesophagectomy and mediastinal dissection. *Laryngoscope* 95 : 156, 1985.
5. Silver CE: Surgical treatment of hypopharyngeal and cervical esophageal cancer. *World J Surg* 5 : 499, 1981.
6. Orringer MB, Sloan H: Esophagectomy without thoracotomy. *J Thorac Cardiovasc Surg* 76 : 643, 1978.
7. Fisher SR, et al: Pharyngoesophageal reconstruction using free jejunal grafts. *Arch Otolaryngol* III : 747, 1985.
8. Orringer MB, Sloan H: Substernal gastric bypass of the excluded thoracic esophagus for palliation of esophageal carcinoma. *J Thorac Surg* 70 : 836, 1975.
9. Watson WL: Cancer of the trachea 15 years after treatment for cancer of the larynx. *J Thorac Surg* 12 : 142, 1942.
10. Postlethwait RW, et al: Colon interposition for esophageal substitution. *Ann Thorac Surg* 12 : 89, 1971.
11. Carrel A: Results of transplantation of blood vessels, organs and limbs. *JAMA* 151 : 1662, 1908.
12. Roeher HD, Horeyseck G: Kirschner bypass operation—A palliation for complicated esophageal carcinoma. *World J Surg* 5 : 543, 1981.

III

REHABILITATION

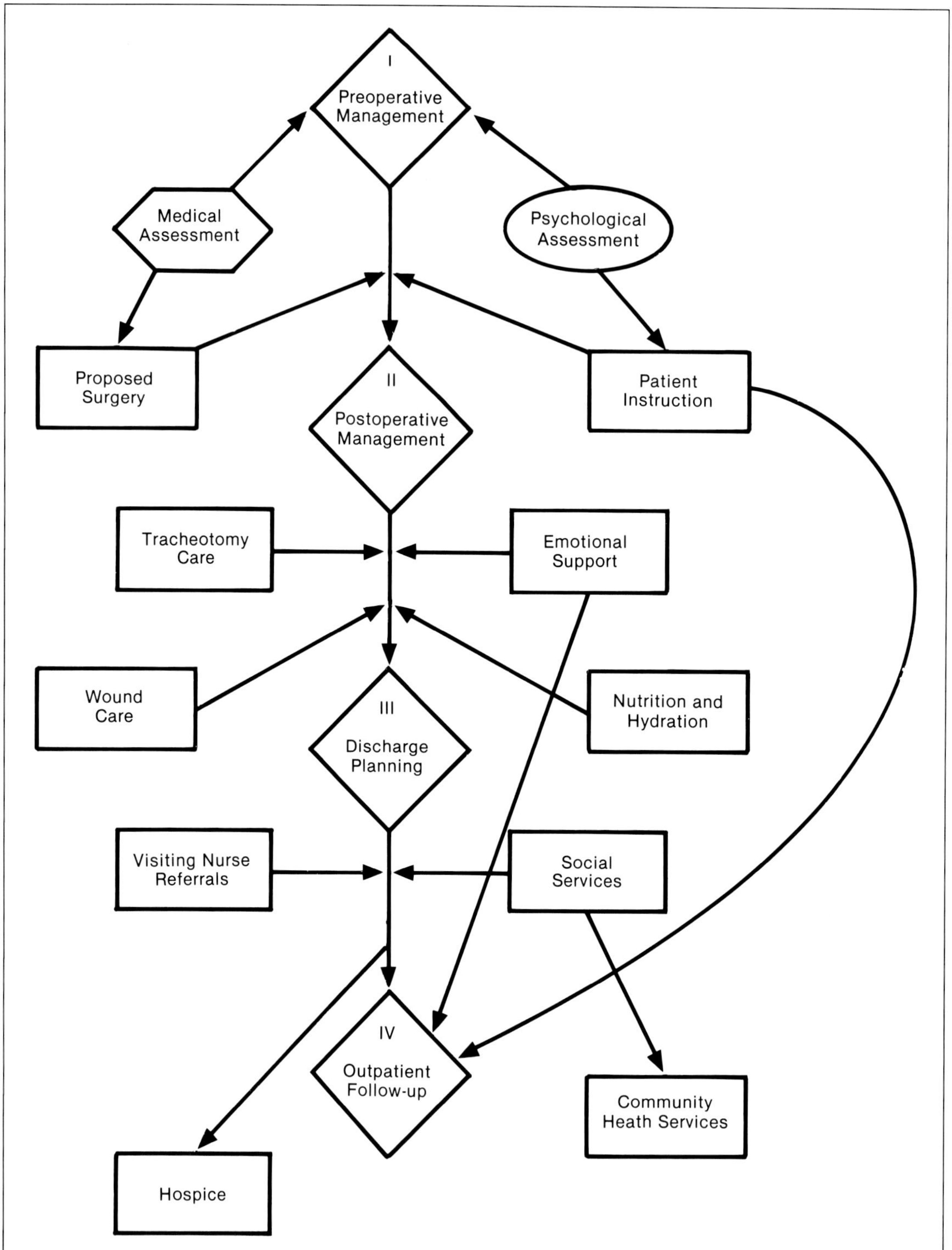

Figure 18-1. The four stages of head and neck surgical nursing.

Table 18-1. Preoperative nursing assessment: high-risk factors

Malnutrition
Cardiovascular system
  Arteriosclerotic cardiovascular disease
  Myocardial infarction: recent versus old
  Hypertension
  Peripheral vascular disease
  Thrombophlebitis
Respiratory system
  Chronic obstructive lung disease
  Restrictive lung disease
  Asthma
  Pneumonectomy
  Lobectomy
  Pulmonary emboli (history)
Neurologic system
  Cerebrovascular accident
  Seizure disorder
  Sensory deficits
    Deafness
    Blindness
    Speech impediment
Gastrointestinal system
  Cirrhosis
  Pancreatitis
Genitourinary system
  Renal insufficiency
  Nephrectomy
  Prostatism
Hematopoietic system
  Anemia
  Coagulopathy
  Acquired immunodeficiency syndrome (AIDS)
Endocrine system
  Diabetes mellitus
  Hypothyroidism
Psyche
  Anxiety
  Paranoia
  Schizophrenia
  Neuroses
Chemical dependency
  Alcoholism: delirium tremens
  Heroin
  Cocaine
Support systems
  Religion
  Family
  Employer
  Spouse or supportive other
  Social worker
  Community health services

2. Assisting the patient to cope with altered body function and image.
3. Helping the patient achieve independent self-care.
4. Returning the patient to both family and society with an optimal level of function.

PREOPERATIVE MANAGEMENT

Psychosocial Status

Preoperatively, the nurse establishes good patient rapport. With proper support and encouragement, patients can develop a more receptive attitude toward therapy. The nurse reinforces and clarifies the physician's explanation of the illness and treatment. The patient and family are encouraged to verbalize their fears and anxieties associated with hospitalization and treatment [4]. The patient's personality, culture values, needs, coping mechanisms, and support systems are assessed [3,5,6]. There must be an understanding of the illness and what it means to both patient and family (Table 18-1).

All involved parties are encouraged to express their expectations and fears. Fear of the unknown is the leading cause of anxiety. The patient and family may be fearful of pain, disfigurement, surgery, dependency, and abandonment. These fears may be manifested by withdrawal, anger, and depression (see Chapters 19 and 30) [7].

Medical Assessment

Preoperative medical assessment identifies risk factors and alerts the nursing staff to potential

Table 18-2. Preoperative nursing assessment of high-risk factors: therapy (past and future)

Preoperative therapy
  Radiotherapy
  Chemotherapy
Anticipated surgical therapy
  Glossectomy (total versus partial)
  Laryngectomy (total versus partial)
  Neck dissection
  Tracheotomy
  Mandibulectomy (total versus partial)
  Flaps
  Grafts

PATIENT NEEDS	DEGREE OF DEPENDENCY ON NURSING SERVICES PERSONNEL					
NEED FOR OBSERVATION	Routine		Moderate		Maximum	
COMMUNICABILITY	No Problem		Needs Assistance		Unable to communicate	
EMOTIONAL APPEARANCE	Normal		Moderate depression or apprehension		Maximum depression or apprehension	
MENTAL ACURITY	Normal		Moderately decreased confused		Unconscious semi-conscious state	
MEDICATIONS	Less than 2 Meds		2-5 meds		6 meds or more	
			Pre-op meds		Multiple PRN, cont. IVs	
			Meds req. freq. sympt. obs.		IV solu-sets or piggy back	
	Instillations BID		Instillations QID		Instillations more than QID	
SPECIAL FUNCTIONS	Obtain specimens		Specimen testing		Hypothermia	
			Sitz bath		Hemorrhage Control	
			Pacemaker		Monitor	
			Periodic aspirating		Aspirating more than q3h	
			Tracheotomy		Rotating tourniquet	
			Intake and Output		Chest Tubes	
RESPIRATORY ASSISTS	IPPB, humidity		Oxygen PRN		Cons. oxygen, respirator	
VITAL SIGNS, TPR	Required BID		Required QID		Required more than QID	
NEUROSENSORY CHECKS	Required BID		Required QID		Required more than QID	
DRESSINGS, K-Pac. ACE BANDAGE, BINDERS, TED	Self care		Re-inforce, assist patient or M.D.		Apply q4hrs or more freq.	
PROSTHESIS OR TRACTION	Self applied		Assist—1 person		Assist—2 people	
CIRCLE-ELECTRIC BED			Stationary		Turned—2 people	
IRRIGATIONS, RECORD DRAINAGE	Nurse provides equip. Patient does proced.		Foley, levine wound less than q4hrs.		Foley, levine wound more than q4hrs.	
			Hemavac, gastrostomy, t-tube less than q4hr		Hemavac, gastrostomy t-tube more than q4hr	
			Blakemore, Miller Abbott less than q4hr		Blakemore, Miller Abbott more than q4hr.	
FOOD, FLUIDS (NPO leave blank)	No assist required		Assistance required fluids forced		Fed by personnel tube feedings	
PERSONAL HYGIENE	Self care		Assistance required		Total care required	
ELIMINATION	B.R.P.		Assist required		Incontinent	
ACTIVITY IN BED	Self care		Needs assistance		Turned q2hr, complete bed rest, passive exercise	
TEACHING	Minimal		Moderate		Maximum	
	TOTAL CHECKS X 1		TOTAL CHECKS X 5		TOTAL CHECKS X 10	
NAME						

SCORE	CLASS
0-40	I
41-80	II
81+	III

Score Record

DATE	SCORE

Add 20 Points for STRICT Isolation

Figure 18-2. Patient classification assessment.

complications (Table 18-2, Figures 18-2 and 18-3). Baseline data is obtained by chart review, observation, and listening. Since many head and neck cancer patients are heavy drinkers and smokers, they may present in a nutritionally depleted state with compromised respiratory function. A careful assessment identifies these and other potential medical problems. It is also important to determine the patient's learning and reading skills.

Patient Education

Patient education begins with admission and is a continuous process throughout the hospitalization. Anticipated pre- and postoperative changes are discussed with both patient and family. The topics include suctioning, nasogastric tubes, drainage tubes, tracheotomy, Foley catheters, intravenous fluids, and communication. It is emphasized that pain is usually minimal and analgesia is provided. Turning, cough-

DATE ___/___/___ UNIT________

	YES	NO		YES	NO
I.D. Band on and correct			Jewelry removed secured safe/home		
O.R. Permit signed, witnessed and dated			Hairpins, makeup, nail polish removed		
History and Physical completed			Clothing removed		
Nameplate and MAR on chart			N.P.O. since midnight		
Dentures removed			Voided Time: Catheterized--Foley inserted Time:		
Contact lenses or glasses removed			Enemas given		
Other Prosthesis removed			Prep-op medication given and charted		
Bath and oral hygiene			Shave prep done		

	DONE	ON CHART	NORMAL	ABNORMAL	DOCTOR NOTIFIED YES	DOCTOR NOTIFIED NO	WHOM?	TIME	COMMENTS AND/OR ACTION TAKEN
BLOOD WORK									
URINALYSIS									
EKG									
X-RAY									
CONSULTATIONS									

MENTAL STATUS BEFORE PRE-OP MEDICATION: ORIENTED________ DISORIENTED________

T____ P____ R____ BP____ To O.R. Time______ AM PM Pre-op Teaching ____Class ____Individual

ADDITIONAL PATIENT CARE INFORMATION:

DATE:____________ UNIT NURSE:____________

PATIENT IDENTIFICATION

Figure 18-3. Preoperative checklist.

ing, and deep breathing, to prevent respiratory complications, are stressed. A clear explanation of all phases of surgery and hospitalization is provided. Posters, models, videos and diagrams are very useful for preoperative and postoperative teaching. Diagnostic procedures such as x-rays, scans, or biopsies are explained in simple, understandable language (see Chapter 7).

Preoperative teaching has definite advantages: more rapid recuperation, decreased use of analgesics, fewer complications, and shorter hospital stays. Most importantly, patient education develops independence and self-confidence and expedites recovery.

POSTOPERATIVE MANAGEMENT

General Considerations

Postoperative nursing care depends largely on the type of the surgery, incision, absence, or presence of a tracheotomy and the patient's ability to talk and swallow. After a major head and neck procedure, the patient invariably returns from the recovery room or intensive care unit with drainage tubes, nasogastric tube, tracheotomy, multiple intravenous lines, arterial lines, and a Foley catheter. Postoperatively, the immediate nursing interventions are airway maintenance and vital signs, head elevation, intake and output, closed wound suction, analgesia, and pulmonary toilet.

Vital Signs
Vital signs (temperature, pulse, respiration, blood pressure) are closely monitored, every 4 hours for 48 hours and then 4 times a day to detect early complications. Airway maintenance is a primary concern (see Chapter 10). The patient is observed closely for subtle signs of hypoxia such as restlessness, apprehension, and disorientation.

Head Elevation
Head elevation in the semi-Fowler's position increases lymphatic and venous drainage.

Nasogastric Tubes
Nasogastric tubes are inserted intraoperatively to prevent oral contamination and aspiration and to enhance suture-line decompression.

Humidification
Humidification is delivered by nebulizers or portable humidifiers. This is particularly important in tracheotomized patients. If the secretions are tenacious or crusty, several drops of sterile normal saline solution are instilled to thin the secretions.

Closed Wound Suction
Closed wound suction provides continuous wound drainage and promotes healing. Drains decrease the risk of hematomas, collapse dead space, and enhance skin flap viability. Drainage varies from 100 to 300 ml (serosanguineous fluid) for the first postoperative day but usually decreases to 30 ml or less by the fourth or fifth postoperative day. It is not unusual for the drainage to be predominately bloody in the first 48 to 72 hours. However, if excessive sanguineous drainage is associated with unstable vital signs, the physician is notified immediately.

Analgesia
Since many sensory nerves are transected during surgery, postoperative pain is minimal. However, if major flaps or skin grafts are used, relief may require opiates (see Chapter 20). Respiratory rate, blood pressure, and pulse are assessed critically, since narcotics depress respiratory function and inhibit coughing. The patient is assigned close to the nurse's station for frequent observation and assessments. A method of patient communication is developed (e.g., writing pad, flash cards, or Magic Slate).

Pulmonary Toilet
Blow bottles, adequate hydration, and early ambulation are important to prevent atelectasis and pneumonia. The patient is encouraged to turn, cough, and breathe deeply. Ambulation begins 24 to 48 hours after surgery.

Tracheotomy
Cuffed tracheotomy tubes prevent aspiration and permit ventilatory assistance. Low-pressure cuffs minimize the risk of tracheostenosis (see Chapter 10). Only minimal pressure is used to seal the trachea. If the patient is not on the ventilator, the cuff is deflated. While the patient is on the ventilator, the cuff is deflated routinely usually for 3 to 5 minutes every hour to relieve intraluminal pressure and discourage pressure necrosis. Prior to cuff deflation, the oropharynx is suctioned to prevent aspiration of secretions collected above the cuff. Oral suctioning follows tracheal suctioning to prevent catheter contamination.

Tracheotomy care is performed at least once each shift or as needed. If there are copious secretions, the tracheotomy tube (inner cannula) is cleaned every 4 hours or every shift. Usually, secretions decrease about the fourth postoperative day.

Tracheotomy Care
The following protocol is recommended:

1. Wash your hands.
2. Assemble all equipment and supplies.
3. Open the tracheotomy care kit on a clean surface; use one drape for the patient.
4. Place two basins on the sterile field; fill one basin with hydrogen peroxide, the other with sterile saline.
5. Discard the soiled tracheostomy dressing, and put on sterile gloves.
6. Remove the inner cannula, and submerge it in hydrogen peroxide. Clean it with the pipe cleaner and brush. Check to see if the tracheostomy tube lumen is clean.
7. Rinse the inner cannula with sterile saline and allow it to drain on sterile 4- × 4-in. pads.
8. Clean the skin and neck wound with hydrogen peroxide, using sterile cotton-tipped applicators. Rinse with sterile normal saline, and dry with sterile gauze.
9. Suction the outer cannula; reinsert the inner cannula and lock in place.
10. Apply new dressing and tape ties. Secure the tapes with a double knot at the side of the neck (not too tight).

Suctioning

The following protocol is recommended:

1. Wash your hands.
2. Open the suction kit on a clean surface, using the inside of the wrapper as a sterile field.
3. Place a sterile glove on the dominant hand; the other hand is used to handle unsterile items.
4. Set up the disposable sterile cup on a sterile field, and fill with normal saline (some suction kits have sterile saline).
5. Attach a sterile suction catheter to the suction tubing by holding the catheter in the gloved hand and the tubing in the ungloved hand.
6. Suction a small amount of saline to test the equipment.
7. Instruct the patient to cough to mobilize secretions.
8. Lubricate the suction catheter tip with normal saline, and with the suction off, gently insert it through the tracheostomy.
9. Pull the catheter back about 1 to 2 cm to free the tip from the tracheal wall.
10. Rotate the catheter 360 degrees back and forth between the gloved fingers, and slowly withdraw. Suction intermittently by placing the thumb over the catheter valve.
11. Remove the catheter within 10 to 15 seconds to prevent hypoxia.
12. Flush the catheter with saline, and then repeat the process as needed.
13. Offer mouth care.
14. Turn off the suction device.
15. Ventilate the patient with oxygen and humidity prior to and after each suctioning attempt to limit hypoxia.

Complications

Complications of tracheotomy include the following (see Chapter 10):

1. Obstruction—caused usually by mucus plugs secondary to inadequate humidification or tube displacement.
2. Decannulation—accidental tube removal. Always keep a replacement tracheostomy tube of the same size and type at the bedside in case of accidental decannulation.
3. Hemorrhage—call the attending physician immediately.
4. Tension pneumothorax—if there is any doubt, call the physician immediately.
5. Wound infection.
6. Tracheostenosis.
7. Tracheoesophageal fistula.

Wound Care

Healing

The factors associated with good wound healing are as follows (see Chapters 12 and 22):

1. Adequate drainage.
2. Head elevation (30–45 degrees) to decrease suture-line tension and discourage edema.
3. Oxygenation (hematocrit at least 30%).
4. Hemostasis.
5. Antibiotics.

lymphatics. Preoperative radiation and surgical edema are other predisposing factors. Adequate nutrition, appropriate hydration, early ambulation, head elevation, and avoidance of tight dressings and tracheotomy ties help reduce this troublesome and at times depressing problem. Given time, normal facial contour returns.

Fistula

The predisposing factors of fistula are infection, poor nutrition, inadequate wound care, residual tumor, and preoperative radiation therapy (see Chapters 12 and 17). Most fistulae heal with good wound care. If a fistula develops, it is cleaned and packed to prevent wound soilage and excoriation. Large fistulae require constant evacuation with drainage bags. If the fistula is small, a stomal bag suffices. Fistulae are cleaned with dilute hydrogen peroxide and dressed with bulky, absorbent pressure dressings.

Chyle Leak

Chyle leak from the transected thoracic duct is characterized by a milky or clear drainage. A significant chyle leak results in fluid and electrolyte imbalance; its composition is similar to plasma and tissue fluid. Therefore, chyle drainage, output, and color are monitored closely.

Flap Slough

Skin flap necrosis occurs usually secondary to ischemia or fistulization. These conditions are ripe for carotid catastrophe.

Carotid Blowout

Carotid artery exposure is a prodrome to vascular catastrophe secondary to thrombosis or rupture. This acute, life-threatening complication is associated with poor wound healing, fistula, previous irradiation, or tumor growth. Fistulae, with copious secretions bathing the carotid artery, are dangerous. Overlying skin necrosis and slough enhance the possibility of a massive hemorrhage. Hemorrhaging may occur within the oropharynx, through the tracheotomy site, or from the neck wound. When a carotid artery ruptures, quickly apply firm pressure with gauze sponges. The basic bedside supplies are suction equipment, gloves, parenteral analgesia, absorptive dressings, and a vascular tray. Until the physician arrives, pressure is applied, and the patient is comforted and monitored constantly.

Neural Complications

The most commonly injured neural structures are the brachial plexus and spinal accessory nerves. Spinal accessory injury produces a shoulder drop and permanent forward shoulder curvature. There is decreased ability to raise the arm above the shoulder level. This occurs in about 30 percent of all patients having a radical neck dissection (spinal accessory nerve sacrifice) (see Chapter 16). Shoulder exercises lessen this problem if started soon postoperatively. These exercises are wall climbing, shoulder swings, the pully motion, and other shoulder movements to strengthen and preserve function.

NUTRITION

Optimal nutrition promotes healing, maximizes function, prevents weight loss, and improves well-being. Protein depletion and malnutrition are common in head and neck patients. Patients with head and neck cancer often are malnourished secondary to alcoholism, dysphagia, or odontophagia. A decrease in protein, calories, and essential nutrients leads to immunosuppression and increased susceptibility to infection. Also the patient's nutritional state may be affected detrimentally by preoperative radiation and chemotherapy.

Tube Feedings

After surgery, tube feedings are the mainstays of optimal protein and caloric intake (see Chapter 21). The extent of surgery and the recovery rate determine their duration (Table 18-3).

The nasogastric tube (Salem-sump) is utilized in the immediate postoperative stage. This is replaced by a softer and more pliable tube (Dobbhoff, Keofeed) for prolonged tube feeding. The presence or absence of swallowing is considered when determining bolus feeding volume. Continuous pump feedings are better tolerated. If a pump is unavailable or if the

Table 18-3. Tube feedings: delivery systems

Type	*Duration*	*Advantages*	*Disadvantages*
Nasogastric tube	1–2 weeks	Gastrointestinal decompression Large lumen Longevity	Discomfort Gastroesophagitis Laryngitis Socially unacceptable
Dobbhoff, Keofeed	Weeks	Tolerance Ease of placement	Small lumen
Cervical esophagostomy, gastrostomy, jejunostomy	Months	Tolerance Socially acceptable Permanence	Surgical procedure Complications Skin excoriation Regurgitation/reflux Obstruction (tube)

patient is semi-independent, bolus feedings, 400 to 500 ml every 4 hours, are administered.

Formulas

An appropriate formula is selected by the dietitian or hyperalimentation team. The choice depends on composition, patient tolerance, and gastrointestinal function. Elemental diets are complete formulas nutritionally, containing proteins and other nutrients in an easily digestible form (Vivonex, Flexical, and Jejunal). Tube feedings are started on the first postoperative day after overnight low gastric suction. Sustacal is a milk-based formula, with a low lactose content that discourages diarrhea. Tube feedings may also include blenderized regular diets, soy bean–based formulas, and elemental diets. They are given by mouth, gastrostomy, jejunostomy, or cervical esophagostomy [13,14].

Management

Initially, the patient is started on water and progressed gradually to full-strength formula. Additional liquids are encouraged to improve hydration and to prevent viscous tracheal secretions. Prior to feeding, the patient is placed in the semi-Fowler's position and suctioned.

The following guidelines are suggested:

1. Check feeding tube patency and placement.
2. Elevate the head 30 degrees.
3. Maintain strict oral hygiene.
4. Monitor intake and output accurately; provide supplemental water as needed.
5. Give feedings at room temperature.
6. Rinse the tubes with water after each feeding.
7. Plug the tubes between feedings.
8. Check tube position periodically.
9. Monitor electrolytes and albumin.
10. Measure urine fractionals.
11. Be alert for gastrointestinal disturbances, such as cramping, nausea, vomiting, and diarrhea.
12. If an infusion pump is used, set at a slow rate.
13. If the patient does not tolerate a particular formula, dilute and decrease the volume. Intolerance is manifested by nausea, vomiting, diarrhea, cramping, or epigastric pain.

Total Parenteral Nutrition

Total parenteral nutrition (TPN) is the intravenous infusion of hypertonic solutions of glucose, amino acids, vitamins, and minerals through a central line. The typical patient has inadequate gastrointestinal function.

Solution guidelines

TPN solutions are prepared sterilely and refrigerated. The bottle is checked for cracks, leaks, or particulate matter before administration. TPN solutions are infused soon after preparation. Each bottle is hung at room temperature no longer than 12 to 18 hours. The solution is individualized to the patient's nutritional needs [15].

Administration

The average adult requires 2 to 3 liters over 24 hours. This is increased according to the patient's tolerance. If infused too rapidly, osmotic diuresis can result, causing dehydration, convulsions, or even death. Only an infusion pump is used to administer TPN solutions. If the TPN solution falls behind schedule, do not speed up the rate.

Complications

Patients on TPN are predisposed to infection as a result of malnutrition, broad-spectrum antibiotics, and the presence of existing infections (Table 18-4). The indwelling subclavian catheter is a potential source of infection, since TPN is a rich culture medium for bacterial growth. To prevent technical complication, the catheter is placed by an experienced surgeon. A chest x-ray is performed after insertion to confirm the proper placement and to rule out possible pneumothorax.

Monitoring

While administering TPN, the nurse monitors the following:

1. Vital signs, every 4 to 6 hours.
2. Daily body weights.
3. Intake and output each shift to assess fluid balance.
4. Fractional urines for glucose and acetone every 6 to 8 hours.
5. Blood urea nitrogen, glucose, serum electrolytes, and proteins weekly.

Table 18-4. Complications associated with TPN

Septicemia
Hypo/hyperglycemia
Catheter embolus
Hematomas
Arteriovenous fistula
Pneumothorax

Catheter Care

Sterile catheter dressing changes over the central catheter are very important, since the danger of infection and air embolism is great. The dressings are changed daily and the site inspected for inflammation. An antibiotic ointment is applied, followed by an occlusive dressing. The catheter is checked and the tubing is changed with each new bottle. A central line is not used for transfusions, medications, central venous pressure measurements, or blood samples.

DISCHARGE PLANNING

Discharge planning begins with admission (see Chapter 30). Adequate time is allowed for both family and patient to express fears and concerns before discharge. At first, all patients are anxious and overwhelmed with the home nursing tasks and equipment. Beginning early in the hospitalization, both patients and family are trained to assume more responsibility gradually. Reassurance, encouragement, and consistent reinforcement by the nurse are initiated before discharge. When appropriate, patients are referred to community health services and supplies are ordered well in advance.

The laryngectomy patient should be informed that there will be changes in the following areas: (1) loss of smell and taste; (2) inability to blow the nose; (3) inability to lift heavy objects; and (4) inability to blow air from the mouth, sip, suck, gargle, or whistle. The patient is introduced to the speech pathologist before discharge to begin relearning verbal communication (see Chapter 26). These new methods include: (1) esophageal speech; (2) electrolarynx; and (3) Blom-Singer or Pauje prostheses. Referrals to the Lost Chord Club, New Voice Club, American Cancer Society, International Laryngectomy Association, and Visiting Nurse Association are initiated early.

Patients are encouraged to wear medical identification, such as a necklace, wallet card, or bracelet. In certain cases, the nurse and social worker collaborate for a home visit prior to discharge. Upon discharge, the patient is given written instructions regarding self-care, where to purchase medical supplies, and specific dates and times of follow-up appointments.

(In short, the primary discharge goals are: assistance to both family and patient; promotion of home care and self-reliance; and identification of outpatient resources. Together, they ensure a smooth transition from hospital to home.)

Rehabilitation

The nursing staff and other health team members all play an important role in the rehabilitation. After surgery many patients require extended care. Ongoing quality care, education, support, and assessment are mandatory. To achieve these goals, the nurse works closely with the patient and other members of the health team. The availability of other health disciplines ensures a smooth transition from the hospital to the outpatient environment.

The aim is rehabilitation of the head and neck cancer patient to the optimal level of functioning. The factors influencing rehabilitation are:

1. Age.
2. Extent of disease.
3. Tissue loss.
4. Previous therapy.
5. Reconstruction.
6. Motivation and attitude.
7. Occupation
8. Performance status.

Outpatient Clinic

The patient usually is seen by the physician in the clinic or office every month the first year, every 2 months the second year, every 3 months the third year, and eventually every 6 months. Once discharged, the patient notifies the physician immediately if any new problems arise.

Equipment

A tracheotomy requires proper home equipment. Humidifiers and portable suction machines are purchased or rented. They are usually covered by most insurance companies. Suction catheters, tracheotomy kits, feeding tubes, and bags are also required. The nurse makes sure that both patient and family are capable of using and maintaining the equipment.

Home Visits

Homebound patients may require the assistance of a visiting nurse. Home nursing care is directed toward wound care, prevention of infection, nutrition, and emotional support. However, follow-up physician appointments still are maintained. Emotional support is a must for the patient with physical deformities or disfigurement. Hospital support groups are also available for patients and families to enhance understanding and provide encouragement after surgery.

Tube Feedings

While the patient is at home, nutrition still remains an important concern. Home tube feedings are administered with careful nursing supervision. Instructions for bolus feedings or the use of feeding pumps are initiated in the hospital and reinforced during home visits. The instructions are kept simple and concise. Family members of loved ones are instructed, prior to discharge, if the patient is unable to perform the tasks. Home feeding requires patience and understanding by both family and patient to feel comfortable with home feedings.

Home TPN

Home parenteral nutrition has greater risks; however, it can be administered safely with proper supervision (see Chapter 21). TPN patients receive infusions for 5 to 7 days, depending on the requirements. Success with home parenteral nutrition requires intensive instruction to patients and families. Some companies provide full services, including supply, delivery, and nurses. Follow-up is by a visiting nurse until the services are no longer needed.

Hospice

Hospice care in the United States is a recent phenomenon for terminally ill patients (see Chapter 30). Hospice emphasizes supportive care for pain and other symptoms of terminal illness. The patient and family, as a single unit, are able to receive hospice services. Hospice employs a broad spectrum of professionals and volunteers to deliver social, psychological, medical, and spiritual services.

Requirements

The requirements vary from program to program; there are no uniform state or federal regulations governing hospices. In general, a patient with a confirmed terminal disease is eligible.

Coordination

Hospice care is coordinated prior to discharge by both the nurse and social worker. The nurse provides the information concerning the patient's present condition, the extent of the disease, patient abilities, and limitations. With this information, the social worker plans assistance to family members and loved ones. Hospice care cannot be overemphasized. It is the difference between dying hopelessly and awaiting death with dignity.

REFERENCES

1. McGuire DB: Familial cancer and the role of the nurse. *Cancer Nurs* 2 : 443, 1979.
2. Keith CF: Wound management following head and neck surgery. *Nurs Clin North Am* 14(4) : 761, 1979.
3. Thomas BJ: Coping with the devastation of head and neck cancer. RN 34(10) : 25, 1974.
4. Daly KM: Oral cancer: Everyday concern. *Am J Nurs* 8 : 1415, 1979.
5. Ostchega YGA: Providing safe conduct: Help your cancer patient find his style of coping. *Nursing* 14 : 42, 1984.
6. Rosillo RH, Welty MJ, Graham WP: The patient with maxillofacial cancer: Psychosocial aspects. *Nurs Clin North Am* 8 : 153, 1973.
7. *Adult Patient Education in Cancer: Office of Cancer Communications.* National Cancer Institute—U.S. Department of Health and Human Services—Public Health Service National Institutes of Health, Sept 1982. Pp 10–17.
8. Trowbridge JE: Caring for patients with facial or intra-oral reconstruction. *Am J Nurs* 11 : 1930, 1973.
9. Daeffler R: Oral hygiene measures for patients with cancer, III. *Cancer Nurs* 4 : 29, 1981.
10. Marina R: *Cancer Nursing.* St. Louis: Mosby, 1981. Pp 276–277.
11. Trowbridge JE, Carl W: Oral care of the patient having head and neck irradiation. Am J of Nurs 12: 2146, 1975.
12. Bersani G, Carl W: Oral care for cancer patients. *Am J Nurs* 83(4): 533, 1983.
13. Donoghue M, Yasko J, Nunnally C: Nutritional needs of cancer patients. *Nurs Clin North Am* 17 : 567, 1982.
14. Burkaltler P, Donley D: *Nutrition: Dynamics of Oncology Nursing.* New York: McGraw-Hill, 1978. Pp 96–99.
15. Metheny NM, Snively WD: *Nurses Handbook of Fluid Balance* (4th ed). Philadelphia: Lippincott, 1980. Pp 151–155.
16. Wiley T: Dealing with depression after radical surgery. *Nursing* 79 : 47, 1979.

GLOSSARY

Airway obstruction The presence of a foreign body, growth, or swelling that occludes the air passageways and interferes with normal breathing.

Biopsy The removal of a sample of tissue for pathologic analysis.

Cauterize The burning of tissue with heat or chemical.

Dead space A cavity that remains after the incomplete closure of a surgical or traumatic wound; a potential area that collects blood, serum, etc., and delays healing.

Debridement Removal or trimming of devitalized tissue.

Decannulation Removal of a tracheostomy tube.

Dehiscence The separation of the layers of a surgical wound; it may be partial, superficial, or complete (total disruption).

Dysphagia Difficulty in swallowing.

Fistula A small opening along or near the incision, creating an opening from the oral cavity, larynx, or pharynx to the skin.

Flaps Tissue that includes skin or muscle, partially removed from one part of the body, to retain its blood supply during transfer to a new location; used to repair defects in an adjacent or distant part of the body.

Hematoma A localized collection of blood, usually clotted, in an organ, space, or tissue.

Hemostasis The cessation of bleeding, either by pressure vasoconstriction, coagulation, ligature, or clamping.

Hypoxia Oxygen deficiency caused by reduced oxygen carrying capacity.

Intraluminal pressure The pressure within the lumen of a viscus.

Ischemia Decreased blood supply to a body organ or tissue.

Lesion A visible or local abnormality that may be described as benign or cancerous.

Metastasis Tumor cell migration to local or distant parts of the body.

Mucositis Inflammation of a mucous membrane.

Neck dissection Removal of lymphoid tissue from the ramus of the jaw down to the clavicle; it usually includes the internal jugular vein and deep cervical fat pad.

Necrosis Tissue death in individual cells, groups of cells, or in localized areas.

Neoplasm Any new and abnormal growth.

Nonocclusive A dressing applied in a fashion that is not too tight or constrictive.

Odontophagia Pain when chewing.

Pulmonary toilet Tracheobronchial hygiene; i.e., coughing, deep breathing, suctioning.

Purulence Consisting of or containing pus.

depression in head and neck cancer patients [5]. This relationship seems especially valid for patients with advanced and long-term disease.

DISFIGUREMENT

Several studies have established the impact and stigma associated with disfigurement [6]. Facial defects have consequences not only for others but also for self-perception. Even persons who suffer from relatively mild facial defects related to aging may experience psychological and social changes [7]. A face altered drastically by surgery or radiation is devastating.

Disfigurement or body image subversion is a powerful force. Changes in appearance, eating, breathing, or communication in the head and neck cancer patient have direct psychological effects. To counteract these changes, patient care emphasizes maintenance of self-esteem and independence (see Chapter 18). There is a need to provide ego support techniques, enhance identifiable strengths, and downplay weaknesses. Changes in eating patterns and the impact on table etiquette also lead to profound psychological pressures. Patients with head and neck cancer are maintained initially with tube feedings. The alteration in body function associated with feeding tubes produces embarrassment and withdrawal. Care is focused on feeding tube acceptance by the family and patient participation in the feeding process (see Chapters 18, 21 and 25). Changes in breathing (e.g., tracheotomy, tracheostomy) also lead to profound hypersensitivity. Patience and understanding are a must; again, family participation is very helpful.

Anticipated changes in communication are discussed preoperatively, and expected limitations are analyzed. Alternative methods of communication are suggested after surgery. In addition, it is very helpful to establish the patient's level of literacy. If the patient is illiterate, audiovisual communication methods such as pictures or charts are used. Failure to maintain communication results in postoperative isolation and ultimately depression. All avenues are explored including esophageal speech, electrolarynx, and so on. A speech therapy consultation is mandatory in the appropriate patient (see Chapters 25 and 26). Equally important is an audiologic evaluation to determine if the patient hears at an acceptable level. If these four areas (appearance, eating, breathing, and communication) are addressed openly, the impact and effects of disfigurement are minimized [8].

PHYSICAL LOSSES

Physical change or loss is associated intimately with depression. In this section, physical losses are analyzed in regard to the primary sites of head and neck cancer (Tables 19-2 and 19-3).

Vision (Sites 1 and 2)

If improperly prepared, the patient's initial reaction to blindness is immobility and expressionless depression. He becomes preoccupied with the fear of total dependency and loss of freedom. This period of shock and grief is normal. Assuming the shock dissipates, the patient usually becomes concerned with the possible social and economic impact. The goal of rehabilitation of the visually impaired or the blind is the restoration of independence and social reintegration.

Fortunately, total blindness is rare in head and neck cancer, and the loss of vision in one eye is relatively easy to accept.

Taste (Sites 1–7)

There are few clinical investigations regarding the impact of dysgeusia; however, an astute head and neck oncologist observes significant anorexia as the result of "food not tasting the same." Radiation has a direct effect on the salivary glands and taste buds as the patient undergoes fractionation. After irradiation, taste usually returns almost to normal. If partial glossectomy or palatectomy is planned, the end organs of taste are affected directly.

Hearing (Sites 1 and 2)

Whereas blindness is defined as less vision than 20/200, deafness is defined more nebulously. However, hearing losses greater than 70 or 80 decibels generally are accepted as profound. Most patients accept this handicap with stoicism

Table 19-2. **Physical and psychological changes versus site***

Site	*Vision*	*Taste*	*Hearing*	*Smell*	*Communication*	*Swallowing*	*Breathing*	*Eating*	*Disfigurement*	*Change in libido*
1. Nasopharynx	++	++	+++	+++	–	–	+/–	–	–	–
2. Sinuses/nose	+++	++	+/–	+++	+/–	–	+/–	–	+/–	–
3. Salivary glands	–	+	–	+	–	–	–	–	–	–
4. Lips	–	–	–	–	++	–	–	+	++	++
5. Oral cavity	–	++	–	–	+++	++	+/–	+++	++	+/–
6. Oropharynx	–	++	–	–	+++	++	+/–	+++	++	+/–
7. Hypopharynx	–	–	–	–	++	+++	++	+++	+/–	+/–
8. Larynx	–	–	–	–	+++	+	++	+	+/–	++
9. Thyroid/parathyroid	–	–	–	–	+/–	–	+	+/–	+/–	–
10. Esophagus (cervical)	–	–	–	–	+	+++	++	+++	+/–	+/–

\+ Possible.
++ Probable.
+++ Likely.
+/– Equivocal.
– Unlikely.
* The impact is dependent on stage and treatment plan.

Table 19-3. Illness versus changes

Physical changes
- Disfigurement
- Dysphonia/aphonia
- Tracheostomy/tracheotomy
- Eating
- Weight loss
- Feeding tube

Psychological
- Self-esteem
- Dignity
- Daily routine
- Impotence and sexual disinterest

Social changes
- Vocation and profession
- Finances
- Interpersonal relationships

and ultimately adapt. Partial loss in the adult has little effect on language or communication and does not result in major economic or social upheaval. Generally, a good outcome is achieved with supportive therapy and appropriate rehabilitative measures (see Chapter 27 and 28).

Smell (Sites 1, 2, and 8)

Few physicians consider the impact of anosomia on head and neck cancer patients. For example, a patient with a craniofacial resection has the olfactory nerves destroyed directly, while a patient undergoing total laryngectomy will be unable to inhale, thus indirectly affecting smell. Together, the two senses, taste and smell, give foods nuance and flavor. Nasogastric feedings totally bypass taste and smell—another impediment in the management of anorexia and nutrition.

Scars (Sites 4–6)

With surgery, scarring is always a concern. Early in the planning stage, the attending surgeon openly discusses this possibility with the patient (see Chapter 7). The proposed incisions are outlined, with every effort made to disguise their placement. Although adding considerable time to ablative surgery, the advantage of simultaneous reconstruction is the immediate restoration of form and function (see Chapter 22). To minimize scarring, everyone on the surgical team should be as aware of cosmesis as well as ablation.

Sexuality (Site 4 and 8)

A physical change in sexuality rarely is discussed in the head and neck oncology literature. However, the questioning of patients, especially men, results in some unpleasant surprises. For example, partial or total laryngectomy eliminates the Valsalva maneuver and breath control, important components of male sexual control. Frank interviews with men after head and neck cancer surgery reveal a high incidence of postoperative impotence. The origins usually are psychological. The effects of actual or perceived disfigurement drastically affect sexuality. The presence of scars, altered speech, and a tracheotomy have an accumulative effect on sexuality. In time, with support from family and loved ones, the patient can return to normal function. If uncorrected, chronic sexual dysfunction undermines self-esteem, self-confidence, and self-image.

DEATH AND DYING

A review of cancer psychology is incomplete without discussing death and dying. Despite our best efforts, approximately one-third of all head and neck cancer patients die within months of their diagnosis. Unfortunately, the experienced and perceptive oncologist often can predict this fate after the initial examination and diagnosis. Therefore, many patients are prepared to ultimately succumb to their illness [9–12]. The following are presented merely as guidelines when discussing death or dying:

1. If the patient does not volunteer the question, do not broach the subject.
2. If the patient asks, explain the prognosis, but maintain hope throughout the discussion.
3. Ethical dilemmas are anticipated in patients with terminal stage III and IV cancers (see Chapter 7).
4. If the patient is suicidal, honesty is tempered with pragmatism.
5. Frank discussions include both patient and family; only in rare instances should either not be informed.
6. Family discussions are not conducted without patient approval.
7. The possibility of hospice care, home or hospital based, is an invaluable and viable alternative.
8. In the terminal stage of disease, do not withhold any reasonable medical therapy—even high doses of addictive pain medication.
9. Palliative therapy and anything that eases the dying process are always considered.
10. Finally, do not withhold treatment without documented approval from the patient, family, or proxy (see Chapter 7).

MEDICAL MANAGEMENT

Anxiety

Anxiety is the unpleasant feeling of tension and apprehension. It is fear's first cousin. Whereas fear is an emotion focused on immediate danger, anxiety is the anticipation of future danger [13].

Anxiety is a common component of depression. Usually it subverts the accommodation to illness, and when persistent, it is a barrier between the patient and the physician. Resistance to anxiety varies with mental alertness, since it is influenced by waning powers of analysis and failing discrimination. Anxiety produces three basic changes: tension, disturbances of intellect, and autonomic visceral and endocrine changes.

Daily dosages of diazepam (Valium), 5 to 40 mg/day, or chlordiazepoxide (Librium), 15 to 100 mg/day, are usually adequate treatment for anxiety. Addiction and potentiation with sedatives are the main side effects.

Insomnia

Insomnia is a classic component of the depression triad. Tranquilizers may suffice as sedatives. However, the following medications induce a more natural sleep: flurazepam hydrochloride (Dalmane), 15 to 30 mg; triazolam (Halcion), 0.125 to 0.5 mg; and chloral hydrate,

500 to 1000 mg. These drugs are supervised carefully in view of the risk of overdose and drug dependency.

Depression

If the depression evolves into actual withdrawal, the patient requires psychiatric intervention and antidepressants (Tables 19-4 and 19-5) [4]. Most medications require at least 3 weeks before attaining a therapeutic effect.

The following tricyclic antidepressants are suggested: imipramine (Tofranil), 75 to 250 mg/day, or amitriptyline (Elavil), 50 to 200 mg/day. The major side effects are xerostomia, a skin rash, and motor weakness. The most potent side effects of the tricyclic antidepressants are anticholinergic complications. Narrow-angle glaucoma, dry mouth, constipation, incontinence, and increased heart rate are potential side effects. Tricyclic antidepressants should be prescribed with caution for patients on medications for hypertension and prostate disorders.

In many instances, dosage reduction or substitution of an alternative antidepressant, such as the monoamine oxidase inhibitors, is recommended. However, the alternatives also are not problem-free.

Table 19-5. Treatment of tricyclic side effects

Side effect	*Treatment*
Sedation	After waiting 3 days, decrease dosage or change medication if sedation persists
Dry mouth	Lozenges; artificial saliva; peripheral cholinergics
Constipation	Fluids and roughage; stool softeners
Agitation	Decrease dosage or change medication
Tremor	Add propranolol (Inderal), 10–40 mg bid
Hypotension (orthostatic)	Change medication; elastic stockings; salt pills

Source. Data from Gelenberg AJ, Donaldson SR: Treating depression. A primer for the nonspecialist. *Med Times* 114 : 33, 1986.

PATIENT EDUCATION

There are several approaches to treating psychological conditions. The options depend on the premorbid personality, illness, interaction between individual and illness, personality traits, and available support systems. By and large, psychotherapy is (1) exploration of resources, (2) growth of the self, (3) habit change, (4) change in concepts and values, and (5) insight and emotional reorganization. With these perspectives, psychotherapy for the oncologic patient is merely adaptation of traditional psychiatric problem-solving.

Ventilation

The devastating psychological effects of head and neck cancer are overcome if the health team

Table 19-4. Tricyclic antidepressants

Drug		*Side effects*			
Generic name	*Brand name*	*Sedation*	*Anticholinergia*	*Hypotension*	*Stimulation*
Amitriptyline	Elavil	+ +	+ + +	+ +	+
Desipramine	Pertofrane	+ +	+	+	+ + +
Doxepin	Sinequan	+ + +	+ + +	+ +	0
Imipramine	Tofranil	+	+ +	+ + +	+ +
Nortriptyline	Aventyl	+	+	+	+ + +

\+ Mild.
\+ + Moderate.
\+ + + Pronounced.
Source. Data from Gelenberg AJ, Donaldson SR: Treating depression. A primer for the nonspecialist. *Med Times* 114 : 33, 1986.

recognizes the various psychological forces. Patient education begins at the time of diagnosis and planning. Patients' fears are anticipated, and they are allowed to express these fears. They are confronted with the fear of disfigurement, grief, and so on. Once confronted, most patients overcome their fears. Patients are encouraged to express their concerns, no matter how trivial they seem. A patient education program addresses the following four psychosocial needs: open communication, information, honesty, and hope.

Family Counseling

Family counseling is very helpful. The family is involved, and time is allotted for their verbalization of fears and expectations associated with the illness. All assistance is given to both patients and family. It is essential that everyone comes to terms with the anticipated changes. Uncertainty about the future and treatment is discussed openly. The facts are presented, and fantasies are dispelled. The anxiety associated with head and neck cancer, be it real or irrational, is recognized and controlled. The anticipated changes in regard to economic status and the patient's role in life are clarified. Patients may become hostile, egocentric, or hypochondriacal, but these reactions are expected and usually temporary. Recognition and understanding of the psychological forces are essential first steps toward rehabilitation. For everyone, the treatment of head and neck cancer creates great emotional demands. Moreover, the distinction between curing and caring assumes concern beyond mere eradication of the disease.

REFERENCES

1. Price JH, et al: Black American's perceptions of cancer: A study utilizing the health belief model. *J Nat Med Assoc* 80 : 1297, 1988.
2. Selye H: *The Stress of Life*. New York: McGraw-Hill, 1948.
3. Hart K: Stress encountered by significant others of cancer patients receiving chemotherapy. *J Death Dying* 17(2) : 151, 1987.
4. Gelenberg AJ, Donaldson SR: Treating depression: A primer for the nonspecialist. *Med Times* 114 : 33, 1986.
5. Westin T, et al: Mental depression and its association with malnutrition in patients with head and neck cancer. *Arch Otol Head Neck Surg* 114 : 1449, 1988.
6. Goffman E: *Stigma: Notes on the Management of Spoiled Identity*. Englewood Cliffs, NJ: Prentice Hall, 1963.
7. Graham JA, Kligman AM: Cosmetic therapy for the patient with facial disfigurement. *Ear Nose Throat J* 66 : 4, 1987.
8. Gates GA: Current Status of Laryngectomee Rehabilitation. In Chretien Johns ME, et al (eds): *Head and Neck Cancer*. Philadelphia: Decker, 1985. Pp 513–516.
9. Brown JG, et al: Nursing Management of the Patient with Total En Bloc Resection of the Temporal Bone. *J Neurosurg Nurs* (G) : 349, 1986.
10. Conley J: The meaning of life-threatening disease in the area of the head and neck. *Acta Otolaryngol* 99 : 201, 1985.
11. Simmons RC and Pardes H: *Understanding Human Behavior in Health and Illness* (2nd ed). Baltimore: Williams & Wilkins, 1981.
12. Schoenberg B, et al: *Loss and Grief: Psychological Management in Medical Practice*. New York: Columbia University Press, 1970.
13. Miller JF: *Coping with Chronic Illness: Overcoming Powerlessness*. Philadelphia: Davis, 1983.

20

Pain

ERNEST M. MYERS

KEY CONCEPTS

Pain Theory; Anatomy and Physiology; Pain Regimens; Morphine Receptors; Morphine Pump

MILESTONES

1500–2000 B.C.	Opium	Assyria
200 B.C.	Hashish	India
1803	Morphine	Serturner
1853	Hypodermic Needle	Pravaz
1860	Cocaine	Neimann
1898	Heroin	Germany

Pain is the unpleasant sensation evoked by noxious stimuli from injured or threatened tissue damage. It is described as prickly, stabbing, tearing, stinging, burning, or throbbing. Cancer causes pain by invasion, pressure, inflammation, traction, and muscle spasms.

Pain control is an important component of head and neck cancer rehabilitation. In all phases of head and neck oncology (diagnosis, treatment, or rehabilitation), patient well-being is affected detrimentally by poor pain control. Although pain intensity varies according to age, sex, culture, and personality, uncontrolled pain emotionally incapacitates and psychologically deteriorates. Fortunately, pain is minimal in the early stages of head and neck cancer. However, as the disease progresses to involve the deep cervical musculature or skull base, pain management becomes crucial. Finally, for the terminally ill, the only solice is pain control.

BASIC ANATOMY AND PHYSIOLOGY

Pain, originating from a complex pattern of stimuli generated at the pain site, is transmitted to the brain by a series of pathways [1]. Its perception in the subcortical or cortical level is the result of many different inputs that are modulated by the psyche and the physical (Figure 20-1).

Spinal Cord

The physiologic basis for pain is the dorsal root ganglion in the spinal cord. At this level, pain is an intimate component of the avoidance reflex. Basically, nociception is conveyed centrally by group III and IV afferent peripheral fibers. In fast pain, short, well-localized nociception is conveyed by group III afferent fibers. In slow pain, throbbing, burning, or aching is conveyed by group IV afferent fibers.

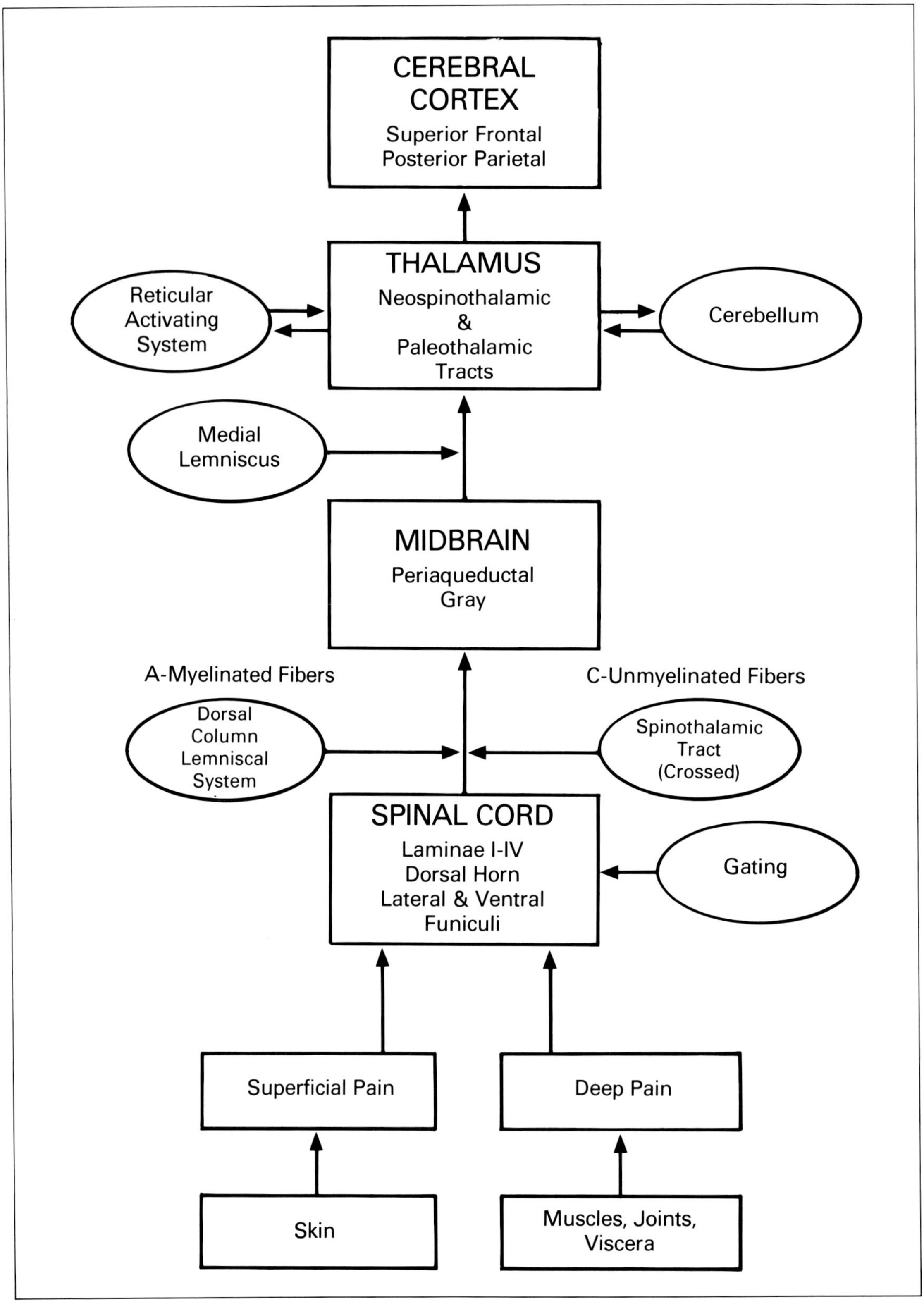

Figure 20-2. Basic neuroanatomy of pain.

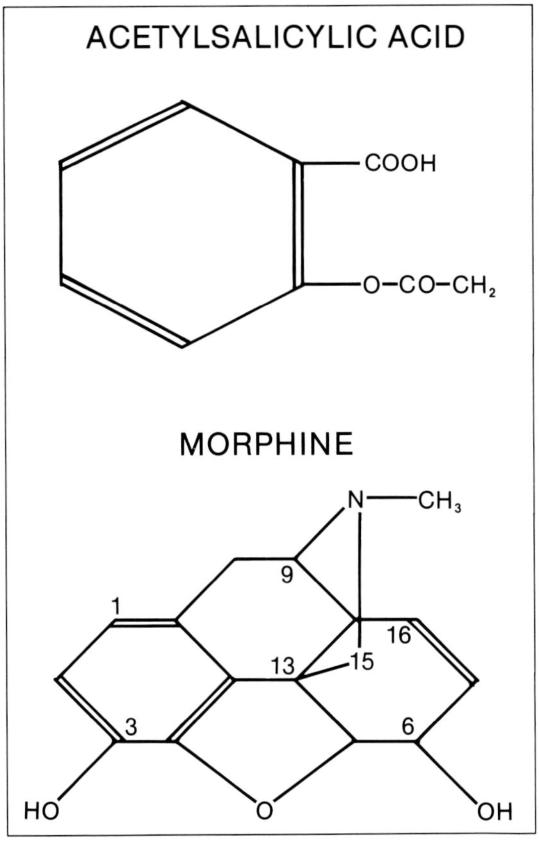

Figure 20-3. Chemistry of acetylsalicylic acid and morphine.

3. Mechanism of action: centrally, on the hypothalamus; peripherally, inhibition of prostaglandins.
4. Systemic effects:
   a. CNS: analgesia and antipyresis.
   b. Cardiovascular: prolonged bleeding time (large doses).
   c. Gastrointestinal: nausea and vomiting; gastritis.
   d. Anti-inflammation.
5. Derivatives: salicylic acid, methysalicylate.

Morphine

Morphine is administered for moderate to severe pain.

1. Origin: unripe seed capsules of *Papaver somniferum* (opium poppies).
2. Chemistry: alkaloids, phenanthrene (Fig. 20-3).
   a. Phenanthrene nucleus (three rings, A, B, C).
   b. Piperidine ring with tertiary amine nitrogen at C-9 and C-13 to C-16.
   c. Modifications: any change of three or six hydroxyl groups alters the pharmacologic activity; changes in the substituent on the nitrogen also change activity.
3. Mechanism of action: analgesia is largely secondary to cerebral, calming effects; it also stimulates endogenous endorphine receptors.
4. Systemic effects
   a. Central nervous system: sedation, nausea, vomiting.
   b. Autonomic: decreases acetylcholine; increases epinephrine.
   c. Respiratory: depression.
   d. Cardiovascular: hypotension.
   e. Gastrointestinal: constipation
   f. Genitourinary: increased antidiuretic hormone resulting in decreased urine production.
5. Derivatives
   a. Semisynthetics: heroin, hydromorphone, codeine.
   b. Synthetics: meperidine, methadone, propoxyphene.

MANAGEMENT

Each patient's needs and pain thresholds differ. Protocol management is discouraged; every patient must have an individual pain regimen (Table 20-2) [6,7]. Due to the complexity of pain, the first step is a clear understanding of the patient's entire problem. This requires a complete patient evaluation followed by appropriate analgesia. Throughout treatment, this regimen must be reassessed constantly and modified when indicated.

The two objectives of pain control are suppression and clear mentation. Narcotics are avoided until the pain becomes too intense. Once pain becomes intractable or chronic, the best control is round-the-clock narcotics given before the pain is perceived.

Table 20-2. Suggested pain regimens

Generic name	Brand name	Dosage: Oral	Dosage: IM	Dosage: Other	Advantages	Disadvantages
Aspirin	Bayer St. Joseph	650 mg	N/A	Suppository	Cost-effective Available Bone pain	Gastritis Masks fevers
Acetaminophen	Tylenol	650 mg	N/A	Suppository	Cost-effective Available	Hypersensitivity Nausea Vomiting Gastritis
Acetaminophen with codeine	Tylenol #3 Tylenol #4	30 mg 60 mg	N/A	Elixir	Cost-effective Available	Hypersensitivity Nausea Vomiting Constipation Habituation
Oxycodone with aspirin	Percodan	1–2 tablets q4h	N/A	N/A	Cost-effective Available	Codeine sensitivity Habituation
Oxycodone with acetaminophen	Percocet	1–2 tablets q4h	N/A	N/A	Cost-effective Available	Codeine sensitivity Habituation
Methadone	N/A	20 mg q4h	8–10 mg q4h	N/A	Oral absorption	} Availability Constipation
Morphine sulfate	Roxanol	20–30 mg q4h	10 mg q4h	N/A	Drug of choice for chronic pain	Hypersensitivity Respiratory depression
Hydromorphone hydrochloride	Dilaudid	7.5 mg q4h	1.5 mg q4h	2–4 mg q4h	High oral absorption	CNS irritability Cough suppression
Meperidine hydrochloride	Demerol	300 mg q2–3 h	80–100 mg q2–3 h	Elixir Suppository q2–3 h	High oral absorption	Seizures Aggravation of intracranial pressure Habituation }

General Measures

Abscess drainage and appropriate antibiosis eliminate many causes of pain. If inflammation or infection is under control, many pain sources can be eliminated or attenuated. Vigorous but gentle oral hygiene is emphasized to discourage mucositis. Adequate intake and hydration also are important for maximal overall comfort.

Pharmacology

Psychotropic Medication

Phenothiazine tranquilizers and tricyclic antidepressants are important analgesia adjuncts (see Chapter 19). These drugs interact with brain neurotransmitters, notably serotonin and dopamine, to alter pain perception by producing a form of "depersonalization" or disassociation. Phenothiazines and haloperidol are used in low doses or in combination with tricyclics. These neuroleptics are administered carefully, since they are associated with a number of side effects, notably extrapyramidal complications.

Aspirin

Aspirin is the non-narcotic analgesic of choice for cancer pain [7]. Effective and readily available, alone or in combination with other medications, aspirin is used in the early stages of head and neck cancer. Aspirin is also invaluable for the management of bony metastasis, a common cause of intractable chronic pain. Bony metastases produce prostaglandins, resulting in osteolysis and lowered peripheral pain thresholds by sensitizing nerve endings. Aspirin and other anti-inflammatory agents (indomethacin and phenylbutazone) suppress prostaglandins and improve pain control.

Narcotics

A review of Table 20-2 clearly reveals the importance of narcotics for pain control. Narcotic usage requires an understanding of side effects. Empiric titration must be balanced with regard to incapacitating side effects.

Surgery

In a select group of patients, the surgical management of intractable pain is very rewarding [8,9]. Morphine receptors in the substantia gelatinosa are of major importance in pain control. These receptors moderate pain when saturated by morphine, epidurally or intrathecally.

Patient Selection

Despite being on high dosages of narcotics, patients who fail to respond to transcutaneous electrical nerve stimulation (TENS), chemotherapy, or radiotherapy are considered candidates for surgical management of pain (Figure 20-4). Morphine infusions are successful and less risky than rhizotomy and cordotomy.

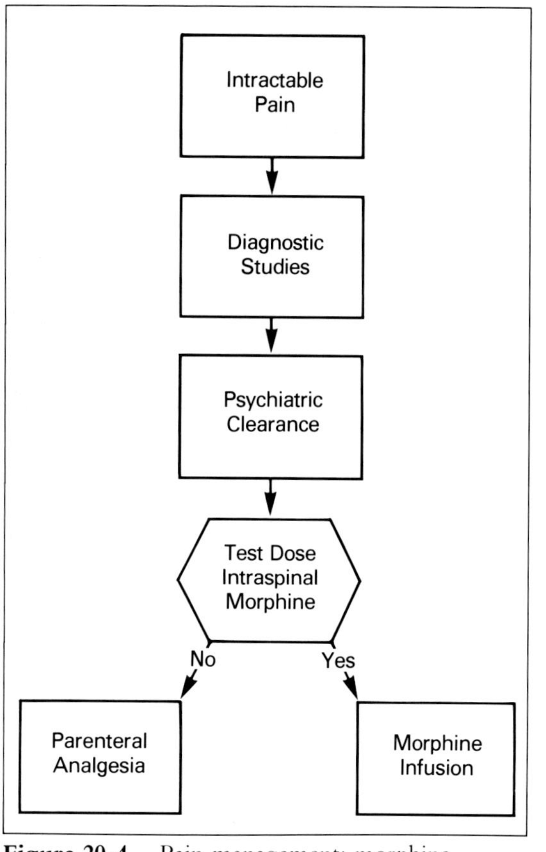

Figure 20-4. Pain management: morphine pump. (Adapted from Dennis GC, Dewitty RM: Management of intractable pain in cancer patients by implantable morphine infusion systems. *J Natl Med Assoc* 79 : 9, 1987.)

Operative Approach

A subcutaneous pocket is formed in the paramedian midabdomen for the pump insertion (Figure 20-5). A second, longitudinal incision between L2 and L5 is carried down to the lumbar fascia. A 14-gauge Thomy needle introduces a Cordis lumbar catheter into the subarachnoid space. The catheter is advanced for optimal placement and connected to the pump through a subcutaneous tunnel (flank incision). The entire procedure is performed under general or local anesthesia.

Advantages

Low-dose, round-the-clock morphine infusion allows 70 to 80 percent of the patients to be ambulatory and free of parenteral injection. Cerebrospinal morphine concentrations are much higher than plasma concentrations. Administering morphine intrathecally prolongs its effectiveness and reduces analgesia requirements. The net result is decreased drug intolerance with lower plasma concentrations. Intrathecal morphine decreases side effects and immeasurably improves the quality of life. The pump automatically administers the drug around the clock, thus controlling pain before it is consciously experienced. Since the pump reservoir is filled every 2 to 3 weeks, the patient is mobile and resumes normal activities. Finally, the improvement in overall morale is tremendous.

SUMMARY

Most head and neck pain is relieved by a combination of physiotherapy and pharmacology. It is important to know the patient's personality and reaction to pain. The patient is followed closely in regard to infection, hydration, and other conditions that decrease pain threshold.

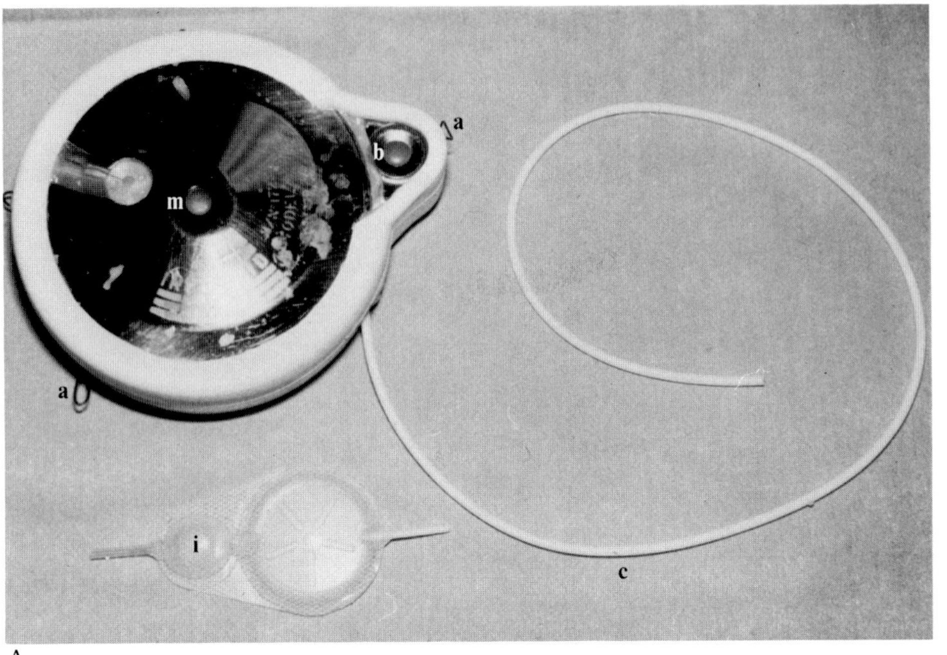

A

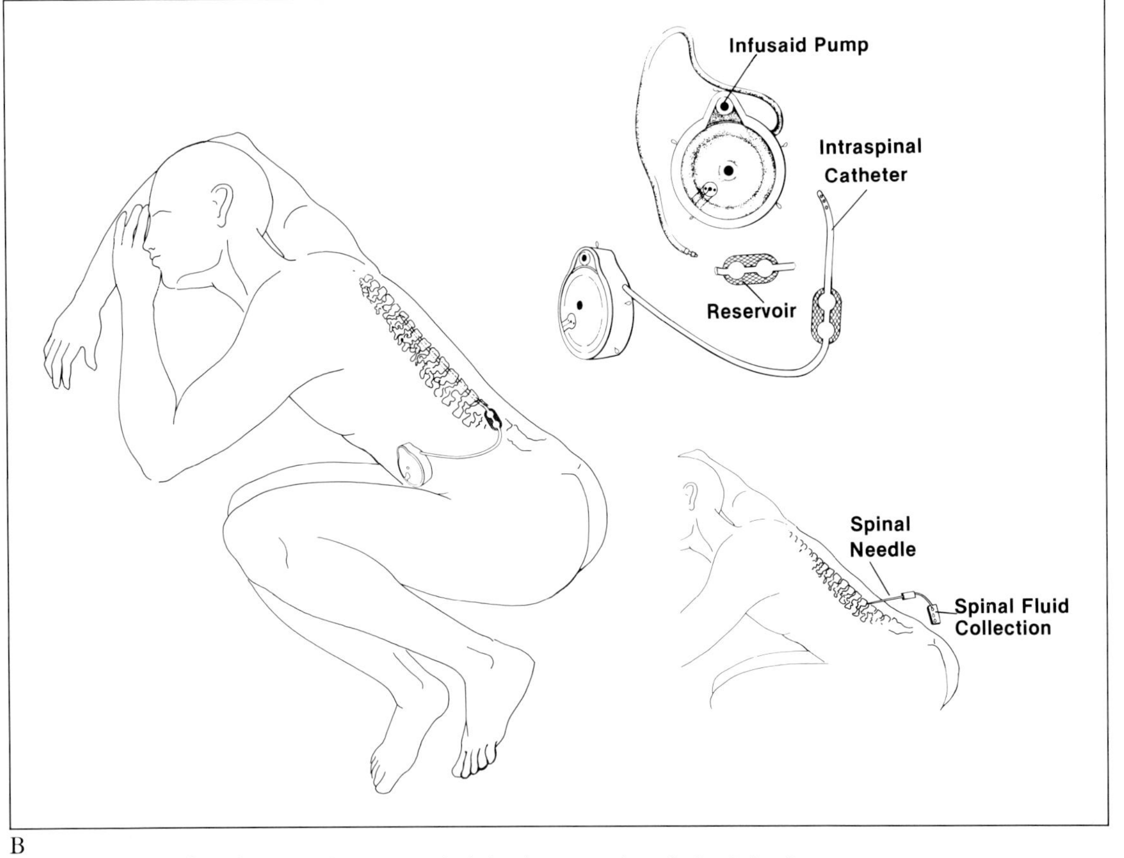

B

Figure 20-5. Infusaid pump. A. *m* = main injection port; *b* = bolus injection port; *a* = anchor wires; *c* = catheter; *i* = inspection reservoir. B. Abdominal-lumbar implantation.

Pain management is a dynamic process with analgesia requirements changing over time. Aspirin is the drug of choice. If aspirin is ineffective or not tolerated, several regimens including narcotics are available. Finally, if routine pharmacologic control is poor, the morphine pump is very effective.

REFERENCES

1. Nauta WJH: Anatomical organization of pain pathways in the central nervous system. In Synder SH, Matthysse S (eds): Opiate Reception Mechanisms. *Neurosc Res Program Bull* 13 : 84, 1975.
2. Melzack R, Wall RD: Pain mechanism: A new theory. *Science* 150 : 971, 1965.
3. Yaksh TL, Reddy SVR: Studies in the primate on the analgetic effects associated with intrathecal actions of opiates, adrenergic agonist and baclofen. *Anesthesiology* 54 : 451, 1981.
4. Catalano RB: The medical approach to the management of pain caused by cancer. *Semin Oncol* 2 : 379, 1975.
5. Shimm DS, et al: Medical management of chronic cancer pain. *JAMA* 241 : 2408, 1979.
6. Boop WC, Fisher JA: Methods of Pain Control. In EN Myers, JY Sueu (eds): *Cancer of the Head and Neck.* New York: Churchill Livingstone, 1981. Pp 821.
7. Tuttle CB: Drug management of pain in cancer patients. *J Can Med Assoc* 132 : 121, 1985.
8. Dennis GC, DeWitty RM: Management of intractable pain in cancer patients by implantable morphine infusion systems. *J Natl Med Assoc* 79 : 9, 1987.
9. Dennis GC, DeWitty RL: Longterm intraventricular infusion of morphine for intractable pain in cancer of the head and neck. *Neurosurgery* 26 : 404, 1990.

21

Nutrition

HAILE MEZGHEBE and S. M. SIRAM

KEY CONCEPTS

Nutritional Assessment; Enteral Feedings; Total Parenteral Nutrition; Complications

MILESTONES

2000 B.C.	Nutrient Enemas	Egypt
1793	First Enteral Feeding	Hunter
1843	Sugar, Milk, and Egg White Solutions	Bernard
1867	Flexible Orogastric Tube	Kussmani
1870	Asepsis	Lister
1877	Bacteria and Infection	Pasteur
1887	Intravenous Glucose Solutions	Landerer
1891	Intravenous Saline Solutions	Matas
1984	Rubber Feeding Tube	Holt
1904	Casein Hydrolysates (Animals)	Aberhalden, Roma, Funk
1912	Vitamins	Funk
1915	Intravenous Fat Emulsions (Animals)	Murlin, Riche
1918	Jejunostomy Tube	Anderson
1920	Intravenous Fat Emulsions (Humans)	Yamakawa
1932	Urine Nitrogen Loss	Cuthbertson
1939	Intravenous Casein Hydrolysates (Humans)	Elman
1940	Crystalline Amino Acids	Shohl, Blackfan
1947	Nitrogen Balance	Riegel, Rhoades
1952	Subclavian Catheterization	Aubaniac
1969	Chemical Defined Diets	Stephens, Randall
1973	Total Parenteral Nutrition	Dudrick
1977	Nutritional Assessment	Blackburn

Although most patients can tolerate brief periods of catabolism, some are affected more adversely than others. Malnutrition in hospitalized patients is estimated to be as high as 50 percent [1–3]. Some patients enter the hospital malnourished, while others become catabolic after admission due to surgery, sepsis, or both. The major determinants of hospital-acquired malnutrition are the severity of stress and the degree of dietary restriction. Deteriorating nutritional status is associated with increased morbidity, mortality, and prolonged hospitalization [4].

Carbohydrates, proteins, and fats are the three sources of energy [5]. Carbohydrate is stored in the liver and skeletal muscle as glycogen; total glycogen stores can be depleted in less than 24 hours. Protein is a larger source of fuel, but when depleted during stress it adversely affects essential functions, such as enzymes, visceral organs, and the musculoskeletal system. Fat, the most efficient and largest source of energy, provides the most amount of calories per gram of tissue. When diet is inadequate, fuel is obtained primarily from fat, but with stress, sepsis, or starvation as components, protein loss is accelerated.

NUTRITIONAL ASSESSMENT

A nutritional assessment identifies deficits that adversely affect therapy (Table 2-1) [6–8]. Ideally, each patient is evaluated by a nutritional team that consists of a dietician, nurse, pharmacist, and physician (Figure 21-1). A nutritional history includes weight change, quality and quantity of food intake, level of appetite, and food intolerance. The patient's initial height and weight are measured and recorded (Table 21-2 and Figure 21-2). Established standard protocols and the team approach reduce complications and cost. This leads to improved care [9,10].

Nutritional Requirements

The standard intravenous solution in most hospitals is 5% dextrose and water. This totals less than 200 kcal/liter, although the average nonstressed adult requires about 1800 kcal/day or greater. A patient solely on 5% dextrose solutions develops progressive caloric debt, mobilization of fuel reserves, and the breakdown of essential body proteins.

Energy expenditure can be estimated using the Harris-Benedict formula:

$$\text{BEE} = \text{Basal Energy Expenditure}$$

$$\text{BEE (males)} = 66.5 + (13.7 \times W) + (5.0 \times H) - (6.7 \times A)$$

$$\text{BEE (females)} = 65.5 + (9.5 \times W) + (1.8 \times H) - (4.7 \times A)$$

where
W = Weight in kg
H = Height in cm
A = age in years

Table 21-1. Nutritional assessment

	Good	*Fair*	*Poor*
Weight (% of ideal)	90–100	80–90	<80
Triceps skinfold (mm)			
Men	>9–24	6–8	<6
Women	>24–36	11–23	<11
Mid-forearm circumference (cm)			
Men	>30	26–29	<26
Women	>29	25–28	<25
Hemoglobin (gm %)			
Men	14–17	11–13	<11
Women	12–15	10–11	<10
Serum albumin (gm %)	3.5–4.5	3.0–3.4	<3.0
Serum transferrin (mg %)	>200	150–199	<150
Delayed hypersensitivity (mm induration)			
Mumps	>10	5–10	<5
PPD	>10	5–10	<5
Candida	>10	5–10	<5

Source: Adapted from Goodwin W J: Nutritional Management of Head and Neck Cancer. In Cummings C W, et al (eds): *Otolaryngology, Head and Neck Surgery*. St. Louis: Mosby, 1986. Vol I, pp 101–113.

DATE	TIME	☐ INITIAL	☐ FOLLOW-UP	SEE NOTE DATED _______

S: ____

O: DIAGNOSIS | AGE | SEX ☐ M ☐ F

☐ TPN ☐ ENTERAL ☐ DIET
ORDER

HT (cm)	ADM WT (kg)	PRESENT WT (kg)	USUAL WT (kg)	DESIRABLE BODY WT (kg)	%DESIRABLE BODY WT

RECENT WT CHG (kg) | %WT CHG ____________% | SIGNIFICANT? ☐ YES ☐ NO

TRICEPS SKINFOLD (mm) | %OF STD | MIDARM CIRC (cm) | %OF STD

MIDARM MUSCLE CIRCUMFERENCE (cm) | %OF STD | CREATININE – HEIGHT INDEX | %OF STD

FEEDING PROBLEMS ☐ NONE ☐ SORE MOUTH ☐ DYSPHAGIA ☐ POOR DENTITION ☐ OTHER__________

G.I. PROBLEMS ☐ NONE ☐ NAUSEA ☐ VOMITING ☐ DIARRHEA ☐ CONSTIPATION ☐ OTHER__________

FOOD ALLERGIES/ INTOLERANCES ☐ NONE LIST IF ANY:

VITAMIN/MINERAL SUPPLEMENTS ☐ NONE LIST IF ANY:

PERTINENT MEDICATIONS

PERTINENT LAB DATA

OTHER

A: ESTIMATED DAILY REQ'MTS __________ Kcal __________ gm Pro

☐ TPN ☐ ENTERAL ☐ DIET AS ORDERED PROVIDES _______ Kcal _______ gm Pro _______ ml H_2O | Additional H_2O Req'd __________ | UUN _______ (gm) | N bal _______

CURRENT DIETARY INTAKE (3 day Avg) ________ Kcal ________ gm Pro | Adequate to meet needs ☐ Yes ☐ No (See Below)

NUTRITIONAL STATUS ☐ Marasmus ☐ Kwashiorkor ☐ Marasmus-Kwashiorkor ☐ Not Compromised

	Degree of Depletion	Preserved	Unable to Assess
Visceral Protein Stores	☐mild ☐mod ☐severe	☐	☐
Somatic Protein Stores	☐mild ☐mod ☐severe	☐	☐
Fat Stores	☐mild ☐mod ☐severe	☐	☐

CODE: N/A – NOT AVAILABLE
N/R – NOT REQUIRED

(Cont'd on other side)

PATIENT'S IDENTIFICATION

Figure 21-1. Nutritional assessment form used by the Department of Nutrition and Food Service, Howard University Hospital, to evaluate nutritional status comprehensively.

Table 21-2. 1983 Metropolitan height and weight tables for adults*

				Small Frame		*Medium Frame*		*Large Frame*	
	Feet	*Inches*	*Cm*	*Pounds*	*Kilograms*	*Pounds*	*Kilograms*	*Pounds*	*Kilograms*
Men	5	1	154.9	128–134	58.2–60.9	131–141	59.5–64.1	138–150	62.7–68.2
(allow 5 lb for	5	2	157.5	130–136	59.1–61.8	133–143	60.4–65.0	140–153	63.6–69.5
indoor clothing)	5	3	160.0	132–138	60.0–62.7	135–145	61.4–65.9	142–156	64.5–70.9
	5	4	162.6	134–140	60.9–63.6	137–148	62.3–67.2	144–160	65.5–72.7
	5	5	165.1	136–142	61.8–64.5	139–151	63.2–68.6	146–165	66.4–74.5
	5	6	167.6	138–145	62.7–65.9	142–143	64.5–70.0	149–168	67.7–76.4
	5	7	170.2	140–148	63.6–67.2	145–157	65.9–71.4	152–172	69.1–78.2
	5	8	172.7	142–151	64.5–68.6	148–160	67.2–72.7	155–176	70.5–80.0
	5	9	175.3	144–154	65.5–70.0	151–153	68.6–74.1	158–180	71.8–81.8
	5	10	177.0	146–157	66.4–71.4	154–166	70.0–75.5	161–184	73.2–83.6
	5	11	180.3	149–160	67.7–72.7	157–170	71.4–77.3	164–188	74.5–85.5
	6	0	182.9	152–164	69.1–74.5	160–174	72.7–79.1	168–192	76.4–87.3
	6	1	185.4	155–168	70.5–76.4	164–178	74.5–80.9	172–197	78.2–89.5
	6	2	188.0	158–172	71.8–78.2	167–182	75.9–82.7	176–202	80.0–91.8
	6	3	190.5	162–176	73.6–80.0	171–187	77.7–85.0	181–207	82.3–94.1
Women	4	9	144.8	102–111	46.4–50.0	109–121	49.5–55.0	118–131	53.6–59.6
(allow 3 lb for	4	10	147.3	103–113	46.8–51.4	111–123	50.0–55.9	120–134	54.5–60.9
indoor clothing)	4	11	149.9	104–115	47.3–52.3	113–126	51.4–57.2	122–137	55.5–62.3
	5	0	152.4	106–118	48.2–53.6	115–129	52.3–58.6	125–140	56.8–63.6
	5	1	154.9	108–121	49.1–55.0	118–132	53.6–60.0	128–143	58.2–65.0
	5	2	157.5	111–124	50.5–56.4	121–135	55.0–61.4	131–147	59.5–66.8
	5	3	160.0	114–127	51.8–57.7	124–138	56.4–62.7	134–151	60.9–68.6
	5	4	162.6	117–130	53.2–59.0	127–141	57.7–64.1	137–155	62.3–70.5
	5	5	165.1	120–133	54.5–60.5	130–144	59.0–65.5	140–159	63.6–72.3
	5	6	167.6	123–136	55.9–61.8	133–147	60.5–66.8	146–167	66.4–75.9
	5	7	170.2	126–139	57.3–63.2	136–150	61.8–68.2	146–167	66.4–75.9
	5	8	172.7	129–142	58.6–64.5	139–153	63.2–69.5	149–170	67.7–77.3
	5	9	175.3	132–145	60.0–65.9	142–156	64.6–70.9	152–173	69.1–78.6
	5	10	177.8	135–148	61.4–67.3	145–159	65.9–72.3	155–176	70.5–80.0
	5	11	180.3	138–151	62.7–73.6	148–162	67.3–73.6	158–179	71.8–81.4

Source: Metropolitan Life Statistical Bulletin, Jan–June 1983, Build Study, 1974. Society of Actuaries and Association of Life Insurance, Medical Division of America.

*These tables correct the 1983 Metropolitan tables to height without shoe heels.

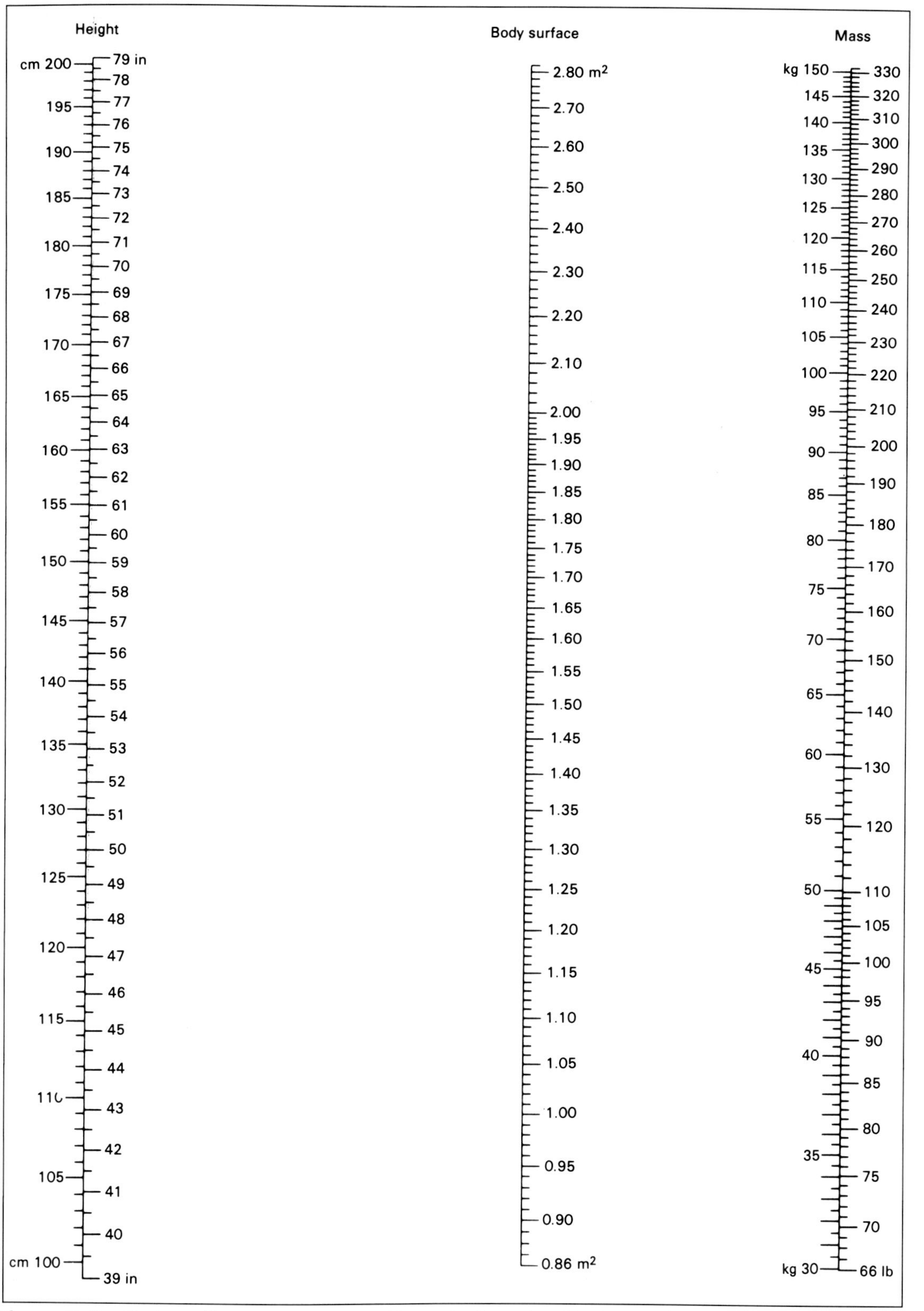

Figure 21-2. Body surface area nomogram. From the formula of DuBois and DuBois, *Arch Intern Med* 17 : 863, 1916: $S = W^{0.425} \times H^{0.725} \times 71.84$, or $\log S = \log W \times 0.425 + \log H \times 0.725 + 1.8564$ (S = body surface area in cm^2, W = weight in kg, H = height in cm).

$$\text{Total energy requirements (TER)} = \text{BEE} \times (\text{activity factor}) \times (\text{injury factor})$$

ACTIVITY FACTORS	INJURY STRESS FACTORS
Confined to bed: 1.2	Starvation: 0.7
Ambulatory: 1.3	Surgery: 1.1–1.2
	Trauma: 1.35–1.60
	Infection, mild: 1.2; moderate: 1.4
	Sepsis: 1.6–1.8

Body Weight

Weight loss is the most common measurement of malnutrition. Ten- to 15-percent loss over a period of 3 to 6 months is clinically significant. A 30-percent loss is associated with significant morbidity, and a 50-percent weight loss is generally incompatible with life.

Triceps Skinfold and Forearm Circumference

The triceps skinfold is an estimate of the fat reserves, whereas the mid-arm circumference estimates somatic protein reserves. Both measurements are obtained on the nondominant arm. These values are compared to a standard table.

Creatinine Height Index

The creatinine height index is a reliable measure of body mass present as active muscle [11]. An index deficit between 5 and 15 percent is mild, whereas 15 to 30 percent is considered moderate.

Immune Status

Failed delayed hypersensitivity reaction is associated with increased morbidity and mortality [12]. A multitest device, loaded with several different antigens, is applied on the forearm. Indurations greater than 5 mm are indicative of immune competency.

Nitrogen Balance

Determination of nitrogen balance is an effective and rapid means of measuring nutritional adequacy. In healthy individuals, anabolism and catabolism are in equilibrium and the nitrogen balance is zero. However, during catabolism (e.g., surgery, trauma, sepsis), protein turnover and losses increase. Unless adequate protein is provided, the patient goes into negative nitrogen balance. Nitrogen balance is calculated by subtracting nitrogen loss from nitrogen intake. Intake is derived by dividing the total protein intake in 24 hours by a factor of 6.25 (1 gm of nitrogen = 6.25 gm of protein). Loss is determined by measuring total urine urea nitrogen (UUN) in a 24-hour urine collection and adding a factor of 4 gm to account for the nonurea nitrogen losses [13].

Miscellaneous Parameters

Serum albumin, total protein, transferrin, retinol binding protein, prealbumin, and total lymphocyte count assess visceral body protein. Albumin's long half-life (20 days) limits its usefulness for acute nutritional assessment. Serum transferrin, with a shorter half-life (8–10 days) better reflects catabolism in the hospitalized patient. Normal values range from 200 to 400 mg/dl. Prealbumin has a half-life of less than 2 days, whereas retinol binding protein has a half-life of a few hours. Both studies are good reflections of acute protein changes; however, they are expensive and are not considered cost-effective for routine screening. Total lymphocyte count, obtained by multiplying white blood cells by the percentage of lymphocytes, is another useful method of nutritional assessment. A total lymphocyte count less than 1800 is abnormal.

ENTERAL FEEDING

Indications

Considerably cheaper, enteral feeding is the method of choice for the patient who has a functioning gastrointestinal tract (Tables 21-3 and 21-4; Figure 21-3) [14]. It includes oral and enterostomy feedings.

Advantages

Enteral nutrition has been shown to decrease hypermetabolism, cause fewer septic complications, maintain gut mucosal integrity, maintain immunologic function of the gut, and decrease biliary stasis. Enteral feedings also

Table 21-3. Enteral feeding indications

Enteral feeding indications
Nasogastric feeding
Head and neck surgery
Coma or altered mental status
Physical impairments:
Conditions affecting mastication (i.e., mandibular fracture, oral lesions, dental surgery)
Conditions affecting swallowing (i.e., obstructive lesions of the esophagus or pharynx, cerebrovascular accident)
Severe anorexia
Severe mental depression
Upper alimentary tract obstruction (i.e., hypopharynx, esophagus)
Hypermetabolism (i.e., major burns, hyperthyroidism, cancer, trauma, sepsis)
Orogastric feeding
Nasoseptal deviation
Nasopharyngeal malignancy
Maxillofacial trauma

Table 21-4. Enteral feeding contraindications

Enteral feeding contraindications
Absolute
Adynamic ileus
Intractable vomiting
Alimentary tract obstruction
Relative
Oral feedings are impractical
Diarrhea
Gastric distention

improve glucose tolerance and enhance nitrogen retention [15–18]. In addition, enteral feedings cause small-bowel villous growth with increased production of crypt cells and regeneration of absorptive epithelium. Food encourages pancreatic biliary secretions, and stimulates epithelial growth and regeneration. Finally, enteral nutrition has few complications.

Requirements

Enteral feeding requires careful selection of the most appropriate preparation for each patient.

Protein

Amino acids are derived from intact protein, hydrolyzed protein (mixture of amino acids and short peptides), or crystalline amino acids.

Intact Protein

Intact protein includes normal foodstuffs, protein isolates (casein), soybean protein or egg albumin. Complex or intact proteins are contraindicated for patients with pancreatic insufficiency or short-bowel syndrome.

Hydrolyzed Protein

Smaller peptide fragments and protein hydrolysates are used when there is reduced gastrointestinal absorptive surface area, such as in celiac sprue or short-bowel syndrome.

Crystalline Amino Acids

Pure crystalline amino acids, not requiring an intact gastrointestinal tract, are absorbed through an active transport mechanism. Amino acids significantly contribute to solution osmolarity. They also have an unpleasant bitter taste, which discourages oral use.

Carbohydrate

Forty-five to 50 percent of the calories in the American diet are derived from starch, sucrose, and lactose. Oligosaccharides are used extensively in place of simple sugars to reduce osmotic load. Approximately 50 percent of black and 10 percent of white patients have recurrent gastroenteritis from lactose deficiency. Milk-based formulas and many mixed food preparations contain significant amounts of lactose. A lactose-free preparation is substituted if nausea, distention, or diarrhea develops.

Fat

Composing 30 to 35 percent of the calories in the normal American diet, fat is mainly in the

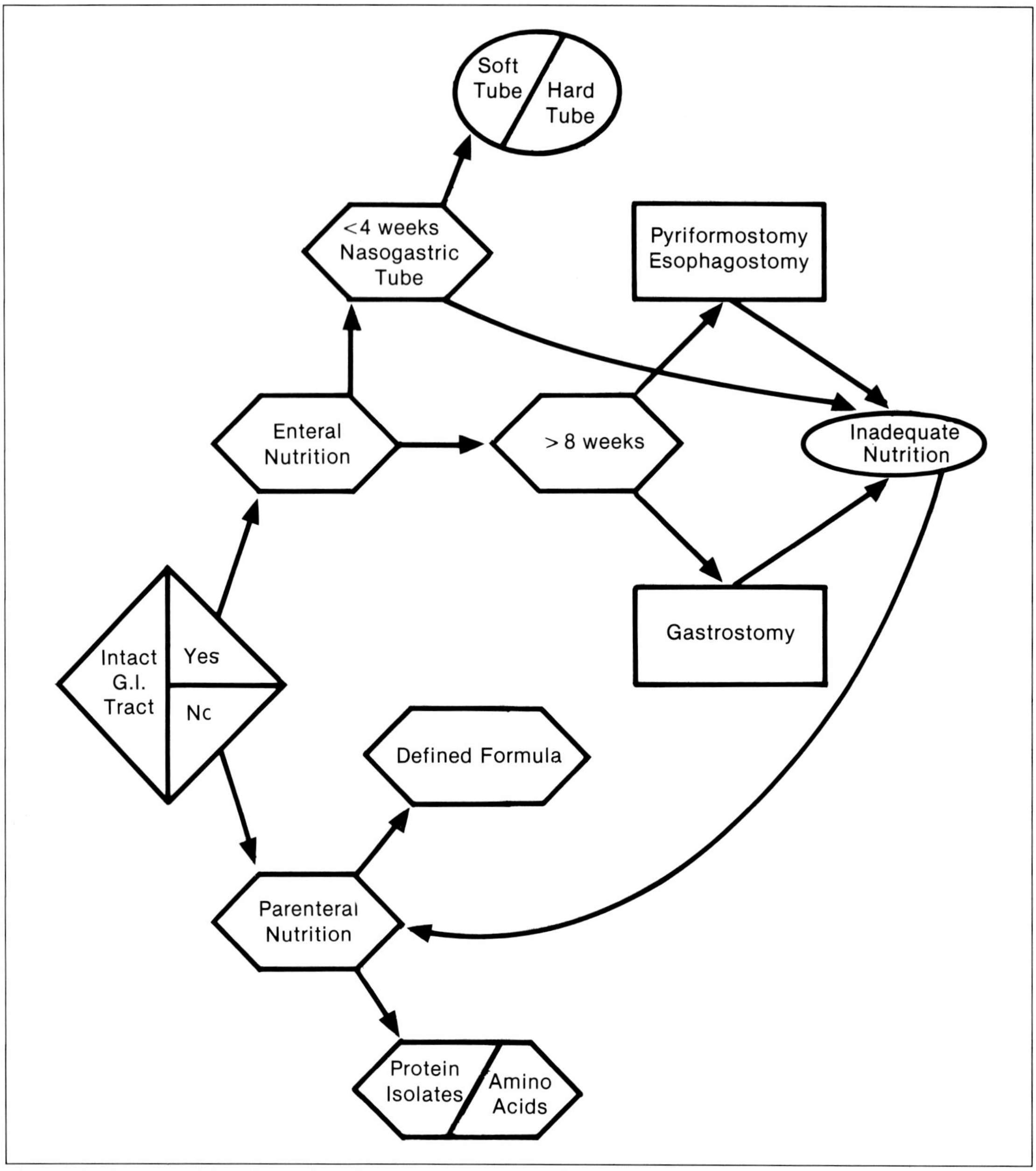

Figure 21-3. Nutrition dynamics. *G.I.* = gastrointestinal.

form of long-chain triglycerides. Fat is a palatable concentrated energy source (9 kcal/gm). Long-chain triglycerides need adequate intestinal surface area for digestion. Medium-chain triglycerides however, require little pancreatic lipase or bile salts for absorption. Medium-chain triglycerides are transported directly into the blood stream through the portal system, thus eliminating complex digestion and absorption. Triglycerides containing linoleic acid meet the essential fatty acid requirements.

Vitamins and Trace Elements
Nutritionally complete commercial formulas provide adequate vitamins and minerals.

Fiber
Some intact protein formulas derived from mixed food contain moderate amounts of fruit and vegetable fiber. The milk-based and lactose-free formulas are very low in fiber. Even a fiber-free diet does not eliminate stooling, since normal stool contains desquamated epithelial cells.

Fluids
Most full-strength formulas are 1 kcal/ml. When fluids are restricted, a higher caloric formula is indicated, such as Isocal HCN or Magnacal. The majority of preparations (1 kcal/ml) provide approximately 900 ml of water/liter. At least 50 to 100 ml of water/day is required to irrigate the feeding tube and prevent free water deficiency.

Preparations
The general categories of enteral preparations are milk-based, lactose-free, defined formulas, special formulas, and supplements (Tables 21-5 and 21-6).

General Formulas
Home blenderized and commercially prepared formulas can be nutritionally complete. A blenderized diet is appropriate for the patient with a functional intestinal tract. The advantages are availability, normal bowel movements, and reasonable cost. Poor passage through small feeding tubes and high viscosity can be troublesome. Compleat Modified is an example of a commercially available formula.

Table 21-5. Enteral feeding guidelines

1. The formula is determined after the nutritional assessment.
2. Containers and tubing are changed every 24 hours.
3. Opened feedings are refrigerated and discarded after 24 hours.
4. When intubated, nasal and oral hygiene is provided at least every 4 hours.
5. A blocked feeding tube is irrigated, flushed, or changed.
6. Infusion pumps are obligatory for continuous drip feedings.

Milk-Based Formulas
There is a wide variety of milk-based (lactose) products. Reasonable cost, palatability, and high nutritional value make these products acceptable. The principal disadvantages are related to gastrointestinal complaints due to lactose intolerance.

Lactose-Free Products
Lactose-free products are complete nutritionally, inexpensive, and regarded as ideal tube-feeding formulas. If flavored, these formulas may be suitable for oral use. Products in this category include Isocal, Osmolite, Ensure, and Isocal HCN. The calorie-dense formulas such as Isocal HCN require administration of free water to prevent hyperosmolar syndrome.

Defined Formulas
Virtually residue-free and requiring minimal digestion, defined formulas vary in their protein and fat contents. Those products with minimal fat contain crystalline amino acids and cause minimal pancreatic stimulation and biliary and small intestinal secretions. Such formulas are invaluable for managing gastrointestinal fistulae, pancreatitis, and radiation enteritis. The disadvantages are expense, high osmolality, and bitter taste. Feeding tube delivery rather than by mouth is appropriate for long-term feedings. Some examples are Vivonex Ten, Vivonex HN, and Criticare.

Special Formula Diets
Special formulas are designed for specific organ failure. Amin-Aid is formulated for patients with renal failure, and Hepatic-Aid is suggested for patients who have hepatic encephalopathy. Amin-Aid is a calorically dense supplement (2.0 cal/ml) containing little or no sodium and potassium. Hepatic-Aid, high in branched-chain amino acids and low in aromatic amino acids, helps minimize hepatic encephalopathy.

Table 21-6. Common enteral feedings

	General	*Milk-Based*		*Lactose-Free*				
	Compleat-B	***Meritene***	***Carnation Instant Breakfast***	***Sustacal***	***Isocal***	***Osmolite***	***Ensure***	***Ensure Plus***
Calories/cc	***1***	***1***	***1***	***1***	***1***	***1***	***1***	***1.5***
Carbohydrate source	Maltodextrin, lactose, sucrose	Lactose, corn syrup, sucrose	Sucrose, corn syrup, lactose	Sucrose, corn syrup	Glucose, oligosaccharides	Corn syrup	Corn syrup, sucrose	Corn syrup, sucrose
Protein source	Beef, skim milk, vegetable	Skim milk	Milk, sodium caseinate, soy protein isolate	Skim milk, calcium and sodium caseinates, and soy protein isolates	Calcium and sodium caseinate, soy protein isolate	Calcium and sodium caseinate, soy protein isolate	Sodium and calcium caseinate, soy protein isolate	Sodium and calcium caseinate, soy protein isolate
Fat source	Corn oil, beef fat	Corn oil	Whole milk	Partially hydrogenated soy oil	Soy oil, MCT oil	MCT oil, corn oil, soy oil	Corn oil	Corn oil
Protein (gm/liter)	40	60	58	60	34	35	37	55
Fat (gm/liter)	40	33	31	23	44	34	37	53
Carbohydrate (gm/liter)	120	115	135	138	130	138	145	197
mOsm/kg	390	550		625	300	300	450	600
Na/K (mEq/liter)	68/33	40/42	41/70	39/53	22/33	22/23	32/32	46/48
Residue	High	Med	Med	Low	low	low	low	low
Vitamin content	yes	yes	yes	yes	yes	yes	yes	yes
Producer	Doyle	Doyle	Carnation	Mead Johnson	Mead Johnson	Ross	Ross	Ross
Flavors	Natural flavor	Varied	Varied	Varied	Unflavored	Unflavored	Varied	Varied
Form	Ready to use	Ready to use	Powder	Ready to use	Ready to use	Ready to use	Ready to use	Ready to use
Uses/Features	Blenderized tube feeding, requires digestion and absorption	High protein supplemental tube feeding, requires digestion and absorption	Supplemental, easily available, requires digestion and absorption	High protein supplemental tube feeding, requires digestion and absorption	Tube feeding, requires digestion and absorption, low Na, lactose free	Supplemental tube feeding, lactose free, low Na, requires digestion and absorption	Supplemental tube feeding, lactose free, low Na, requires digestion and absorption	Supplemental tube feeding, lactose free, low Na, requires digestion and absorption

Source: Adapted from Steffee W P, Krey S H: Enteral hyperalimentation for patients with head and neck cancer. *Otolaryngol Clin North Am* 13(3):437, 1980.

Chemically defined formulas			*Elemental*		*Special formulas*		*Additives*		
Precision LR	***Precision HN***	***Flexical***	***Vivonex***	***Vivonex HN***	***Amin-Aid***	***Hepatic Aid***	***Microlipid***	***Polycose***	***Polycose***
1	***1***	***1***	***1***	***1***	***1.9***	***1.6***	***4.5***	***4 cal/gm***	***2 cal/cc***
Malto-dextrin, sucrose	Malto-dextrin, sucrose	Corn syrup, modified tapioca starch	Glucose, oligosaccharides	Glucose, oligosaccharides	Malto-dextrose, sucrose	Malto-dextrins, sucrose	—	Hydrolysis of corn starch	Hydrolysis of corn starch
Egg albumin	Egg albumin	Casein hydrolysate crystalline amino acids	L-Amino acids	L-Amino acids	Crystalline essential amino acids	Branch chain and aromatic amino acids	—	—	—
Soy oil	Soy oil	Soy oil, MCT oil	Safflower oil	Safflower oil	Partially hydrogenated soy oil	Soy oil, lecithin, mono and diglycerides	Safflower oil, soy lecithin	—	—
26	44	23	21	42	19	43	—	—	—
0.8	0.5	34	1	1	66	36	500	—	—
249	218	152	226	210	330	287	—	—	500
525	557	550	550	844	900	900	32	—	570
30/22	43/23	15/32	37/30	34/18	<8/<8	—	—	—	27
low	low	low	low	low	low	low	low	low	low
yes	yes	yes	yes	yes	no	no	no	no	no
Doyle	Doyle	Mead Johnson	Eaton	Eaton	McGaw	McGaw	Organon	Ross	Ross
Varied	Citrus	Varied	Varied	Varied	Varied	Varied	Unflavored	Unflavored	Unflavored
Powder	Powder	Powder	Powder	Powder	Powder	Powder	Ready to use	Powder	Liquid
Supplemental tube feeding, lactose free, absorbed in upper gut	Supplemental tube feeding, lactose free, absorbed in upper gut, high protein	Supplemental tube feeding, lactose free, absorbed in upper gut	Supplemental tube feeding, lactose free, no pancreatic stimulus, absorbed in upper gut	Supplemental tube feeding, lactose free, absorbed in upper gut, high protein	Supplemental tube feeding, low electrolytes, essential amino acids, lactose free, indicated for renal disease	Supplemental tube feeding, high branch chain amino acid formula, low electrolytes, lactose free, indicated for liver disease	Supplemental pure fat emulsion, low osmolarity, low electrolytes, lactose free	Supplemental, lactose free	Supplemental, lactose free

Patient's Name: ______________________ Location: ______________________

Administration Method: ☐ Central Line ☐ Peripheral Line RATE: ____________ ml/hr. Patient's Weight: ________

This form is designed for dosage regimen based on content per liter. An order should cover a 24 hour period. The quantity of amino acid and dextrose solutions should total 1000ml (ie. amino acid 8.5% . . 500ml plus dextrose 50% . . 500ml is equal to 1000ml of base solution. This 1000ml provides approximately 1kcal per ml. The additives are ordered in dose per liter.

NOTE: ALL TPN ORDERS FOR THE DAY MUST BE IN THE PHARMACY BY 1:00 p.m. LATE ORDERS WILL BE PREPARED ON THE FOLLOWING DAY. PLEASE CONTACT PHARMACY IF THERE ARE ANY QUESTIONS OR PROBLEMS. PHARMACY EXT 1321.

BASE SOLUTIONS

☐ Amino Acid 5.5% . . . . . . 500ml (Provides 28.9gms Protein—4.6gm Nitrogen)	☐ Dextrose 10% . . . . . . 500ml (Provides 170kcal)
☐ Amino Acid 8.5% . . . . . . 500ml (Provides 44.7 gms Protein—7.15gm Nitrogen)	☐ Dextrose 20% . . . . . . 500ml (Provides 340kcal)
☐ Amino Acid 10% . . . . . . 500ml (Provides 52.6gms Protein—8.4gm Nitrogen)	☐ Dextrose 50% . . . . . . 500ml (Provides 850kcal)
Other: ☐ Renal Amino Acid solution ________ ml ☐ Other ________ ml	☐ Dextrose ____ % ________ ml

SOLUTION ADDITIVES

ADDITIVES

	Normal/L	Amt/L
Sodium Chloride	25-60mEq/L	____
Potassium Chloride	30-50mEq/L	____
Potassium Phosphate	10-15mmoles	____
Magnesium Sulfate	4-8mEq	____
Calcium gluconate (will be added to first liter only unless otherwise indicated)	0-4.7mEq	____
Heparin Sodium	1000 units	____
Sodium Acetate (prn acidosis)	Max 40m Eq/L	____
Insulin (Regular)		____

PHARMACY STANDING ORDERS*

TO BE PLACED IN 1st LITER ONLY

MVI-12, 10ml

Trace Elements:
Zinc 4mg
Copper 1mg
Chromium 10mcg
Manganese 0.5mg

* Pharmacy standing orders will be followed as above unless indicated otherwise.

Comments: ______________________

☐ I.V. FAT EMULSION 10% ____________ ml/day at ________ ml/hr

RECOMMENDATION: Initial dose 1ml/min for 15 to 30 minutes. If no complications administer at the above rate three times weekly to prevent essential fatty acid deficiency. May be administered via piggyback on the central subclavian line at the distal injection port below the filter.

Please addressograph here with patient's plate

OTHER COMMUNICATION ______________________

Date: ____________ Time: ____________

Ordering Physician: ______________________ M.D.

Nurse Signature: ______________________ R.N.

Figure 21-5. Parenteral nutrition form.

DOCTOR'S ORDERS (SIGN ALL ORDERS)

THE DOCTOR SHALL RECORD DATE AND TIME FOR EACH SET OF ORDERS.
(TO BE UPDATED BY M.D. EVERY MONDAY)

(If you do not wish to have one or all of the following orders, please mark NO next to the order.)

_____ 1. Chest x-ray to confirm catheter location.

_____ 2. Use D-5% W at 30cc/hr for infusion until subclavian cathether tip position confirmed by x-ray.

_____ 3. Vital signs and temperature every 4 hrs. Notify M.D. if sudden change.

_____ 4. Test urine glucose every 6 hours

_____ 5. Weigh patient daily and record

_____ 6. Maintain strict daily intake and output records

_____ 7. Maintain a constant infusion rate with an IVAC pump for infusion. DO NOT TRY TO CATCH UP. If rate varies 20% from prescribed flow, notify M.D. Have label and time strip on bottle at all times.

_____ 8. Monitor flow rate and bottle level every shift, and record sequential H.A. bottle number on the I & O records.

_____ 9. Nurse to inform M.D. to execute a physical therapy consult to P.M. & R. Department for active and passive exercise q day.

_____ 10. Notify M.D. and H.A. nurse if leaking occurs around catheter site or any problem with the catheter dressing.

_____ 11. Keep line open with D10W at same rate if Hyperalimentation solution is not available.

_____ 12. Change administration set, extension and filter every day when disconnecting and attaching administration set, have patient perform Valsalva Maneuver.

_____ 13. Aqua Mephyton 10mg IM every Wednesday

_____ 14. Laboratory Test
- A.) C.B.C. (with differedtial), platelet count P.T.T., & P.T. every Monday
- B.) Serum Magnesium, Serum Transferrin, T.I.B.C. every Monday.
- C.) S.M.A.-6 daily for first (1st) 5 days, then repeat every Monday, Wednesday and Friday.
- D.) S.M.A.-12 every Monday and Friday
- E.) Obtain Serum triglyceride level prior to starting intralipid(s), then repeat serum triglyceride (note LIPEMIA) every Monday.

_____ 15. Collect 24-hour urine specimen for Urinary Urea Nitrogen (U.U.N.) and creatinine starting from Sunday 7:00am to Monday at 7:00am.

_____ 16. Notify H.A. nurse to apply skin test antigen:
Mumps P.P.D. Candida

_____ 17. Nurse will notify the Dietician assigned to the unit to perform nutritional assessment

_____ 18. Notify PHARMACY for any problems with the T.P.N. solution Ext. 1321.

Please addressograph here with patient's plate.

Date:__________ Time __________

Signature__________ M.D.

Transcribed by__________ R.N. Time:__________

HUH 0448

Figure 21-6. Total parenteral nutrition (TPN) general orders.

Infusate Contamination
Infusate contamination is minimized by sterile preparation under a laminar flow hood and refrigeration. The substitution of protein hydrolysates with crystalline amino acids also decreases bacterial contamination.

Fever of Unknown Origin
Patients who become febrile while on TPN require a methodical search for the source. The catheter insertion site is inspected, the TPN solution and tubing are changed, and blood cultures are obtained from a peripheral site. If the septic source is not identified, the catheter is removed and its tip sent for culture and sensitivity. When vascular access is limited, the catheter is changed over a sterile guidewire.

Patients with an infected catheter or positive blood cultures require intravenous antibiotics. Candidemia often resolves after catheter removal, but some immunocompromised patients require systemic antifungal therapy.

Table 21-9. Total parenteral nutrition complications

Technical
Pneumothorax
Air embolism
Catheter tip malposition
Subclavian artery laceration
Brachial plexus injury
Phrenic nerve injury
Venous thrombosis
Tracheal injury
Septic
Catheter contamination
Infusate contamination
Fever of unknown origin
Metabolic
Hyper/hypoglycemia
Glucosuria
Hyperosmolar coma
Cholestasis
Electrolyte imbalance
Vitamin deficiency
Trace element deficiency
Free fatty acid deficiency

Metabolic Complications

Glucose
Hyperglycemia, glucosuria with osmotic diuresis, hyperosmolar coma, and rebound hypoglycemia are the common metabolic complications. Most patients achieve glucose tolerance after pancreatic adaptation [19]. Increases in osmolar input, sepsis, or surgical trauma can lead to metabolic imbalance. Hyperosmolar coma is associated with rapid infusion of hyperosmolar solutions. The primary central nervous system effect, if not recognized and treated promptly, leads to irreversible brain injury. When suspected, the hyposmolar solution is stopped, isotonic solutions are administered to correct intracellular dehydration, and an insulin drip is started. Hypoglycemia implicates excessive insulin or abrupt TPN withdrawal.

Hepatic Abnormalities
Cholestasis or elevated liver function enzymes are not unusual. In the majority of patients, this is self-limited and resolves spontaneously after stopping TPN. In patients with significant liver disease however, formulas enriched with branch-chain amino acids are preferred.

Electrolyte Imbalance
Electrolyte imbalances are avoided by regular monitoring and correction as indicated. Unrecognized hypophosphatemia leads to extreme muscle fatigue and respiratory arrest. Hyperchloremic acidosis is treated by substituting acetate for chloride. Serum potassium levels must be monitored closely.

Water and Vitamins
Water and fat-soluble vitamins added routinely to TPN solutions prevent vitamin deficiency. Intramuscular vitamin K is given weekly.

Trace Elements
Zinc, copper, chromium, and manganese are given daily to prevent trace element deficiency. Sporadic cases of selenium deficiency are being reported and selenium may need to be added during long term TPN administrations.

Free Fatty Acids

Routine administration of fat emulsions prevents free fatty acid deficiency; 250 ml of 20% Intralipid is administered once or twice a week. Fat emulsions are withheld in patients with bleeding disorders and severe thrombocytopenia.

In patients who are ventilator dependent, substituting fat for glucose as a primary source of calories may facilitate weaning from the ventilator by decreasing carbon dioxide production. Increased ventilatory work is required to remove accumulated carbon dioxide.

REFERENCES

1. Shils, ME: How to nourish the cancer patient. *Nutrition Today* 16(4), 1981.
2. Bistrian RR, et al: Protein status of general surgical patients. *JAMA* 230 : 856, 1974.
3. Hill S, Smith T, Carle A: Hospital malnutrition. *Lancet* 1 : 689, 1977.
4. Weisner RL, et al: Hospital malnutrition: A prospective evaluation of general medical patients during the course of hospitalization. *Am J Clin Nutr* 32 : 418, 1979.
5. Goodwin WJ: Nutritional Management of Head and Neck Cancer. In Cummings CW, et al (eds): *Otolaryngology, Head and Neck Surgery*. St. Louis: Mosby, 1986. Vol I, Pp 101–113.
6. Lang CE: *Nutrition Support in Critical Care*. Silver Spring, MD: Asperin, 1987.
7. Long C, et al: Metabolic response to injury and illness: Estimation of energy and protein needs from indirect calorimetry and nitrogen balance. *JPEN* 3 : 457, 1979.
8. Schneider HA, Anderson CE, Coursin CE: *Nutritional Support of Medical Practice* (2nd ed). New York: Harper & Row, 1983.
9. Nehme AE: Nutritional support of the hospitalized patient: The team concept. *JAMA* 243 : 1906, 1980.
10. Friedman MH, Higa AM, Davis AJ: A unique team to optimal nutritional support with minimal cost. *Nutr Support Serv* 3(3) : 27, 1983.
11. Bistrian BR, et al: Therapeutic index of nutritional depletion in hospitalized patients. *Surg Gynecol Obstet* 141 : 512, 1975.
12. Meakins JL, et al: Delayed hypersensitivity: Indicator of acquired failure of host defense in sepsis and trauma. *Ann Surg* 186 : 241, 1977.
13. McKenzie T, Blackburn GL, Flatt JP: Clinical assessment of nutritional states using nitrogen balance. *Fed Proc* 33 : 683, 1974.
14. Steffee WP, Krey SH: Enteral hyperalimentation for patients with head and neck cancer. *Otolaryngol Clin North Am* 13(3) : 437, 1980.
15. Mochizvki H, et al: Mechanism of prevention of postburn hypermetabolism and catabolism by early enteral feeding. *Ann Surg* 200 : 297, 1984.
16. Moore, EE, Jones TN: Benefits of immediate jejunostomy feeding after major abdominal trauma: A prospective, randomized study. *J Trauma* 26 : 874, 1986.
17. Dominioni L, et al: Enteral feeding in hypermetabolism: Nutritional and metabolic effect of different levels of calorie and protein intake. *J Parenter Enter Nutr* 9 : 269, 1985.
18. Alverdy J, Sang H, Sheldon G: The effect of parenteral nutrition on gastrointestinal immunity: The importance of enteral stimulation. *Ann Surg* 202 : 681, 1985.
19. Dudrick SJ, Long JM: Application and hazards of intravenous hyperalimentation *Annu Rev Med* 28 : 517, 1977.
20. Coppa GF, Gonge TH, Hofstetter SR: Air embolism: A lethal preventable complication of subclavian vein catheterization. *JPEN* 5 : 166, 1981.
21. Goldman DA, Maki DG: Infection control in total parenteral nutrition. *JAMA* 223 : 1360, 1973.
22. Bjornson HS, et al: Association between microorganism growth at the catheter insertion site and colonization of the catheter in patients receiving total parenteral nutrition. *Surgery* 92 : 721, 1982.
23. Sanderson I, Dietel M: Insulin response in patients receiving concentrated infusion of glucose and casein hydrolysate for complete parenteral nutrition. *Ann Surg* 179 : 387, 1974.

22

Reconstruction Overview

ERNEST M. MYERS and ETIENNE MASSAC

KEY CONCEPTS

Assessment; Preparation; Grafts; Flaps; Tissue Expanders; Myocutaneous Flaps; Free Tissue Transfer

MILESTONES

1600 B.C.	Treatise, Reconstructive Surgery of Ears and Nose	Elbers Papyrus (Egypt)
600 B.C.	Partial and Total Nasal Reconstruction (Forehead)	Samhila Texts (India)
25–50 A.D.	Advancement Flap Closure	Celsus
400 A.D.	Cheek Flap Rhinoplasty	Vagbat
1470s	Facial Proportions	de Vinci
1597	Total and Partial Nasal Reconstruction	Tagliacozzi
1842	Nape of Neck Flap	Mutter
1942	Cervical Skin Flap Reconstruction	Wookey
1955	Compound Sternocleidomastoid Flap	Owens
1963	Forehead Flap for Oral Cavity Reconstruction	McGregor
1965	Deltopectoral Flap	Bakamjian
1972	Flap Physiology	McGregor
1976	Identification of Myocutaneous Flap Territories	McGraw
1979	Pectoralis Myocutaneous Flap	Ariyan
1980s	Microvascular Surgery	Ariyan

According to Conley [1], the two basic reasons for reconstruction are esthetic gratification and functional improvement. These laudable goals are difficult in the small, compact, anatomy of the head and neck. Moreover, any reconstruction method must not impinge on adjacent vital organs (i.e., aerodigestive tract, cervical spine, and great vessels). Tumor ablation in such a confined area easily produces cosmetic and functional deformities. Therein is the challenge: to ablate, functionally preserve, and reconstruct among multiple vital structures (Table 22-1).

The history of head and neck reconstruction parallels the development of effective tumor ablation. Before the turn of the century, less than half the patients were cured. Surgery was in its infancy, and radical neck dissection remained to be conceptualized. The explosive development of radiotherapy, effective general anesthesia, and a better understanding of metabolism led to more aggressive, curative head and neck surgery. This has greatly increased the need for quality reconstruction to enhance complete patient rehabilitation. In short, it is impos-

Table 22-1. Reconstruction goals

Anatomic restoration
Functional restoration
Acceptable donor site morbidity
Durability & permanence

sible to manage head and neck cancer properly without a thorough knowledge of modern reconstruction [1,2].

ASSESSMENT

Preoperative assessment and planning include the past medical history, habits, and occupation as well as an analysis of specific ablative procedures. In regard to the medical history, the following are especially important: pre- or postoperative radiotherapy, chemotherapy, diabetes mellitus, renal disease, hepatic disease, and cardiovascular disease.

PATIENT PREPARATION

Nutrition

The nutritional status must be optimal. A nutritional assessment and correction of deficiencies are the first preparatory steps (see Chapter 21).

Antibiotics

Antibiotics play a major role in the prophylaxis and alleviation of infection, especially from the contaminated aerodigestive tract (see Chapter 12). The antibiotics of choice are penicillins or cephalosporins with or without other drugs for gram-negative coverage. Postoperative infection is managed by specific antibiotics as determined by culture and sensitivity.

Skin Preparation

Donor site toilet helps decrease infection by decreasing skin bacterial count. Showers the night before and the morning of surgery with povidone-iodine (Betadine) or chlorhexidine gluconate (Hibiclens) are effective.

PLANNING

When possible, skin and mucosal defects are closed primarily. If the defect is too large or unsuitable for direct closure, other means are utilized: grafts, local or distant flaps, composite or free flaps. These various techniques require an understanding of sound physiologic principles and their practical application (Table 22-2).

Table 22-2. Planning sequence

1. Establish realistic goals
2. Choose the optimal donor site:
   - Skin graft
   - Skin flap (local versus distant)
   - Myocutaneous flap
   - Free flap
3. Immobilization
4. Soft-tissue reconstruction: to minimize donor site dysfunction
5. Physical therapy: to enhance psychological and functional rehabilitation
6. Occupational therapy

The Principles of Reconstruction

Sir Harold Gillies [3], an early pioneer of reconstruction techniques, proposed the following dictums:

1. Keen observation is the basis of diagnosis.
2. Know the normal and its variations.
3. Diagnosis must precede therapy.
4. Formulate a primary and secondary plan of reconstruction.
5. Always have a backup option.
6. Treat the primary defect first.
7. Losses must be replaced in kind: replace what is normal in normal position.
8. Never discard any tissue.
9. Document your results for critical analysis and improvement.

The Available Options

The extensive list of options includes direct closure, grafts, flaps, fasciocutaneous flaps, muscle flaps, myocutaneous flaps, visceral flaps, compound flaps, and free tissue transfer.

The Chosen Option

The chosen reconstructive option is predicated upon cosmesis, preservation of function, patient cost, length of stay, the anticipated gain in function, and the need for further corrective surgery.

SKIN GRAFTS

Skin grafts consist of epidermis and a variable amount of dermis. Full-thickness skin grafts contain the entire thickness of the dermis, whereas split-skin grafts contain a portion of the dermis.

Technique

Full-thickness grafts are harvested with the scalpel; split-skin grafts usually are obtained with a dermatome or Humby knife. A full-thickness skin graft, leaving no epidermal structure in the donor area for resurfacing, must be closed primarily. Primary closure of the donor site limits the practical size of a full-thickness skin graft. In contrast, the split-skin graft leaves adnexal remnants as foci for donor site resurfacing. Moreover, the split-skin graft donor site requires little care.

The advantage of skin grafts is the effective coverage of large areas, especially when the graft is meshed or quilted. The disadvantages are poor color match, thinness, and the need for a vascular, clean recipient site.

Take

During transfer, a free skin graft is detached completely from the body. While detached it is viable for only a limited period. This limited viability depends on ambient temperature. Permanent survival requires establishing a fresh blood supply at the recipient site. The reattachment and revascularization of a skin graft is called a *take* [4].

Nutrition

The graft initially adheres by fibrin, and its metabolic requirements are sustained by defusion. However, capillary ingrowth quickly establishes graft vascularity. In optimal circumstances, this occurs rapidly after grafting. Simultaneously, fibrin, infiltrated by fibroblasts, increases the strength of this attachment. Lymphatic and imperfect neural reconstitution occurs more slowly.

Vascularity

Blood supply and fibrous tissue fixation are the most important factors for a take. Its effectiveness and speed are determined by the graft bed, graft characteristics, and technique. The graft bed must have a rich blood supply and the capacity to provide the necessary fibrin anchorage. The following are graftable surfaces in the head and neck: muscle, fascia, fat, cartilage (covered with perichondrium), bone (covered with periosteum), dura mater, mucoperiosteum, and mucoperichondrium.

FLAPS

In head and neck reconstruction, at times, the choice between a graft or flap is difficult. The fundamental choice depends on vascularity. A flap has two basic advantages: immediate wound coverage and restoration of physiology and function [1]. For large defects, these advantages include great-vessel protection and augmentation of large defects [2]. A graft must establish a new blood supply, whereas the flap, carrying its own blood supply, is more reliable. If the recipient surface is incapable of sustaining vascularity, a flap is chosen.

Flap Physiology

The dominant blood supply in the head and neck is the perforating branches of the temporal branch of the external carotid artery, the internal mammary arteries, and the pectoral arteries [1]. The secondary blood supply is the branches of the external carotid and axillary arteries. The strong flaps have a dominant blood supply; conversely, the weak flaps have a random blood supply.

Survival

Ultimately, skin flap survival is dependent on adequate surface circulation (Table 22-3). Segmental artery pressure is in the range of 90 to 100 mm Hg, whereas distal arteriole pressure is 30 mm Hg. Skin blood flow is determined by arteriole resistance that is regulated by a variety of neural, hormonal, and local factors. The distal skin blood flow is regulated in a longitudinal fashion.

Vascularity

In general, the body's blood supply is organized on three levels. Segmental major vessels arising

Table 22-3. Flap failure: etiology

Suboptimal patient preparation
Malnutrition
Diabetes mellitus (hyperglycemia)
Anemia
Prerenal azotemia
Dental caries/periodontal disease
Suboptimal preoperative antibiosis
Suboptimal planning and execution
Flap design
Elevation
Vascular compromise
Torsion
Kinks
Mobilization
Stretch
Tension
Transfer
Compression
Edema
Gravity
Closure (leaks)
Suboptimal postoperative care
Malnutrition
Anemia
Dehydration
Strangulating tracheotomy tube ties
Inadequate wound drainage
Compression dressing (exaggerated)

from the aorta are accompanied by large veins and nerves, such as axial extremity vessels. Perforating vessels or muscle branches conduct the blood supply from the segmental major vessels to the cutaneous vessels. Finally, the cutaneous vessels or skin branches consist of musculocutaneous and direct cutaneous vessels whenever skin overlies muscle [2].

Gillies and Millard [3] amplify this scheme and emphasize the importance of the deep fascia blood supply. Organized in a random fashion overlying muscle, the deep fascia has many more vessels than the muscles.

1. Perforating arteries—vessels that leave the muscle or intermuscular septa through the deep fascia to branch freely on the fascia surface and anastomose with the superficial plexus.
2. Subcutaneous arteries—vessels that are found in areas devoid of perforators; they run deeply in the fat in all directions, anastomosing with each other and the superficial fascial plexus.
3. Subfascial arteries: the arterial system within the loose alveolar tissue immediately beneath the deep fascia.

Delay

Technique

Initially, the flap is partially incised and mobilized. It then is placed immediately back into its original position. For unknown reasons, these simple maneuvers encourage distal circulation. Ten to 14 days later, the flap is mobilized and transferred completely.

This technique is indicated when there is tenuous vascular territory. Its advantage is avoidance of distal flap necrosis, and its disadvantages are additional procedures and time.

Theory

In effect, the delay augments skin capillary blood flow and distal perfusion. This phenomenon does not depend on angioneogenesis, adaptation to ischemia, or arterial venous shunting secondary to circulating catecholamines. Instead, it is theorized that the delay releases neurohumoral substances [4]. Guillane and Heeneman [2] suggest that distal blood flow is encouraged by the closure of arteriovenous shunts by sympathetic denervation. This reverses the pooling and decreased perfusion associated with shunts [5]. Whatever the mechanism, ultimate flap survival is determined by the equilibration between perfusion pressure and intravascular resistance.

Flap Geometry

There are two basic skin flaps, axial and random flaps, each with a distinctive geometry imposed by its vascular anatomy [2,5,6].

Axial Flap

The axial flap is designed on a definite arteriovenous system. There is a recognized circulation parallel to the flap with branches to the dermal-subdermal plexus. Such strong vascularity makes it possible to construct a flap at least as long as the axial artery territory with minimal regard for width. In short, there is an unrestricted length versus width ratio.

Random Flap

Random flaps are nourished by indistinct random dermal-subdermal vascular communications.

Advantages

The success of random flaps depends on a pattern of horizontal vessels with adequate vascular caliber for a given local territory. Fortunately, the entire head and neck area has rich networks of significant vessels capable of sustaining viable circulation. These plexuses appear also to cross the midline freely.

Disadvantages

The maximum viable length of a random flap is related to its width and the number of vessels incorporated within its base. Such a flap has no preexisting bias in its vascular pattern. Therefore, there are limits to its dimensions, particularly the ratio between length and breadth. The design depends on the richness of the subdermal vascular plexus. Thus, there are stringent restrictions regarding length versus width ratios, that is, 1 : 1 for the trunk, 4 : 1 for the face.

Flap Technique

Basically, a skin flap is mobilized with variable amounts of subcutaneous tissue that is transferred to fill in a defect. This transfer, while still attached partially, results in a secondary defect that is closed primarily or with a skin graft. During transfers, a flap never is detached completely from the body. This preserves its vascularity. Adequate circulation is crucial at every stage of the transfer.

Classification

1. Local flap: a flap developed from tissue adjacent to a defect.
   a. Indications: small defects.
   b. Advantages: one stage; similar color and texture.
   c. Disadvantages: scarring and distortion; large defects.
2. Distant flap: a flap developed from tissue removed from a defect.
   a. Indication: large defects.
   b. Advantages: size; healthy nonirradiated tissue.
   c. Disadvantages: increased risks; prolonged anesthesia; multiple procedures; different color and texture.

Design

The basic principle is borrowing from areas of surplus and transferring to areas of scarcity. Possible areas for borrowing include the glabella, upper eyelid, nasolabial fold, preauricular region, angle of the mandible, and upper neck [7].

Essentially, each flap is designed to include a superficial subdermal and deep suprafascial plexus [1]. A flap should adhere to the following basic principles:

1. Plan: incorporation of a blood supply to support transfer.
2. Design: proper recipient-site configuration and fit.
3. Mobilization: transfer without vascular compromise.
4. Position: secure closure without vascular compromise.
5. Support: maintenance of position with drains and dressings.

Methods

Since skin immediately adjacent to a defect is similar in texture, whenever possible, local flaps are preferable to distant flaps. The shifting of local tissue is predicated on the natural elasticity of skin. A variety of techniques are utilized. They are summarized as follows (Figure 22-1):

1. Advancement flaps: the undermining of wound edges, followed by mobilization and approximation. When indicated, the excess tissue in the flap base is excised in a triangular fashion (Burow's triangle) to prevent puckering.
   a. Advantages: simplicity, predictability.
   b. Disadvantages: hyperelasticity; skin tightly adherent to underlying tissues, such as the jaw or posterior neck.
2. V-Y flap: a variation of undermining, where a V-shaped incision and defect are advanced to form a Y closure.
   a. Advantages: wound elongation; closure of secondary defects.
   b. Disadvantages: noticeable scar.

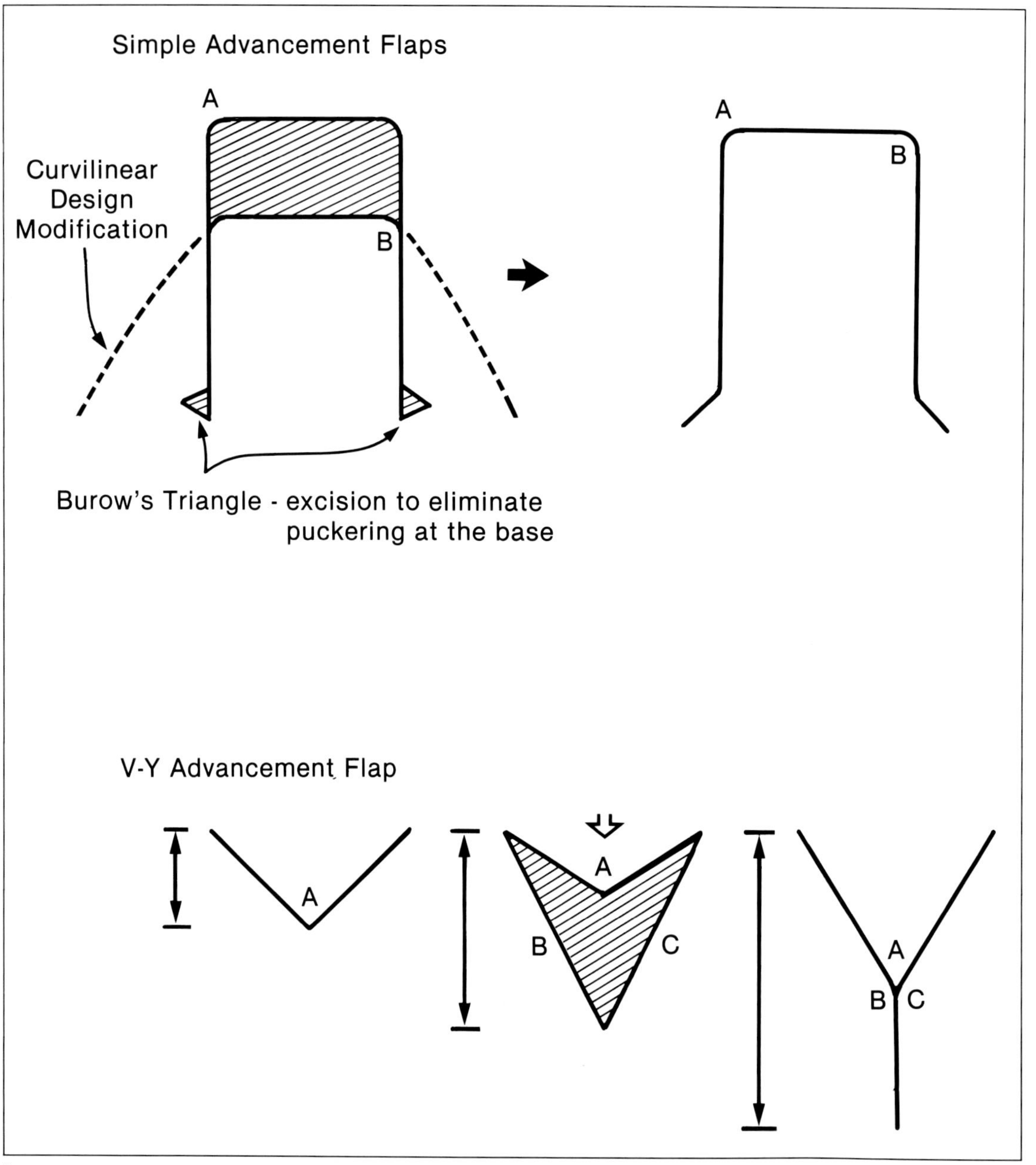

A
Figure 22-1. Local flaps.

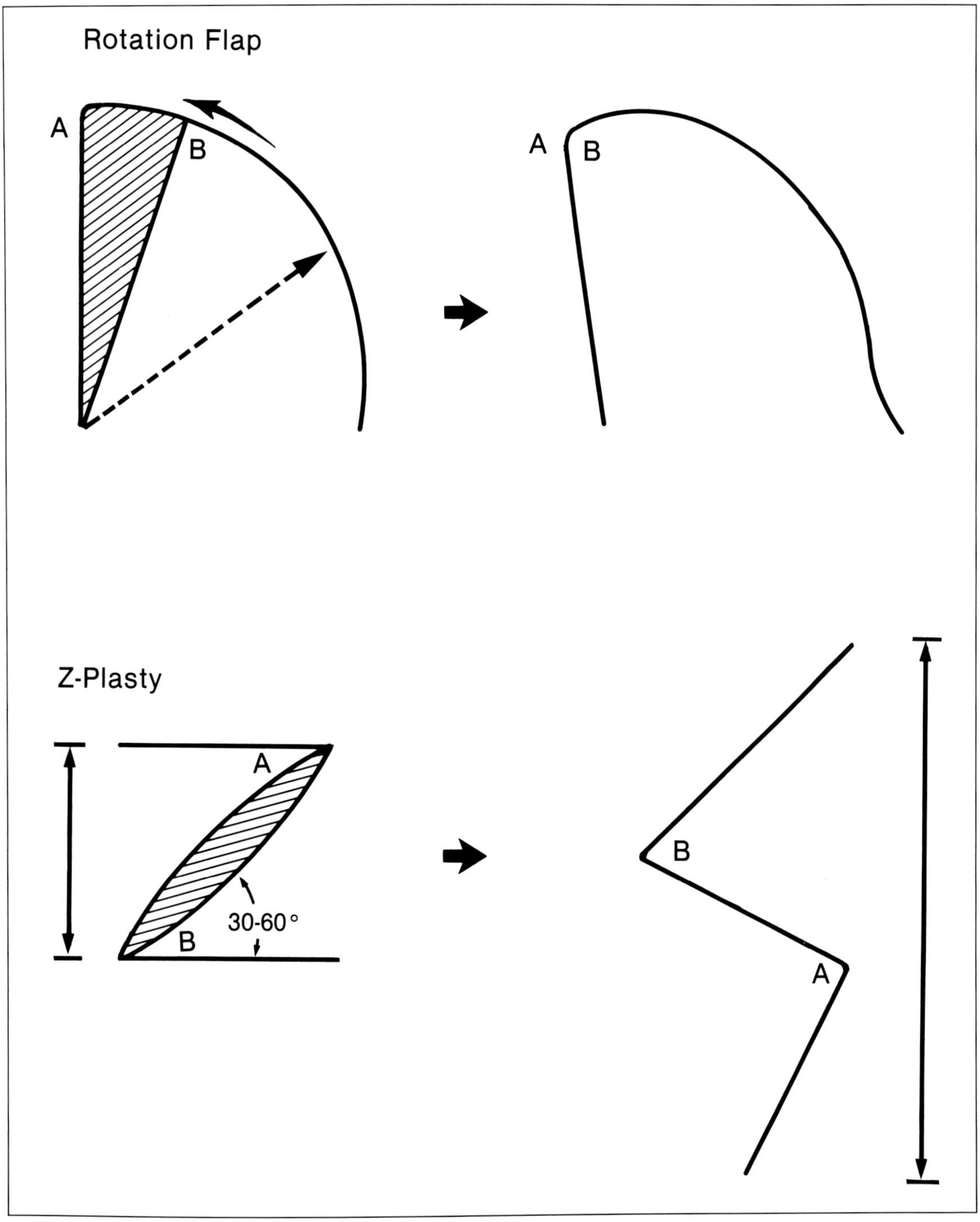

B

1. Dehiscence: suture-line disruption usually is secondary to tension (hematoma, seroma, devascularity) or poor healing. Early recognition and intercession can salvage many flaps.
2. Necrosis: the most common causes are devascularity and infection. The former is predicated usually on poor design and execution. The latter may be due to technical or patient factors.
3. Infection: aside from patient factors, infection is rarely the sole cause of flap death.

In summary flap failure may be singly due to any of these causes aggravated by the underlying medical conditions. There is generally a dynamic interplay of various conditions (Table 22-5).

BASIC FLAPS

Local Flaps

The areas of frequent tissue availability are the mandibulomasseteric jowl, nasolabial fold, glabella, and temple (posterior to the lateral canthus (Figures 22-2 through 22-6). To a lesser degree, the midline forehead has some limited tissue availability (see Figure 22-4). Advancement, rotation, or transposition techniques are utilized in these areas. Two of the common local flaps are as follows:

1. Nasolabial flap: local flaps, inferiorly or superiorly based on the facial artery, that are derived from the nasolabial fold (see Figures 22-2 and 22-3) [12].
   a. Advantage: provides thin local tissue for coverage of small facial or intraoral defects.
   b. Disadvantages: beard transfer in men limits available tissue; requires multiple stages.
   c. Clinical applications: nasal coverage; labial and sulcus defects; floor of mouth.
2. Temporal forehead temporalis muscle flap: a lateral forehead flap based on the superficial temporal artery (Figures 22-4 and 22-7)
   a. Advantages: well vascularized; one stage; thinness; suitable for external or internal transfer; pattern baldness extends useful territory.
   b. Disadvantages: donor site deformity requires secondary closure; hair transfer.
   c. Clinical applications: complete or partial nasal reconstruction; floor of mouth; buccal defects.

Table 22-5. Complications: prevention

Patient preparation
Nutrition
Pulmonary toilet
Diabetes mellitus control
Prophylactic antibiotics
Dental extractions
Pharmacologic preparation
Insulin
Dilantin
Digoxin
Aminophylline
Preoperative counseling
Patient
Family
Preoperative consultations
Anesthesiology
Cardiology
Endocrine
Radiotherapy
Speech pathology
Physical therapy
Maxillofacial prosthodontics
Postoperative radiotherapy
Precise surgical planning and execution

Figure 22-2. Nasolabial flap (right) in a 57-year-old man with stage III carcinoma of the anterior floor of the mouth, treated initially with chemotherapy. A. Proposed flap outline. B. Elevation and intraoral transfer. C. Right floor-of-mouth defect with mandibular involvement. D. Floor-of-mouth resection and partial mandibulectomy. E. Flap sutured into defect. F. Closure of donor site. G. Donor site appearance after a 2-week flap delay. H and I. Closure (donor and recipient sites) after completion of second stage.

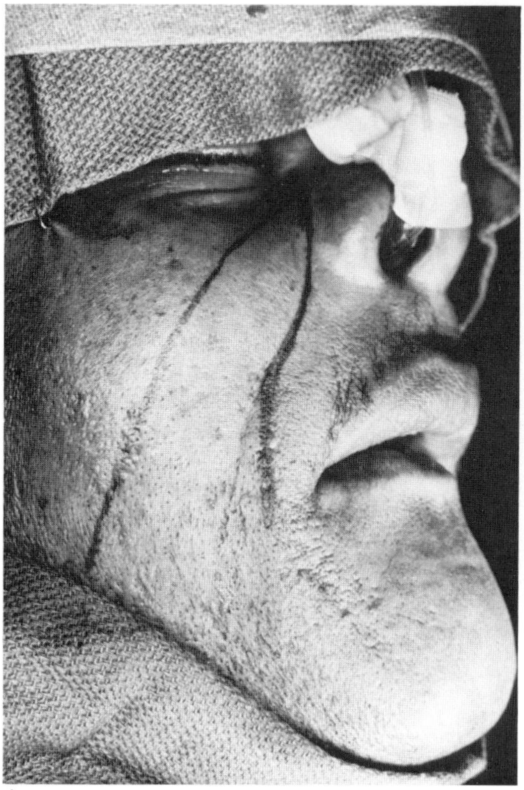

A

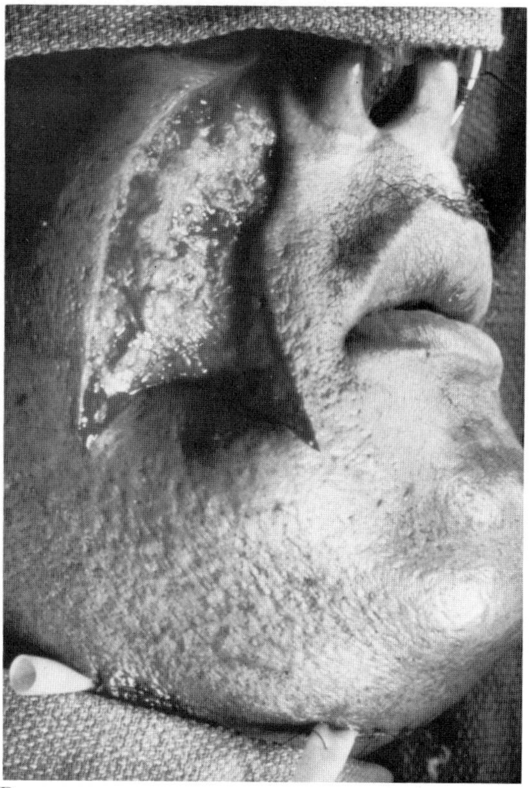

B

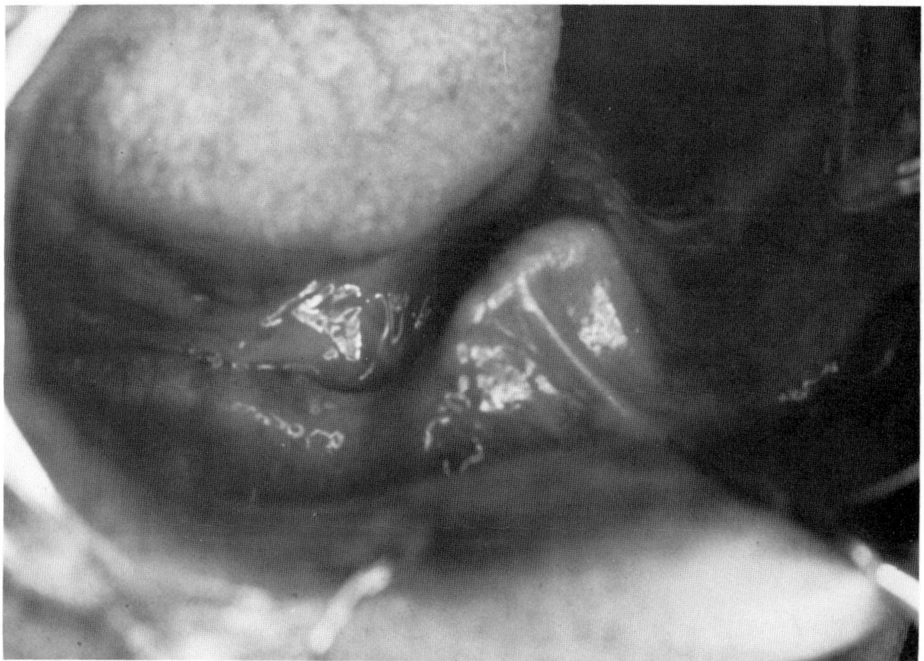

C

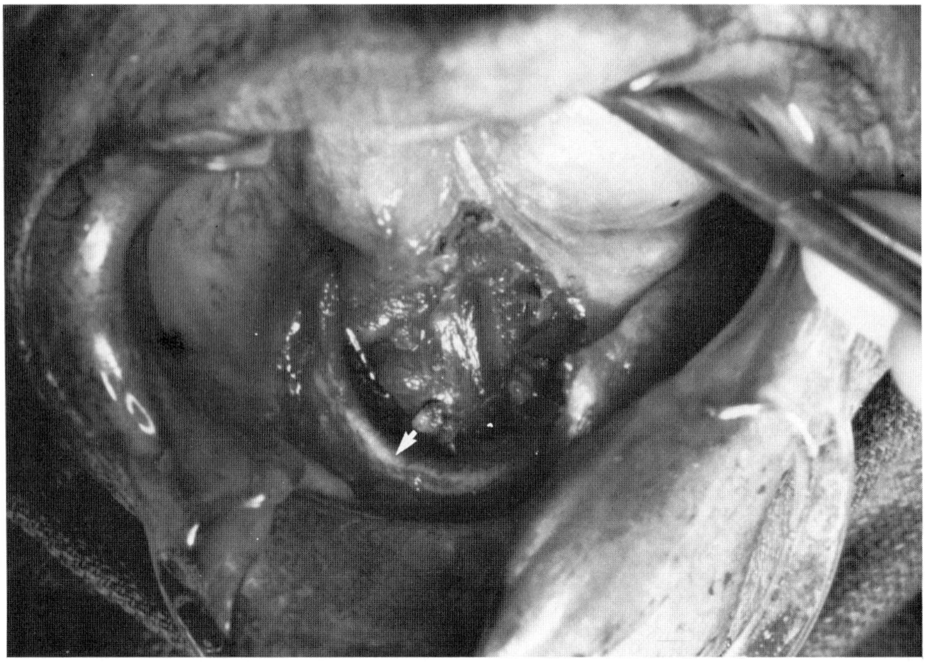

D

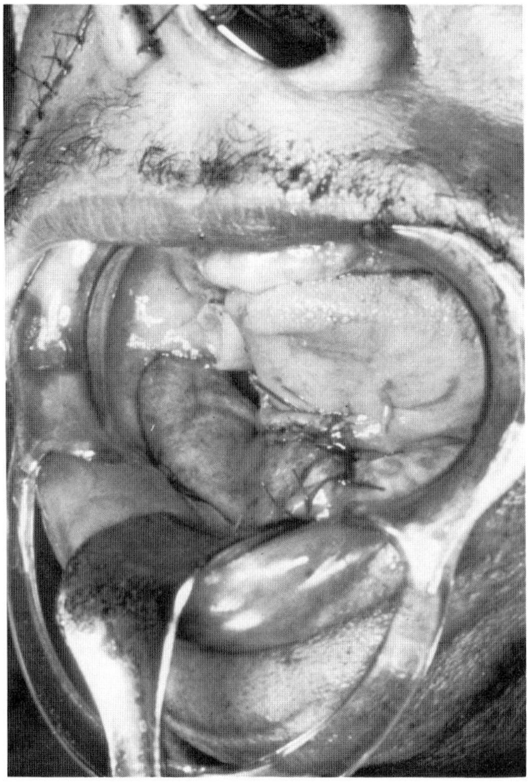

E

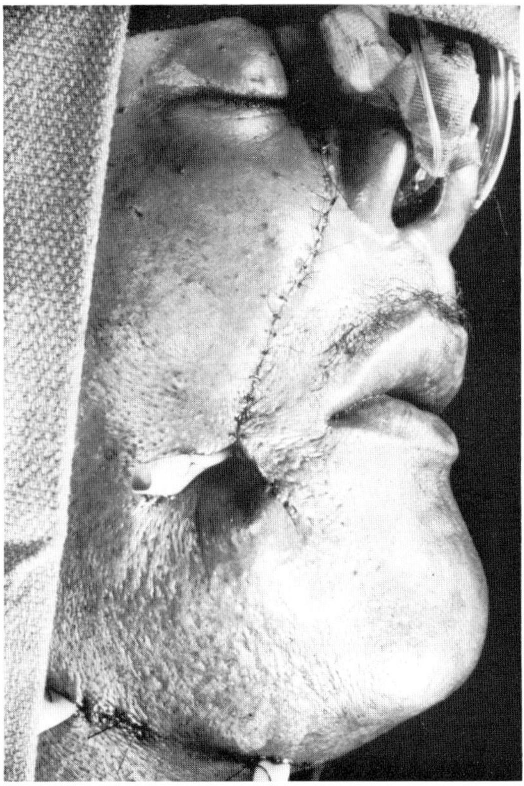

F

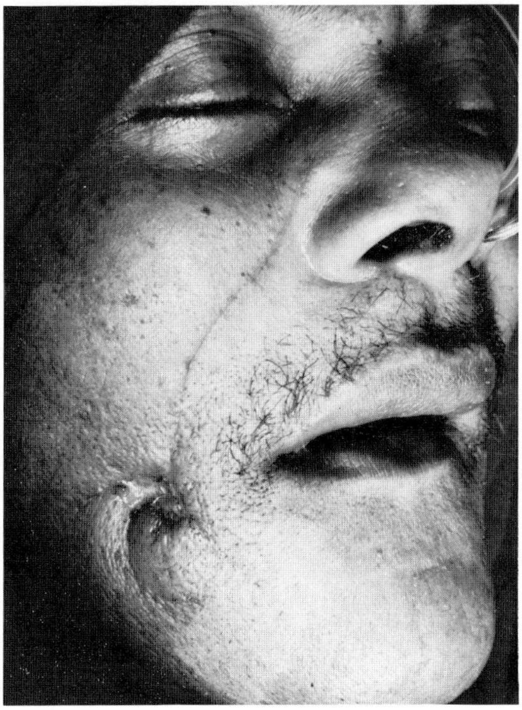

G

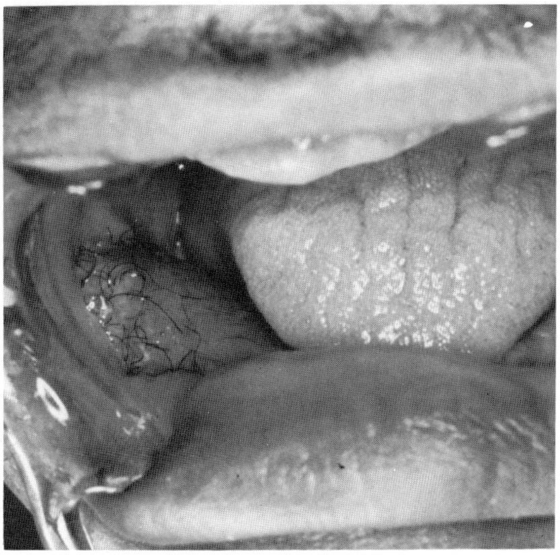

H

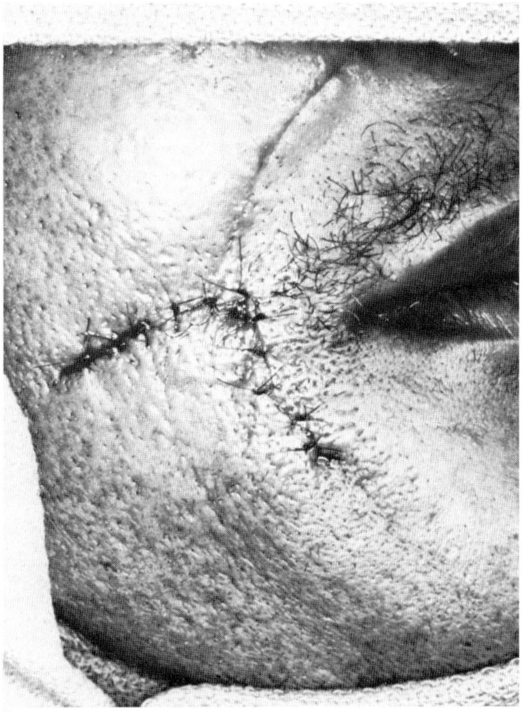

I

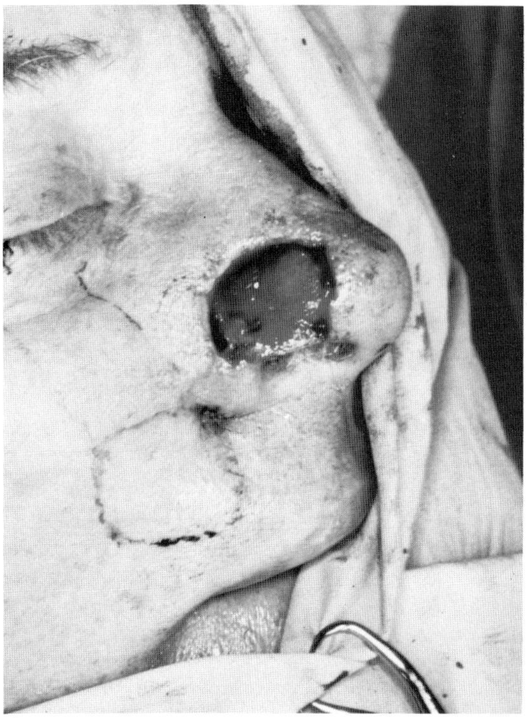

A

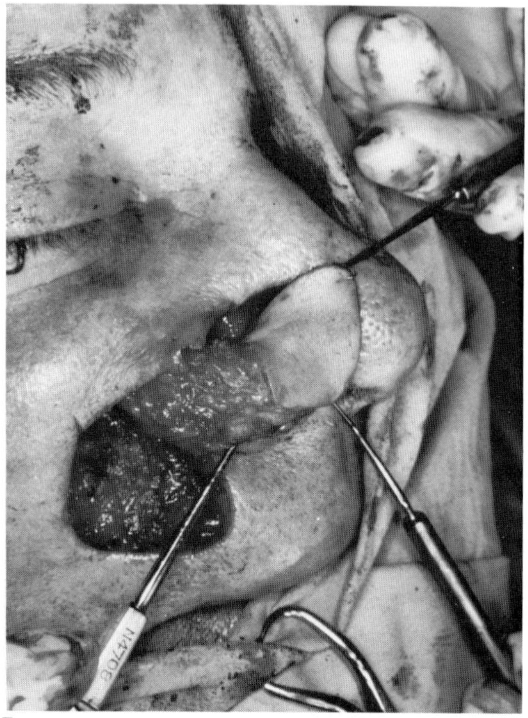

B

Figure 22-3. Subdermal nasolabial flap based on infraorbital vessels. A. Excision of basal cell carcinoma of the right ala. B and C. Transfer of flap into the recipient site. D and E. Postoperative appearance. F. Normal left ala.

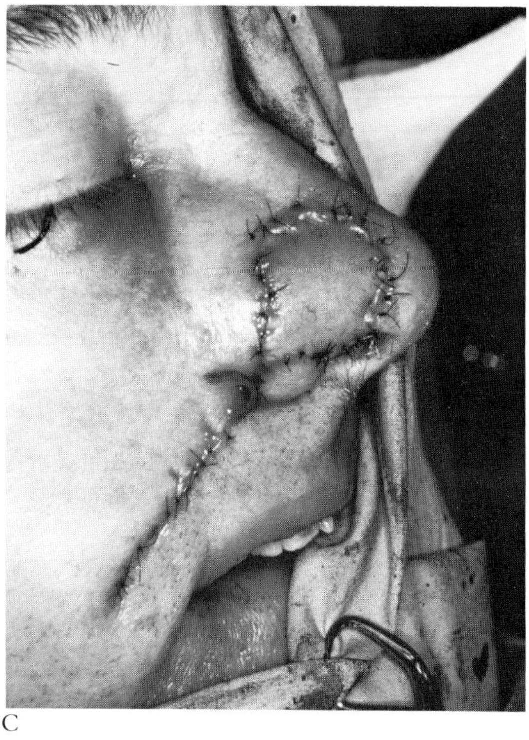

C

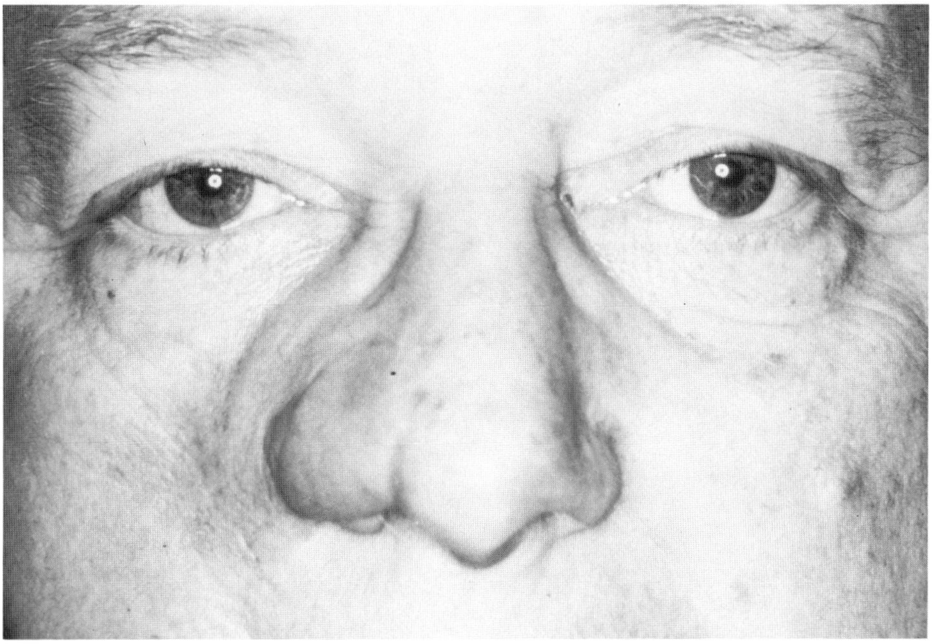

D

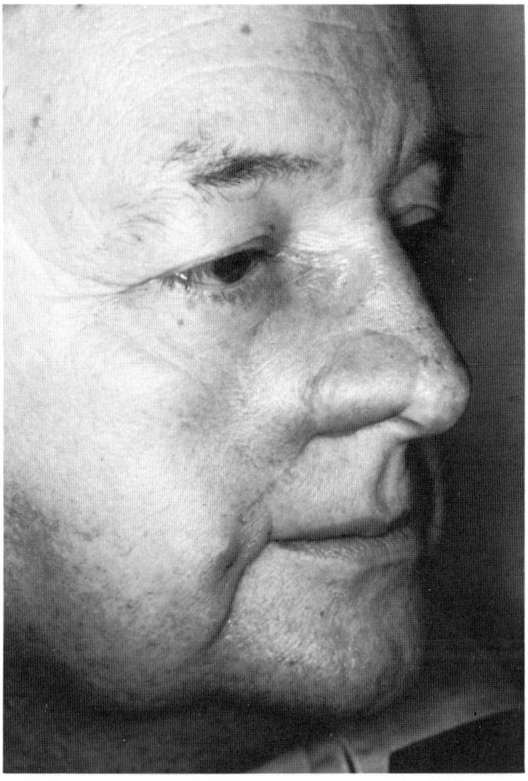

E

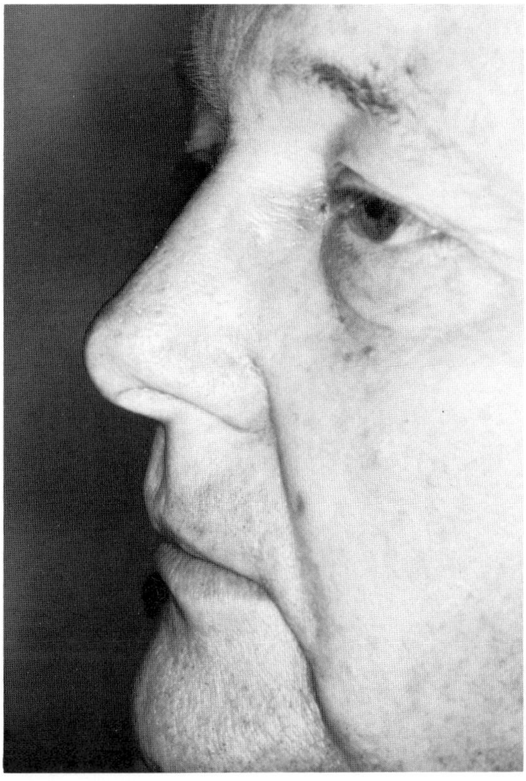

F

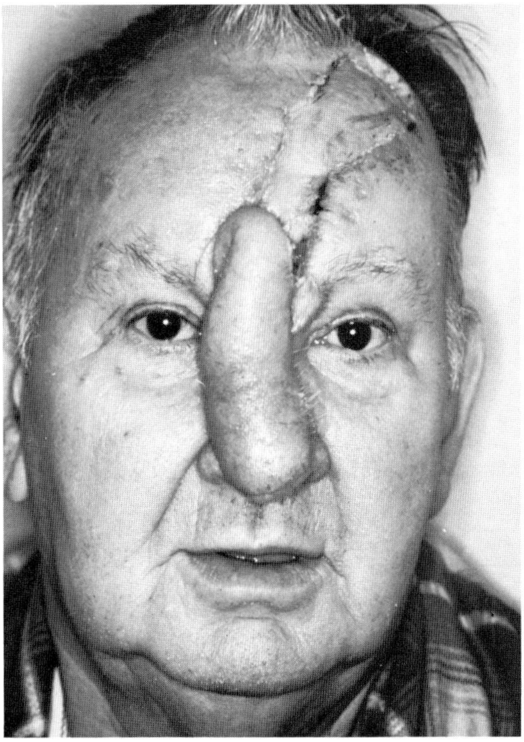

A

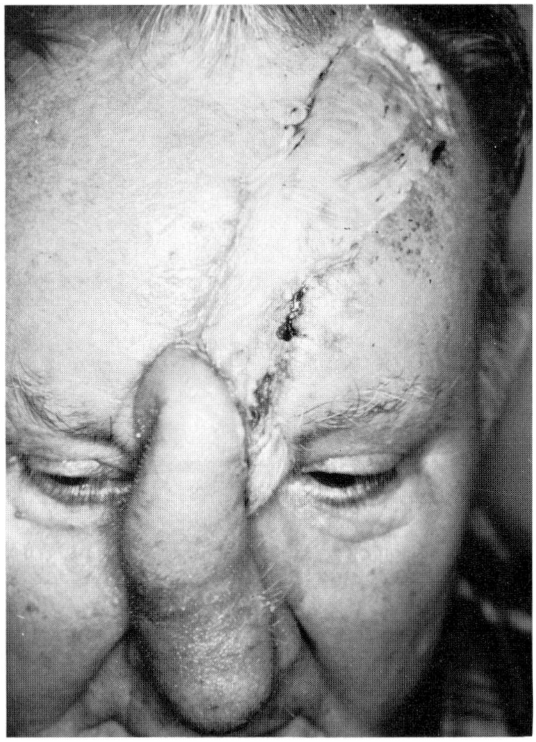

B

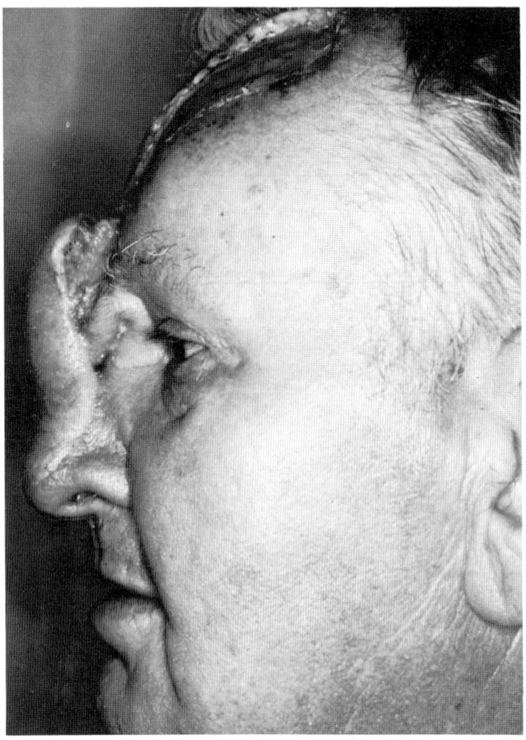

C

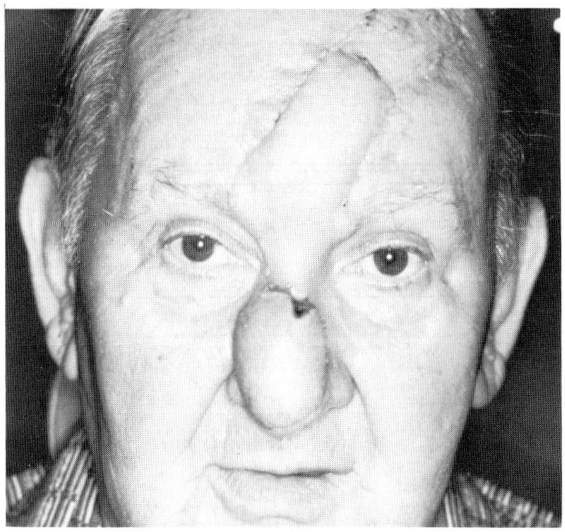

D

Figure 22-4. Frontal-glabella-scalp flap reconstruction of dorsal nasal defect in a 66-year-old man with squamous cell carcinoma. A–C. Appearance 2 weeks after first stage. D. Appearance after second stage: split-thickness skin graft to donor site; dorsal contour will require minor defatting.

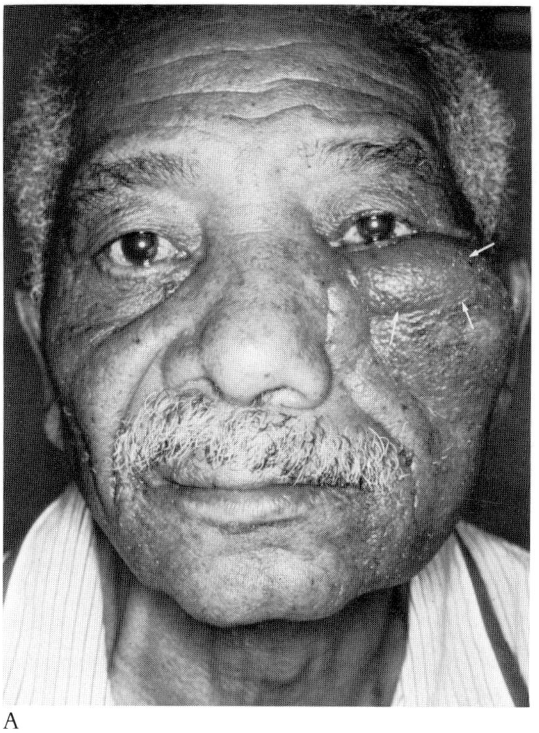

A

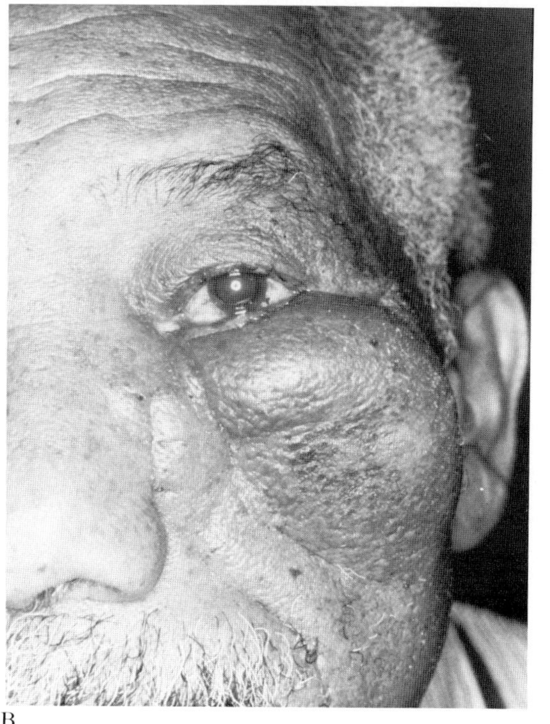

B

Figure 22-5. Preauricular simple transposition flap. A and B. 58-year-old man with recurrent basal cell carcinoma involving the left cheek. C. Remaining defect and proposed transposition flap. (continued)

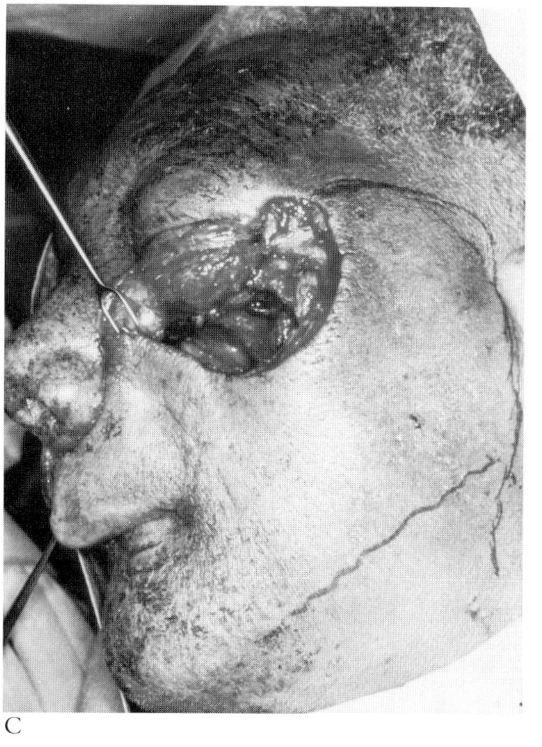

C

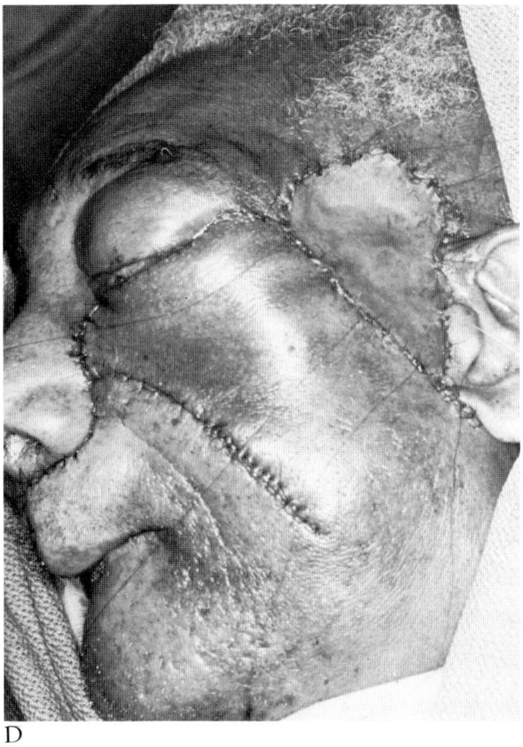

D

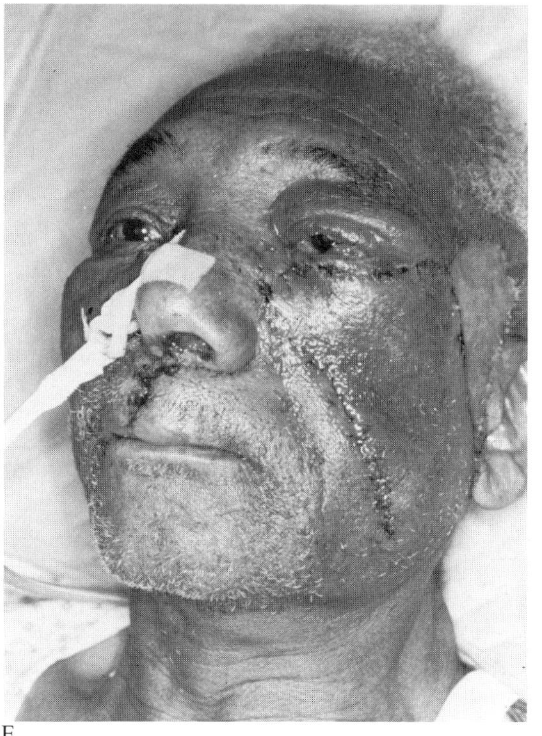

E

Figure 22-5. (continued) D and E. Flap rotated into the defect with a split-thickness skin graft covering the donor site.

Figure 22-6. Cervical rotation flap in a 53-year-old man with (*mucoepidermoid carcinoma*) post full-course radiotherapy and deep recurrence in the right parotid gland. A and B. Flap outline for total parotidectomy and partial facial resection. C. Closure after resection. D and E. Appearance 2 months later: right facial paralysis and scar hypertrophy along posterior border.

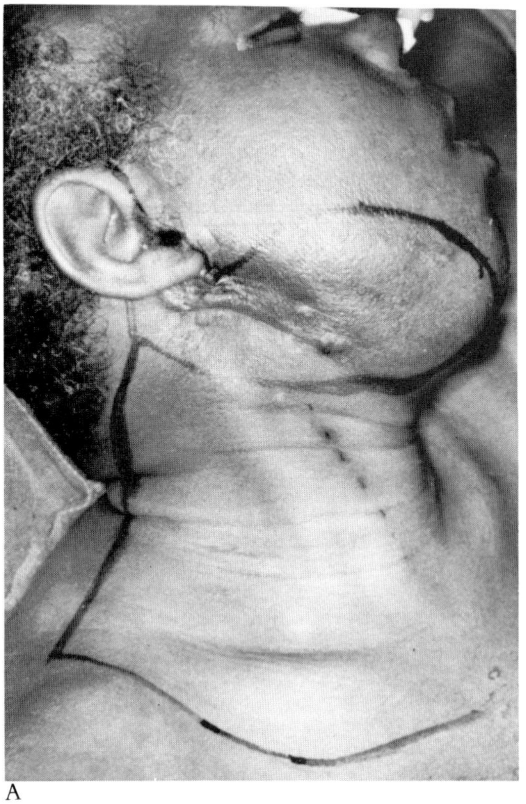

A

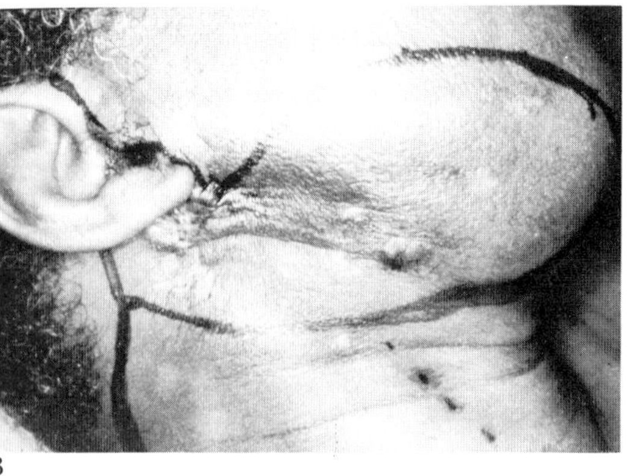

B

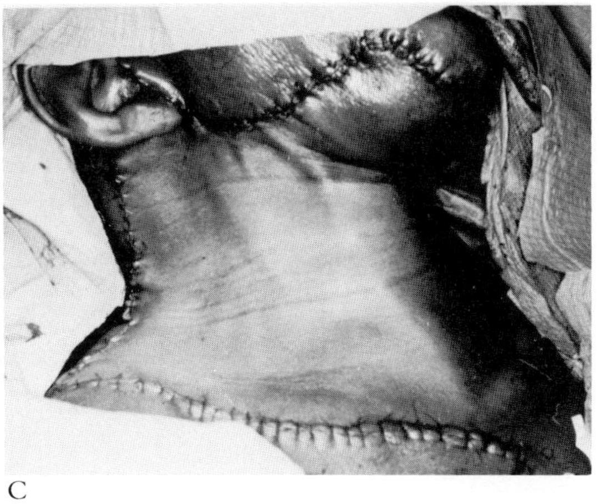

C

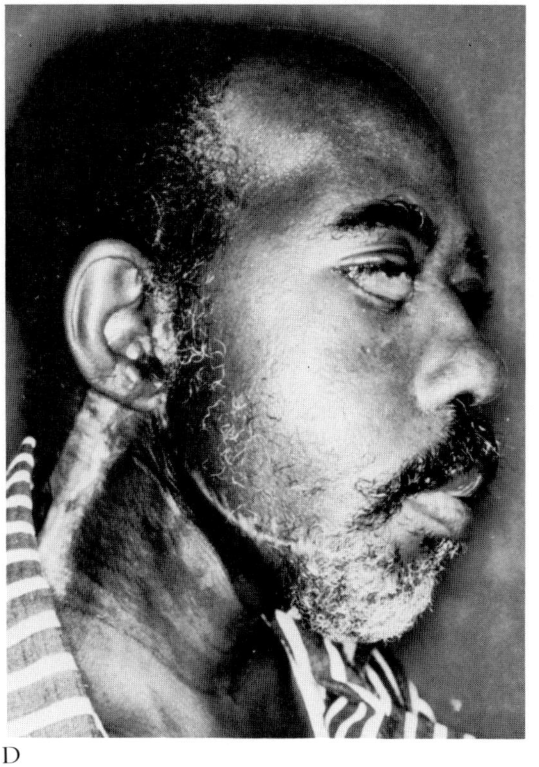

D

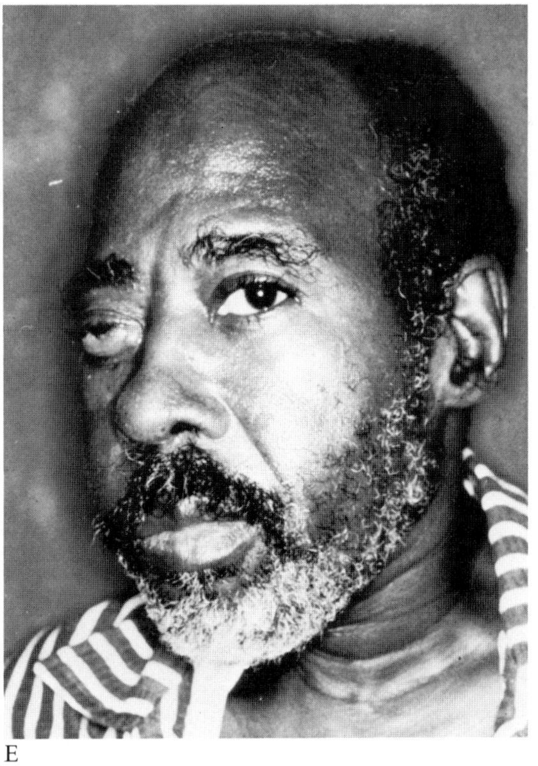

E

Figure 22-7. Temporalis muscle flap. A. Intraoperative view of the squamous cell carcinoma of the right tonsil with palate, tongue, and retromolar trigone extension. B. The proposed incision incorporates the upper component of the McFee incision. C. The flap is elevated from the temporal fossa. D. Immediate postoperative view of the donor site; note the Hemovac drain. E and F. Postoperative views of the donor site. The shadow accentuates the supratemporal fossa defect.

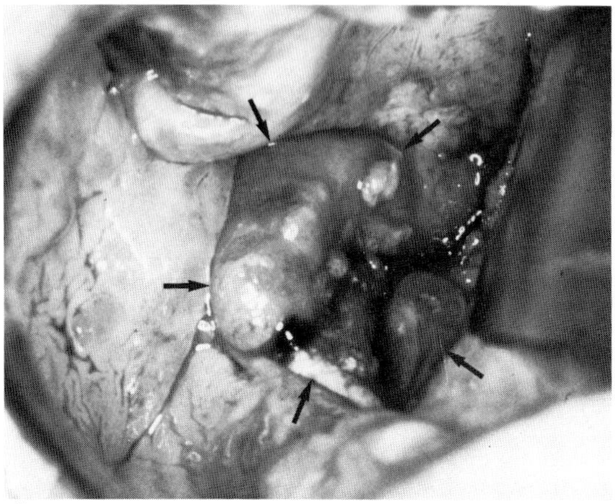

A

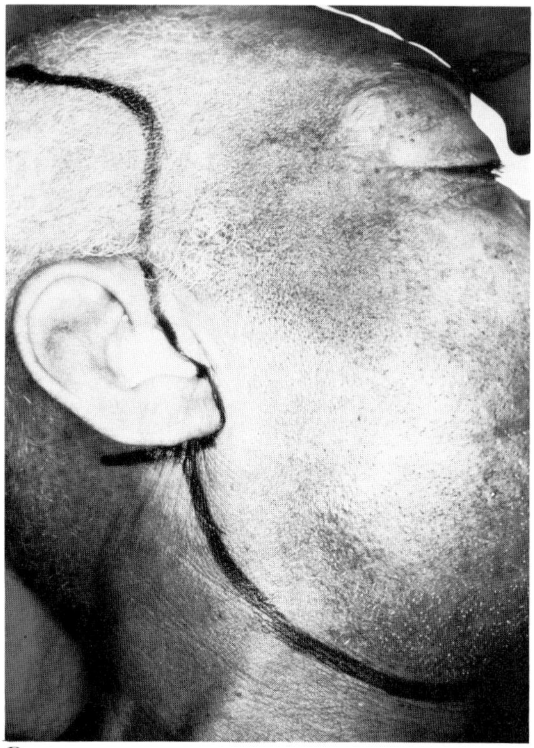

B

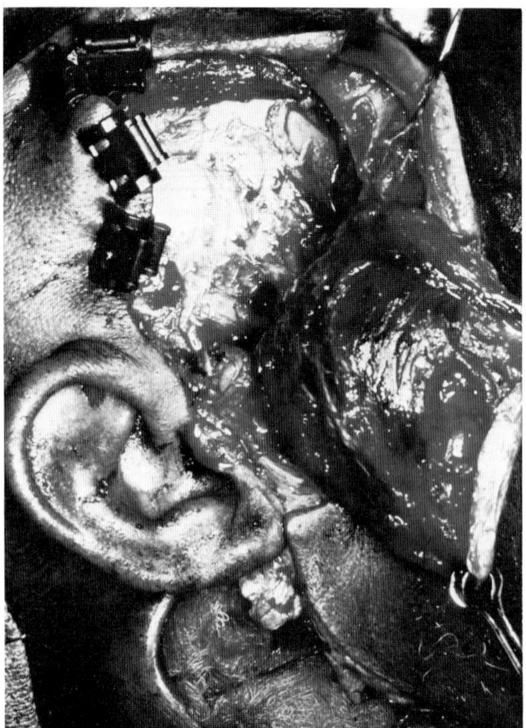

C

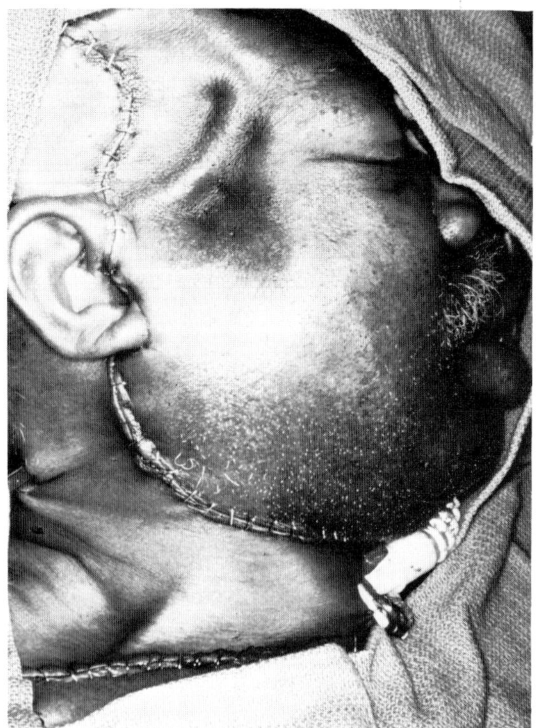

D

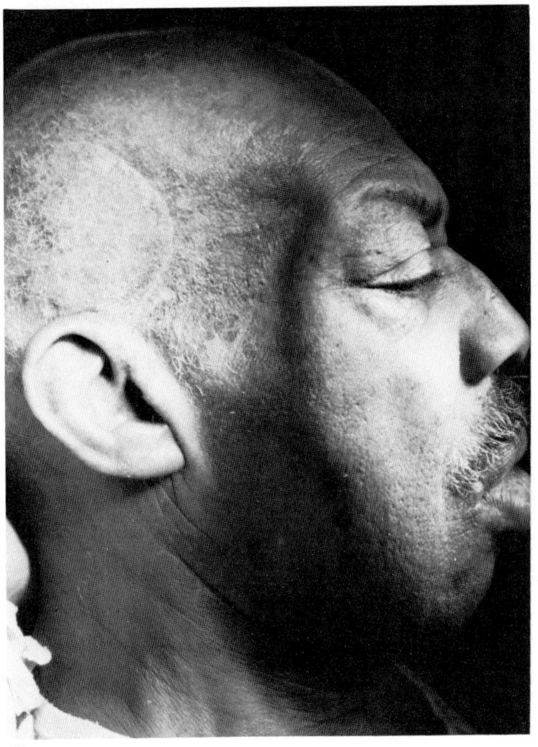

E

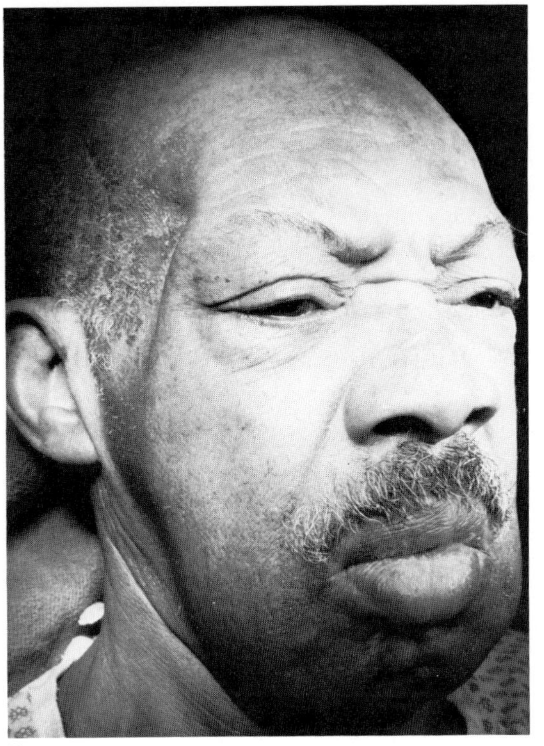

F

Regional Flaps

Although many distant skin flaps have been described for head and neck reconstruction, for many years the deltopectoral flap was the primary regional flap for head and neck reconstruction. It has the following advantages: speed, versatility, reliability, convenience, and a low incidence of complications. The secondary distant flaps are the cervical and trapezius flaps. However, they are less reliable and require multiple delays to enhance viability.

1. Deltopectoral flap
   a. Advantages: simple to elevate; thin and well vascularized.
   b. Disadvantages: donor site requires skin graft; delay suggested in old and medically marginal patients.
   c. Clinical applications: reconstruction of the floor of the mouth; exposed mandibular coverage.
2. Trapezius apron flap [13]
   a. Advantages: large amount of thin skin; sturdiness; major neck and facial coverage.
   b. Disadvantage: frequently requires multiple stages and skin grafts for donor site.

Tissue Expanders

The basic principle of tissue expanders is the creation and development of local donor tissue with the use of a temporary expander [14]. In essence, local skin is stretched to create a redundant skin pouch capable of transfer to a regional location. Most expanders are Silastic bags or pouches locally implanted. Over time, normal saline is injected into a gel-filled valve system. Internal pressure forceably expands the flap, thus creating more available tissue.

The advantages of tissue expanders are donor tissue of the same color, texture, and thickness with minimal scar formation and minor donor site morbidity. The disadvantages are the multiple stages required and unpleasant interim protrusions.

MYOCUTANEOUS FLAPS

Physiology

Myocutaneous flaps are based on the principles of the three-tiered vascularity outlined previously [13]. The body has numerous myocutaneous territories based on musculocutaneous vessels lying between the muscles and overlying skin. This rich, extensive vascularity between the skin and muscle permits the development and transfer of a compound flap (skin and muscle) without regard to length or width.

In the head and neck, there are five major myocutaneous flaps: platysma, sternocleidomastoid, pectoralis major, trapezius, and latissimus dorsi (Table 22-6). Each of these flaps has the following advantages: (1) one-stage reconstruction, (2) primary donor site closure, (3) long arcs of rotation, (4) excellent survival, and (5) nonirradiated tissue transfer [14].

Head and Neck Applications

1. Platysma [16]
    a. Advantages: thin; immediate availability.
    b. Disadvantages: may be (underdeveloped) or attenuated and therefore unreliable; contraindicated in irradiated necks.
    c. Clinical applications: coverage of small wounds in and around the mouth and lips.
2. Sternocleidomastoid [17,19]
    a. Advantages: minimal functional deficit; donor site can be closed primarily.
    b. Disadvantages: tenuous flap; limited arc of rotation; neck contour deformity.
    c. Clinical applications: reconstruction of mouth, floor of mouth, intraoral cheek, etc.
3. Pectorialis major [1,17,20–23]
    a. Advantages: reliable for single-stage reconstruction; coverage of irradiated tissue; restores neck symmetry.
    b. Disadvantages: hair-bearing tissue in men; may cause breast asymmetry in women; bulk in obese or muscular patients.
    c. Clinical applications: intra- and extracervical coverage; bulk from the zygomatic arch to the thoracic inlet (Figure 22-8).
4. Trapezius [24–26]
    a. Advantages: one-stage reconstruction; restores contour; bone may be transferred with the muscle; primary closure of donor site.
    b. Disadvantages: limited arc of rotation; functional loss (shoulder syndrome); patient may have to be repositioned; spinal accessory denervation.
    c. Clinical applications: skin-muscle flap (transverse flap) to resurface the neck, face, or chin; occipital temporal or cranial coverage; intraoral coverage; pharyngeal or mandibular reconstruction.
5. Latissimus dorsi [27–29]
    a. Advantages: large flap; long arc of rotation; sturdy and reliable.
    b. Disadvantages: patient repositioning; tenuous, long vascular pedicle.
    c. Clinical applications: same as for pectoralis major muscle; suitable for women or those patients with an absent pectoralis flap.

FREE TISSUE TRANSFER

Any tissue can be transferred freely provided there is a suitable recipient and donor artery and vein [30,31]. Above all, however, there must be reliable microvascular anastomosis.

Indications

The indications, similar to other flaps, include restoration of external skin, scalp, mandible, and cervical esophagus (Figures 22-9 through 22-11).

Table 22-6. Myocutaneous flaps

Flaps	*Region*	*Blood supply*	*Arc of rotation*	*Indications*	*Features*	*Pitfalls*
Pectoralis	Anterior trunk	Thoracoacromial artery and anterior branch of the second portion of the axillary artery	20 cm Entire sternum Contralateral rib cartilages Midface Skull base	Composite resection of oral cavity and oropharynx Reconstruction of cervical esophagus and hypopharynx	Most reliable and versatile myocutaneous flap	Pendulous breasts Highly developed pectoralis major Neck dissection Injury to axillary vein
Trapezius	Posterior trunk	Transverse cervical artery Descending branches of occipital artery	Head and neck Upper thorax Skull Posterior neck Chest wall Shoulder	Parietal, temporal, orbital reconstruction Intraoral reconstruction	Second most reliable	Spinal accessory denervation Ipsilateral radical neck dissection
Latissimus dorsi	Posterior trunk	Subscapular artery Third portion of axillary artery, divides into circumflex scapular and thoracodorsal arteries	Lateral abdomen Head and neck Posterior neck Lumbar, thoracic, and cervical vertebrae	Same as pectoralis myocutaneous flap	Requires patient repositioning for head and neck transfer	Poor bulk in malnourished and postmastectomy patients Long vascular pedicle Winging of scapula High incidence of seroma formation
Temporalis	Upper face	Internal maxillary, superficial temporal arteries	8 cm Anterior face Inferior, lateral face	Palatectomy Maxillectomy Jaw-neck dissection, Posterior pharynx	Often used with skin and muscle	Male pattern baldness Temporal fossa depression
Sternocleidomastoid	Head and neck	Occipital artery Posterior auricular artery Bunches from thyrocervical trunk	Anterior neck Face Forehead Posterior neck Skull	Mobile tongue Tonsil Floor of mouth Buccal area	The most tenuous myocutaneous flap (30% complication rate) Limited arc of rotation	Internal jugular vein injury Ipsilateral modified neck dissection Spinal accessory denervation Preoperative radiotherapy
Platysma	Neck	Facial artery	8–10 cm Anterior midface Anterior and lateral floor of mouth Angle of mandible	Lower face Floor of mouth	The second most tenuous	Preoperative radiotherapy Carotid artery exposure Ipsilateral neck dissection

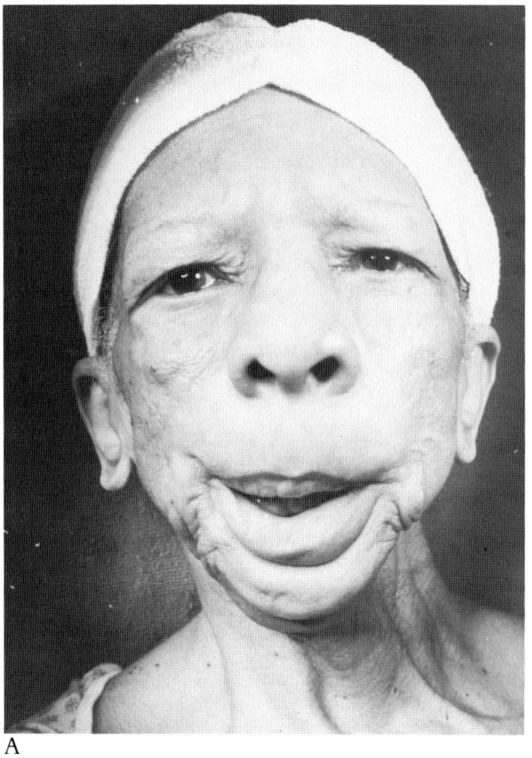

A

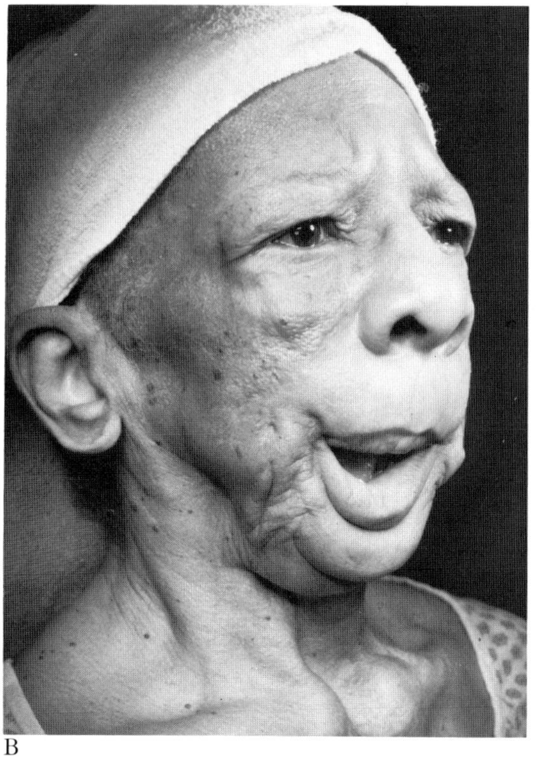

B

Figure 22-9. This elderly woman is 1½ years post–subtotal mandibulectomy for recurrent carcinoma of the floor of the mouth. A and B. Preoperative views. The original reconstruction consisted of bilateral nasolabial flaps and a left pectoralis myocutaneous flap reconstruction. C. The profile demonstrates the drooping chin and lack of lip closure Functionally, she only swallows liquids. D–F. The left foot is the donor site for a dorsalis pedal free tissue transfer. 1 = dorsalis pedal vessels; 2 = skin paddle; 3 = second metatarsal. G. The donor site is covered with a meshed split-thickness skin graft.

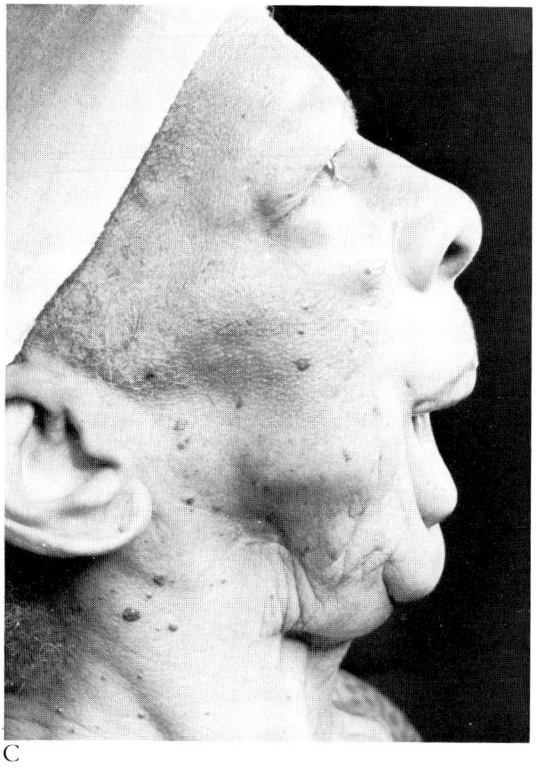

C

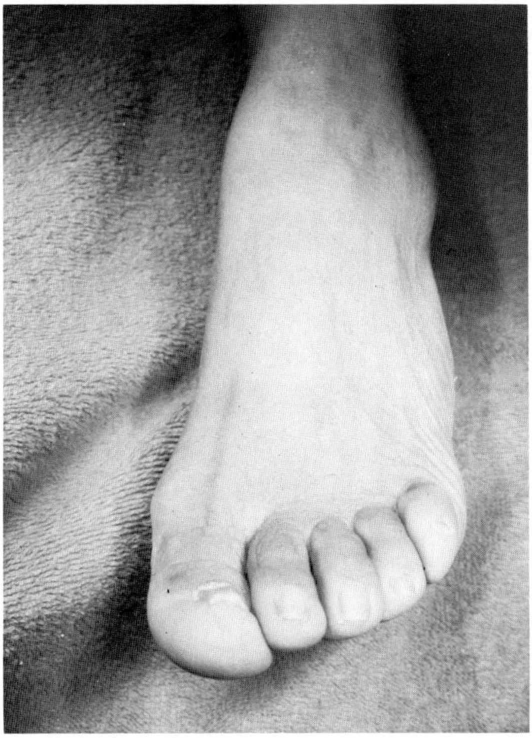

D

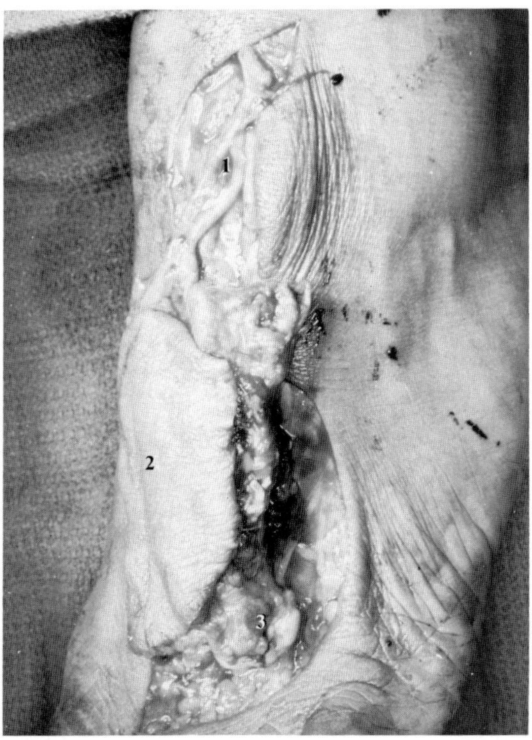

E

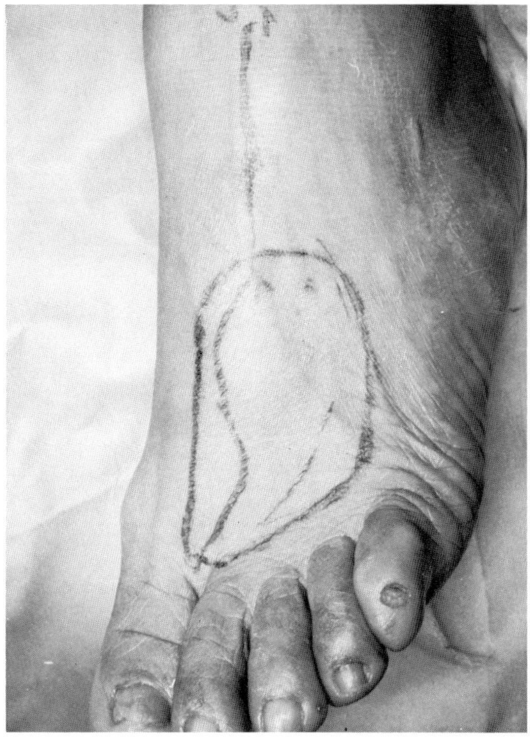

F

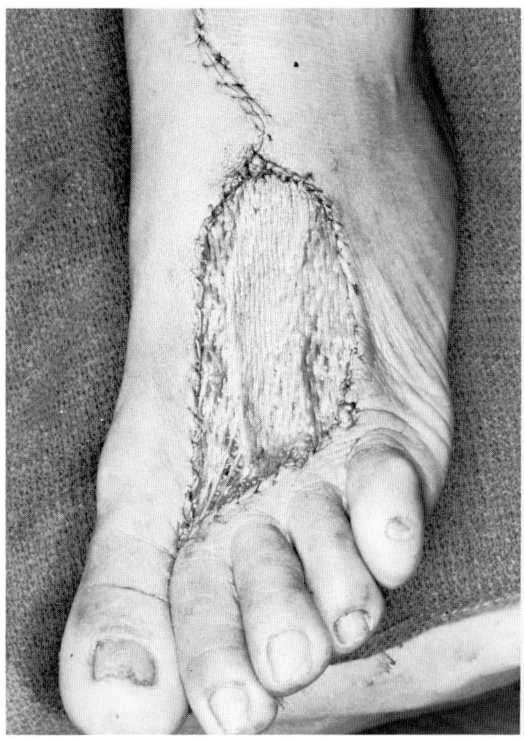

G

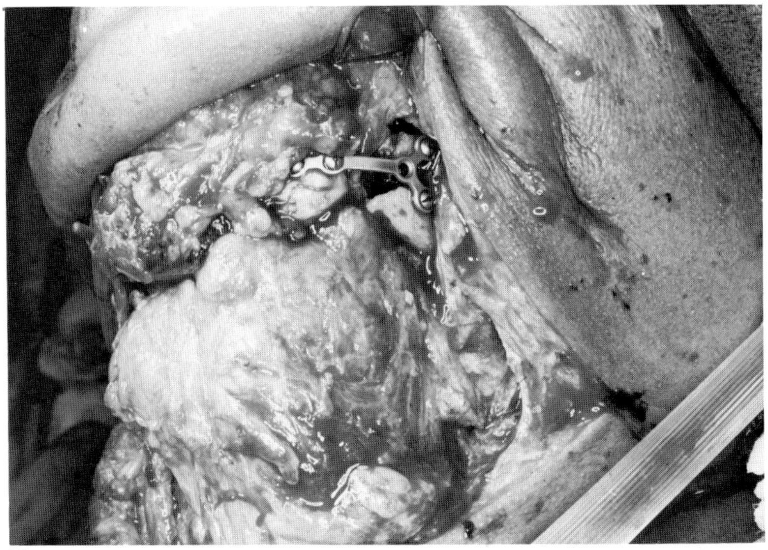

H

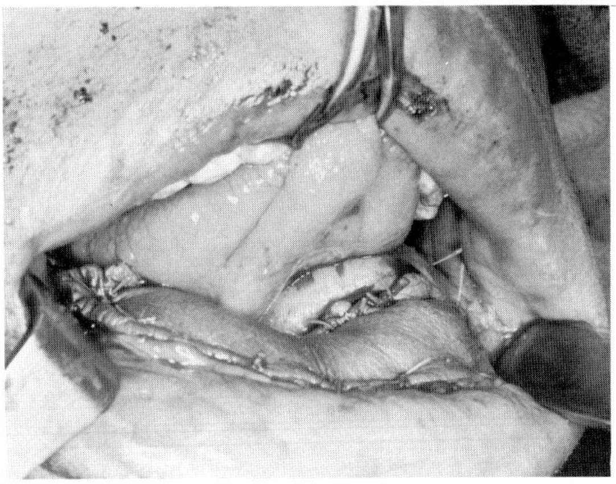

I

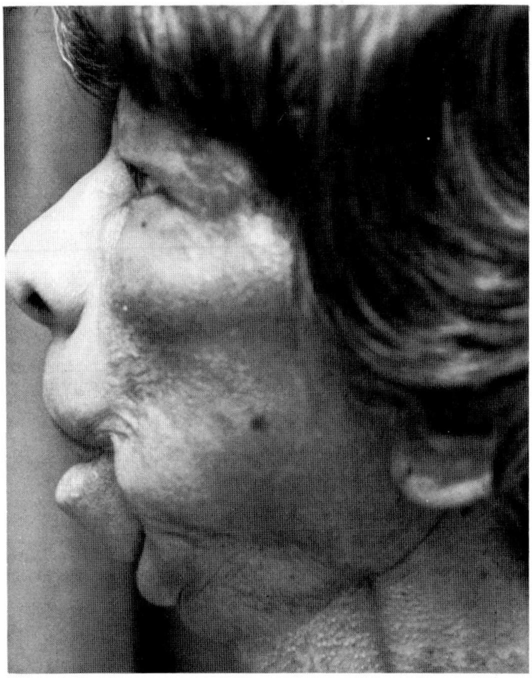

J

Figure 22-9. (continued) H. The second metatarsal is fashioned into a V and secured bilaterally to the residual body of the mandible with titanium miniplates. I. The skin paddle augments the previous soft-tissue reconstruction. J. Postoperative profile view.

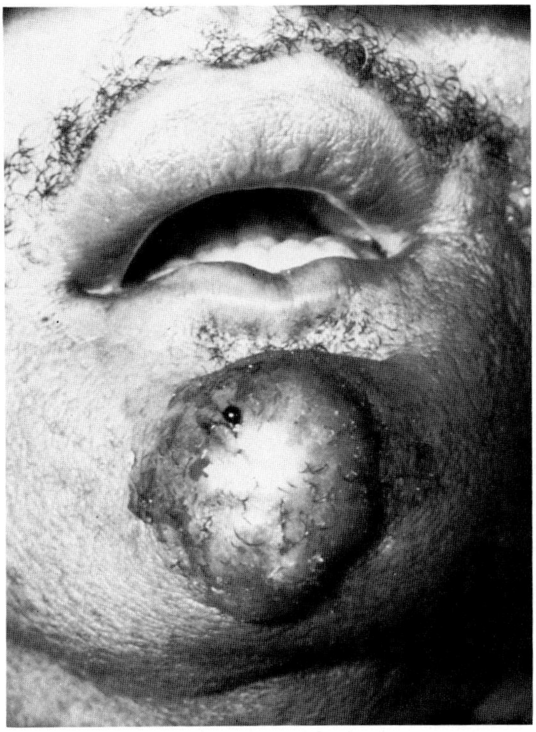

A

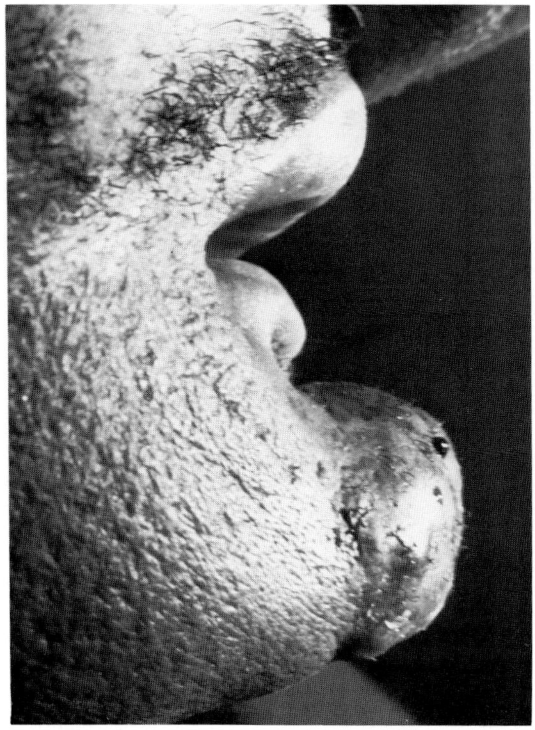

B

Figure 22-10. This middle-aged man has recurrent floor-of-mouth cancer 24 months after floor-of-mouth resection, partial mandibulectomy, bilateral submandibular triangle dissections, and bilateral nasolabial flap reconstruction. A and B. The tumor not only involves the floor of the mouth but also has invaded the symphysis and mentum. C. The proposed resection is a symphysectomy and subtotal mentectomy. (continued)

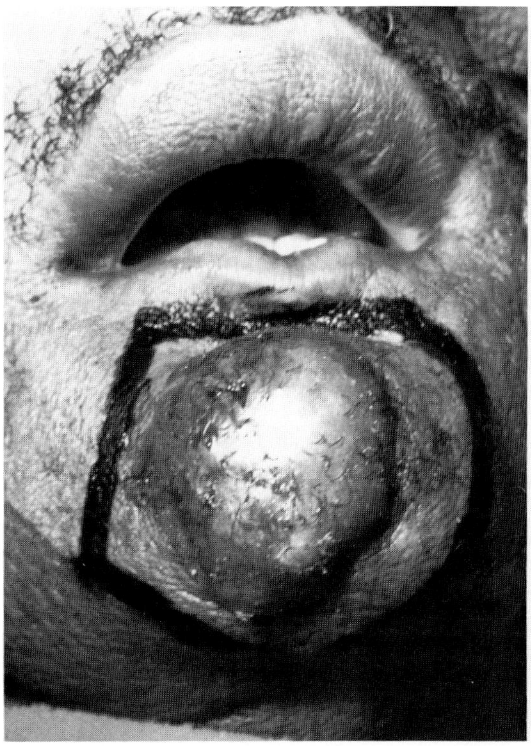

C

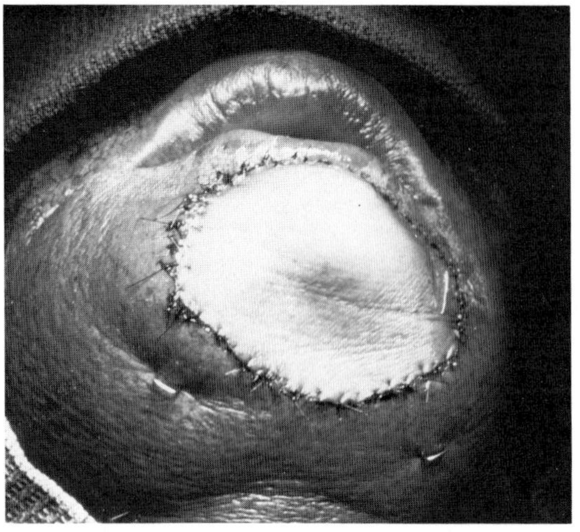

D

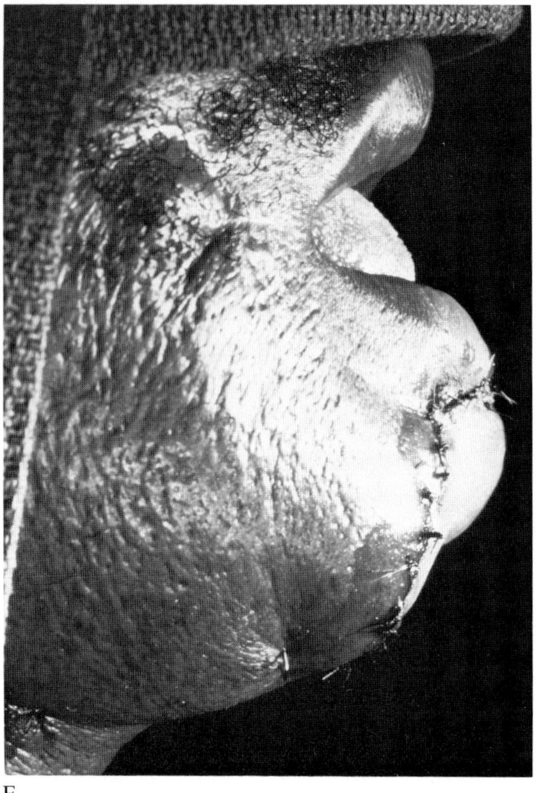

E

Figure 22-10. (continued) D and E. Bilateral dorsalis pedal flaps reconstruct the defect. The pale skin paddle appears pale. F. Within 1 week, the external skin paddle became obviously necrotic. Note both the exposed dead second metastarsal and titanium miniplate. G and H. After local wound toilet and debridement, a left composite free scapular tissue transfer was placed. The massive flap congestion was treated with leeches. (Same patient as in Figure 22–2.)

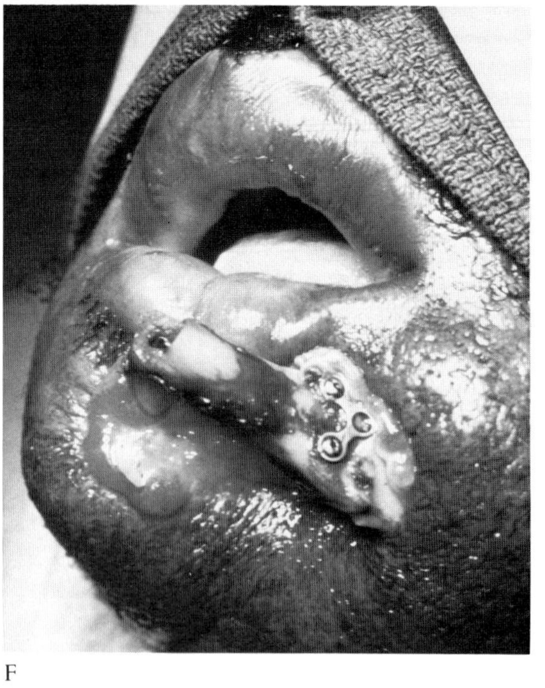

F

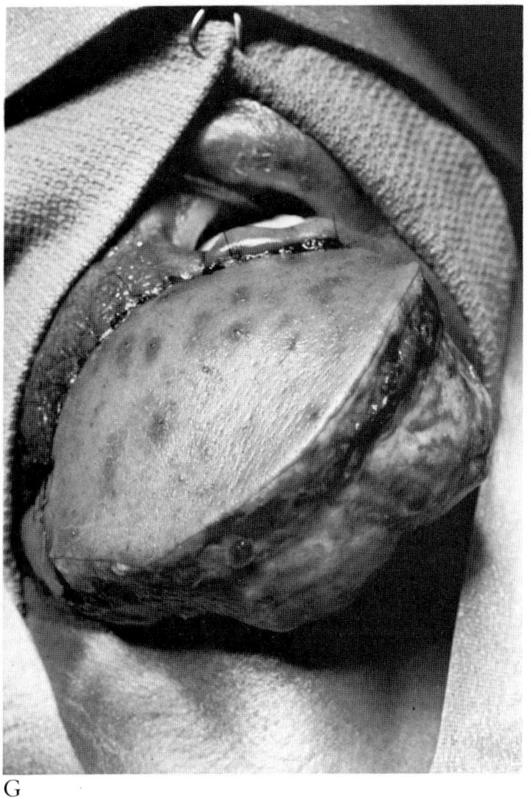

G

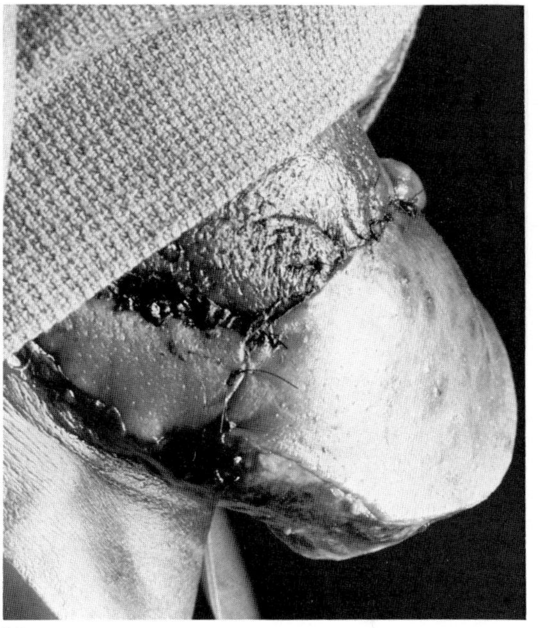

H

Figure 22-11. Free jejunal transfer. A. After total laryngopharyngectomy, a 10-cm jejunal segment is anastomosed to the base of the tongue and esophagus. *jt* = jejunal transfer; *mv* = microvascular pedicle; *cc* = common carotid artery; *sl* = sentinel loop. B. Exteriorization of a small sentinel loop allows for easy monitoring of flap viability. *t* = tracheostoma; *s* = skin staples.

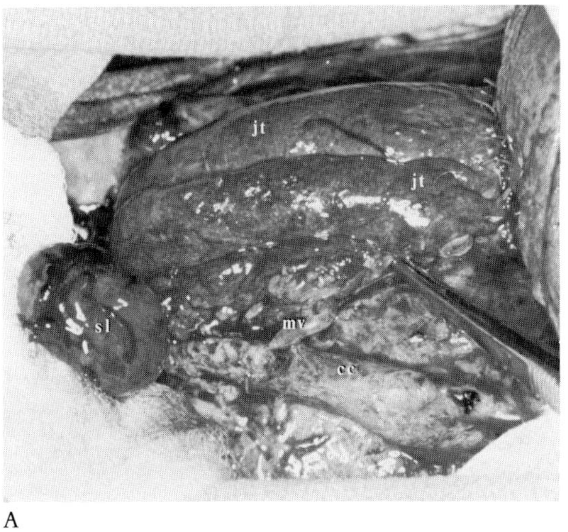

A

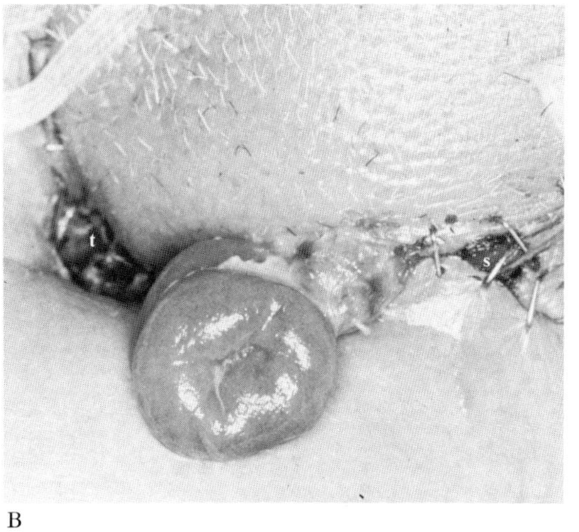

B

Table 22-7. Free tissue transfers

Classification	*Tissue*	*Transfer*	*Indications*	*Pitfalls*
Single tissue	Skin	Groin Dorsalis pedis Median forearm	Bulk, lower jaw lining of oral cavity, oropharynx	Obesity Peripheral vascular disease
	Muscle	Temporalis Latissimus dorsi	Oral cavity oropharynx	Pattern baldness Malnutrition Previous mastectomy
	Bone	Scapula Rib Iliać crest Second metatarsal	Mandibular reconstruction	Winged scapula Pneumothorax Chronic hip pain Peripheral vascular disease
	Nerve	Superficial peroneal	Facial nerve graft	Regional hypesthesia
	Intestine	Jejunum	Esophageal reconstruction	Previous abdominal surgery
Compound tissue	Myocutaneous	Latissimus dorsi Rectus abdominis	Oral cavity Oropharynx	Malnutrition Obesity
	Osseocutaneous	Temporalis calvarium Dorsalis pedal (2nd metatarsal) Groin-iliac crest	Mandibular reconstruction	Skull defect Gait difficulties

Contraindications

The biggest contraindication is nonavailability of healthy recipient vessels, especially suitable veins. It appears that the most reliable anastomoses are end-to-side grafts to the carotid artery and the internal jugular vein.

Material and Methods

Unlike other forms of head and neck reconstruction, with free tissue transfer there is a more intense commitment of time, expertise, and instrumentation (Table 22-7). Microsurgery requires an operating microscope, trained assistants, microinstruments, and microsutures. In particular, the microsurgeon must have reliable skills honed after hours of practice in the microvascular laboratory.

1. The tissue transfer must be entirely nourished by pedicled vessels of sufficient diameter, that is, greater than 0.6 mm
2. The tissue transfer must be predictable in its location and vascular territory.
3. The tissue transfer must be harvested with little donor site cosmetic or functional deformity.
4. The tissue transfer must be adequate for both coverage and function.

REFERENCES

1. Conley J: *Regional Flaps of the Head and Neck.* Philadelphia: Saunders, 1976.
2. Gullane PJ, Heeneman H: *Regional Flaps in the Head and Neck: Self-Instructional Package.* Rochester, MN: American Academy of Otorhinolaryngology Foundation 1986.
3. Gillies HD, Millard DR: *The Principles and Art of Plastic Surgery.* Boston: Little Brown, 1957.
4. Cutting, C: Skin Physiology. In: *Otolaryngology: Head and Neck Surgery* St. Louis: Mosby, 1986. Pp 89–99.
5. McGregor IA, Morgan G: Axial and random pattern flaps. *Br J Plast Surg* 26 : 202, 1973.
6. Milton SH: Pedicled skin flaps: The fallacy of the length-width ratio. *Br J Surg* 57 : 502, 1973.
7. Converse JM: *Surgical Treatment of Facial Injuries.* Baltimore: Williams & Wilkins, 1975, Pp 486–529.

8. Kerrigan CL, Daniel RK: Monitoring acute skin-flap failure. *Plast Reconstr Surg* 71(4) : 519, 1983.
9. Davidson TM, Webster RC: *Scar Revision: Self-Instructional Package*. Rochester, MN: American Academy of Otorhinolaryngology, Head and Neck Surgery, 1977.
10. Silverman DG, et al: Monitoring tissue elimination of fluorescein with the perfusion fluorometer: A new method to assess capillary blood flow. *Surgery* 90 : 409, 1981.
11. Nolan J, et al: The acute effects of cigarette smoke exposure on experimental skin flaps. *Plast Reconstr Surg* 75(4) : 544, 1985.
12. Rubin LS, Mishriki Y, Lee G: Anatomy of the nasolabial fold: The keystone of the smiling mechanism. *Plast Reconstr Surg* 83(11) : 1, 1989.
13. Owens N: Compound neck pedicle designed for repair of massive facial defects: Formation development and application. *Plast Reconstr Surg* 15 : 369, 1955.
14. Radovan C: Tissue expansion in soft-tissue reconstruction. *Plast Reconstr Surg* 74(4) : 482, 1984.
15. McCraw JB, Dibbell DG, Carraway JH: Clinical definition of independent myocutaneous flap territories. *Plast Reconstr Surg* 60 : 341, 1977.
16. Cantrell RW: Myocutaneous Flaps. In: Symposium 1983 On Reconstruction in Head and Neck Surgery. *Otolaryngol Clin North Am* 16 : 353, 1983.
17. Coleman JJ, et al. The platysma musculocutaneous flap: Experience with 24 cases. *Plast Reconstr Surg* 72(3) : 315, 1983.
18. Larson DL, Goepfert H: Limitations of the sternocleidomastoid musculocutaneous flap in head and neck cancer reconstruction. *Plast Reconstr Surg* 72(3) : 328, 1981.
19. McGaw J, Magie WP, Kalwaic A: Uses of the trapezius and sternomastoid myocutaneous flaps in head and neck reconstruction. *Plast Reconstr Surg* 63 : 49, 1979.
20. Baek SM, Lawson WL, Biller HF. An analysis of 133 pectoralis major myocutaneous flaps. *Plast Reconstr Surg* 67(3) : 460, 1982.
21. Little, JW, McCullock PT, Lyons JR: The lateral pectoral composite flap in one-stage reconstruction of the irradiated mandible. *Plast Reconstr Surg* 71(3) : 326, 1983.
22. Tobin GR: Pectoralis major segmental anatomy and segmentally split pectoralis major flaps. *Plast Reconstr Surg* 75(6) : 814, 1985.
23. Ariyan S: The pectoralis major myocutaneous flap: A versatile flap for reconstruction in the head and neck. *Plast Reconstr Surg* 63 : 73, 1979.
24. Rosen HM: The extended trapezius musculocutaneous flap for craniorbital-facial reconstruction. *Plast Reconstr Surg* 75(3) : 318, 1985.
25. Guillamondegui OM, Larson DL: The lateral trapezius musculocutaneous flap: Its use in head and neck reconstruction. *Plast Reconstr Surg* 67(2) : 143, 1981.
26. Baek SM, et al: The lower trapezius island myocutaneous flap. *Ann Plast Surg* 5 : 108, 1980.
27. Quillen CG: Latissimus dorsi myocutaneous flaps in head and neck reconstruction. *Plast Reconstr Surg* 63 : 644, 1979.
28. Dinner MI, Peters CR: The arc of the latissimus dorsi myocutaneous flap. *Ann Plast Surg* 3 : 425, 1979.
29. Bartoy FE, Spicer TE, Byra HS: Head and neck reconstruction with the latissimus dorsi myocutaneous flap: Anatomic observations and report of 60 cases. *Plast Reconstr Surg* 71(1) : 199, 1983.
30. Harii K, et al: Pharyngoesophageal reconstruction using a fabricated forearm free flap. *Plast Reconstr Surg* 75(4) : 463, 1985.
31. Harii K, et al: Microvascular free skin flap transfer. *Clin Plast Surg* (5)2 : 239, 1978.
32. Brent B, et al: Experience with the temporoparietal fascial free flap. *Plast Reconstr Surg* 76(2) : 177, 1985.

23

Mandibular Reconstruction

NEAL BECKFORD

KEY CONCEPTS

Defect Classification; Planning; Alloplasts; Cancellous Bone; Osseomyocutaneous Grafts; Microvascular Grafts

MILESTONES

Pre–World War I	Cortical Bone Grafts for Mandibular Reconstruction	
1915	Superiority of Cancellous Iliac over Cortical Bone Grafts	Lindermann
1944	Fractured Cancellous Bone	Mowlem
1969	Inert Metallic Trays	Boyne, Hahn, and Corgill
1979	Osseous Microvascular Free Grafts	Taylor

PLANNING

Restoration of mandibular continuity after an ablative head and neck procedure is extremely difficult (Table 23-1, Figure 23-1) [1]. There are many options whose techniques are somewhat controversial. Furthermore, the myriad possibilities often confuse the basic issues: (1) patient benefit, (2) morbidity, (3) integration within a treatment plan, (4) timing, and (5) method [1,2]. Obviously, careful preoperative analysis is essential for successful restoration (see Chapters 7 and 22). This chapter explores the options available for mandibular reconstruction (Table 23-2, Figure 23-2).

Classification

There are three postoperative mandibular defects, depending on the site and amount of bone removed (Figure 23-3).

1. Segmental body: excision between the mental foramen and the angle.
2. Posterior mandible and ramus: excision from the mental foramen to the mandibular notch.
3. Anterior segment: resection of the mandibular arch.

What to Reconstruct

Posterior Segment

Posterior segment resections are the most common defects. Since the functional deficit is minimal, they usually are not reconstructed. Patients have more difficulty adjusting to the loss of function after oral and oropharyngeal soft-tissue resection than from the mandibular resection. Esthetically, the defect can be significant. However, after successful rehabilitation, most patients are satisfied and hesitant to undergo further surgery. In fact, reconstruction of the posterior body and ramus may cause even more disability, such as trismus.

Body

Mandibular arch and segmental body resections cause considerable morbidity and deserve con-

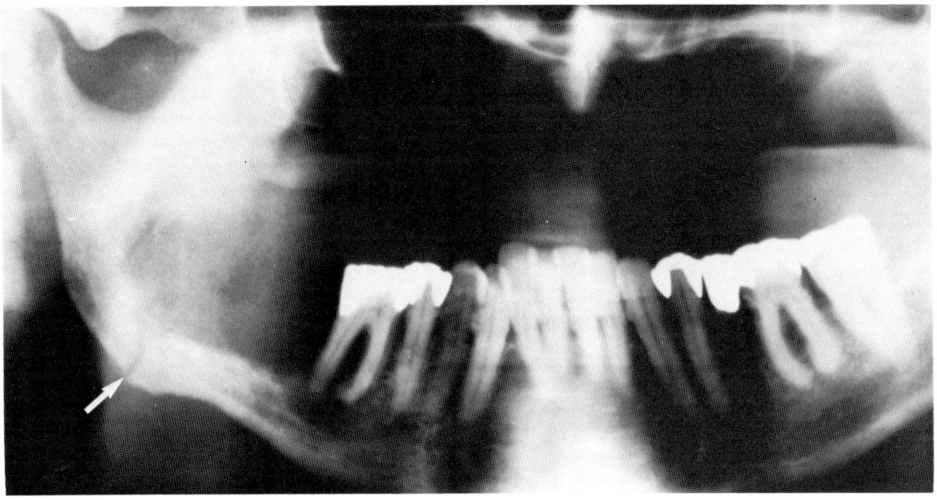

Figure 23-1. Panorex of the mandible. A large invasive lesion occupies the right body. There is an associated pathologic fracture.

sideration for reconstruction. Segmental body resections produce significant dysfunction and cosmetic deformity. Unless corrected early, severe malocclusion develops between the maxillary and mandibular teeth secondary to mandibular drift. Mandibular drift is caused by the unopposed action of the ipsilateral muscles of mastication, postoperative scarring, and the type of oral cavity reconstruction. If reconstruction is not anticipated, then the remaining posterior body and ramus are removed to facilitate primary closure [3].

Anterior Segment

Arch resections are debilitating, both functionally and esthetically. The arch stabilizes the hyoid bone and facilitates anterior and posterior tongue movement via the genioglossus muscle. It also serves as the point of attachment for the mylohyoid muscle, a dynamic contributor to the floor of the mouth. Loss of the arch collapses the oral cavity, compromises oral competence, and affects tongue protrusion. Ultimately, speech, swallowing, and esthetics are compromised severely. Thus, reconstruction is beneficial and is recommended strongly.

Immediate Versus Delayed Reconstruction

Historically, delayed mandibular reconstruction is the preferred method [4]. Immediate reconstruction has a higher incidence of intraoral graft exposure, wound infection, graft loss, extrusion, and fistulization. Graft exposure to contaminated saliva is the most common cause of rejections or failures. Higher success rates are obtained by delayed reconstruction when the oral cavity defect is well healed. The subsequent reconstruction, being extraoral, decreases the risk of contamination. Although radiation inhibits graft healing, delayed reconstruction facilitates timely and appropriate radiation therapy. Waiting for confirmation of surgical margins and adequacy of resection also is prudent. Finally, with immediate reconstruction, there is the unconscious temptation to compromise the surgical ablation to accommodate the anticipated reconstruction.

Radiation

Most lesions that require mandibulectomy are best treated by combined therapy (see

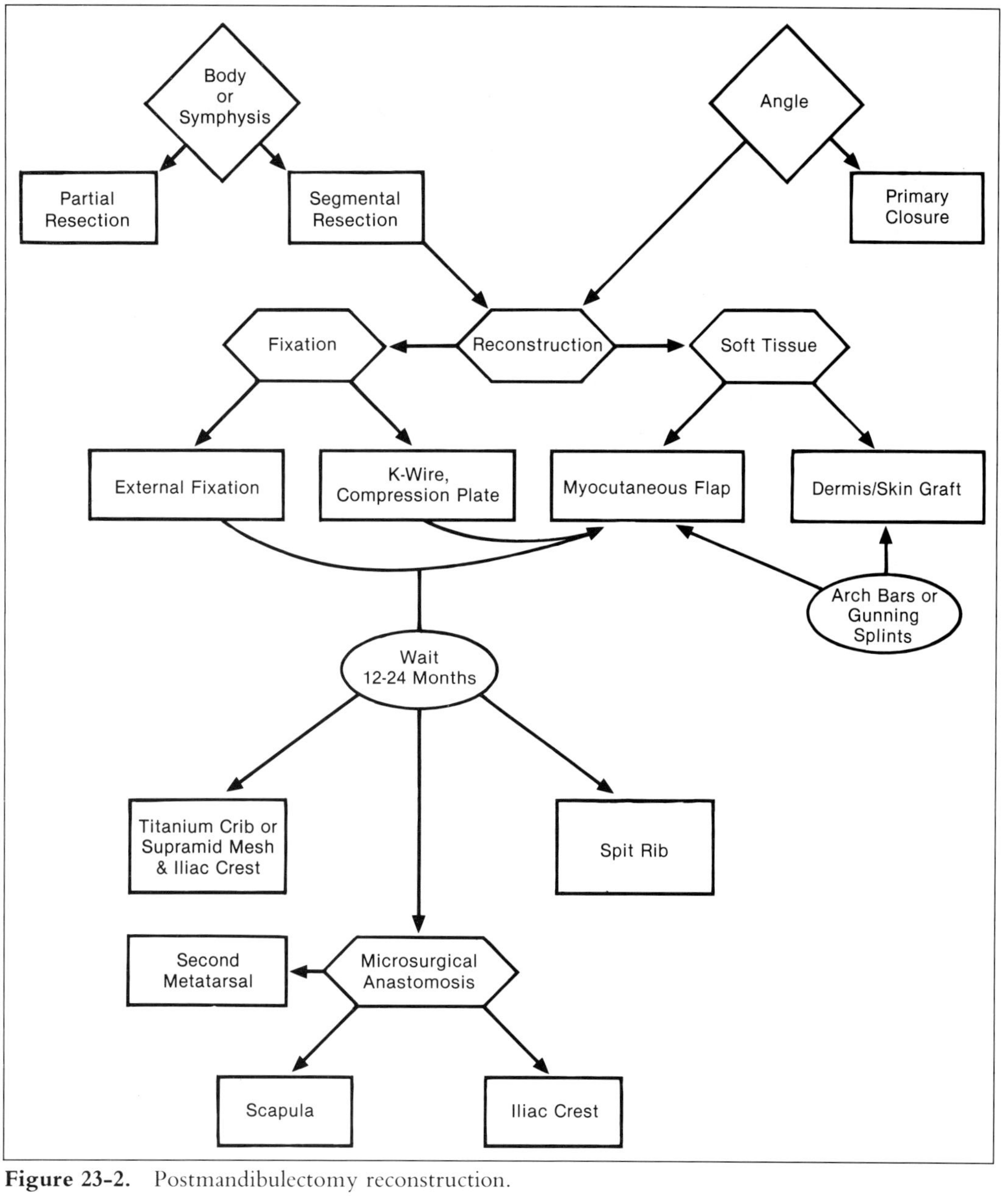

Figure 23-2. Postmandibulectomy reconstruction.

Chapter 7). Post operative radiation therapy generally is more effective when administered within 6 weeks after surgery [5]. A procedure should be completed within this grace period. Thus, reconstruction that has a high incidence of postoperative complications precludes the administration of timely radiation therapy.

Metal compression plates or trays may create problems by generating secondary electrons that affect irradiation dosimetry. Dosimetric miscalculations are implicated in some treatment failures. If possible, metallic appliances in the treatment field are avoided. External fixation devices are less problematic.

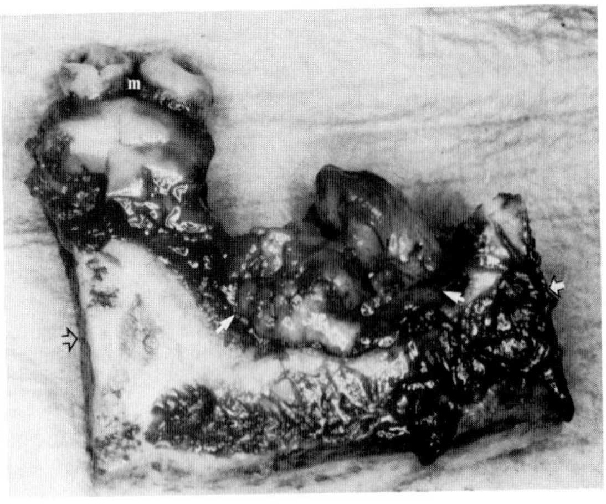

A

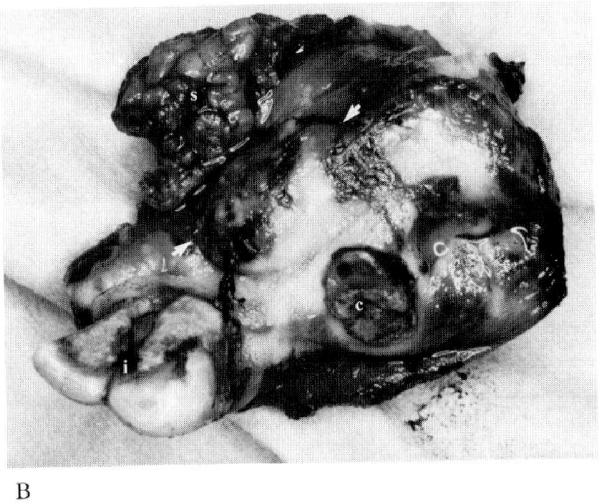

B

Figure 23-3. Typical surgical pathologic specimens. A. Right body resection for invasive squamous cell carcinoma. *m* = molars; *white arrows* = tumor; *open arrows* = osteotomy cuts. B. Symphysectomy for invasive squamous cell carcinoma (*arrows*). *i* = incisors; *s* = right sublingual gland; *c* = canine.

Table 23-1. Mandibular reconstruction goals

Arch continuity
Maintenance of oral function
Articulation
Mastication
Swallowing
Airway
Preservation of facial contour

Table 23-2. Reconstruction prerequisites

Stable patient
Negative surgical margins
Healthy mandibular remnants
Clean wound bed

OPTIONS

Prerequisites

Versatility

Choosing an appropriate method for mandibular reconstruction given the many available options is confusing (Tables 23-3, 23-4; Figure 23-2). This cornucopia reflects that no one option is perfect. The surgeon should be acquainted with a number of techniques and choose a method that technically is both feasible and most appropriate for the given clinical situation (Figure 23-4).

Vascularity

Adequate vascularity of the recipient bed is a must for any nonvascularized graft, especially in the symphysis and parasymphyseal areas. Obviously, vascularity is not as important when free grafts or osseomyocutaneous grafts are utilized. The presence of nonvital teeth, hematomas, foreign bodies, and wound dehiscence also contributes to poor vascularity and postoperative graft failure.

Table 23-3. Reconstruction options

Primary closure
Soft tissue
Soft tissue with stabilization
A-O compression plates
Interdental fixation
External splint
K-wire
Soft tissue with bone
Nonvascular bone
Iliac crest
Split calvarium
Split rib
Vascularized bone
Trapezius osseomyocutaneous flap
Pectoralis osseomyocutaneous flap
Free vascularized bone
Iliac crest
Rib
Scapula

Table 23-4. Mandibular reconstruction

	Advantages	*Disadvantages*	*Complications*
Iliac crest	Good for small defects Can be bridged for larger defects Easy access Moderate morbidity	Slow remineralization Longer immobilization Needs a good vascular bed Donor site defect may be significant	Nonunion, delayed union Malunion Bone resorption Infection Osteomyelitis
Cancellous bone and marrow	Abundant graft material Great osteogenic ability Less donor site defect Tray provides good support Shorter immobilization	Large amount of foreign material in graft site Limited vertical height of tray limits osteogenic potential Tray may need removal	Infection/fistula Nonunion Malunion
Osseomyocutaneous grafts	Familiar techniques Soft-tissue coverage possible Suited for immediate reconstruction	Vascular supply of graft segment tenuous Cartilage resorption Awkward positioning for trapezius flap	Cartilage resorption Graft slough Orocutaneous fistula Malunion, nonunion
Vascular free grafts	Best for immediate reconstruction Excellent after radiation or with compromised vascular beds	Microvascular expertise necessary Prolonged operating time Results in inexperienced hands are poor	Vascular compromise Graft slough Orocutaneous fistula Malunion, nonunion

Figure 23-4. Dermal-pouch reconstruction (*white arrows*). Post left jaw-neck dissection. *da* = anterior belly of digastric and *dp* = posterior belly of digastric muscle; *dg* = dermal graft over carotid artery. The pouch is stuffed with antibiotically impregnated cotton balls.

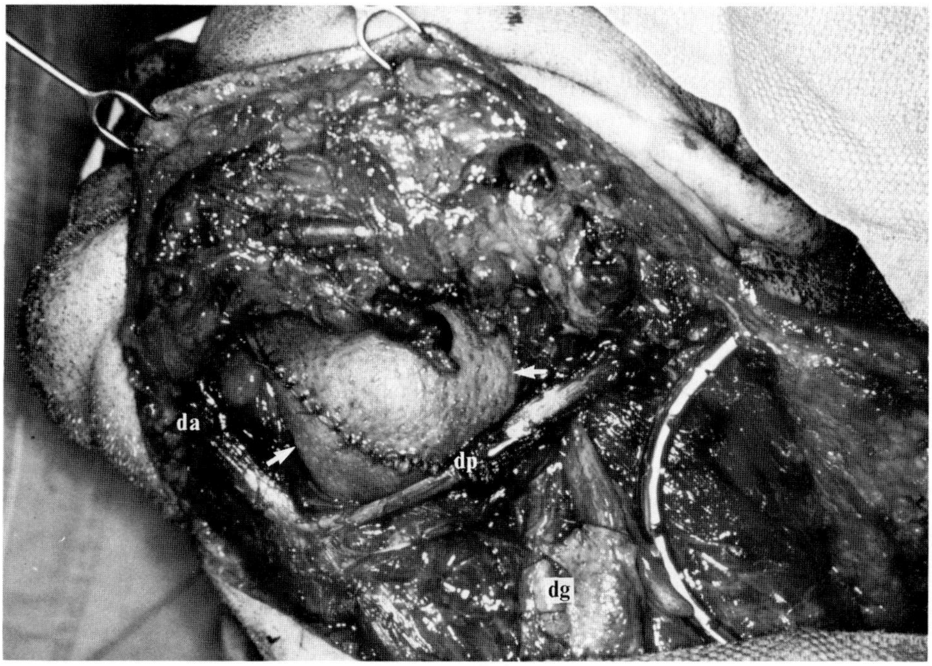

Table 23-5. Osseomyocutaneous flaps

Muscle	*Bone*	*Artery*	*Advantages*	*Disadvantages*
Trapezius	Spine of scapula	Transverse cervical artery	Low donor site morbidity	Resection of acromion leads to shoulder dysfunction; variable origin of artery
Pectoralis major	Sternum (outer table)	Thoracoacromial artery	No need to turn patient	Thin bone makes fixation difficult
Pectoralis major	Anterior rib	Thoracoacromial artery	No need to turn patient	Curvature of rib requires rotation of pedicle
Serratus anterior	Anterior rib (sixth)	Thoracodorsal artery	Prevent dysfunction of serratus by using only inferior slips	May require division of clavicle
Latissimus dorsi	Posterior rib	Thoracodorsal	Patients with pendulous breasts	Patient reposition Long vascular pedicle
Sternocleidomastoid	Clavicle	Occipital & transverse cervical	Same field as most primary head and neck tumors	Field of resection for radical neck dissection Limited arc of rotation Tenuous musculocutaneous perforators

Source: Courtesy of Lisa Fox, M.D.

Trapezius Grafts

A trapezius myocutaneous flap with attached scapular spine is popular for anterior mandibular defects. Based on the transverse cervical artery, these flaps offer 10 to 12 cm of vascularized bone that is usually 2 cm in height. Bone cuts or small wedges are removed on the proposed lingual surface to mold an arch. Although this flap has a vigorous vascular supply, some surgeons report problems with graft viability. In addition, patient positioning for ablation and reconstruction is cumbersome [10].

Pectoralis Grafts

Pectoralis major myocutaneous flaps with attached rib are somewhat successful. The fourth or fifth rib is harvested, carefully maintaining continuity between the undersurface of the muscle and the anterior rib periosteum. There is no attempt to harvest the posterior periosteum, as this increases the risk of pneumothorax. The graft is attached to the previously stabilized mandibular segments with interosseous wiring. Theoretically, the well-vascularized pectoralis muscle increases the likelihood of viability. Varying amounts of cartilage in the rib segments, high rates of resorption, and pneumothorax are the unattractive features [11].

Sternocleidomastoid and Latissimus Dorsi Grafts

Superiorly based sternocleidomastoid flaps, with attached clavicle, and latissimus dorsi myocutaneous flaps, with attached posterior rib, are recommended for experienced surgeons. Sternocleidomastoid flaps have the highest rate of myocutaneous flap failure. As for latissimus dorsi myocutaneous flaps, patient positioning and flap mobilization are tedious. In addition, mechanical problems with the long vascular pedicle during its transfer from its donor site to a relatively distant recipient site contribute to graft failure.

Microvascular Free Grafts

Advantage

Microvascular surgery creates exciting possibilities for mandibular reconstruction. Free microvascular bone grafts have many advantages over other methods (Table 23-6, Figure 23-9). Being highly vascular, these grafts are more resistant to infection, extrusion, and radiation therapy. Free iliac crest, scapular spine, and rib grafts are all successful microvascular techniques [12,13].

Disadvantages

Free tissue transfers also have distinct disadvantages. Although head and neck surgeons are becoming more proficient with microvascular skills, many remain untrained. Often a second team is necessary for reconstruction. Microvascular reconstruction adds 4 to 6 more hours of operative time. Graft survival is related directly to successful vascular anastomosis and microvascular team expertise. Finally, vascular access is a problem after neck dissection and irradiation. Arterial anastomosis is performed commonly to the stump of the facial or superior thyroid arteries. When necessary, an end-to-side anastomosis is created directly to the carotid artery. Venous access is more difficult. Most microvascular surgeons prefer the internal jugular vein for venous access; this is a problem when florid neck metastasis dictates internal jugular sacrifice. If venous access is inadequate, free flaps are abandoned.

Table 23-6. Free osseocutaneous flaps

Bone	*Artery*	*Advantages*	*Disadvantages*
Radius (portion)	Radial artery	Up to 14 cm of bone available	Potential for pathologic fracture of forearm Anesthesia over radical nerve distribution Possible hand ischemia
Iliac crest	Deep and/or superficial iliac artery	14 cm of bone available Well-hidden scar	Late hernia Osteotomies needed for contour Bulky flap in obese patients Gait disturbance Numbness in anterior thigh
Scapula (lateral border)	Circumflex artery	No functional loss Up to 14 cm of bone available	Osteotomies needed for contour Patient reposition
Second metatarsal	Dorsalis pedis artery	No gait problems Minimal cosmetic deformity Efficient two team utilization	Average 7 cm of bone available Osteotomies needed for contour

Source: Courtesy of Lisa Fox, M.D.

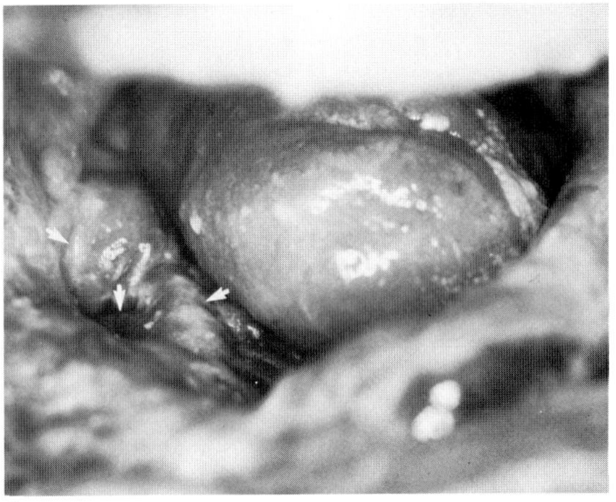

A

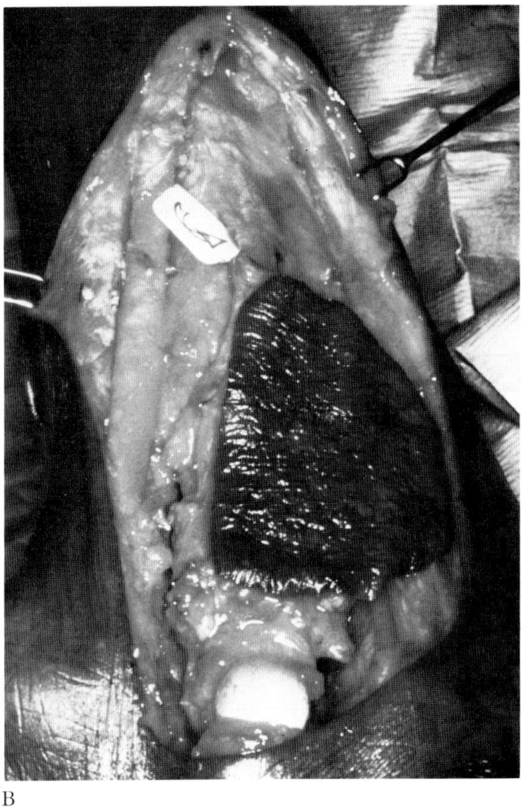

B

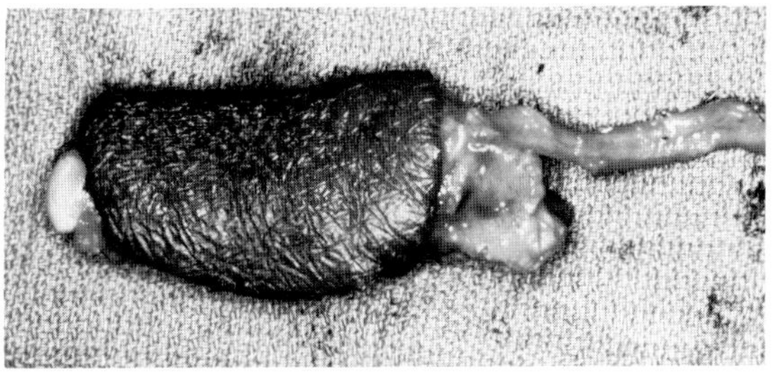

C

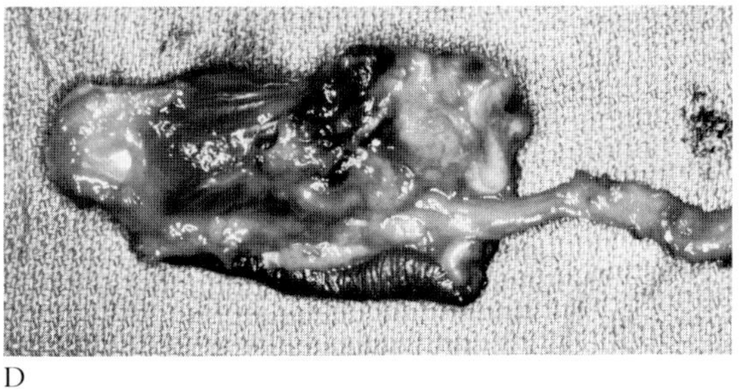

D

Figure 23-9. Reconstruction of the body with free osseocutaneous transfer. A. The preoperative intraoral view shows a postradiotherapy and postsurgical recurrence in the right alveolar process associated with a fistula (*arrows*). B. A right second metatarsal osseocutaneous transfer based on the dorsalis pedal artery (*arrow*) is developed. C and D. The dorsal and ventral surfaces of the free transfer with the artery and vein. E. The transfer spans the defect: titanium miniplates (*mp*); dorsalis pedal vessels (*dpv*); hypoglossal nerve (*hy*); and posterior belly of the diagnostic muscle (*pd*). F. Intraoral view of the osseocutaneous transfer. G–I. Postoperative views demonstrate only subtle facial asymmetry.

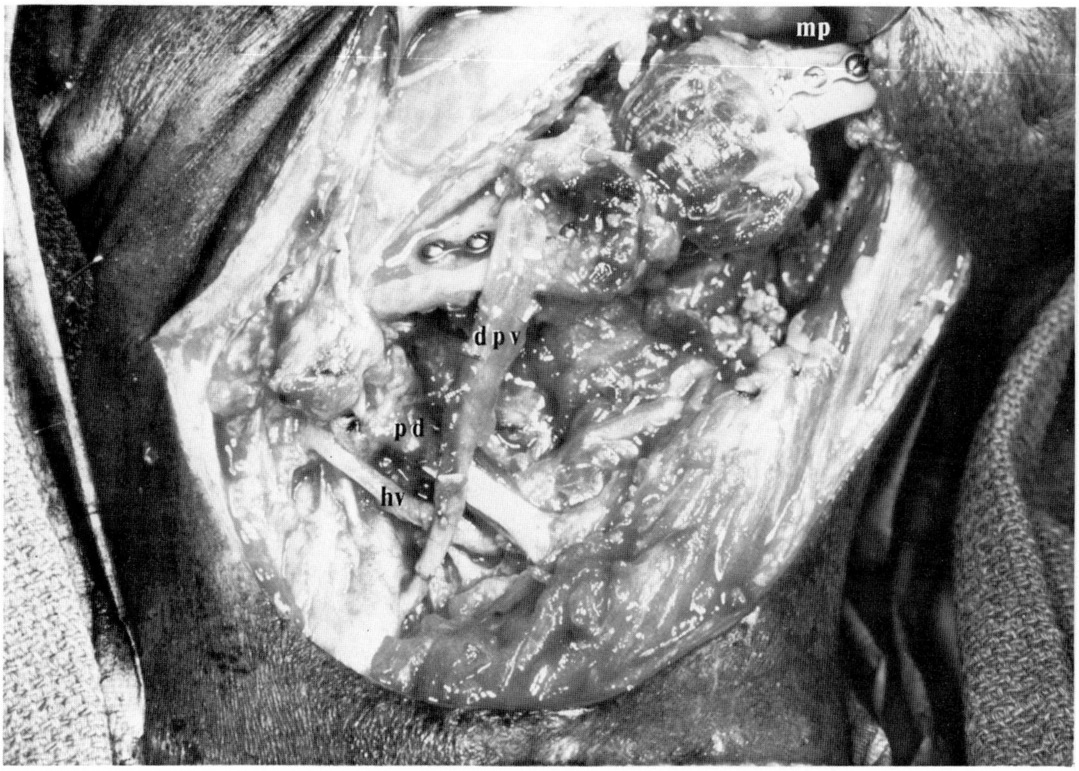

E

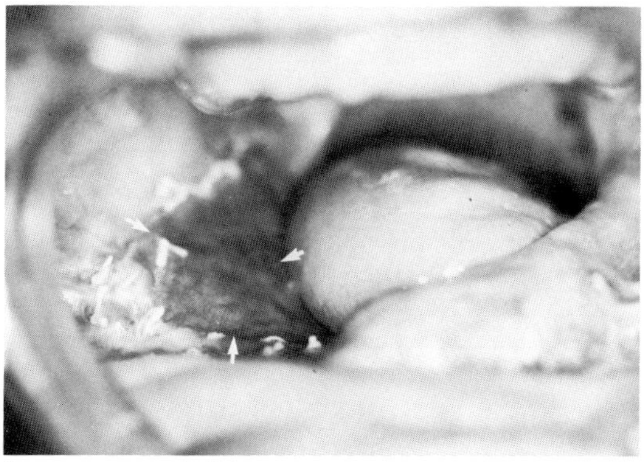
F

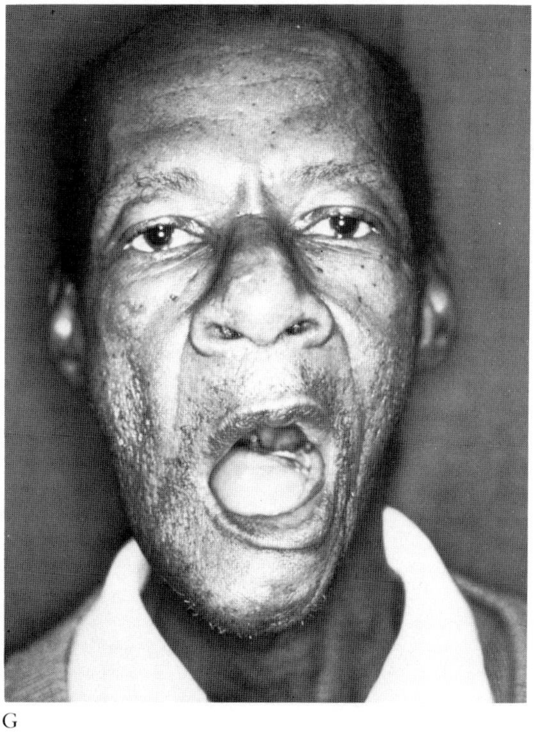
G

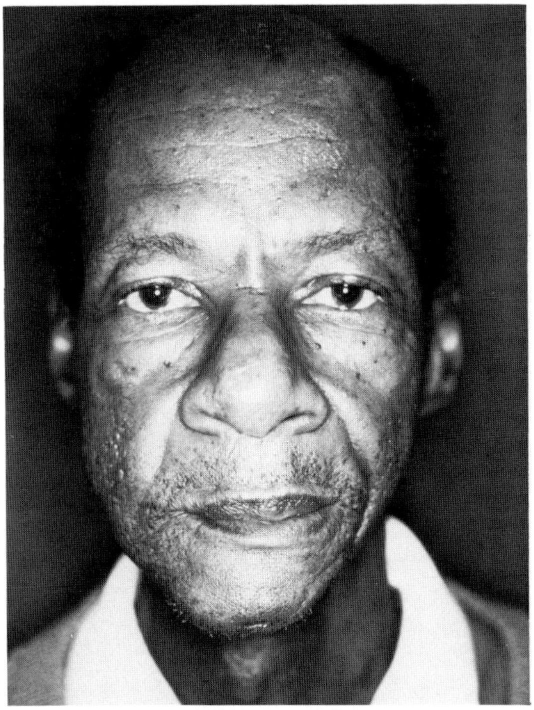

H

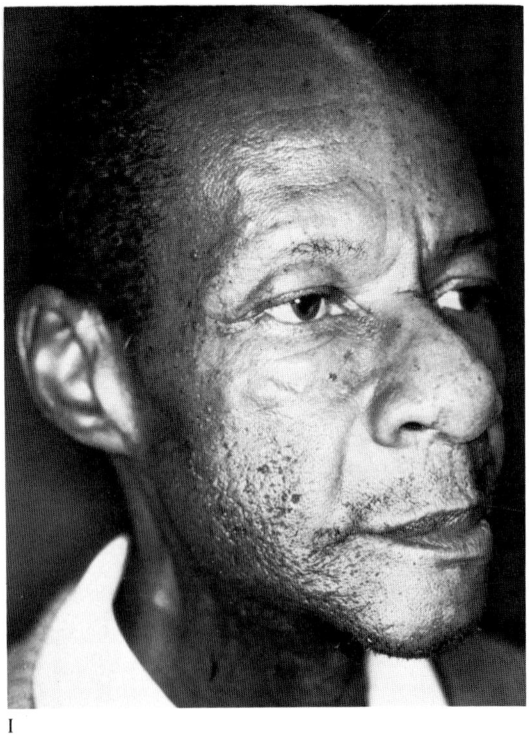

I

Conclusions

1. The numerous options available for mandibular reconstruction suggest that no one method is appropriate for all situations.
2. Delayed reconstruction is more successful than immediate reconstruction.
3. For immediate reconstruction, well-vascularized bone segments are advocated.
4. External fixation of mandibular remnants after ablation facilitates reconstruction.

REFERENCES

1. Maisel RH, Hilger PA: Mandibular Reconstruction. In Cumming CW (ed): *Otolaryngology Head and Neck Surgery*. St. Louis: Mosby, 1986. Pp 1555–1570.
2. Donald PJ: Oral Cavity. In Donald PJ (ed): *Head and Neck Cancer: Management of the Difficult Case*. Philadelphia: Saunders, 1984. Pp 1–39.
3. Taylor DT, LaVelle WF: Dental Management and Rehabilitation. In Thawley SE (ed): *Comprehensive Management of Head and Neck Tumors*. Philadelphia: Saunders, 1987. P 596.
4. Lawson W, et al: Experience with immediate and delayed mandibular reconstruction. *Laryngoscope* 92 : 5, 1982.
5. Vikram B: Importance of the time interval between surgery and postoperative radiation therapy in the combined management of head and neck cancer. *Int J Radiat Oncol Biol Phys* 5 : 10, 1979.
6. Lawson W, Biller H: Mandibular reconstruction: Bone graft techniques. *Otolaryngology* 9 : 589, 1982.
7. Hilger P, Adams G: Mandibular reconstruction with the A-O plate. *Arch Otolaryngol* 111 : 469, 1985.
8. Ariyan S: The pectoralis major myocutaneous flap. *Plast Reconstr Surg* 63 : 73, 1979.
9. Baek S, et al: The pectoralis major myocutaneous flap for reconstruction of the head and neck. *Head Neck Surg* 1 : 293, 1979.
10. Panje WR: Mandibular reconstruction with the trapezius osteomusculocutaneous flap. *Arch Otolaryngol* 111 : 223, 1985.
11. Maisel R, Adams GL: Osteomyocutaneous reconstruction of the oral cavity. *Arch Otolaryngol* 109 : 731, 1983.
12. Swartz WM, et al: The osteocutaneous scapular flap for mandibular and maxillary reconstruction. *Plast Reconstr Surg* 77(4) : 530, 1986.
13. Miyamoto Y, Tani T: Reconstruction of mandible with free osseocutaneous flap using deep circumflex iliac vessels as the stem. *Ann Plast Surg* 6(5):, 1981. Pp 354–361.

24

Hypopharyngeal Reconstruction

NEAL BECKFORD

KEY CONCEPTS

Indications; Defect Classification; Primary Reconstruction; Regional Flaps; Myocutaneous Flaps; Visceral Reconstruction

MILESTONES

1877	First Pharyngoesophageal Reconstruction with Cervical Flaps	Czermy
1942	Cervical Skin Flaps for Hypopharyngeal and Cervical Esophageal Reconstruction	Wookey
1958	Visceral Transpositions and Autografts	Seidenberg
1965	Deltopectoral Flaps for Pharyngoesophageal Reconstruction	Bakamjian
1979	Pectoralis Major Myocutaneous Flap	Ariyan
1980s	Microvascular Surgery and Free Graft Reconstruction	

Hypopharyngeal reconstruction is indicated for extensive lesions involving the esophagus, postcricoid area, pyriform sinus, posterior pharyngeal wall, and larynx. The closure of these defects is a technical challenge that must surmount postoperative stricture, infection, and fistulization. Often the extent of resection is predictable; however different reconstruction techniques should be available for the unexpected. Despite unforeseen difficulties, complications can be minimized with meticulous preoperative planning. The old adage of primary repair with only enough mucosa to enclose a nasogastric tube is outmoded. Additional tissue is readily available and should be used when indicated (Table 24-1; Figure 24-1).

Primary hypopharyngeal resections and the resultant defects are categorized into three general empirical classes: class I—30 percent or less, class II—30 to 70 percent, and class III—greater than 70 percent.

PRIMARY RECONSTRUCTION

Hypopharynx

During the resection attempts are made to conserve as much normal mucosa as possible without compromising appropriate surgical margins. Lesions that require mucosal resections of 30 percent or less are closed primarily. In selected cases, total laryngectomy facilitates primary closure. Small pyriform sinus lesions that are amenable to partial larynogopharyngectomy are closed primarily with minimal dysfunction. Defects greater than 30 percent have a higher incidence of postoperative stricture and dysphagia. Therefore, large hypopharyngeal resections require additional tissue for closure.

Table 24-1. **Hypopharyngeal reconstruction**

Technique	*Advantages*	*Disadvantages*	*Complications*
Primary closure	Easiest technique Eliminates the need for flap reconstruction Procedure of choice for small lesions	Limited to small lesions Inappropriate use can result in stricture	Pharyngocutaneous fistula Infection Stricture
Tongue flap	Well vascularized Easy Access	Limited to anterolateral defects	Pharyngocutaneous fistula Hypoglossal nerve damage
Regional flaps	Reliable alternative for repair of primary closure failures Circumferential closure possible	Multistaging necessary Prolonged hospitalization Aesthetically inferior to other methods	Pharyngocutaneous fistula Great-vessel exposure
Myocutaneous flaps	Ability to close large defects Reliable, one-stage reconstruction Carotid coverage	Excessive bulk at times Sternocleidomastoid and latissimus dorsi have high failure rate	Flap failure Pharyngocutaneous fistula
Visceral transfers	Best for circumferential replacement One-stage procedure Easily replaces long segments	Special skills necessary May require two or more surgical teams Strictures not uncommon with jejunal grafts Decreased tolerance to post operative radiotherapy	Compromised vascular supply causing graft, intestinal necrosis Peritonitis Death

Posterior Pharynx

Small posterior pharyngeal wall defects are exteriorized for granulation, whereas large defects are covered with split-thickness skin or dermal grafts. The grafts are sewn to adjacent mucosa (3-0 Vicryl) in a vertical mattress fashion. A protective tie-over bolus consisting of Xeroform gauze is removed endoscopically after 5 to 7 days.

LOCAL AND REGIONAL FLAPS

Defects not amenable to primary closure are reconstructed using local or regional flaps. Although numerous options are available, the reconstruction technically should be feasible, functional, and accomplished in one stage.

Tongue Flaps

Laterally based tongue flaps repair anterolateral defects. A musculomucosal horizontal tongue-base flap is developed preserving the lingual artery. The flap is rotated inferiorly, without tension, to fill the hypopharyngeal defect. Due to an abundant blood supply, vascular compromise is unusual. Defects up to 5 to 6 cm are closed with this technique. This convenient flap has good epithelial coverage and closes moderate size defects. Donor site epithelialization is rapid and unassociated with speech or swallowing problems if vascularity is preserved [1].

Skin and Chest Flaps

Regional skin flaps first were popularized by Wookey [2] in the early 1940s (see Chapter 22) [2]. A laterally based rectangular cervical skin flap is interposed between the oropharyngeal and hypopharyngeal remnants at the time of resection. The neopharynx is established by tubing at a second stage. Flap-tip necrosis, fistula, multiple stages, and extended hospitalization are disadvantages of this technique. The Bakamjian or deltopectoral flap is a more reliable alternative (Figure 24-2) [3,4]. Based on the

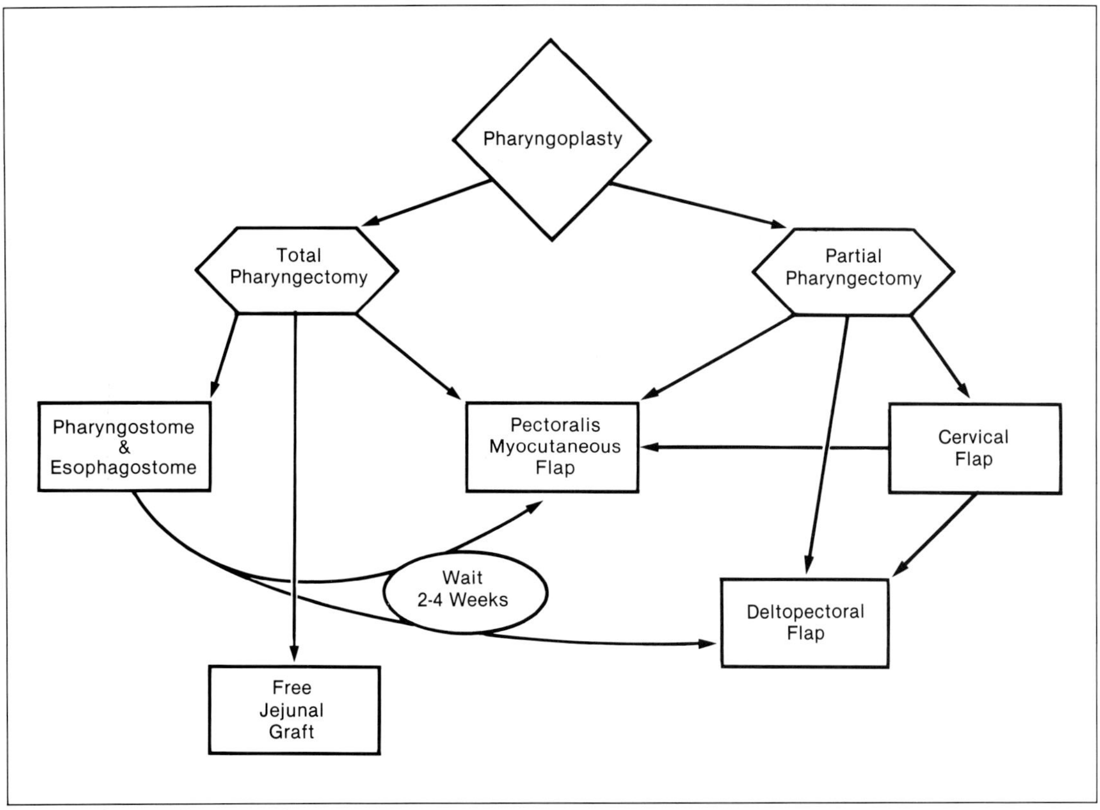

Figure 24-1. Pharyngoplasty.

perforators of the internal mammary artery, this medially based, well-vascularized chest flap is suitable for cervical esophageal reconstruction. The pliable chest skin, when tubed, bridges the hypopharyngeal defect. The inferior aspect of the tube remains open to create a pharyngocutaneous fistula, diverted away from the tracheostomy site.

The donor site is covered with split-thickness skin graft. Three to 4 weeks after the initial procedure, the base is transected and the flap is closed upon itself, thus completing the reconstruction. Flap vascularity and survival are enhanced by delay techniques. Although more viable than the Wookey flap, the deltopectoral flap shares many of the same problems and inconveniences. However, under certain circumstances, cervical and chest flaps are invaluable options.

MYOCUTANEOUS FLAPS

Advantages

The myocutaneous flap, introduced by Ariyan and Baek in the early 1970s, has revolutionized head and neck reconstruction (Figure 24-3). These flaps are versatile and reliable methods of one-stage reconstruction. Well-vascularized skin paddles, up to 10 cm × 10 cm, are developed to close large defects. Additional skin with a random blood supply is obtained, when necessary.

Technique

When outlining the incisions for a pectoralis major myocutaneous flap, the superior chest skin is preserved for a future deltopectoral flap. Surprisingly, in most cases, the donor site is closed primarily. The pectoralis muscle pro-

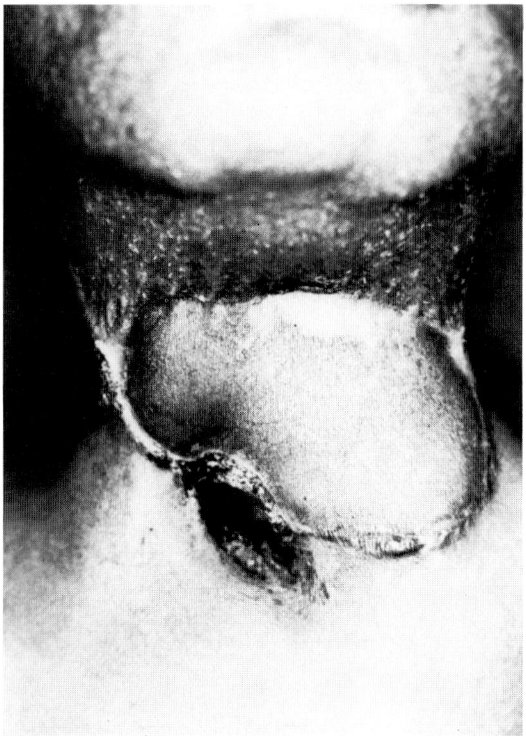

E

Figure 24-3 (continued) C. Two weeks later the wound appears mature. D. Second stage: reconstruction. The entire area including both stomas is outlined to develop the cervical flaps for the inner lining. A left pectoralis myocutaneous flap is mobilized for the external lining and skin coverage. E. The final appearance is a skin-lined (cervical flap) conduit covered by muscle and skin (pectoralis flap).

vides excellent carotid artery coverage and obviates the need for dermal grafts. Failures are less than 25 percent, and subsequent radiation therapy is well tolerated. The following suggestions decrease flap loss: suture the muscle to dermis to minimize the shearing of perforator vessels; prevent vascular pedicle kinks at all times; and avoid occlusive dressing and tight tracheotomy ties. Be aware that excessive flap bulk in well-developed or obese patients prohibits circumferential reconstruction. Pectoralis major and trapezius myocutaneous flaps are preferred for hypopharyngeal reconstruction [5]. Latissimus dorsi flaps are not recommended because of difficult patient positioning, unacceptable failure rates, and excessive bulk.

VISCERAL RECONSTRUCTION

The previously mentioned techniques are not suitable for all circumferential hypopharyngeal and cervical esophageal reconstruction. Other techniques rely on segments of the gastrointestinal tract (see Chapter 17) [6]. Jejunal microvascular free grafts, gastric pull-up, and colon interpositions are excellent reconstruction methods [7].

Free Jejunal Interposition

Free jejunal interposition is a free transfer of jejunum with its vascular arcade. Large defects can be spanned from the nasopharynx to the mediastinum. These grafts are useful especially after full-course radiation salvage and for hypopharyngeal and cervical esophageal stenosis. A small bowel segment with a large feeding vessel from the superior mesenteric artery is harvested by a second surgical team. Graft survival depends largely on successful microvascular anastomosis to appropriate cervical vessels identified during tumor resection. Arterial access is obtained easily from one of the branches of the external carotid system. The more tenuous venous anastomosis is end-to-end (external jugular vein) or end-to-side (internal jugular vein). As the graft bridges the pharyngeal defect, the jejunal segment is reversed to avoid antiperistalsis. These free grafts are reliable one-stage reconstructions. High success rates are obtained, and barring complications, patients are discharged in 10 to 14 days. The disadvantages are abdominal surgery and graft survival dependent on microvascular expertise. Although visceral strictures may develop, especially after administration of radiation therapy, the results unquestionably are superior to local and regional flaps [7].

Gastric Pull-up

Gastric mobilization and direct anastomosis to the proximal pharyngeal remnant requires two teams, one for resection and the other for gastric mobilization. The stomach is mobilized, based on the right gastric and right gastroepiploic arteries, and tunnelled through the posterior mediastinum. Since skin lesions are common in the thoracic and lower esophagus, a blunt (closed-chest) total esophagectomy is performed. Success depends on the degree of tension-free gastric mobilization. When its vascular supply is intact, the gastric pull-up is the most dependable visceral reconstruction method. A single anastomosis and reliable patency are the prime advantages. However, postoperative morbidity is significant. Complications include uncontrolled air leaks from tracheobronchial tears, hemorrhage, mediastinitis, anastomotic leaks, pharyngocutaneous fistula, gastric necrosis, and death. Gastric regurgitation, endocrine abnormalities, and poor alaryngeal speech are other long-term problems. In short, pharyngogastroplasty is a formidable procedure and is reserved for patients in good medical condition.

Colon Interposition

If gastric mobilization is impractical, an alternative is colon interposition. Left colon transposition with its greater length is preferred. The transposed segment, based on the left colic artery, is mobilized, brought behind the stomach through the posterior mediastinum, and delivered into the neck. The proximal colon is anastomosed to the oropharyngeal remnant while the distal segment is reanastomosed to the antrum. A pyloroplasty facilitates gastric emptying. The major problems are vascular compromise and graft failure [7,8].

CONCLUSIONS

1. Efforts are directed at establishing a wide conduit for effective alimentation.
2. Resection is never compromised for reconstruction.
3. A knowledge of several methods is necessary.

REFERENCES

1. Calcaterra TC: Tongue flap repair of postlaryngectomy hypopharyngeal stenosis. *Laryngoscope* 96 : 617, 1986.
2. Wookey, H: The surgical treatment of the pharynx and cervical esophagus. *Surg Gynecol Obstet* 75 : 499, 1942.
3. Bakamjian VY: A two state method for pharyngoesophageal reconstruction with a primary pectoral skin flap. *Plast Reconstr Surg* 36 : 176, 1955.
4. Ramadan MG, Stell PM: Reconstruction after pharyngolaryngoesophagectomy using delto pectoral flap. *Clin Otolaryngol* 4 : 5, 1979.
5. Panje WR: Myocutaneous trapezius flap. *Head and Neck Surgery* 206, 1980.
6. Seidenberg B, et al: Immediate reconstruction of the cervical esophagus by a revascularized isolate jejunal segment. *Ann Surg* 149 : 162, 1959.
7. Silver CE: Surgical treatment of hypopharyngeal and cervical esophageal cancer. *World Journal of Surgery* 5 : 499, 1981.
8. McConnel FMS: Rehabilitation of patients with tumors of the pharynx. In Thawley et al (eds), *Comprehensive Management of Head and Neck Tumors*. New York: Saunders. Pp. 813–857, 1987.

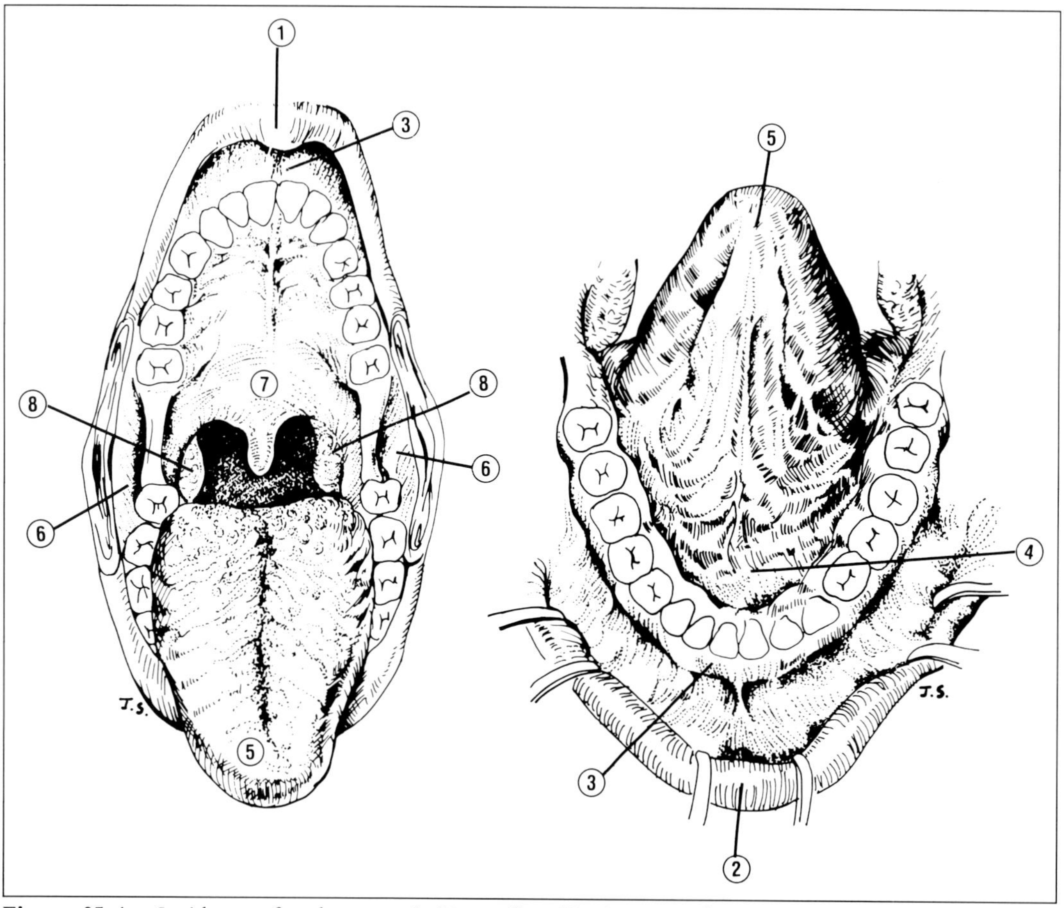

Figure 25-1. Incidence of oral cancer. 1. Upper lip, 4%. 2. Lower lip, 38%. 3. Gingiva, 6%. 4. Anterior floor of mouth, 17%. 5. Anterior tongue, 22%. 6. Buccal mucosa, 2%. 7. Soft palate, 6%. 8. Tonsil, 5%.

terminates when the bolus is propelled posteriorly past the faucial pillars, triggering the involuntary pharyngeal phase. The oral stage requires (1) intact labial musculature to prevent drooling, (2) adequate mandibular movement for mastication, (3) intact lingual functioning for lateralization and posterior bolus propulsion, and (4) functional palatal musculature to prevent nasal regurgitation.

Pharyngeal Stage

The tongue releases the bolus as the elevated soft palate produces palatopharyngeal closure. Simultaneously, the suprahyoid muscles contract to elevate the larynx while the vocal folds adduct to protect the airway. When the bolus enters the pharynx, the involuntary swallowing reflex is activated, transporting it into the esophagus by peristalsis. The pharyngeal stage requires (1) intact palatopharyngeal musculature to prevent nasal regurgitation, (2) adequate laryngeal function to prevent aspiration, and (3) intact pharyngeal musculature to trigger the swallowing reflex.

Esophageal Stage

Peristaltic contractions of the esophageal musculature propel the bolus into the stomach. This stage begins when the bolus passes through the

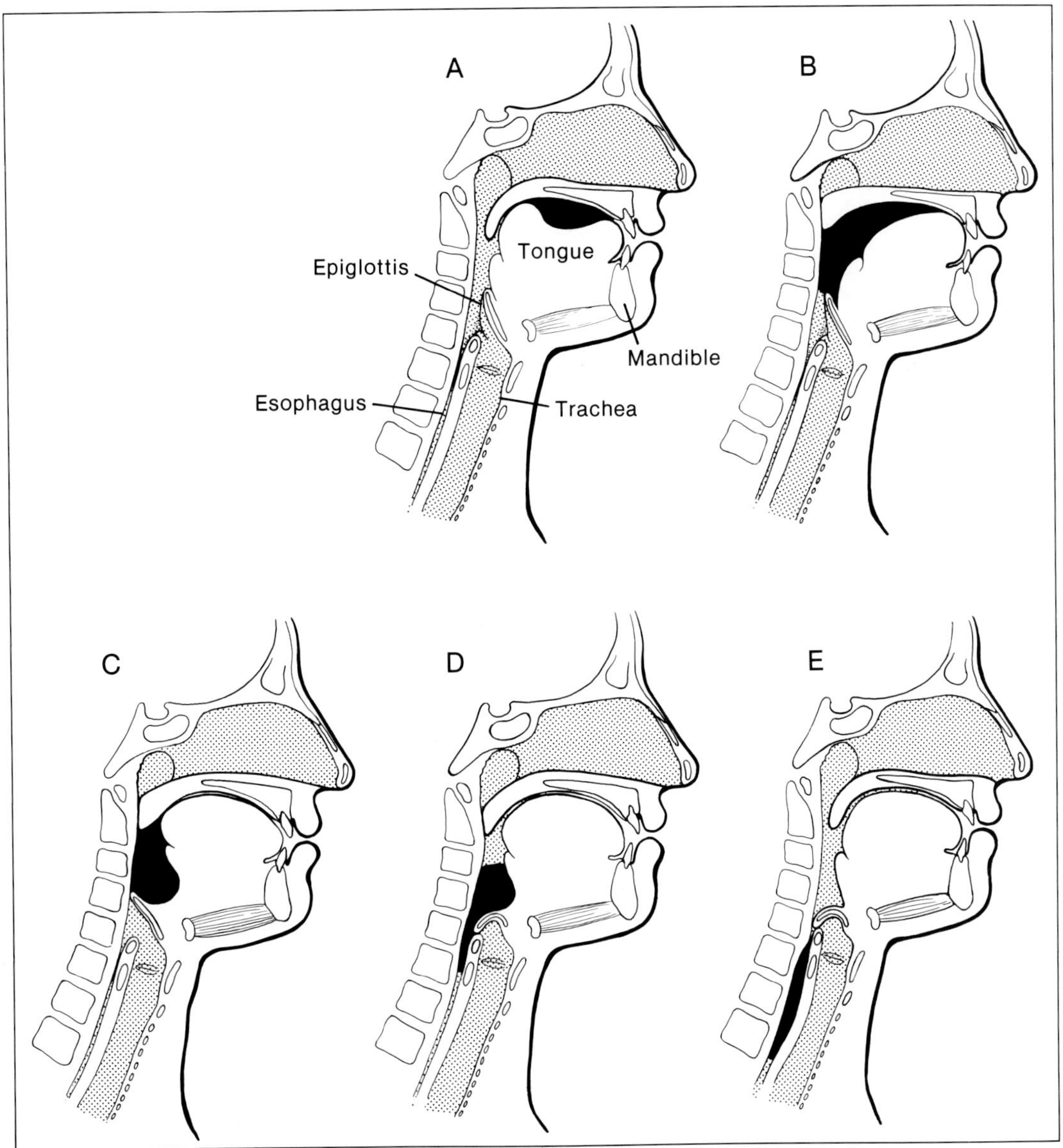

Figure 25-2. The swallowing reflex. A, B, C. Oral stage. D. Pharyngeal stage. E. Esophageal stage.

cricopharyngeal sphincter and continues until it enters the stomach following gastroesophageal relaxation. Intact esophageal musculature is required. Esophageal dysmotility, unlike other motility disorders, is not amenable to rehabilitation. However, medical and surgical management have been effective for the treatment of cricopharyngeal (upper esophageal sphincter) problems.

Postoperative Assessment

The speech pathologist reviews the patient's history and evaluates oral, laryngeal, and respiratory function (Tables 25-1 and 25-2) [3].

Table 25-1. Assessment and rehabilitation procedures

Deglutition	*Speech*
Assessment	
History	History
Onset & etiology	Same as for deglutition
Type & extent of carcinoma	
Surgical treatment	
Radiotherapy	
Chemotherapy	
Oral mechanism examination	Oral mechanism examination
Structural evaluation	Structural evaluation
Functional evaluation	Functional evaluation
Oral sensory skills	
Reflexes	
Laryngeal & respiratory function	Laryngeal & respiratory function
Laryngeal valving efficiency (vowel prolongation)	Same as for deglutition
Respiratory function	
Airflow (s/z ratio)	
Air volume (spirometer)	
Swallowing evaluation	Speech evaluation
Clinical swallowing evaluation	Reading sample
Videofluoroscopy	Conversational sample
	Articulation testing
Rehabilitation	
Oromotor exercises	Range of motion exercises
Compensatory techniques	Compensatory placement
Feeding aids	Maxillofacial prosthetics
Maxillofacial prosthetics	

History

A review of the operative report determines the extent of surgery, reconstruction, pre- and post-operative radiotherapy, and whether induction chemotherapy was given (see Chapters 8 & 9). The potential for dysphagia increases when irradiation is administered postoperatively.

After determining the level of orientation and alertness, the patient is asked to indicate (1) which food consistency—liquid, soft, or solid—is most difficult to swallow and (2) where in the oral cavity and pharynx it collects. Usually, the patient's description is very accurate. For example, if the patient points to the base of the tongue or epiglottis, then food probably is collecting in the valleculae. If the lower neck or area beneath the larynx is identified, then food is collecting in the pyriform sinuses.

Oral Mechanism Examination

Structural Evaluation

The lips, hard palate, soft palate, tongue, faucial arches, and mandible are examined. The presence of asymmetry, atrophy, tremor, and fasciculations is recorded. The soft palate is examined for velopharyngeal insufficiency, a condition that occurs when little residual palate remains. The extent of the surgical resection and scarring is determined. The oral cavity is examined for mucositis, osteoradionecrosis, and the presence of thick, viscous mucus. Tenacious mucus can impair swallowing and increase dental caries.

Functional Evaluation

Functional evaluation is the assessment of the range, speed, accuracy, and strength of the oral

Table 25-2. Deglutitory and articulatory disorders versus site of lesion

Site	*Deglutitory disorder*	*Articulatory disorder*	*Comments*
Lips	Minimal: Oral phase	Minimal: /p,b,f,v,w,m,o,u,au/	Possible increase in drooling with decreased lip hypoesthesia
Maxilla & palate	Severe without prosthesis: Oral and pharyngeal phase	Severe: /t,d,k,g,θ,ð,s,z,ʃ,ʒ,tʃ, dʒ,n,1/	Hypernasal resonance Nasal air emission Nasal regurgitation
Tongue	Mild: < 50% resection with tongue mobility Severe: > 50% resection Impairs lingual peristalsis Increases oral phase Impairs anteroposterior bolus movement	Ablation dependent: can affect /t,d,k,g,θ,ð, s,z,ʃ,ʒ,tʃ,dʒ,n, l,r,i,e,æ,a,ɛ,o,u/	When tongue mobility is severely restricted, severe difficulties with lingual peristalsis and mastication occur Restricted to liquids Restrictions involving the anterior regions of the tongue result in severe impairment to speech intelligibility
Mandible	Severe: Oral and pharyngeal phases are affected	/p,b,f,v,m,w,o,u,au/ with lower lip resection	Depends on site Symphysis> body>angle Difficulty chewing Drooling Phonation may be affected

musculature during speech and nonspeech tasks. Diadochokinetic tasks are administered to evaluate the range, speed, and accuracy of movement, while muscle strength is determined by having the patient move an oral structure against resistance.

Oral Sensory Skills
Due to the tendency for sensory and functional problems to coexist, an evaluation of oral sensory skills is performed. Three areas are evaluated: sensation to light touch, taste, and temperature. A two-point discrimination task evaluates response to tactile stimulation. In this test, the patient indicates whether one or two points within the oral cavity have been stimulated. Taste is evaluated by placing two to three drops of various solutions (sweet, salty, bitter) on the tongue. Temperature discrimination is tested by placing warm and then cold liquids on the tongue.

Reflexes
Finally, the gag and pharyngeal reflexes are elicited. A tongue depressor placed at the posterior pharyngeal wall or base of the tongue triggers the gag reflex. A cold laryngeal mirror on the juncture of the hard and soft palates initiates the pharyngeal reflex.

Laryngeal and Respiratory Function
Before conducting the swallowing evaluation, the patient's ability to protect the airway is determined. Inadequate glottic closure is associated with aspiration. To assess the strength of laryngeal adduction, the patient is asked to cough, prolong a vowel, gradually increase intensity while counting to 10, and read a paragraph. A weak cough or breathy voice indicates possible inadequate laryngeal adduction. When the patient's cough reflex is diminished or absent, physician clearance is obtained before conducting the swallowing evaluation [4].

can alter resonance, impair articulation, and affect the ability to regulate airflow (Table 25-2) [8].

Postoperative Assessment

The medical history is reviewed to determine the extent of resection and type of reconstruction. Secondly, the impact on strength and function of oral structures is determined. When weakness of the oral structures exists, dysarthria often accompanies dysphagia. Moreover, behavioral data are obtained using a variety of production tasks, including vowels in isolation, words containing lingual and nonlingual phonemes, structured sentences, oral reading, and conversational speech. The patient's articulation should be assessed for speed and precision. A detailed analysis of articulatory patterns determines the sites of dysfunction and rates overall intelligibility. Finally, the voice should be examined in terms of quality (breathiness, hoarseness and harshness), pitch and intensity. The presence of hypernasality suggests impaired palatopharyngeal function. These baseline data help to formulate a treatment program, measure progress, and determine prognosis.

Diagnosis

The six major subsites of oral tumors are (1) anterior floor of the mouth or lower alveolar ridge; (2) anterior and lateral tongue; (3) lateral floor of the mouth, lateral alveolar ridge, or tonsils; (4) base of the tongue; (5) hard palate; and (6) soft palate (Figure 25-1) [3]. The most prevalent sites are the lower lip and alveolar ridge [8,9]. The impact of surgical ablation on deglutition and articulation is summarized in Table 25-2.

Lips

Partial labialectomy may affect phonemes requiring labial rounding (o, w) and valving (p, b, m, f, v).

Maxilla

Maxillectomy, partial or total, may affect approximately 17 phonemes, including the labiodental, linguadental, lingua-alveolar, and linguapalatal consonants.

Palate

Palatectomy, partial or total, often causes hypernasal resonance and nasal air emission. These procedures can severely distort speech intelligibility and affect the high-pressure consonants (fricatives and plosives) [10].

Tongue

A glossectomy detrimentally affects lingual shaping and lingual elevation. The former is required to prevent lateral air escape; the latter is involved in the production of lingua-alveolar /t,d/, linguavelar /k,g/, and linguapalatal /tʃ, dʒ/ consonants.

Total Glossectomy

In addition to severe articulatory dysfunction, the imbalance to the resonating cavity created by removal of the tongue produces reduced pitch variability, a guttural voice, impaired antiresonance, and excessive noise.

Partial Glossectomy

The severity of articulatory dysfunction depends on the site of the resection (Figure 25-3). An anterior tongue resection can cause more severe impairment to intelligibility than a hemiglossectomy [11]. The former affects tongue-palate valving during speech because the tongue remnant fails to touch the hard palate. This causes lingua-alveolar and linguapalatal phoneme distortions. Hemiglossectomy patients with mobile tongue remnants achieve adequate tongue palate valving. However, lateral air emission occurs during the production of lingual fricatives (/s, z, ʃ, and ʒ/) and affricates (/tʃ; and dʒ/) due to an incomplete seal around the periphery of the oral cavity.

Mandible

Limited mandibular excursion and movement after partial or total mandibulectomy impairs speech production.

Rehabilitation

Even with massive tissue extirpation, intelligible speech is attainable with the combined skills of the speech pathologist and maxillofacial prosthodontist. However, prosthetics are unneces-

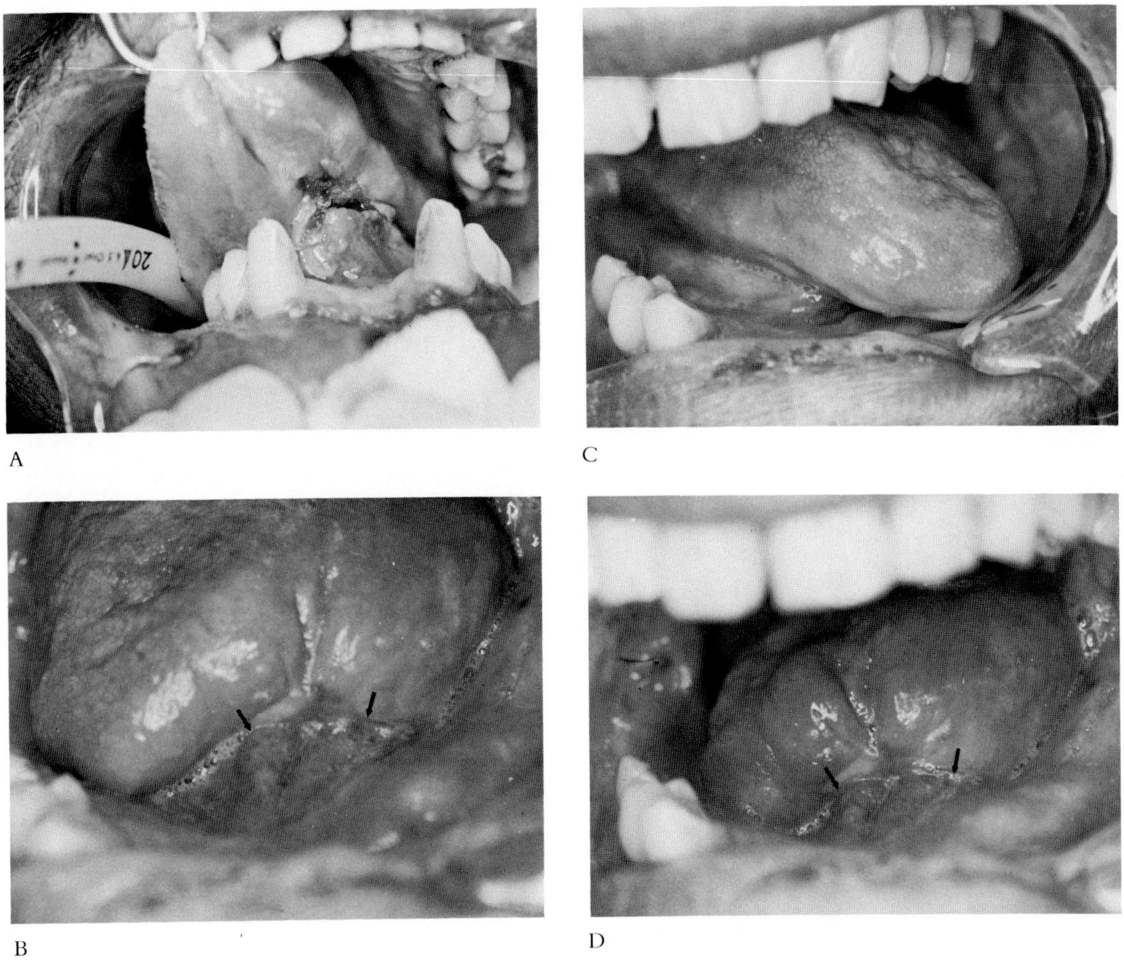

Figure 25-3. Carcinoma of the tongue. A. Left ventral tongue. B. This photograph shows the primary site after partial glossectomy, floor of mouth resection, modified neck dissection, and split-thickness skin graft reconstruction (*arrows*). C and D. Left and right tongue mobility is maintained.

sary if residual mobility permits linguapalatal contact [3]. Rehabilitation normalizes air release patterns and establishes three contrasting places of articulation for bilabial /p,b/, lingua-alveolar /t,d/, and linguavelar /k,g/ plosives.

Range of Motion Exercises

The first goal is to improve the mobility of residual structures with tongue and jaw range of motion exercises 6 to 10 times a day for at least 6 weeks. After postoperative radiotherapy, these exercises are extended for an additional 5 weeks to decrease scar tissue and fibrosis. Each exercise should be limited to four or five repetitions; otherwise, muscle strain or fatigue may occur. With each repetition, the patient extends the structure (i.e., lip, tongue, jaw) as far as possible for 3 to 5 seconds.

Tongue

Maximal tongue extension for 3 to 5 seconds is recommended along with lateralization, protrusion, retraction, posterior elevation, and anterior elevation exercises.

Mandible

The jaw is moved in an exaggerated circular motion and extended in each direction as far as possible. Other exercises include lowering the jaw and moving it from side to side as far as possible.

Lips
Mobility is enhanced by repetitive puckering, smiling, and maximal extensions. Another exercise involves opening and closing the lips while the mouth is closed and the teeth are clinched.

Palate
Palatopharyngeal closure can be improved through exercises designed to increase posterior and lateral pharyngeal wall movement.

Compensatory Articulatory Placements

The patient is trained to utilize articulatory substitutions to compensate for tissue loss and reduced mobility. Compensatory techniques for commonly misarticulated phonemes are shown in Table 25-3.

Lips
To compensate, the affected phonemes are produced by the central incisors or the tongue tip. For example, when the lower lip is ablated, the upper lip contacts the lower incisors to produce labial sounds.

Maxilla
Although many maxillectomy patients receive restorative surgery or prosthetics, compensatory techniques help improve speech intelligibility.

Tongue
Therapy improves air release patterns associated with the production of fricatives (/s,z,θ,ð,ʃ,ʒ/). Also three contrasting places of articulation for plosives (/t,d,k,g/) and affricates (/tʃ, dʒ/) are established.

Maxillofacial Prosthetics and Therapeutic Intervention

Insufficient tongue contact requires a maxillofacial prosthesis. This device lowers the palatal vault to complement the tongue for production of stops and fricatives. The prosthesis is fitted no more than 5 to 7 days after a 6-week range of motion exercise program to prevent the patient from developing undesirable compensatory articulatory patterns [12].

When therapy is initiated, the patient is trained to produce maximum tongue contact at the anterior and posterior borders of the prosthesis. This is accomplished by using minimal pairs to contrast the two places of articulation in the pre-, inter-, and postvocalic positions of words such as /te/-/ke/, /ete/-eke/, and /et/-/ek/. The patient's kinesthetic awareness of the contrasting places of articulation is developed through the production of monosyllabic words while concentrating on either anterior or posterior valving. Production starts slowly to facilitate kinesthetic awareness. As the patient's articulatory competence improves, the production rate is increased to normal.

Next, therapy focuses on establishing adequate valving for the production of alveolar (/s,z/) and palatal (/ʃ,ʒ/) fricatives. The airstream direction depends on the degree of tongue grooving and the narrowness of the airstream over the lower lip. Production of /s/ and /z/ requires that a narrow stream of air flows medially over the tongue and lower lip. The production of the /ʃ/ and /ʒ/ requires a broader release.

Finally, short phrases such as "pass the salt" or "wash this carrot" are used to facilitate coarticulation of the plosive and fricative phonemes. Gradually, the practice material is lengthened until the patient produces the target phonemes in paragraphs and structured conversation.

Hypernasal resonance caused by velopharyngeal insufficiency or impaired palatopharyngeal function may be treated by fitting a palatal lift or obturator. In both cases, palatopharyngeal closure can be improved through exercises designed to increase lateral and posterior pharyngeal wall movement.

PROGNOSIS

Swallowing

When dysphagia is present, the patient's prognosis for recovery is affected by the site and size of lesion. As a general guideline, if less than 50 percent of an oral structure is removed or

Table 25-3. Postoperative articulatory compensation

Cognate pair	*Place/manner*	*Surgical resection*	*Compensatory placement*	*Technique*
/p, b/	Bilabial/ plosive	Labialectomy	Lingual-labial or dental-labial placement	When the upper lip has been resected, valving is achieved by placing the maxillary incisors against the lower lip. Patients who have undergone a resection of the lower lip can produce these phonemes by placing the tongue tip or mandibular incisors against the upper lip. In both cases, the air is built up behind the point of closure, then released to produce a sound that is acoustically similar to the target phonemes.
/t, d/	Lingua-alveolar plosive	Total glossectomy	Labial-dental or labial-alveolar placement	The lower lip, serving as a substitute for the tongue, is placed against the upper teeth or inner surface of the alveolar ridge. Oral air pressure is built up behind the point of contact and quickly released by moving the lower lip forward and down.
/k, g/	Linguavelar	Total glossectomy	Pharyngeal or glottal placement	A pharyngeal constriction is produced by anterior movement of the pharyngeal muscles against the posterior tongue remnant, if present, or epiglottis. Infraglottal air pressure is built up behind the posterior pharyngeal bulge and then suddenly released, resulting in a sound that resembles the glottal stop. Another compensatory technique is the glottal stop, produced by tightly adducting the vocal folds, building up infraglottal air pressure, and rapidly releasing it by abducting the vocal folds.
/f, v/	Labial-dental fricative	Maxillectomy or labialectomy	Bilabial or labial-dental placement	These phonemes may be produced by bilabial constriction or placing the lower incisors against the upper lip (if present). In the former, the upper and lower lips are positioned slightly apart and the airstream forced through a narrow opening, while the latter compensatory technique involves placing the upper lip against the lower incisors. The friction feature of these phonemes is created by buccal compression, allowing the airstream to be directed over the upper or lower lip.
/θ, ʒ/	Linguadental/ fricative	Total glossectomy or maxillectomy	Labial-dental placement	The lower lip is placed posterior to the upper incisors, allowing the airstream to be released by moving the upper lip down and forward against the teeth. If the patient is edentulous, the upper lip can be used instead. In this case, the air is released in a sudden burst by drawing the lower lip down and forward against the upper lip.

(Continued)

Table 25-3. *(Continued)*

Cognate pair	*Place/manner*	*Surgical resection*	*Compensatory placement*	*Technique*
/s, z/	Lingua-alveolar/ fricative	Total glossectomy or maxillectomy	Bilabial or labial-dental placement	The upper teeth and lower lip (or both upper and lower lip in the case of edentulous patients) are positioned slightly apart to allow the airstream to be forced through a narrow opening. The airstream is driven through the slit-like opening by compression of the cheeks. The frication required for this sound appears to be created by directing the airstream over the upper lip.
/ʃ, ʒ/	Linguapalatal/ fricative	Total glossectomy	Pharyngeal fricative placement	These sounds are produced as pharyngeal fricatives. As in production of /k, g/, a pharyngeal constriction is produced by anterior movement of the pharyngeal muscles against the posterior tongue remnant. If a total glossectomy has been performed, these phonemes can be produced by pharyngeal constriction. The friction is created by the airstream moving into the narrow aperture from the infraglottis.
/m/	Bilabial/nasal	Maxillectomy or mandibulectomy	Labial-dental placement	In the case of lip tumors where either lip is surgically resected, the incisors may be used to produce this phoneme. Patients having ablative surgery involving the upper lip can compensate by placing the upper incisors against the lower lip and directing the airstream through the nasal cavity by opening the velopharyngeal port.
/n/	Lingua-alveolar/ nasal	Total glossectomy or maxillectomy	Labial-dental placement	The lower lip is placed against the alveolar ridge and the airstream is directed into the nasal cavity by depression of the soft palate. Patients with impaired lip mobility will experience difficulty producing this phoneme.
/g/	Linguavelar/ nasal	Total glossectomy or palatectomy	Pharyngeal or glottal placement	The soft palate is lowered and a pharyngeal constriction is created to achieve this phoneme. The intelligibility of this phoneme depends on the patient's success in producing /n/ and /g/ using compensatory productions.
/l/	Lingua-alveolar glide	Total glossectomy or maxillectomy	Velar vibration or labial and buccal production	Production of the "light" /l/ following a total glossectomy is virtually impossible for most patients (Skelly 1973). However, production of the "dark" /l/ has been successfully achieved by many glossectomees using one of two techniques. Patients with normal velopharyngeal function may produce the sound by slight vibration of the uvula, while those with inadequate control of the uvula can often produce it using a combination of labial constriction and slight vibration of the cheeks by compression of the buccal cavity.
/r/	Linguapalatal/ glide	Total glossectomy	Buccal retroversion of the anterior mandibular placement	The consonantal /r/ can be produced by retroversion of the upper lip, buccal compression and anterior movement of the mandible. Patients with poor lip mobility can produce /r/ by pharyngeal constriction combined with flattened position of the lips.

Table 25-4. Complications versus surgical procedure

	Deglutition				*Speech*		*Respiratory system*		
Procedure	***Drooling***	***Malocclusion***	***Mastication***	***Swallowing***	***Articulation***	***Phonation***	***Breathing***	***Cough***	***Aspiration***
Floor-of-mouth resection	+ +	+	+		+				
Glossectomy									
Partial	+		+	+ +	+	+	+	+	+ +
Total			+ + +	+ + +	+ +	+ +	+ +	+ + +	+ + +
Mandibulectomy									
Partial	+ +	+ +	+ +	+					
Total	+ + +	+ + +	+ + +	+ + +	+ + +	+ + +	+ + +	+ + +	+ + +
Palatectomy			+ +	+ + +	+ +	+			
Laryngectomy									
Partial				+ +		+ +	+ +	+ +	+ + +
Total				+	+ + +	+ + +			
Neck dissection	+								+
Maxillectomy		+ +	+ +	+ +	+ +				
Tracheotomy				+ +	+ + +	+ + +	+	+ +	+ +

+ Possible. + + Probable. + + + Likely.

affected by reconstruction procedures, the prognosis is favorable, as dysphagia is amenable to rehabilitation (Table 25-4) [7,10,13,14]. Other factors influential in determining prognosis include the patient's pre- and postoperative health, psychological state, level of oral sensation, and ability to learn compensatory placements. Table 25-5 presents several variables relevant to determining a patient's prognosis.

Speech

The prognosis for developing adequate speech intelligibility following surgery depends on several factors. Perhaps the most critical to speech rehabilitation are the specific site and extent of surgical resection or reconstruction. Other prognostic variables are the type of surgical closure, the degree of muscle strength, the function of residual structures, the level of oral sensation, the amount of postoperative radiotherapy, the degree of comprehension, and the level of patient motivation.

Table 25-5. Deglutitory and articulatory prognosis

Psychological Profile
Comprehension
Attitude
Motivation
Medical profile
Age
General health
Laryngeal function
Respiratory function
Muscle strength & function
Sensation
Surgery
Lesion site
Extent of resection
Reconstruction
Graft
Flap
Closure
Postoperative radiotherapy
Xerostomia
Mucositis
Osteoradionecrosis
Maxillofacial prosthesis
Maxilla
Palate
Tongue

SUMMARY

Rehabilitation of the head and neck cancer patient with swallowing and speech disorders requires that the speech pathologist have a thorough knowledge of normal anatomy and physiology as well as techniques for training the use of compensatory placements and procedures for prosthodontic management (Figure 25-4). In speech rehabilitation, compensatory techniques are utilized to improve intelligibility. For patients with dysphagia, muscle strength and function are improved to eliminate aspiration. Team management is critical for effective patient rehabilitation. The speech pathologist works closely with the otolaryngologist, prosthodontist, dietician, and nurses to ensure that the best functioning of residual structures is attained.

REFERENCES

1. *Cancer Facts and Figures.* New York: American Cancer Society, 1988.
2. Lauciello FR, et al: Prosthodontic and speech rehabilitation after partial and complete glossectomy. *J Prosthet Dent* 43 : 204, 1980.
3. Logemann JA: *Evaluation and Treatment of Swallowing Disorders.* San Diego: College-Hill, 1983.
4. Koch DG: Role of the Speech Pathologist in the Rehabilitation of Oral Cancer Patients. In Sklar G. (ed), *Oral Cancer: The Diagnosis, Management & Rehabilitation of the Oral Cancer Patient.* Philadelphia: Saunders, 1984.
5. Skelly M, et al: Compensatory physiologic phonetics for the glossectomee. *JSHD* 36 : 101, 1971.
6. Doberneck R, Antoine A: Deglutition after resection of oral, laryngeal and pharyngeal cancer. *Surgery* 75 : 87, 1974.
7. Groher ME: *Dysphagia: Diagnosis and Management.* Boston: Butterworth, 1984. Pp 65–70.
8. Hufnagle J, Pullon P, Hufnagle K: Speech considerations in oral surgery, parts I & II. *Oral Surg* 46 : 349, 1978.
9. Krolls SO, Hoffman S: Squamous cell carcinoma of the oral soft tissue: A statistical analysis of 14,253 cases by age, sex and race of patients. *JADA* 92 : 571, 1976.
10. Fleming SM, Weaver AW: Clinical management of dysphagia in head and neck cancer patients: Dysarthria, Dysphonia, Dysphagia, 1 : 80, 1982.

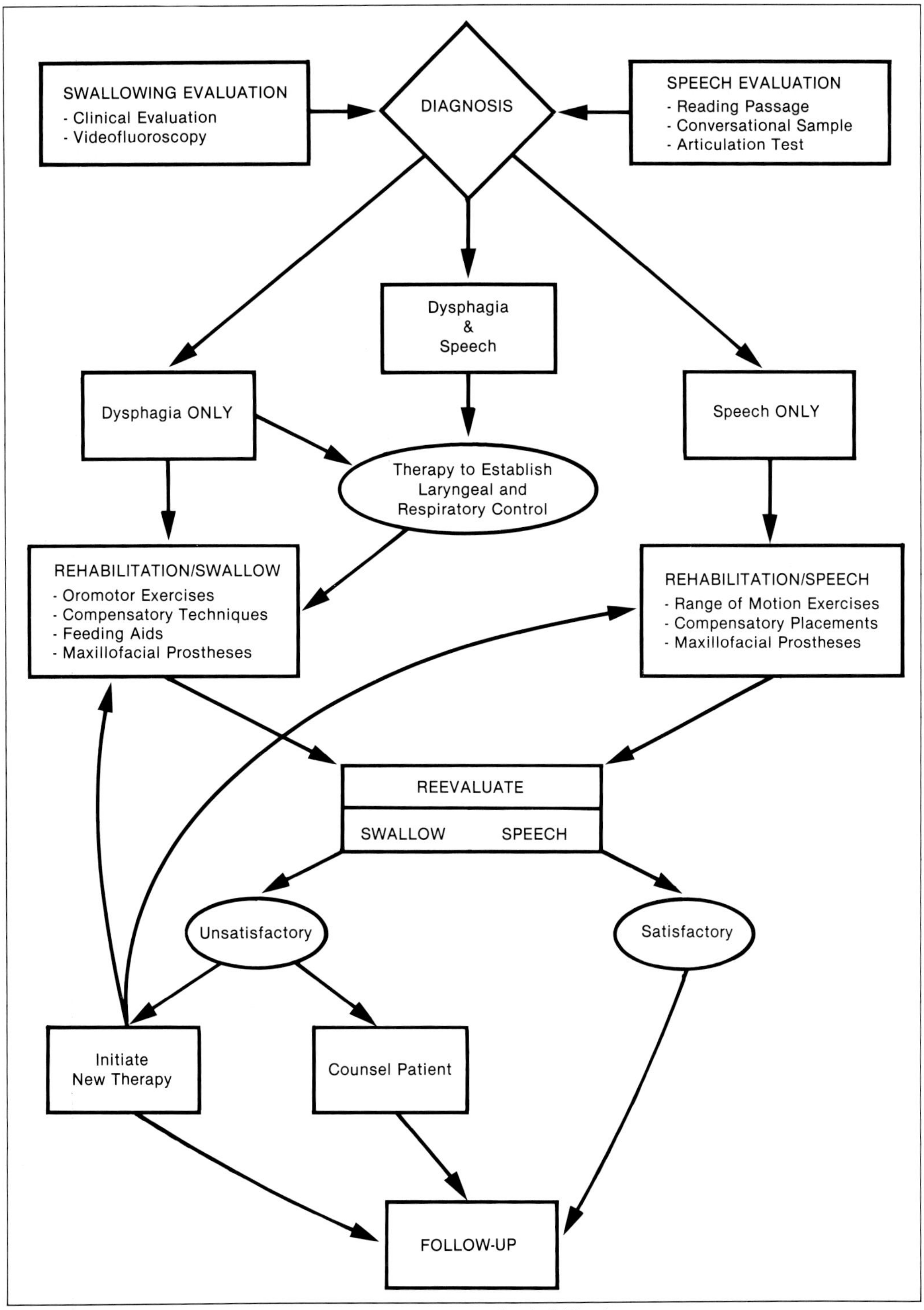

Figure 25-4. The oral cancer patient: assessment and rehabilitation.

Table 26-1. The impact of total laryngectomy

Airway
Permanent tracheostomy
Crust formation
Anosmia & Dysgeusia
Dysphagia
Rhinorrhea
Sphincter
Aphonia
Absent valsalva maneuver
Constipation
Eructation

1. Consultation for esophageal speech or tracheoesophageal puncture.
2. Insufflation test as performed by the speech pathologist.
3. "Lost Chord" club attendance.
4. Visitation from a rehabilitated laryngectomee.

During the preoperative consultation, the speech pathologist obtains information regarding the patient's communication abilities: verbal agility, articulatory patterning, speaking rate, pitch variance, and dialectal differences. The patient and family are provided literature about laryngectomy speech rehabilitation. The handouts, published by the American Cancer Society and the International Association of Laryngectomees, are complete and informative.

Postoperative Evaluation

Three to 5 days post surgery, the patient is revisited by the speech pathologist. This visit usually includes a laryngectomee from one of the Lost Chord clubs. This gives both the family members and patient an opportunity to ask questions and express concerns about vocal rehabilitation and related problems. All questions are answered clearly and discussed to relieve as much anxiety as possible. Finally, a plan for speech therapy as well as possible speech prosthetics is outlined.

ALARYNGEAL SPEECH

The primary objective of post–total laryngectomy speech therapy is to determine the optimal communication production mode for each patient. Some factors that influence the mode of alaryngeal speech selection are (Figure 26-1):

1. Degree of tissue ablation (pharynx and esophagus).
2. Esophageal stenosis.
3. Hearing acuity.
4. Hand-eye coordination.
5. Speech environment.
6. Motivation.
7. Personal preference.

Alaryngeal speech requires a sound source and a vibrating structure. The sound source may be internal or external. The external source is a mechanical or electrical prosthesis. The internal source is a sphincter (pharyngeal or esophageal pseudosphincter), surgical shunt, or prosthetic valve.

Esophageal Speech

Theory

There are several methods for the production of esophageal speech. In general, esophageal speech is produced by esophageal air insufflation, followed by a controlled belch or air release. Sound production is the result of the vibration of the esophagus and modification by the pharynx and oral cavity. Esophageal insufflation occurs when there is sufficient intraoral pressure to override the pharyngeal or esophageal sphincter. This sphincter consists of the cricopharyngeus and the inferior pharyngeal constrictor. The primary objective of esophageal speech is to prevent pharyngoesophageal sphincter closure and to permit sufficient airflow into the esophagus. The entrapped esophageal air is regurgitated voluntarily, thus causing the pharyngoesophageal segment to vibrate. Through relaxation and practice, the adept patient efficiently develops rapid ingestion, expansion, regurgitation, and vibration.

Techniques

There are four techniques of esophageal speech production: the consonant injection method, the glossopalatal or glossopharyngeal press

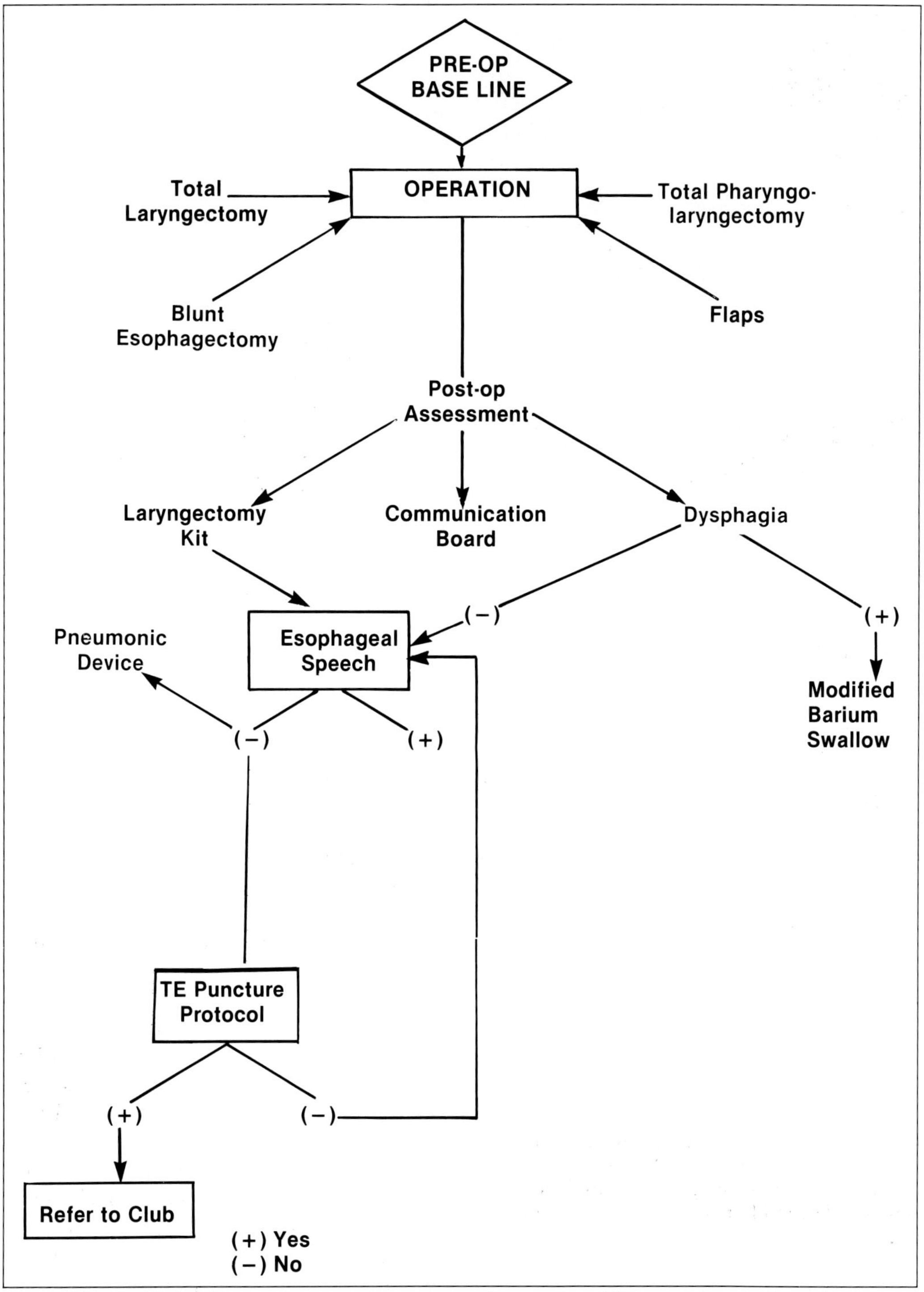

Figure 26-1. Laryngectomee assessment and treatment. *TE* = tracheoesophageal.

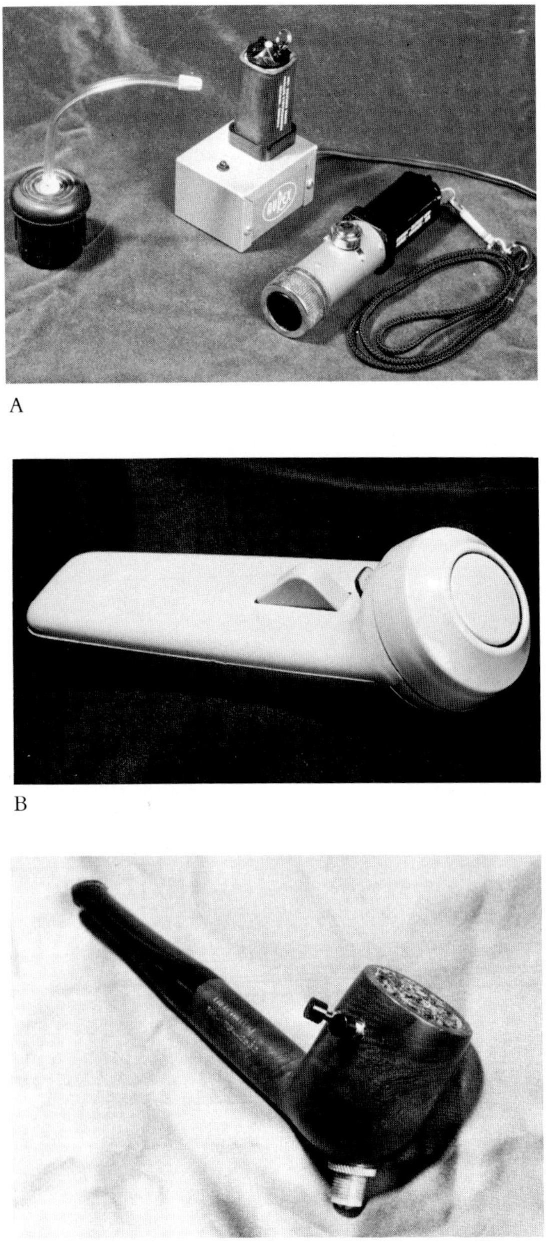

A

B

C

Figure 26-2. Electronic larynges. A. Cooper-Rand Electronic Larynx; Aurex-Neovox Electronic Larynx with charger and spare battery. B. Western Electric Electronic Larynx. C. "Pipe" larynge.

method, the inhalation method, and the swallow method.

The consonant injection method is the most efficient. This method utilizes the intraoral air pressure method of introducing air into the esophagus. Air is injected into the esophagus during intervals and rest periods. With the glossopalatal or glossopharyngeal press method, the patient uses the tongue tip to create a seal against the alveolar ridge, thus allowing the dorsum of the tongue to compress the air trapped in the mouth. The inhalation method differs by increasing intraesophageal pressure and overriding the pharyngoesophageal sphincter, resulting in esophageal insufflation. The swallow method, the least efficient, requires the tongue to move air across the hard palate during swallowing, thus forcing air into the esophagus. In practice it is very difficult to swallow quickly and repeatedly; many patients experience gastric distention.

Disadvantages

Regardless of the method, there are significant problems with any form of esophageal speech: grimacing and excessive body tension, excessive stomal noise, extraneous noises, and air swallowing.

Laryngeal Devices

Realistically, 45 percent of laryngectomy patients will never acquire intelligible esophageal speech [2]. For these patients, a speech prosthesis (pneumatic or electrical) is strongly recommended (Figure 26-2).

Pneumatic Larynges

Pneumatically powered prostheses utilize air from the lungs; pulmonary air enters the voice prosthesis through an airtight cover fitted over the patient's stoma [3]. The speaker simply places the end of the device into the mouth and articulates. There are several models; an example is the Van Humen artificial larynx. One pneumatic artificial larynx uses an air-driven, vibrating reed for tonal production. This device diverts the tone from the vibrating reed directly into the mouth. Patients who use a pneumatic artificial larynx under optimal conditions are capable of producing 95-percent intelligible alaryngeal speech [2].

Electrical Larynges

Electrical larynges interface with either the mouth, teeth, or neck. The vocal quality varies and depends on the acoustic characteristics of the patient's vocal tract. Some devices generate the sound source extraorally with the tone directed intraorally through a plastic tube; other devices generate sound intraorally within a specially designed denture. Other models produce tones that are conducted from the external surface of the neck to the hypopharynx. Examples of electronic larynges are the Western Electric Larynx, Aurex-Neovox Electronic Larynx, Siemens, Servox Electronic Larynx, and Barts Vibrator Electronic Larynx.

Voice Bak Larynge

In 1972, Taub and Spiro described a valved prosthesis called the "Voice Bak." This requires creation of a laterally placed cervical esophagostoma to permit maximum airflow across of the pharyngoesophageal mucosa for sound production. The esophagostoma is selected after preoperative insufflation of the esophagus through a nasal catheter. The Voice Bak Larynge is unsafe for radiated or post–neck dissection patients, a limitation that greatly restricts widespread application [1].

Surgical Shunts

Tracheoesophageal air shunts are created by the staged construction of a skin-lined shunt from the tracheostoma to the pharynx. These procedures were popular in the late 1950s. The surgery is multistaged and involves connecting the trachea to the hypopharynx with a dermal tube. Sound is generated by occluding the stoma with a finger and forcing pulmonary air through the dermal tube into the hypopharynx. Although the voice is good, aspiration and dermal tube stenosis can occur. Today, these procedures rarely are performed in the United States.

Tracheoesophageal Prosthesis

In 1979, Singer and Blom proposed an alternate endoscopic technique, a silicone tracheal valve [4,5]. This simple surgical approach is a tracheoesophageal puncture (TEP) or fistula maintained by a silicone voice prosthesis (Figure 26-3). The Blom-Singer and the Panje Voice Button are small silicone prostheses that are inserted into a surgically created midline tracheoesophageal fistula. The patient insufflates pulmonary air from the trachea into the esophagus through the prosthesis to vibrate the pharyngoesophageal segment.

Esophageal Insufflation

One of the best predictors is a positive response to the esophageal distention test [6]. After transnasal passage of a 14F rubber catheter, air is instilled with a bulb syringe. As air is insufflated, the patient is instructed to regurgitate simultaneously and phonate. Intelligible speech production is considered if a positive insufflation is obtained. However, the TEP is not positive for speech production for all patients. A negative test does not rule out a tracheoesophageal prosthesis, especially if underlying cricopharyngeal spasm is present. Pharyngoesophageal spasm (an occlusive spasm of the pharyngeal constrictors) or cricopharyngeal spasm may be triggered by esophageal insufflation, thus adversely affecting the voice. If the spasm persists, selective myotomy increases the chances of fluent speech production [7].

Candidates

Tracheoesophageal puncture requires a highly motivated patient. The experienced speech pathologist establishes a preoperative screen for such candidates. The following protocol is suggested [8]:

1. Manual dexterity: The patient must have the ability to insert and remove the prosthesis.
2. Stoma size: The patient must be able to occlude the stoma with one finger for voice production.
3. Airflow: The patient must generate adequate pulmonary air pressure.

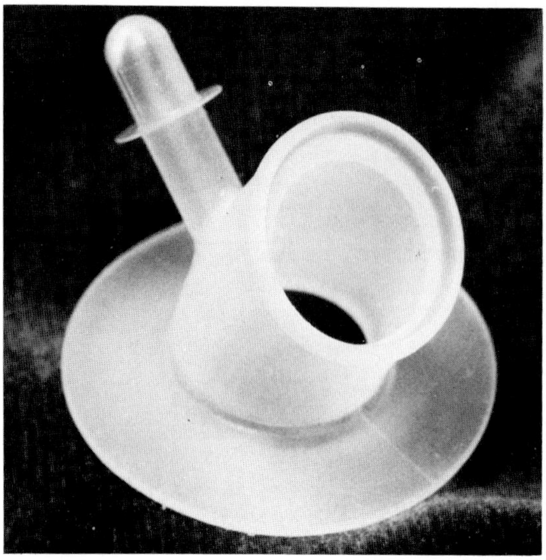

A

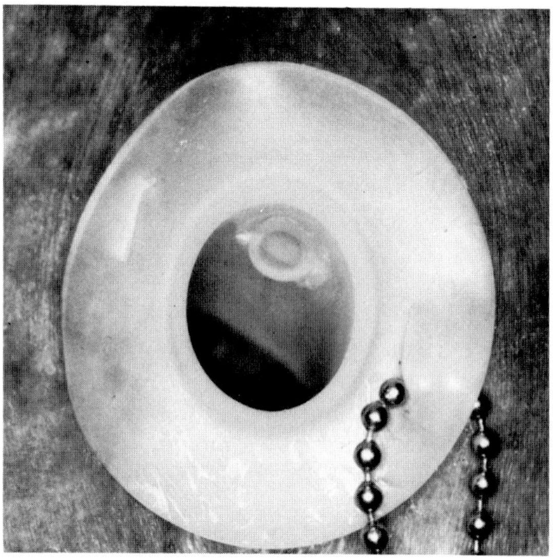

C

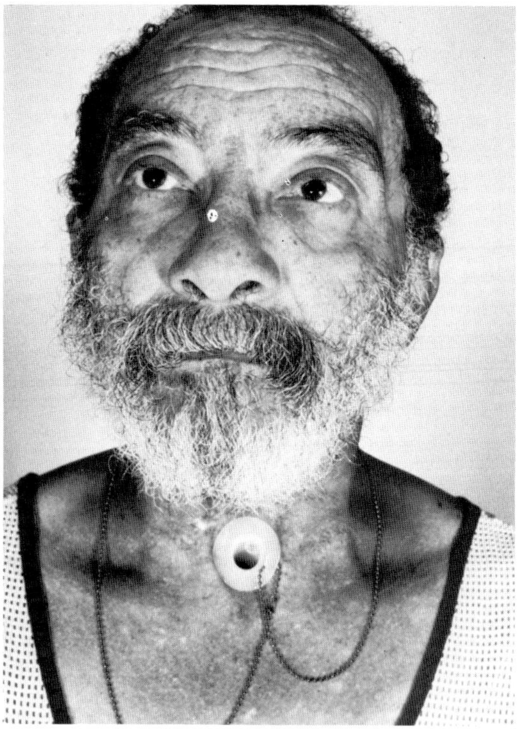

B

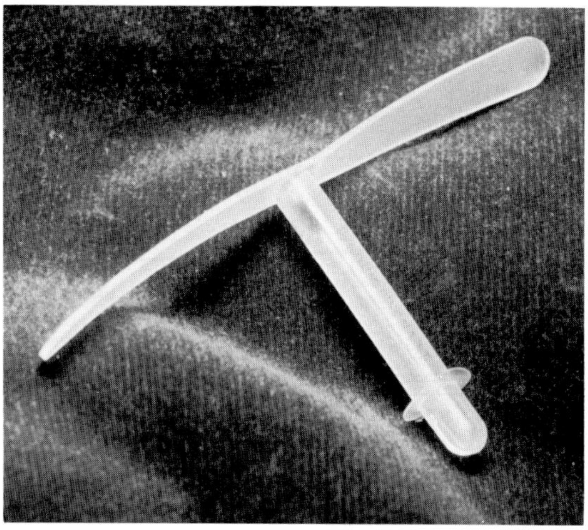

D

Figure 26-3. Tracheoesophageal shunts. A–C. Bivona Colorado prosthesis. D. Bivona Bifold TEP, high resistance.

Timing

Tracheoesophageal puncture is recommended 6 months after either radiotherapy or surgery. This waiting period ensures minimal tissue breakdown and stoma maturity. The prosthesis requires 1 to 4 weeks of practice (catheter removal and reinsertion) before the patient is considered proficient.

Advantages

1. Most patients are potential candidates despite radical neck dissection or full-course radiotherapy.
2. The procedure is reversible; the fistula closes rapidly after removal of the prosthesis.
3. Several voice prostheses are available.

Blom-Singer Versus Panje Voice Prosthesis

The two most popular devices are the Blom-Singer and Panje prostheses (Table 26-2). The Blom-Singer device is cleaned and removed daily, whereas the Panje Button requires monthly removal. Poor manual dexterity is the major cause of failure with the Blom-Singer prosthesis [8]. The Panje Button is secured by two small, easily inserted, internal flanges. This contrasts with the two large retention flanges of the Blom-Singer valve that require taping to the skin.

Other Devices

Both prostheses are being studied to establish the levels of aerodynamic performance. The Blom-Singer prosthesis has 3 to 4 times higher aerodynamic performance characteristics than the resistance offered by the normal larynx [4]. High airway resistance may trigger pharyngoesophageal spasm in some patients. Some researchers have developed a low-resistance, low-pressure voice prosthesis. Others have developed a tracheostoma valve that is used in combination with the various voice prostheses to eliminate digital stomal occlusion while speaking. An example is the Colorado Voice Prosthesis developed by Bivona Surgical Supplies.

REFERENCES

1. Gates GA, Ryan WJ, Cooper JC: Current status of laryngectomee rehabilitation results of therapy. *Am J Oto* 3 : 1, 1982.
2. Keith GL, Darley FL (eds): *Laryngectomee Rehabilitation*. Houston: College-Hill, 1979.
3. Mares MD, Lingeman RE: Primary local rehabilitation using the Blom-Singer and Panje Voice Prosthesis. *Ann Oto Rhinol Laryngol* 91 : 458, 1982.
4. Singer MI: Tracheoesophageal speech: Vocal rehabilitation after total laryngectomy. *Laryngoscope* 93 : 1454, 1983.
5. Weinberg B (ed): *Readings in Speech Following Total Laryngectomy*. Baltimore: University Park Press, 1984.

Table 26-2. Tracheoesophageal laryngeal device comparison

Characteristic	*Bivona (Blom-Singer)*	*Xomed (Panje)*	*Dow Corning (Hec)*
Opening pressure	Low	High	Very low
Airflow	Medium	Low	High
Extrusion rate	High	Low	Low
Stoma obstruction	Yes	Low	No
Valve crusting	High	High	Low
Self-care difficulty	Moderate	Moderate	Minimal
Postoperative visits	Many	Many	Few
Patient training	Moderate	Moderate	Minimal
Speech fluency	Good	Fair	Very good
Speech volume	Good	Fair	Very good
Speech strain	Some	Moderate	Minimal
Device removal	Daily	Daily	2–3 months

6. Singer MI, Blom ED: A selective myotomy for voice restoration after total laryngectomy. *Arch Otolaryngol* 107 : 670, 1981.
7. Singer MI, Blom ED: An endoscopic technique for restoration of voice after total laryngectomy. *Ann Otol Rhinol Laryngol* 89 : 529, 1980.
8. Weinbert B, Moon J: Aerodynamic properties of four tracheoesophageal puncture prostheses. *Arch Otol* P. 110 : 1984.

27

Audiology: Hearing Loss

PATRICIA R. THOMPSON

KEY CONCEPTS

Neuroanatomy/Physiology; Radiotherapy; Tumor Location; Ototoxicity; Patient Assessment

MILESTONES

1791	Animal Bioelectrical Potentials	Galvani
1877	Sodium Salicylate Hearing Loss	Muller
1880	Quinine and Salicylate Hearing Loss	Maillard
1928	X-Rays and Hearing Loss	Thielemann
1940s	Development of Audiometric Testing	Sohmer and Feinmesser
1970s	Clinical Application of Auditory Evoked Potentials	

Many patients with head and neck cancer risk hearing loss due to either the lesion site or its subsequent management (i.e., surgery, radiotherapy, or chemotherapy). The common otologic complaints are ear fullness, hearing loss, tinnitus, and vertigo. To properly manage these patients, audiologic monitoring is an integral component of the treatment plan. This chapter analyzes the impact of head and neck oncology on the auditory system (Figure 27-1).

ANATOMY AND PHYSIOLOGY

Sound Transmission

The ear is divided into three components: outer, middle, and inner. The outer ear, composed of the pinna and external auditory meatus, plays a minimal role in sound transmission (Figure 27-2). It does, however, funnel sound waves to the tympanic membrane and amplifies critical speech sounds in the vicinity of the external auditory meatus' natural resonance frequency of 2700 Hz.

The middle ear consists of the tympanic membrane and three ossicles. The ossicles link the tympanic membrane to the fluid-filled cochlea via the oval window. At the tympanic membrane, sound is transduced from acoustical to mechanical energy and amplified approximately 27 dB by the transformer action of the middle ear. It then is transmitted to the receptor cells in the organ of Corti. Here, mechanical energy is converted to an electrical analog by shearing forces between the tectorial membrane and hair cell cilia (Table 27-1) [1–4].

The electrical response is transmitted neurochemically to the auditory nerve and then to the ipsilateral cochlear nucleus (pontomedullary junction). In the brain stem, the signal is relayed ipsilaterally and contralaterally to higher auditory centers.

Cochlear Anatomy

The inner ear is composed of the cochlea and the vestibular system. Only the former, which contains the end organ of hearing, will be dis-

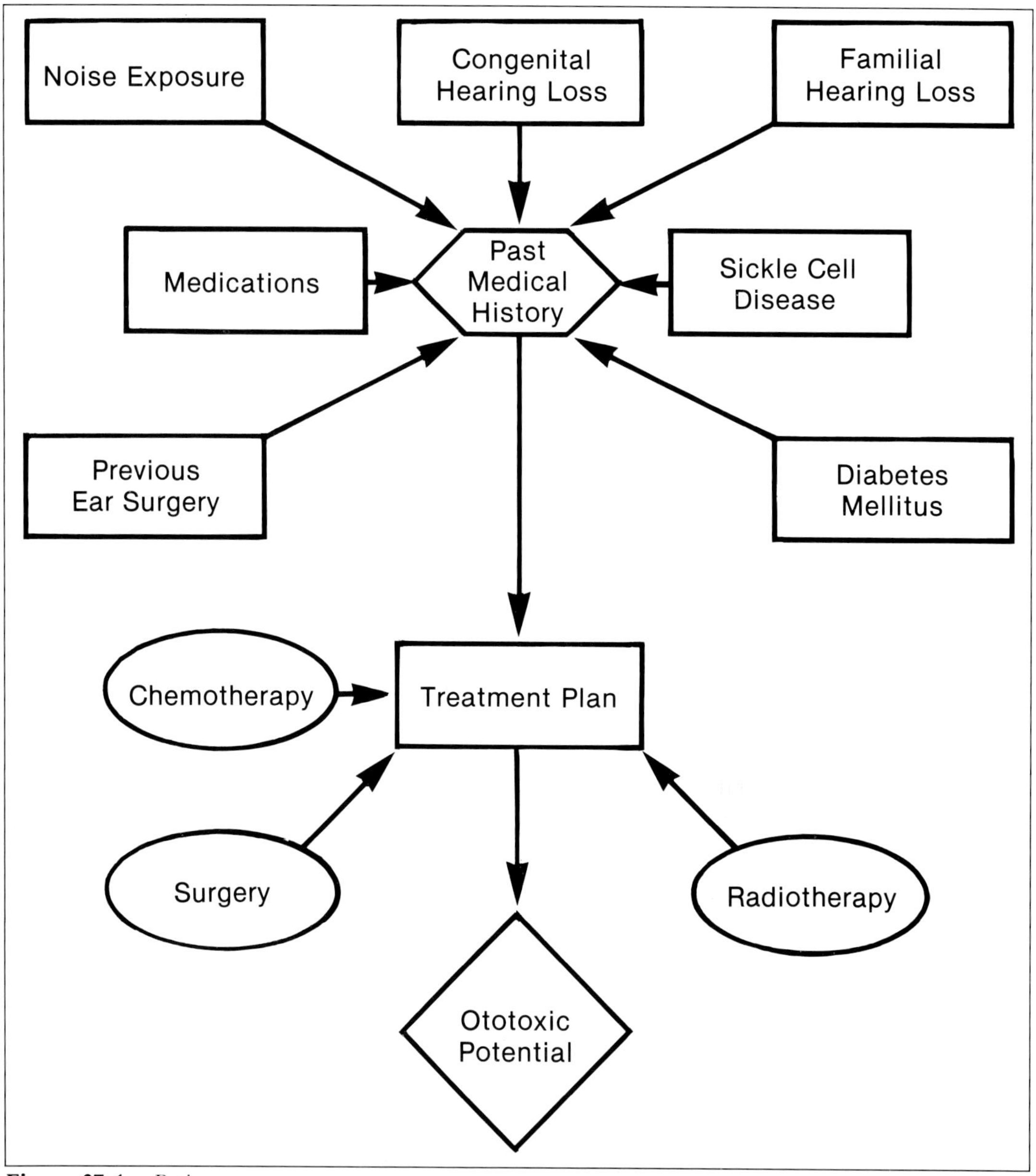

Figure 27-1. Patient assessment.

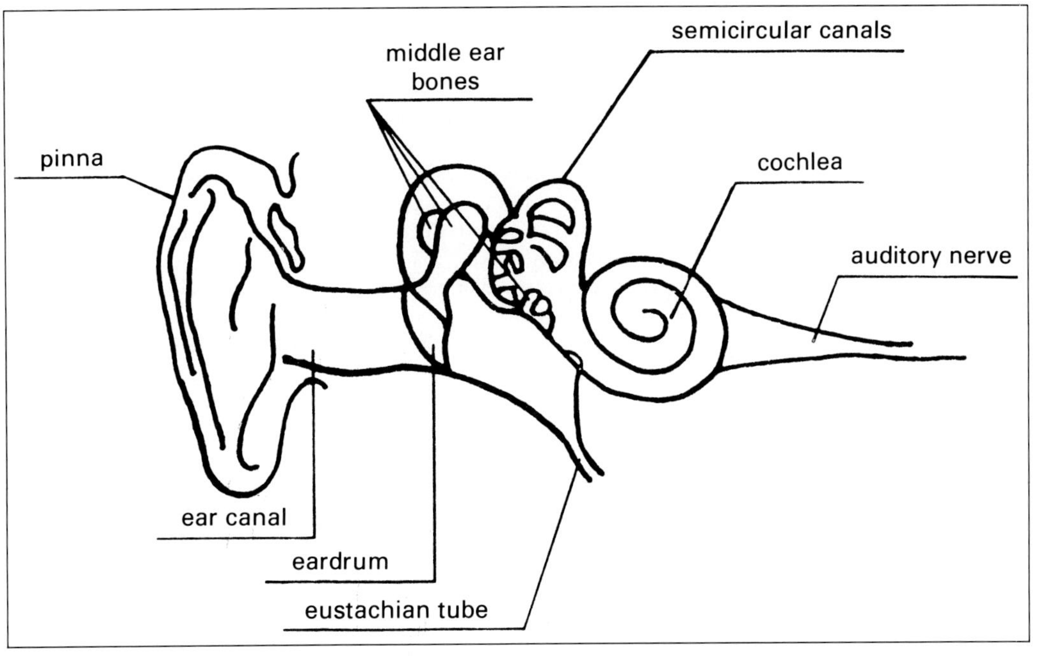

A

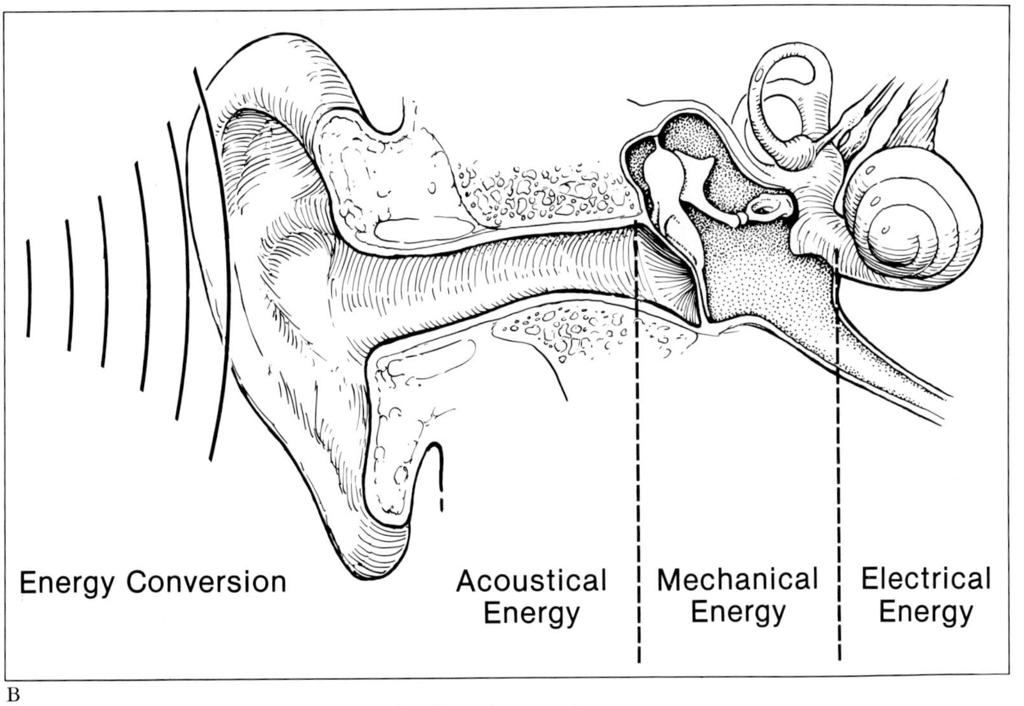

B

Figure 27-2. A. Basic ear anatomy. B. Sound transmission.

Table 27-1. Cochlear structures/potentials

Structure/mechanism	*Function*
Reissner's membrane	Separates perilymph in the scala vestibuli from endolymph in the scala media.
Basilar membrane	Generates the traveling wave phenomenon and makes a significant contribution to the tonotopic organization of the cochlea (i.e., high frequencies encoded basally and low frequencies apically).
Tectorial membrane	The gelatinous membrane that embeds the outer hair cell cilia. Shearing action between the hair cell cilia and membrane generates the receptor potential.
Inner hair cells (IHC)	Flask-shaped cells that encode auditory information for transmission to the afferent auditory nerve fibers. Inner hair cells are passive mechanoreceptors. Note: 95% of these fibers innervate the inner hair cells.
Outer hair cells (OHC)	Cylindric-shaped cells that generate a motile response that sharpen the mechanical properties of the basilar membrane, thus modulating the response of the inner hair cells. This motile response is driven by the receptor potential. Note: 5% of afferent auditory nerve fibers innervate the outer hair cells.
Stria vascularis	This highly vascularized patch of tissue is the cochlea's power plant and is responsible for the generation of the scala media's endocochlear DC potential and endolymph secretion.
Cochlear microphonic	An AC receptor potential generated by the shearing action between the tectorial membrane and cilia of the hair cells. It mimics the acoustic input.
Summating potential	A DC receptor potential that represents distortion in the transducer process of the hair cell and cochlear mechanism.

cussed in detail. Histologically, the cochlea consists of an osseous and membranous labyrinth. A schematic transverse section of the cochlea is displayed in Figure 27-3. Reissner's membrane and the basilar membrane separate the endolymphatic fluid of the scala media from the perilymph in the scala vestibuli and scala tympani. The endolymph is similar in ionic composition to intracellular fluid (high K^+, low NA^+); perilymph is akin to cerebrospinal fluid (high Na^+, low K^+). The organ of Corti, located on the basilar membrane, contains the receptor (hair) cells and the supportive structures. The receptor cells consist of a single row of approximately 3400 inner hair cells and three to five rows of outer hair cells that average 13,500 in number. Bathing the hair cells is a third fluid known as cortilymph, which in composition is similar to perilymph [2].

Hair Cells

The inner hair cell is flask-like in shape. Near the upper surface there is a thick cuticular plate containing two rows of embedded stereocilia. Lateral to the stereocilia is a cuticular-free region where the basal body of the kinocilium is found. Beneath this region is a high concentration of Golgi bodies and mitochondria. This highly metabolic region is the probable site of mechanical to electrical energy conversion [3]. The organelles in the inner hair cell are disseminated throughout the cytoplasm and are like those found in active epithelial cells. The outer hair cell differs from the inner hair cell as follows: it is shaped cylindrically, it has three rows of stereocilia arranged in a W pattern, and its organelles (i.e., the endoplasmic reticulum and mitochondria) are located peripherally.

Supporting Cells

Several supporting cells help stabilize the organ of Corti. For example, Claudius', Hensen's and Deiters' cells lend support to the outer hair cells while the inner hair cells are supported by the inner sulcus cells. Additional support is provided by the inner and outer pillar cells, which

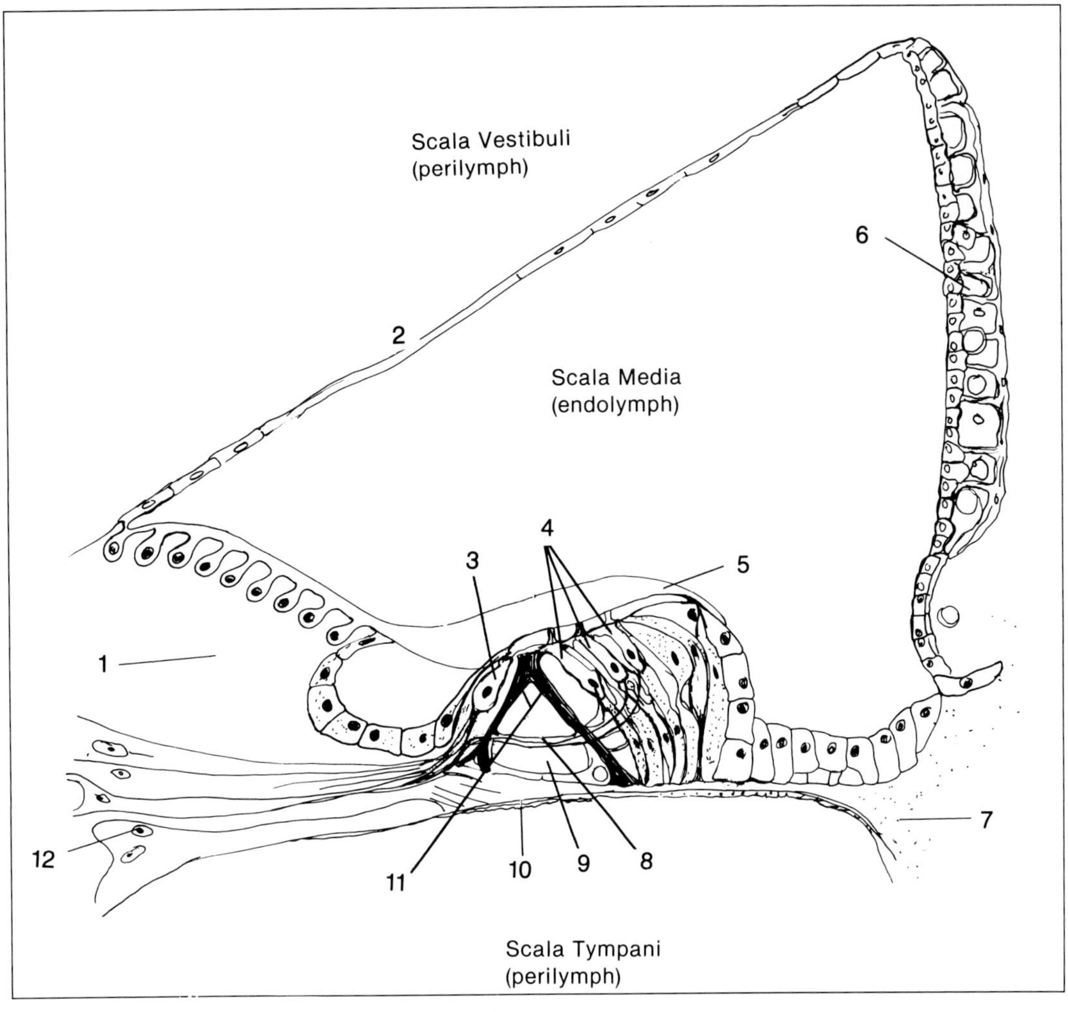

Figure 27-3. The inner ear. 1. Spiral limbus. 2. Reissner's membrane. 3. Inner hair cell. 4. Outer hair cells. 5. Tectorial membrane. 6. Stria vascularis. 7. Spiral ligament. 8. Nerve fibers. 9. Tunnel of Corti. 10. Basilar membrane. 11. Rods of Corti. 12. Spiral ganglion. (Adapted from drawing by Fred M. Harwin in Smith: The Inner Ear: Its Embryological Development and Microstructure. In Tower DB (ed): *The Nervous System: Vol 3. Human Communication and Its Disorders*. New York: Raven, 1975.)

together form the tunnel of Corti. The heads of these cells, along with the cuticular plate and the Deiters' phalangeal processes, collectively form the reticular lamina, which serves as a barrier between the endolymph in the scala media and the cortilymph in the organ of Corti [4].

Transducive Mechanism

Above the organ of Corti is the gelatinous tectorial membrane. One end is attached to the basilar membrane via a structure made of connective tissue called the spiral limbus; the opposite end is loosely connected to Hensen's cells. Embedded in the membrane are outer hair cell stereocilia. This intricate connection between the tectorial membrane, the supporting structures, and the receptor cells establishes an effective transducive mechanism. Movement of the basilar membrane bends the hair cell stereocilia, causing a disturbance of the hair cell membrane, thus resulting in an ionic exchange (current flow). This process converts mechanical energy to electrical impulses. The conversion process is dependent, however, on the electrical potential differences present in the cochlea.

Cochlear Physiology

Resting Membrane Potentials

With the scala tympani as a reference, there are three resting direct current (DC) potentials: the scala media's endocochlear potential (EP) of +80 mV; the hair cell's intracellular potential of −45 to −70 mV; and the scala vestibuli's +2 to +5 mV. Because of the positive EP and negative intracellular potentials, the electromotive force (emf) across the top of the hair cell is between 125 and 150 mV. This large potential difference probably is responsible for the extreme hair cell sensitivity to mechanical stimulation [5]. Electrophysiologic studies have supported this hypothesis by demonstrating that significant decreases in the EP reduce the amplitude of evoked cochlear potentials.

The EP, theoretically, is generated by the stria vascularis [6,7]. In guinea pigs, transmission electron microscopy has shown three cell types within the stria vascularis: marginal, intermediate, and basal cells. The marginal cells, lining the lateral wall of the cochlear duct, are in intimate contact with the scala media's endolymphatic fluid. The intermediate cells are not in contact with endolymph. The large and flat basal cells separate groups of marginal and intermediate cells and also appear to form a barrier between the fluid in the spiral ligament and the stria vascularis [4].

Receptor Potentials

With acoustical stimulation, two receptor potentials are generated in the cochlea: the summating potential (SP) and the cochlear microphonic (CM). The SP is a DC response that is recorded as a baseline shift, whose etiology has been attributed to a complex inner and outer hair cell response. The CM, an electrical analog of the sound wave, is attributed primarily to the depolarization and hyperpolarization of the outer hair cells [8]. Basilar membrane displacement, in response to acoustical stimulation, and the subsequent bending of the hair cell cilia initiate this process.

The receptor potential generated by the hair cells is responsible for stimulating the adjacent auditory nerve fibers. Many suggest that this excitation is transmitted by the release of acetylcholine from hair cell vesicles.

Central Auditory Pathway

Auditory nerve fibers along with fibers from the vestibular system collectively form the eighth cranial nerve. The auditory branch of the eighth nerve enters the brain stem at the pontomedullary junction and terminates ipsilaterally in the brain stem on cochlear nuclei in the upper medulla. The cell bodies of these second-order neurons are found in the anterior and posterior ventral cochlear nuclei and the dorsal cochlear nucleus. Of these three, the anterior ventral cochlear nucleus is a part of the primary ascending auditory pathway. Although some anterior ventral cochlear nucleus fibers ascend ipsilaterally, most course through the ventral acoustic stria (trapezoid body) to synapse on third-order neurons whose cell bodies are in the contralateral superior olivary complex. A few second-order neurons bypass the superior olivary complex completely and synapse at higher levels in the brain stem.

Superior Olivary Complex

The superior olivary complex is located in the lower pons and consists of several nuclei. Those contributing to hearing are the medial superior olive, the lateral superior olive, and the nucleus of the trapezoid body. Of these three, the lateral superior olive and the nucleus of the trapezoid body are not developed well in humans. The medial superior olive, however, is large and is noted to receive major input from second-order neurons that originate from both ventral cochlear nuclei. Because of this binaural input, the superior olivary complex is the first level in the auditory system where binaural integration takes place [9]. The third-order neurons that arise from the medial superior olive course through the lateral lemniscus to synapse on cell bodies in the inferior colliculus located in the mesencephalon. Others terminate in the auditory region of the thalamus.

Inferior Colliculus

The inferior colliculus, considered the most complex nucleus in the auditory system, consists of the central nucleus, the pericentral nucleus, the external nucleus, and intercollicular commissural fibers. Of the three nuclei mentioned, the central nucleus is the major auditory center and the location of fourth-order neuronal cell bodies. The other nuclei are not considered to be directly involved in audition. The commissural fibers in the inferior colliculus are the second major decussation in the auditory system.

Axons from the central nucleus, as well as those from lower auditory regions (i.e., cochlear nucleus, superior olivary complex, and lateral lemniscus), course through the brachium (axonal bundle) of the inferior colliculus and terminate in the auditory region of the thalamus, called the medial geniculate body.

Medial Geniculate Body

The medial geniculate body is the final relay for auditory input destined for the primary auditory cortex. This nucleus is subdivided into dorsal, ventral, and medial regions. It is, however, the ventral portion of the medial geniculate body that receives auditory input from the central nucleus and lower centers. Therefore, it is from this region that the auditory radiations seem to arise.

Auditory Cortex

The auditory radiations from the brain stem synapse within the primary auditory cortex that is hidden inside the Sylvian fissure on the posterior region of the superior temporal gyrus. This is Heschl's gyrus or Brodmann's area 41. Adjacent to area 41 is area 42, which in humans is a part of the primary auditory cortex. From these auditory regions, input is sent to auditory association areas such as Brodmann's area 22, ipsilaterally, and to auditory areas in the contralateral hemisphere through the corpus callosum [10,11].

Other Pathways

This brief summary presents the most direct ascending auditory pathway. Auditory input also can be transmitted through other ipsilateral and contralateral relay networks in the central auditory nervous system. Because of the complexity of the human auditory system, first-, second-, third-, fourth-, and fifth-order neurons do not synapse necessarily at sequential levels in the auditory pathway. Consequently, when the auditory system is stimulated by sound, electrical activity is generated at several levels in the auditory pathway almost simultaneously.

RADIOTHERAPY

Radiotherapy, a commonly recommended treatment modality, can affect hearing (see Chapter 9). The following is a brief review of its impact on the auditory system.

Animal Studies

Between 1928 and 1969, radiotherapists utilized single-dose or nonfractionated radiation. Single-dose irradiation to the otic capsule is associated with hemorrhage, edema, and endolymphatic space compression. These histologic and physiologic changes produce transient or permanent hearing loss, decreased cochlear potentials, and nystagmus [12].

Today, fractionation or multiple-dose radiation is used. In chinchillas, this technique (2 cGy/day, 5 days/week for 5–7 weeks) results in hair cell loss and degeneration of supporting cells and auditory nerve fibers. Stria vascularis degeneration is minimal. More significantly, no middle ear lesions, temporal bone osteonecrosis, or middle/inner ear hemorrhage is observed [13].

Human Studies

In humans, the detrimental effects are auricular desquamation, cerumen gland atrophy, external auditory canal and temporal bone osteonecrosis, serous otitis media, and atrophy of the spiral ligament, stria vascularis, and basilar membrane [13–16]. Associated with these structural changes are tinnitus, fullness, vertigo, mild to moderate hearing loss, and occasionally profound hearing loss [15–17].

Audiologic Management

The radiation effects are dose related. Therefore, with high dosages, the following precautions are recommended: (1) pretreatment baseline audiometry followed by semiannual assessments and (2) appropriate medical treatment and audiologic management of significant hearing loss (see Chapter 28).

NEOPLASMS

Cerebellopontine Angle

Epidermoid cysts, neurofibromas, meningiomas, or acoustic neuromas are located in the cerebellopontine angle or in the internal auditory meatus (see Chapters 4 and 13). These tumors compress the auditory nerve and disrupt the cochlear vascular supply. This reduces the conduction velocity of the remaining auditory nerve fibers and alters the biochemistry of the cochlear fluids [18]. The audiologic profile associated with these tumors is ipsilateral sensorineural hearing loss, reduced word recognition ability, absent ipsilateral stapedial reflexes, and abnormal auditory brain stem evoked potentials (see Chapter 28).

In addition to facial nerve preservation, the ideal treatment goal is tumor ablation with hearing conservation [19]. The latter depends on tumor size, oto-audiologic profile, and intraoperative monitoring techniques.

Tumor Size

If the tumor is less than 2.5 cm and hearing is functional (speech reception threshold less than 50 dBHL and word recognition better than 60%), the middle cranial fossa, transtemporal, or suboccipital surgical approach may preserve hearing. If the tumor is greater than 2.5 cm, hearing preservation is unrealistic. Hence, a lateral or translabyrinthine approach is recommended (see Chapter 13) [19].

Oto-Audiologic Profile

Onset of Hearing Loss

Patients with sudden hearing loss have a poor postoperative prognosis for hearing preservation. The converse is true for patients with gradual hearing loss [18].

Bilateral Tumors

Bilateral hearing loss is devastating. Therefore, when bilateral tumors are present, hearing preservation is a primary consideration [19].

Bilateral Hearing Loss

The audiologic profile (pure tone and speech audiometry) is reviewed to determine the extent of hearing loss bilaterally. When hearing is significantly better in the operative ear, hearing preservation should be considered. If preservation is not feasible (i.e., large tumor), then the postoperative handicap depends on the amount of residual hearing in the nonoperative ear.

MINIMAL IMPAIRMENT

Hearing in the nonoperative ear is normal or minimally impaired (pure tone average < 40 dBHL and word recognition 75% or better). With appropriate postoperative audiologic management (i.e., amplification and counseling), prognosis is excellent.

MODERATE IMPAIRMENT

The nonoperative ear exhibits a pure tone average of 40 to 60 dBHL, a word recognition score of 65 to 75 percent without visual cues and better than 75 percent with visual input. With amplification and follow-up counseling, the prognosis is good.

SEVERE IMPAIRMENT

Hearing in the nonoperative ear is greater than 60 dBHL, and word recognition is less than 65 percent with and without visual cues. The prognosis depends on patient motivation, adjustment to amplification, and benefits obtained from aural rehabilitation (see Chapter 28).

Intraoperative Eighth Nerve Monitoring

Postoperative inner ear damage is due to direct or indirect trauma to the labyrinthine artery, the labyrinth, or the cochlear nerve. Hearing preservation is enhanced by intraoperative eighth nerve monitoring (see Chapter 13). Any intraoperative change of the eighth nerve potential (i.e., amplitude or latency) portends possible eighth nerve damage [18].

Temporal Bone/Middle Ear

Neoplasms in the temporal bone or middle ear, (i.e., glomus tympanicum or jugulare) compromise the middle ear transformer (ossicular adherence or erosion) and result in conductive hearing loss. Treatment includes ablative surgery and probable amplification, and the rehabilitative prognosis is good.

Skull Base and Nasopharynx (Site 1)

Skull base and nasopharyngeal malignancies commonly present with eustachian tube dysfunction secondary to mechanical obstruction or inflammation (see Chapter 4) [12]. Eustachian tube dysfunction impairs middle ear aeration and precipitates the development of serous otitis media. This results in a mild to moderate conductive hearing loss (see Chapters 2 and 4).

Treatment includes myringotomy and tube insertion followed by an audiologic evaluation and amplification, if indicated. The rehabilitative prognosis is good.

OTOTOXIC DRUGS

The treatment of head and neck cancer often requires ototoxic drugs (i.e., chemotherapeutic agents, loop diuretics, and aminoglycosides).

Cisplatin

Indications

Cisplatin, a heavy-metal chemotherapeutic agent, is favored currently by medical oncologists for the treatment of squamous cell carcinoma (see Chapter 8) [20–24]. It usually is included in multiple-drug treatment protocols (i.e., cisplatin and 5-fluorouracil; cisplatin, vincristine, and bleomycin; or cisplatin, 5-fluorouracil, and methotrexate) [12].

Ototoxicity

Nephrotoxicity is the most serious side effect, but hydration and osmotic diuresis (intravenous saline in combination with mannitol) successfully minimizes this problem. Even with hydration, ototoxicity still may occur [25].

Early in the treatment course, tinnitus or high-frequency sensorineural hearing loss may arise. The loss is usually bilateral and irreversible [20,26,27]. Occasionally, moderate to severe sensorineural hearing losses involving the critical speech frequency range (500–2000 Hz) are associated with rapid infusion, high initial or cumulative dose levels, or concurrent ototoxic drugs [28]. Any of these conditions alone or in combination potentiates ototoxicity. Other conditions that predispose the patient to ototoxicity are preexisting hearing loss, advanced age, and renal insufficiency [20,25,29,30].

Histologically, cisplatin damages the outer hair cells and supporting cells at the basal end of the organ of Corti. To a lesser degree, the stria vascularis, Reissner's membrane and the vestibular neuroepithelial hair cells are affected [21–23,29–32]. Inner hair cells and pillar cells seem impervious to injury [24].

Generally, it has been reported that the potential for ototoxicity increases with high infusion rate, total dose exceeding 400 mg, and concomitant use with other ototoxic drugs (i.e., aminoglycosides or loop diuretics such as furosemide or ethacrynic acid).

Audiologic Monitoring

Usually, cisplatin ototoxicity occurs after the first or second treatment [33]. A baseline audiogram prior to treatment in conjunction with a follow-up assessment identifies most susceptible patients (Figure 27-4) [34].

Loop Diuretics

Ethacrynic acid, bumetanide, and furosemide are rapid-acting loop diuretics. They produce large amounts of iso-osmotic urine by (1) inhibiting electrolyte absorption in the ascending loop of Henle, (2) increasing renal blood flow, and (3) stimulating renin release [32]. Although these drugs are potentially ototoxic (alone or in combination with other ototoxic drugs),

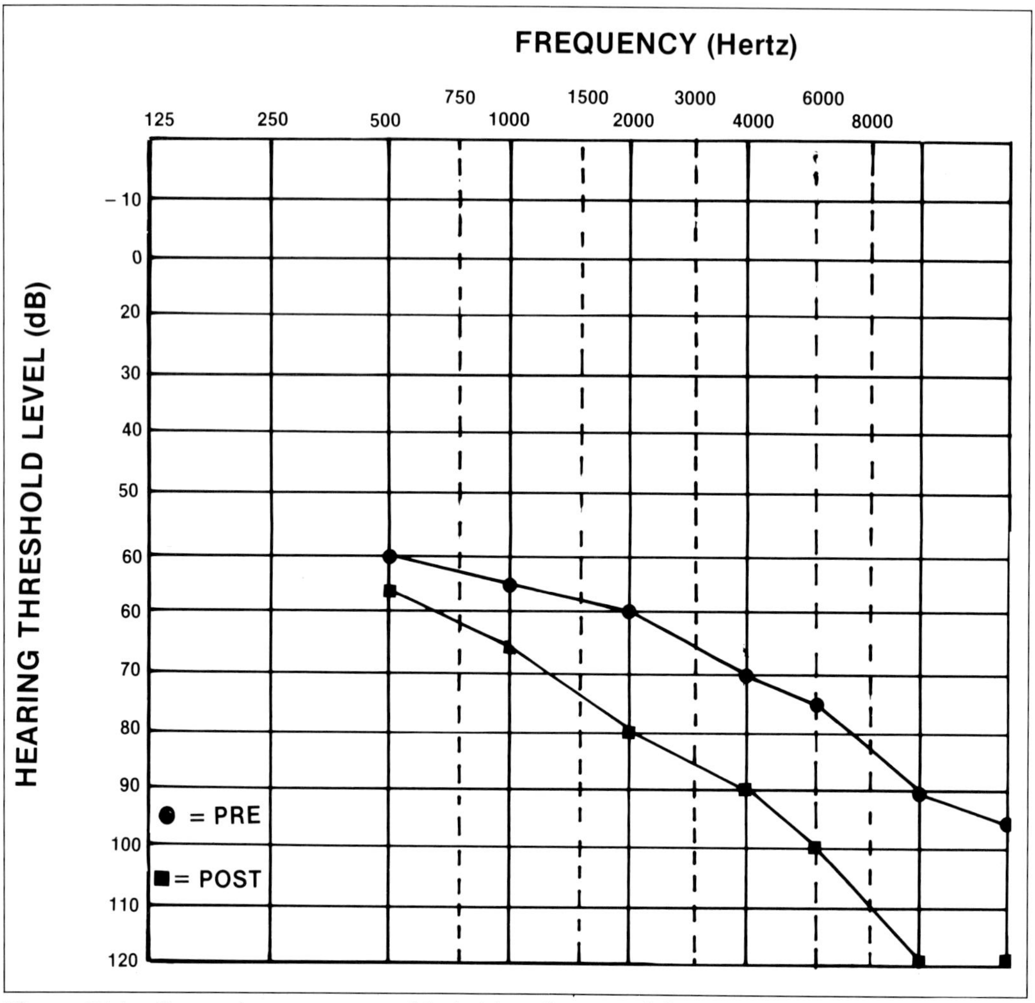

Figure 27-4. Pre- and post-treatment (cisplatin) audiogram of the right ear in a 49-year-old man with metastatic squamous cell carcinoma to cervical nodes and vertebrae.

patients with normal renal function rarely are affected (Table 27-2) [30–39].

Clinical symptoms of ototoxicity consist primarily of transient hearing loss and occasional vestibular disturbances. With excessive drug use, histopathologic studies in animals indicate that the stria vascularis undergoes temporary morphologic changes. Because the stria vascularis is responsible for maintaining the EP, any alteration in its structure may have a detrimental effect on the EP. Electrophysiologic studies suggest that this does occur along with alterations in the CM, action potential (AP), and early brain stem and late cortical potentials [39–46].

Table 27-2. Loop diuretics

Characteristic	*Ethacrynic acid*	*Furosemide*
Indications	Cardiac, hepatic, or renal edema	Congestive heart failure, acute or chronic renal failure, and hypertension
Mode of action	Enzymatic inhibition of cyclic adenosine monophosphate production in stria vascularis; reduction in adenylate cyclase activity in organ of Corti	Actively blocks K^+ transport channels in the marginal cells of stria vascularis, thus decreasing flow of K^+ into endolymph
Histopathology	Strial edema; outer hair cell loss	Strial edema; degenerative changes in intermediate and marginal cells in stria vascularis
Electrophysiologic changes	Reversible EP decline; irreversible CM decrease	Primary effect is EP decrease; secondary effect is CM and action potential reduction
Ototoxicity	Transient hearing loss	Transient hearing loss
Precautions	<1 mg/kg (body weight) with IV administration	Slow IV infusion (<4 mg/min; blood levels $<$ 85–90 μg/ml)
Audiologic monitoring	Baseline and follow-up audiogram	Baseline and follow-up audiogram

Ethacrynic Acid

Ethacrynic acid, a rapid-acting loop diuretic, can produce transient hearing loss. Permanent hearing loss and vestibular dysfunction (i.e., vertigo, dizziness, ataxia, reduced caloric responses) also have occurred but usually in the presence of impaired renal function or the concomitant use of other ototoxic drugs [30].

Electrophysiologic studies reflect a reversible decline in the EP along with an irreversible attenuation of the CM. Biochemical studies suggest that the mode of action for these two phenomena are different. EP attenuation results from an inhibition of the enzyme responsible for cyclic adenosine monophosphate (AMP) production, adenylate cyclase, in the stria vascularis [40]. The CM attenuation is due to a reduction in succinic dehydrogenase activity in the organ of Corti.

Some previous studies concluded that a reduction in the activity of the strial enzyme, sodium potassium adenosine triphosphatase (Na^+K^+-ATPase), is responsible for the transient effect on the EP. However, the work of Kusakari and co-workers [41] demonstrated that ethacrynic acid did not inhibit this enzyme until the concentration level was 500 times greater than the amount needed to decrease the EP. The subsequent work of Horn and associates [35] demonstrated that the inhibition in vitro of the enzyme responsible for cyclic AMP production (adenylate cyclase) occurred at ethacrynic acid concentration levels that were comparable to those affecting the EP, suggesting then that the mode of action within the stria vascularis may be an inhibition of adenylate cyclase rather than Na^+K^+-ATPase. Horn attributed the irreversible decrease of the CM on ethacrynic acid's interference with the oxidative process within the basal hair cells by reducing the activity of adenylate cyclase.

Furosemide

Furosemide, one of the five most frequently prescribed drugs, is the most potent clinically available diuretic. It is used for congestive heart failure, chronic renal failure, and hypertension. With high intravenous or bolus injections, ototoxicity may occur. Clinically, this manifests as transient hearing loss. However, permanent hearing loss and vestibular disturbances have been reported, primarily in patients with impaired renal function.

Electrophysiologic changes are similar to those of ethacrynic acid: a reduction in the EP, the CM, and the AP. Alterations in the EP is suspected to be the primary effect of furosemide use. Reductions in the AP and the CM are secondary. At present, the mechanism behind these effects are unknown. However, Rybak [39] has postulated that furosemide may reduce the EP by differentially blocking potassium transport channels in the marginal cells of the stria vascularis. For example, furosemide may actively block the K^+ channels responsible for the accumulation of K^+ within the marginal cell while simultaneously, but to a lesser degree, blocking the K^+ channels that transport K^+ into the scala media. This event is speculated to reduce the EP by causing a reduction in the flow of K^+ into the endolymph, making more apparent the K^+ diffusion potential alone or in combination with a negative electrogenic potential.

In an attempt to explain the profound effect furosemide has on the AP, Sewell [42] simultaneously monitored the EP and spontaneous discharge rate of the eighth nerve in cats during furosemide use. He found that a reduction in the EP correlated well with a decrease in the auditory nerve neural discharge rate. Based on these findings, it was speculated that the EP modulates the spontaneous release of the inner hair cell's neurotransmitter. A decrease in the EP may then indirectly reduce the discharge rate of the auditory nerve fibers by hyperpolarizing the inner hair cells and consequently reducing the release of neurotransmitter. It is also speculated by some that the slight reduction noted in the CM may be attributed to changes in the electrical activities of specific inner hair cells [43].

Recent histochemical studies suggest that unlike ethacrynic acid, furosemide does not appear to directly alter cyclic AMP production, Na^+K^+-ATPase, or adenylate cyclase activity [44]. Histologic studies support these findings in that no permanent hair cell damage has been noted. However, strial edema and degeneration of the intermediate cells in the stria vascularis as well as marginal cell shrinkage and tight junction changes have been reported [39,45,46].

Aminoglycoside Antibiotics

Aminoglycosides, the most commonly prescribed ototoxic antibiotics, consist of an organic base linked to monosaccharides or disaccharides. They are prescribed for gram-negative infections and require intramuscular or intravenous administration (see Chapter 12). Occasionally, head and neck cancer patients have a history of aminoglycoside use.

Ototoxic Sites of Action

Animal experimentation (guinea pigs, chinchillas, rabbits, and rats) suggests that aminoglycosides reduce cochlear energy by (1) inhibiting basal hair cell succinic dehydrogenase activity [43], (2) decreasing stria vascularis ATPase activity [3], (3) competing with the glucose transport mechanism, and (4) interfering with glycolysis [30]. However, the attractive theory presented by Weiner and Schacht [47] suggests that aminoglycosides adhere to polyphosphoinositides. This is believed to alter membrane permeability and therefore serve as a precursor to detrimental alterations to carbohydrate metabolism and energy utilization.

Histologic studies indicate that the basal outer hair cells are more susceptible to aminoglycoside use. This susceptibility is attributed to their higher metabolism and, therefore, are the first to be affected by a reduction in energy supply.

Specific Aminoglycosides

Streptomycin

Streptomycin was the first aminoglycoside to be isolated and used to treat gram-negative infections. Although largely replaced by more effective agents, it is prescribed to treat tuberculosis. Associated with excessive dose levels, streptomycin is primarily vestibulotoxic. The symptoms and signs are unsteadiness, vertigo, decreased caloric response, spontaneous nystagmus, and ataxia [48]. For histopathologic changes, see Table 27-3 [48–55].

Kanamycin

Kanamycin is used for severe, life-threatening gram-negative infections. More cochleotoxic than vestibulotoxic, it is associated with tinnitus and sensorineural hearing loss. The latter is

Table 27-3. Aminoglycoside antibiotics

Antibiotic	*Histopathology*	*Electrophysiologic changes*	*Ototoxicity*	*Audiologic monitoring*
Gentamycin	OHCs damaged more than IHCs, especially basal region	CM decreases	Primarily vestibulotoxic	Baseline audiogram Follow-up evaluation
Kanamycin	Basal OHC damage; minimal IHC damage; occasional damage to vestibular type I hair; cell in ampulla cristae and striola in utricle	Minimal	More cochleotoxic; tinnitus; permanent and progressive SNHL; SNHL may be gradual or sudden in onset	Because symptoms may occur 3–4 months post treatment, baseline and serial audiograms every 3–6 months for 1 year
Streptomycin	Damage to type I and II cells in ampulla	Minimal	Primarily vestibulotoxic; little effect on hearing; toxic symptoms include unsteadiness, vertigo, spontaneous nystagmus, ataxia	Baseline audiogram
Tobramycin	Basal OHC loss; high dosage causes loss of IHCs, pillar cells, and supporting cells	Attenuation of CM, EP, and AP	Minimal	Baseline audiogram
Bleomycin	No morphologic changes	No functional changes	None	Rarely required
Vancomycin	No significant ototoxic effect	No significant change	Rare	Rarely required
Amikacin	OHC loss only when dosage level far exceeds the clinical amounts	No significant change	Infrequent	Rarely required

OHC = outer hair cell; IHC = inner hair cell; CM = cochlear microphonic; SNHL = sensorineural hearing loss; EP = endocochlear potential; AP = action potential.

either gradual or sudden in onset and usually is permanent with continued drug use [50]. Immediate drug termination with the appearance of ototoxic symptoms may prevent further hearing deterioration, if renal function is normal. However, hearing loss can occur 3 months or more after treatment. Therefore, a baseline audiogram should be obtained, if possible, with audiologic monitoring at 3- to 6-month intervals for a 1-year duration.

Gentamycin

Gentamycin is more toxic than either kanamycin or streptomycin. Most of its damage is to the vestibular mechanism. In some instances, cochleotoxicity occurs in isolation or in combination with vestibular dysfunction. The result usually is permanent. The risk factor increases as the total dosage exceeds 45 mg/kg or a history of previous or current ototoxic drug use exists.

Tobramycin
Although pharmacologically similar to gentamycin, tobramycin is less ototoxic. The toxicity is equally distributed between the vestibular and cochlear mechanisms. Minimal clinical evidence of ototoxicity occurs when renal function is normal [51].

Recommendations
Whenever aminoglycosides are used, maintain safe peak serum levels, monitor renal function, and assess cochlear and vestibular function before, during, and at the completion of parenteral drug treatment, whenever possible [38].

COMBINED USE OF OTOTOXIC DRUGS

When any of the ototoxic drugs (i.e., aminoglycosides, loop diuretics, cisplatin) are used synchronously or metachronously, the ototoxic effect is synergistic, even with nontoxic drug levels [55]. Although the mechanism underlying this effect is unknown, kinetic studies have concluded that loop diuretics, for example, may increase the cell membrane's permeability to aminoglycosides, thus increasing the endolymphatic aminoglycoside concentration. Because peak serum levels remain unchanged, this assay is invalid for monitoring ototoxic potential. Therefore, whenever possible, close audiologic monitoring is recommended.

REFERENCES

1. Lippe WR: Recent developments in cochlear physiology. *Ear Hear* 7(4) : 233, 1986.
2. Durrant JD, Lovrinic JH: *Bases of Hearing Science*. Baltimore: Williams & Wilkins, 1984.
3. Thalmann R: Biochemical Studies of the Auditory System. In Tower DB (ed): *The Nervous System: Human Communication and Its Disorders*. New York: Raven, 1975. Pp 31–44.
4. Smith CA: The Inner Ear: Its Embryological Development and Microstructure. In Tower DB (ed): *The Nervous System: Vol 3. Human Communication and Its Disorders*. New York: Raven, 1975. Pp 1–18.
5. Yost WA, Nielsen DW: *Fundamentals of Hearing: An Introduction*. New York: Holt, Rinehart, and Winston, 1985.
6. Tasaki I, Spyropoulos CS: Stria vascularis as source of endocochlear potential. *J Neurophysiol* 22 : 149, 1959.
7. Davis H: A model for the transducer action in the cochlea. *Cold Spring Harbor Symp Quant Biol* 30 : 181, 1965.
8. Nuttal AL: Transduction and Frequency Tuning in Hair Cells. In Miller JM (ed): *Semin Hear* 7(1) : 27, 1986.
9. Harrison JM: Functional Properties of the Auditory System of the Brain Stem. In Masterton RB (ed): *Handbook of Behavioral Neurobiology*. Plenum Press, NY: 1978. Vol 1, pp 421–423.
10. Jacobson JT, Hyde ML: An Introduction to Auditory Evoked Potentials. In Katz J (ed): *Handbook of Clinical Audiology*. Baltimore: Williams & Wilkins, 1985. Pp 496–533.
11. Harrison JM, Howe ME: Anatomy of the Afferent Auditory Nervous System of Mammals. In Keidel WD, Neff WD (eds): *Handbook of Sensory Physiology: Vol V/1. Anatomy Physiology (Ear)*. Berlin: Springer, 1974.
12. Keleman G: Radiation and Ear. *Acta Otolaryngol [Suppl]* (Stockh) 184 : 1, 1963.
13. Bohne BA, Marks JE, Glascow GP: Delayed effects of ionizing radiation on the ear. *Laryngoscope* 95 : 818, 1985.
14. Dias A: Effect on hearing of patients treated by irradiation in the head and neck area. *J Laryngol* 80 : 276, 1966.
15. Gamble JE, Peterson EA, Chandler JR: Radiation effects on the inner ear. *Arch Otolaryngol* 88 : 64, 1968.
16. Leach W: Irradiation of the ear. *Journal Laryngol Otol* 79 : 870, 1965.
17. Coplan J: Hearing loss after therapy with radiation. *Am J Dis Child* 135 : 1088, 1981.
18. Silverstein H, McDaniel AB, Norrell H: Hearing preservation after acoustic neuroma surgery using intraoperative direct eighth cranial nerve monitoring. *Am J Otol* (Suppl) : 99, 1985.
19. Tator CH, Nedzelski JM: Preservation of hearing in patients undergoing excision of acoustic neuromas and other cerebellopontine angle tumors. *J Neurosurg* 63 : 168, 1985.
20. Aguilar-Markulis NV, et al: Auditory toxicity effects of long-term cis-dichlorodiammineplatinum II therapy in genitourinary cancer patients. *J Surg Oncol* 16 : 111, 1981.
21. Schweitzer VG, et al: Ototoxic and nephrotoxic effects of combined treatment with cis-diamminedichloroplatinum and kanamycin in the guinea pig. *Otolaryngol Head Neck Surg* 92(1) : 38, 1984.
22. Estrem SA, et al: Cis-diamminedichloroplatinum (II) ototoxicity in the guinea pig. *Otolaryngol Head Neck Surg* 89 : 638, 1981.
23. Guthrie TH, Gynther L: Acute deafness. *Arch Otolaryngol* 111 : 344, 1985.

24. Strauss M, et al: Cis-platinum ototoxicity: Clinical experience and temporal bone histopathology. *Laryngoscope* 93 : 1554, 1985.
25. Hong WK: Induction chemotherapy in advanced squamous head and neck carcinoma with high-dose cisplatinum and bleomycin infusion. *Cancer* 44 : 19, 1979.
26. Fleming S, et al: Ototoxicity from cis-platinum in patients with stages III and IV previously untreated squamous cell cancer of the head and neck. *Am J Clin Oncol* 8 : 302, 1985.
27. Stadnicki AW, et al: Cis-dichlorodiammineplatinum (II) NSC-119875: Hearing loss and other toxic effects in rhesus monkeys. *Cancer Chemother Rep* 59(3) : 467, 1975.
28. Weaver A, et al: Cis-platinum and 5-fluorouracil as initial therapy in advanced epidermoid cancers of the head and neck. *Head Neck Surg* 4 : 370, 1982.
29. Schaefer SD, et al: Ototoxicity of low and moderate dose cisplatin. *Cancer* 56 : 1934, 1985.
30. Bhattacharyya TK, Dayal VS: Ototoxicity and noise-drug interaction. *J Otolaryngol* 13(6) : 361, 1984.
31. Nakai Y, et al: Ototoxicity of the anticancer drug cisplatin: An experimental study. *Acta Otolaryngol* 93 : 227, 1982.
32. Moroso MJ, Blair RL: A review of cis-platinum ototoxicity. *J Otolaryngol* 12(6) : 365, 1985.
33. Fausti S: Early detection of cisplatin ototoxicity. *Cancer* 53 : 224, 1984.
34. Reddel J: Ototoxicity in patients receiving cisplatin: Importance of dose and method of drug administration. *Cancer Treat Rep* 66 : 1923, 1982.
35. Horn K, et al: Early effects of ethacrynic acid on cochlear histochemistry. *Arch Otolaryngol* 104 : 42, 1978.
36. Brummett R, et al: The delayed effects of ethacrynic acid on the stria vascularis of the guinea pig. *Acta Otolaryngol* 83 : 98, 1977.
37. Prazma J, et al: Ototoxicity of the ethacrynic acid. *Arch Otolaryngol* 95 : 448, 1972.
38. Shulman JB: Ototoxicity. In Goodhill V (ed): *Ear: Diseases, Deafness & Dizziness*. Hagerstown, MD: Harper & Row, 1979.
39. Rybak LP: Furosemide ototoxicity clinical and experimental aspects. *Laryngoscope* 95 (Suppl. 38) : 1, 1985.
40. Thalmann R: Action of loop diuretics and mercurials upon the cochlea. *Acta Otolaryngol* (Stockh) 83 : 221, 1977.
41. Kusakari J, et al: Effect of ethacrynic acid, furosemide and ouabain upon the endolymphatic potential and upon energy phosphates of the stria vascularis. *Laryngoscope* 88 : 12, 1978.
42. Sewell WF: The relation between the endocochlear potential and spontaneous activity in the auditory nerve fibers in the cat. *J Physiol* 347 : 685, 1984.
43. Miller JJ: *Handbook of Ototoxicity*. Boca Raton, FL: CRC, 1985.
44. Marks SC, Schacht J: Effects of ototoxic diuretics on cochlear NA^+K^+-ATPase and adenylate cyclase. *Scand Audiol [Suppl]* 14 : 131, 1981.
45. Brown CG, et al: High dose furosemide in acute reversible intrinsic renal failure. *Scott Med J* (suppl 19) : 35, 1974.
46. Quick CA, Hoppe W: Permanent deafness associated with furosemide administration. *Ann Otol* 84 : 94, 1975.
47. Weiner ND, Schacht J: Biochemical Model of Aminoglycoside-Induced Hearing Loss. In Lerner SA, Matz GJ, Hawkins JE (eds): *Aminoglycoside Ototoxicity*. Boston: Little, Brown, 1981. Pp 113–121.
48. Nabol JB: Histopathology of Human Aminoglycoside Ototoxicity. In Lerner SA, Matz GJ, Hawkins JE (eds): *Aminoglycoside Ototoxicity*. Boston: Little, Brown, 1981. Pp 409–434.
49. Johnsson L, et al: Aminoglycoside-induced cochlear pathology in man. *Acta Otolaryngol [Suppl]* (Stockh) 383 : 1, 1981.
50. Schuknecht HF: *Pathology of the Ear*. Cambridge, MA: Harvard University Press, 1974.
51. Tablan OC, et al: Renal and auditory toxicity of high doses prolonged therapy with gentamicin and tobramycin in pseudomonas endocarditis. *J Infect Dis* 149(2) : 257, 1984.
52. Dal I, Edsmyr F, Stahle J: Bleomycin therapy and ototoxicity. *Acta Otolaryngol* 75 : 323, 1973.
53. Sorrell TC, Collignon PJ: A prospective study of adverse reactions associated with vancomycin therapy. *J Antimicrob Chemother* 16 : 235, 1985.
54. Kucer A: Vancomycin. *J Antimicrob Chemother* 14 : 364, 1984.
55. Komune S: Potentiating effects of cisplatin and ethacrynic acid in ototoxicity. *Arch Otolaryngol* 107 : 594, 1981.

28

Audiology: Hearing Assessment and Rehabilitation

KAREN L. BEVERLY-DUCKER and PATRICIA R. THOMPSON

KEY CONCEPTS

Audiologic Evaluation; Site-of-Lesion Testing; Aural Rehabilitation

MILESTONES

1855	Earliest U.S. Patent for Hearing Aid	Hyde
1906	Calorics	Barany
1920	Vacuum Tube Hearing Aid	Hanson
1923	Clinical Audiometer	
1942	Binaural Bithermal Caloric Test	Fitzgerald and Hallpike
1940s	Speech Audiometry	Harvard Psycho-Acoustics Lab
1959	Tympanometry	Terkildsen and Thomsen
1964	Hearing Aid Miniaturization	
1971	First Cochlear Implant House	
1977	Federal Drug Administration Hearing Aid Standards	
1978	American National Standards Institute (ANSI) Standards for Audiometry	

As presented in the previous chapter, hearing loss in head and neck cancer patients is secondary to either the disease process or therapy. Effective communication is crucial for comprehensive management (Figure 28-1). Therefore, audiology should be consulted for suspected or anticipated hearing loss during diagnostics, treatment, or rehabilitation.

TUNING FORKS

Initially, when audiologic services are not readily available, tuning forks can screen and evaluate hearing. Although simple to perform, they are subjective and insensitive to subtle hearing loss. Therefore, they are never a substitute for an audiologic evaluation.

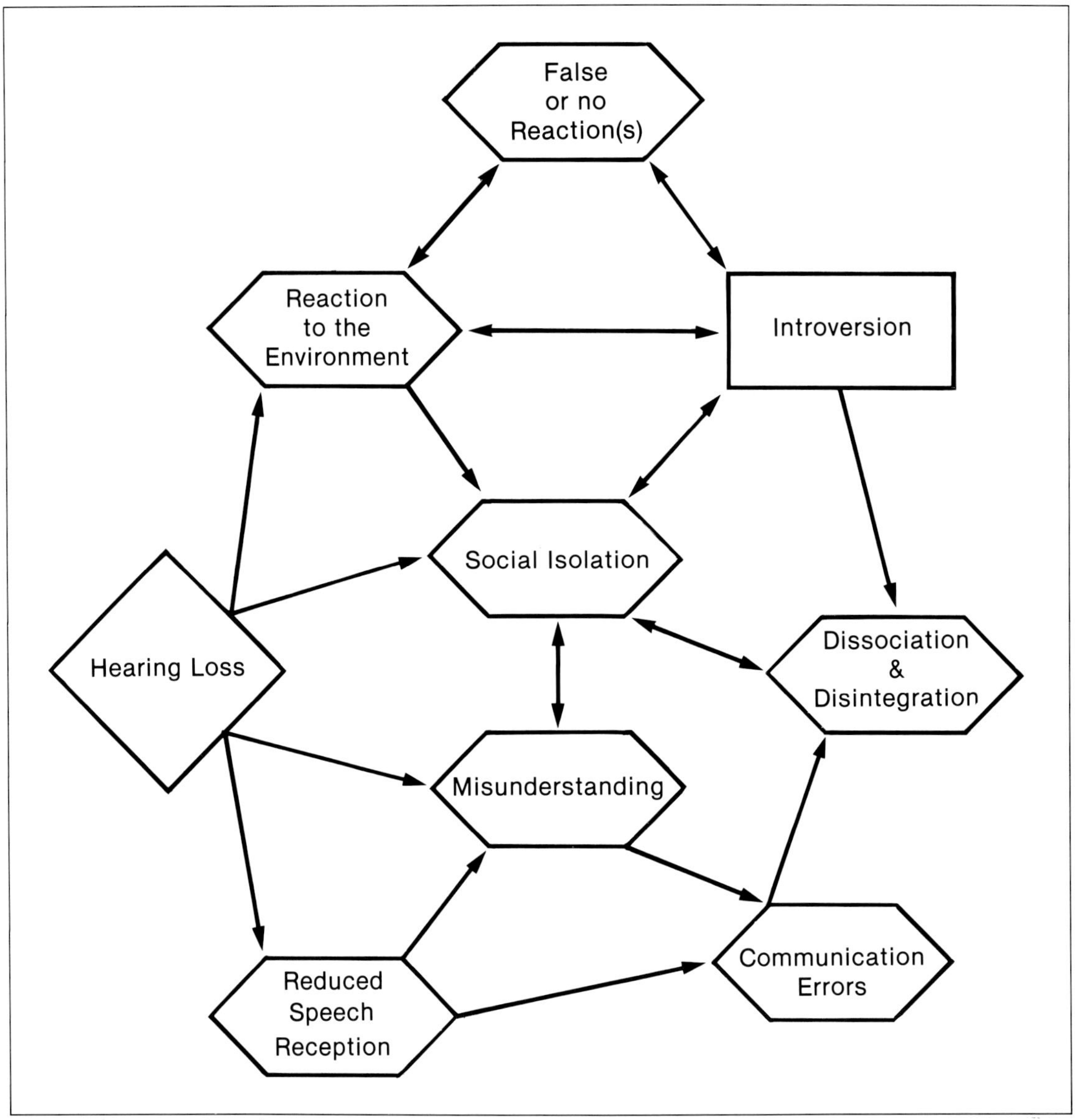

Figure 28-1. Deafness dynamics.

Rinne Test

The Rinne test differentiates between conductive and sensorineural hearing loss. The examiner places a vibrating 512-Hz tuning fork near the external auditory canal (air conduction [AC]). The patient indicates when the tone is no longer heard. The fork then is placed on the mastoid process (bone conduction [BC]).

1. Negative: the patient continues to hear the tone (BC > AC); this suggests conductive loss.
2. Positive: the patient no longer hears the tone (AC > BC); this suggests normal hearing or a sensorineural loss.
3. Limitations: does not detect a slight conductive loss or a unilateral sensorineural loss;

an erroneous conductive loss may be diagnosed.

Weber Test

The Weber test differentiates between conductive and sensorineural loss when the hearing loss is unilateral. After a vibrating 512-Hz tuning fork is placed on the forehead, the patient localizes where the sound is heard best (right, left, or center).

1. Negative: failure to lateralize suggests normal hearing or minimal ear difference.
2. Positive: lateralization toward the better ear suggests sensorineural loss; lateralization toward the poorer ear suggests conductive loss.
3. Limitations: useful only with a unilateral loss; must be correlated with the Rinne test.

Schwabach Test

The Schwabach test predicts the degree of sensorineural loss based on the hearing acuity of the examiner. A vibrating 512-Hz tuning fork is placed on the patient's mastoid process. When the tone is no longer heard, the examiner places the fork on his or her own mastoid bone and counts the number of seconds the tone is heard.

1. Negative: hearing is as good as the examiner's.
2. Positive: hearing is worse than the examiner's.
3. Limitations: examiner must have normal hearing; the exact amount of loss remains unknown; no differentiation between conductive and sensorineural; fails to detect unilateral hearing loss.

BASIC AUDIOMETRY

A thorough audiologic evaluation includes the history, otoscopy, and basic audiometry.

History

The past medical and neuro-otologic history is reviewed with emphasis on ear disease, previous ear surgery, tinnitus, noise exposure, preexisting hearing loss, head trauma, and ototoxic drugs (see Chapter 2).

Otoscopy

Otoscopy, performed before the audiologic evaluation, examines the outer and middle ear (see Chapter 2). When impacted cerumen, infection, foreign bodies, or fluid is present, an otology consultation is obtained.

Pure Tone Audiometry

Conventional pure tone audiometry, consisting of air and bone conduction testing, determines hearing thresholds between 125 Hz and 8000 Hz. The results are charted on an audiogram. Audiometric interpretation indicates the degree and type of hearing loss (Tables 28-1 and 28-2; Figure 28-2).

Speech Audiometry

Speech audiometry quantifies the ability to receive and understand speech. Two test measures are obtained: the speech reception threshold (SRT) and the word recognition score. The former indicates the decibel (dB) level that spondaic words (Table 28-3) are identified correctly 50 percent of the time. When the SRT is greater than 20 dBHL, a significant hearing loss exists. Often word recognition is measured using a phonetically balanced monosyllabic word list (Table 28-4). The percent correct (0–100%) indicates how well speech is understood when it is sufficiently loud. It also serves as a prognostic indicator for aural rehabilitation. For example, if the score falls between 70 and 100

Table 28-1. Degree of hearing loss derived from audiometric findings

Degree of hearing loss	*Air condition thresholds (dBHL)**
Normal	0–15
Slight	16–25
Mild	26–40
Moderate	41–55
Moderately severe	56–70
Severe	71–90
Profound	>90

*Air conduction thresholds determine the degree of hearing loss.

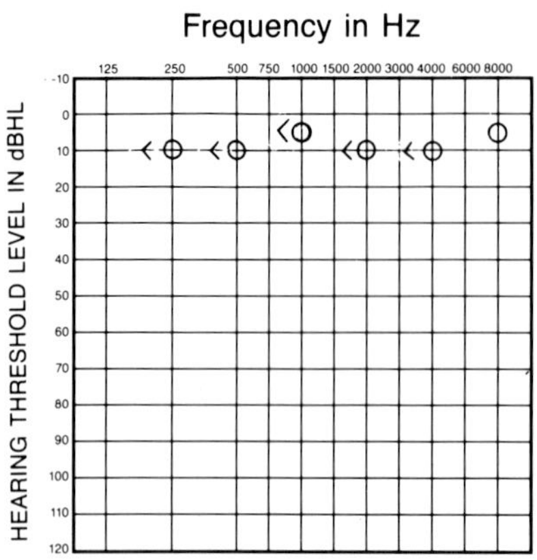

AD: Normal hearing

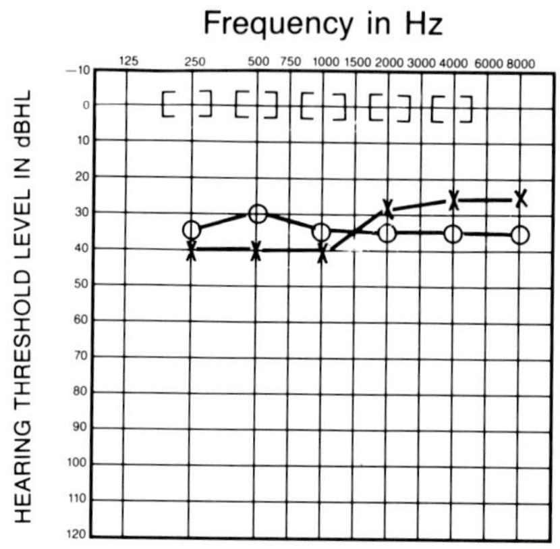

A mild conductive hearing loss bilaterally

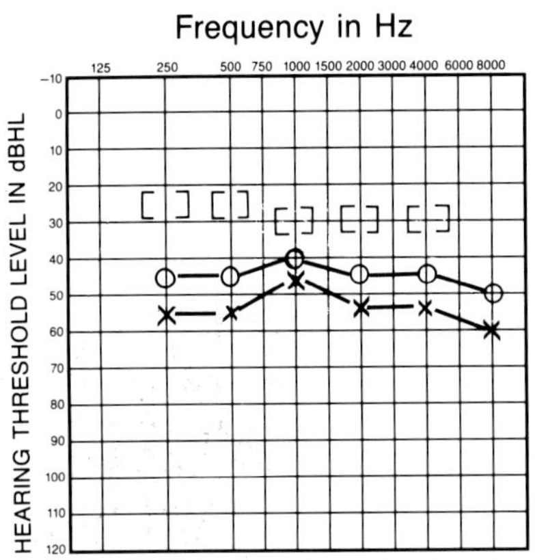

A moderate mixed hearing loss bilaterally

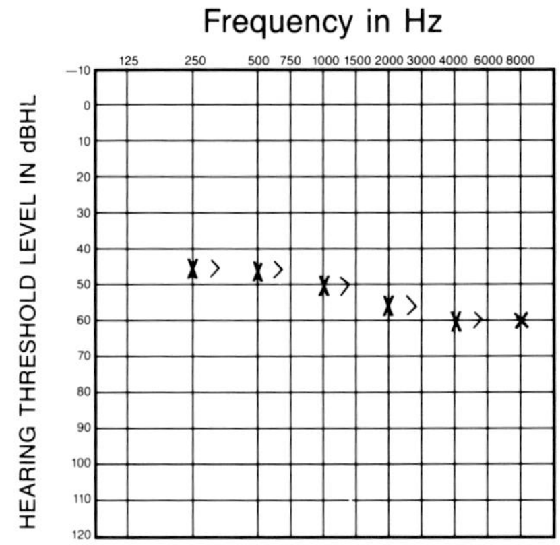

AS: A moderate sensorineural loss

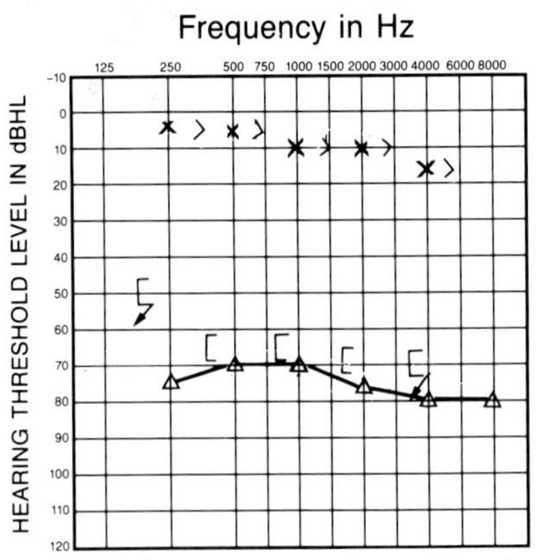

AD: A severe sensorineural hearing loss
AS: Hearing is within normal limits

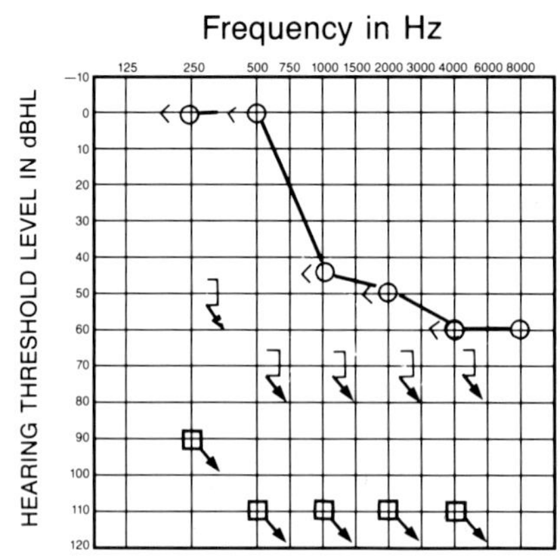

AD: Normal hearing at 250 Hz-500 Hz with a moderate sensori-neural loss at 1k-8k Hz

AS: A profound sensorineural loss

A

Table 28-2. Hearing loss and lesion site

Type of hearing loss	*Lesion site*	*AC/BC relationship*
Conductive	Outer and/or middle ear	BC score ≤ 15 dBHL AC score > 15 dBHL AC/BC gap > 10 dBHL
Sensorineural	Inner ear and/or auditory pathway	AC = BC AC score > 15 dBHL AC score > 15 dBHL
Mixed	Outer and/or middle ear **and** inner ear and/or auditory pathway	BC score > 15 dBHL AC score > 15 dBHL AC/BC gap > 10 dBHL

*By comparing air conduction (AC) and bone conduction (BC) thresholds at a given frequency, the type of hearing loss and lesion site are determined.

Table 28-3. Spondee CID W-1 word list*

hothouse	hotdog
armchair	farewell
inkwell	playground
headlight	eardrum
grandson	sidewalk
northwest	woodwork
schoolboy	doormat
hardware	stairway
greyhound	workshop
pancake	toothbrush
daybreak	railroad
mushroom	padlock
airplane	iceberg
cowboy	oatmeal
drawbridge	baseball
duckpond	birthday
sunset	mousetrap
horseshoe	whitewash

*Spondaic words are two-syllable words where equal stress is placed on each syllable. These words are used to establish the patient's speech reception threshold or spondee threshold.

Table 28-4. Word recognition tests*

CID W-22 List 1A		*NU Auditory Test #6 List 1A*	
an	you	laud	love
yard	as	boat	sure
carve	wet	pool	knock
us	chew	nag	choice
day	see	limb	hash
toe	deaf	shout	lot
felt	them	sub	raid
stove	give	vine	hurl
hunt	true	dime	moon
ran	isle	goose	page
knees	or	whip	yes
not	law	tough	reach
mew	me	puff	king
low	none	keen	home
owl	jam	death	rag
it	poor	sell	which
she	him	take	week
high	skin	fall	size
there	east	raise	mode
earn	thing	third	bean
twins	dad	gap	tip
could	up	fat	chalk
what	bells	met	jail
bathe	wire	jar	burn
ace	ache	door	kite

*Each 50-word list has been designed to contain familiar words and encompass all of the sounds found in spoken English with the same frequency of occurrence.

AUDIOGRAM KEY

	UNMASKED		MASKED		EX. OF NR
	AC	BC	AC	BC	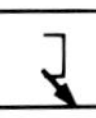
AD	O	<	Δ	[	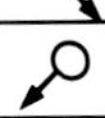
AS	X	>	□	]	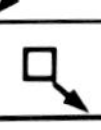

B

Figure 28-2. A. Audiometric profiles. *AD* = right ear; *AS* = left ear; *AC* = air conduction; *BC* = bone conduction. B. NR means no response at the output limits of the audiometer. The output limits in dBHL is less for bone conduction than air conduction. (See diagram on bottom row, right column, p. 492.)

High-Level Short-Increment Sensitivity Index

The high-level short-increment sensitivity index (SISI) measures the perception of subtle increases in intensity at a high stimulus level. A continuous 75-dBHL pure tone is presented and periodically a 1-dB increment is superimposed on the steady-state tone. The patient indicates each time the 1-dB increment is perceived. Ten trials are administered. Patients with normal hearing or cochlear hearing loss can detect the intensity change with 70- to 100-percent accuracy. Patients with retrocochlear pathology generally perform poorly (0–20%) [5].

Central Auditory Test Battery

The auditory nerve enters the brain stem at the level of the pontomedullary junction and synapses on cell bodies in the cochlear nucleus. Cochlear nucleus afferents travel predominately contralaterally but also ipsilaterally en route to higher auditory centers. Because the central auditory nervous system is highly redundant, patients with high brain stem or cortical lesions have normal findings on routine audiometry (i.e., pure tone and speech audiometry). Therefore, more sophisticated tests are needed.

Auditory tasks using speech stimuli may detect central auditory nervous system dysfunction if the stimuli are degraded so that the number of speech cues available (i.e., sound length, syntax, semantics) are reduced. Filtered speech, binaural fusion, synthetic sentences with a competing message and other types of stimuli are used for this purpose (see Glossary). The results generally are scored as a percentage, with performance deficits being site dependent. For example, patients with cortical lesions involving the temporal lobe frequently exhibit contralateral ear deficits on certain types of central auditory nervous system tests, while patients with low brain stem disorders, such as extra-axial tumors involving the cochlear nucleus or eighth cranial nerve, display an ipsilateral ear effect on other tests in the battery. Intra-axial brain stem lesions, however, typically exhibit either a bilateral performance deficit or a contralateral ear effect. In normals, no deficit is noted. Therefore, a performance deficit exhibited by a central auditory test battery is a soft sign that must be confirmed by other diagnostics.

Brain Stem Auditory Evoked Response Audiometry

The brain stem auditory evoked response (BAER) test determines auditory nerve and low brain stem integrity. The BAER is generated by clicks or brief pure tones. Surface electrodes, strategically placed on the scalp and earlobes, along with a computer-linked auditory evoked response system, respectively detect and record the response. A typical BAER readout is shown in Figure 28-4. With loud stimulation, the wave I latency approximates 1.5 msec. Each subsequent wave, identified by Roman numerals, generally occurs at 1-msec intervals [6]. Because there are no uniform standards, each clinical laboratory establishes its own normative data for test interpretation. When hearing is normal, absolute and interwave latencies exceeding the established norms by more than 2 standard deviations implicate possible retrocochlear pathology [7]. BAER is the most sensitive and diagnostic of all the special audiometric tests.

Electronystagmography

Anatomic and Functional Considerations

The vestibular system consists of three orthogonally arranged semicircular canals and the otolith organs known as the utricle and saccule. The otolith organs respond to linear acceleration, while the semicircular canals are sensitive to angular acceleration of the head. Like the cochlea, the membranous vestibular labyrinth is filled with endolymph. Also contained within the ampullated end of the semicircular canals and the otolith organs are the vestibular receptor (hair) cells. These cells differ from cochlear hair cells in that each cell has two types of cilia, a large kinocilium and several smaller stereocilia. Sensory input from these receptor cells is relayed to the vestibular branch of the eighth cranial nerve and then is transmitted primarily to the four (superior, inferior, medial, and lateral) vestibular nuclei. Here second-order neurons project to the cerebellum, the spinal cord,

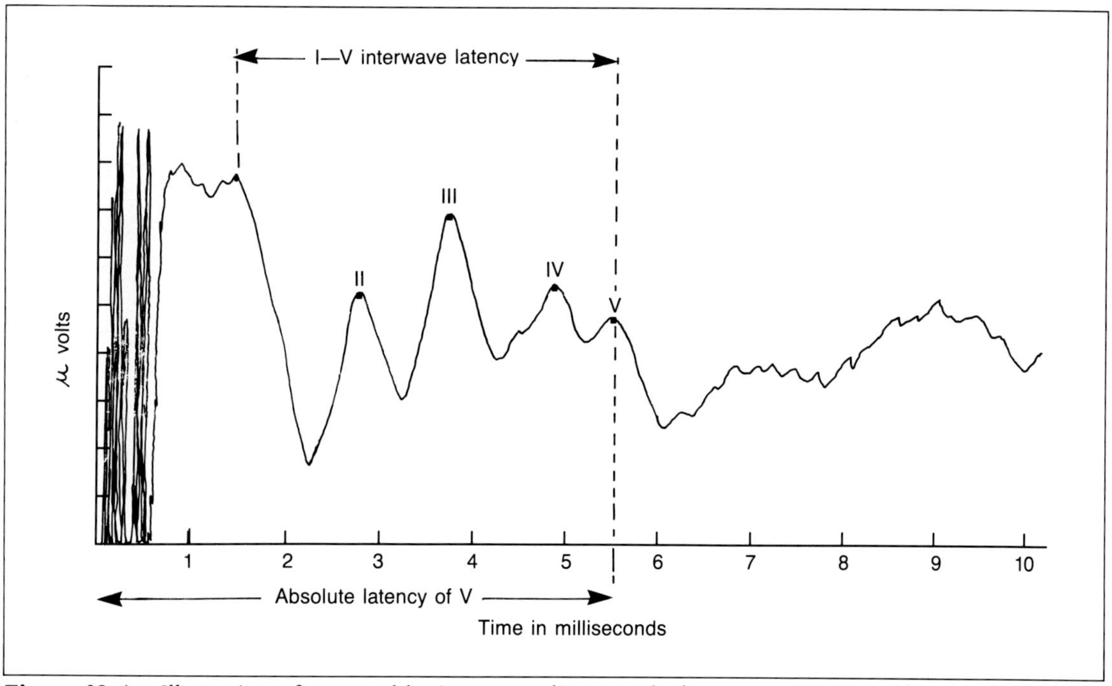

Figure 28-4. Illustration of a normal brain stem auditory evoked response (BAER). The measurement of the absolute wave V latency and the I–V interwave latency also is displayed.

the reticular nuclei, and cranial nerves III, IV, and VI through the ascending medial longitudinal fasciculus (MLF). The MLF, because of the significant role it plays in conjugate eye movement, is fundamentally important to electronystagmography.

Hair Cell Polarization During Angular Acceleration

Under static conditions (i.e., inactivity or cessation of acceleration), the hair cells in the vestibular system generate a basal or resting discharge. During angular acceleration, the cilia are displaced. If the cilia are displaced toward the kinocilium, the cell is depolarized; movement away from the kinocilium hyperpolarizes the cell. These responses are relayed to the extrinsic eye muscles through a three-neuron pathway called the vestibulo-ocular reflex arc. A summary of this pathway and the resulting compensatory eye movement is presented in Figure 28-5 [8].

Nystagmus

Prolonged angular rotation, caloric stimulation, or a unilateral vestibular lesion can elicit a rapid to-and-fro involuntary vestibular nystagmus. It consists of a slow (compensatory) and fast (reflexive) phase. The direction of the fast component indicates whether the nystagmus is right or left beating. The slow component determines the degree of compensatory eye movement that results from vestibular stimulation. Nystagmus also can be induced through visual stimulation.

Examination of Vestibular Function

Patients who are referred for an electronystagmogram (ENG) typically present with one or more of the following: vertigo, dizziness, nystagmus, nausea, vomiting, and ataxia. In some cases, auditory symptoms also are present (i.e., hearing loss, tinnitus, ear fullness). Peripheral nystagmus often is suppressed by visual fixation, thus making documentation difficult. Hence, the ENG is a valuable diagnostic modal-

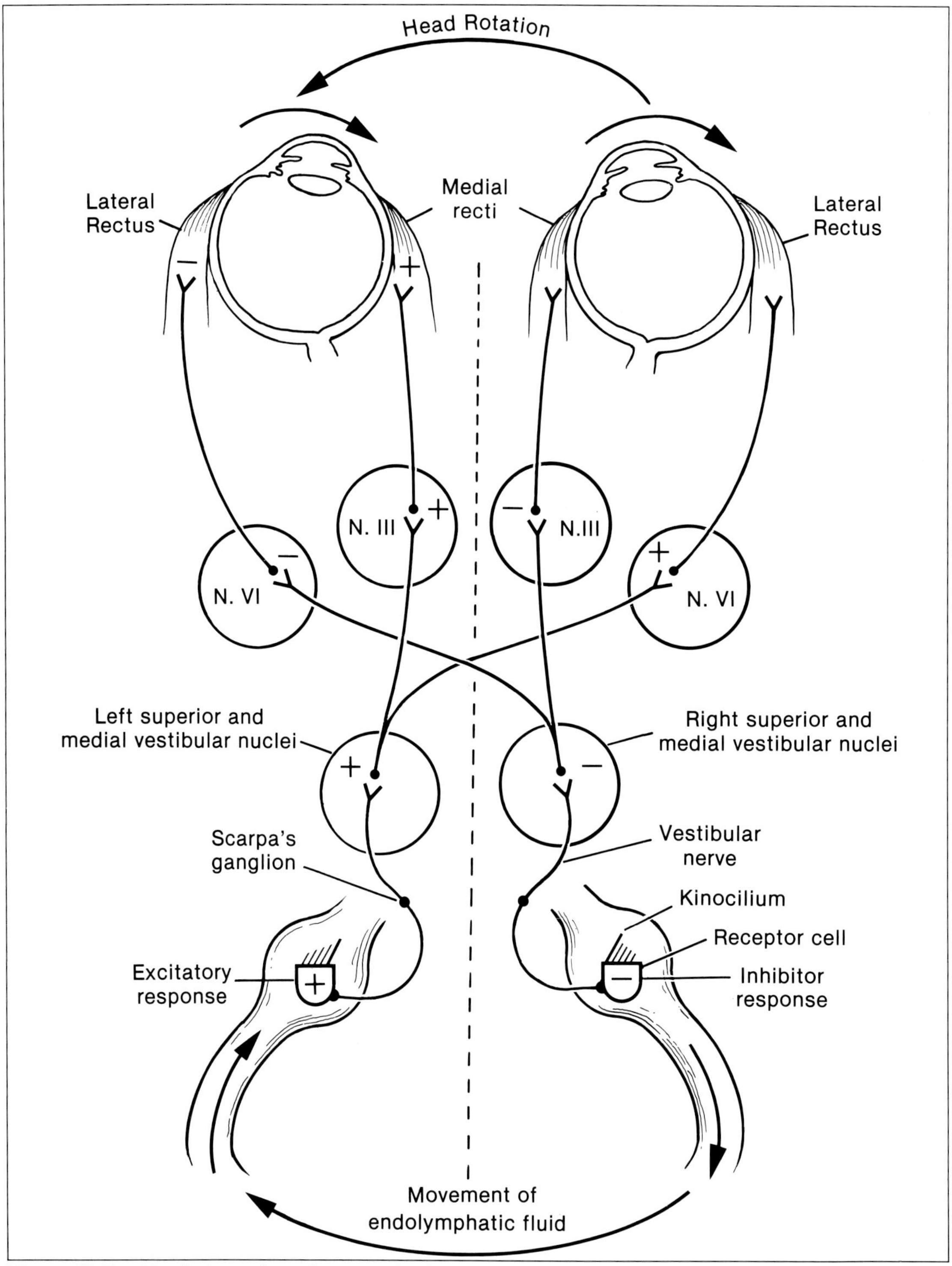

Figure 28-5. Vestibulo-ocular reflex arc. The functional axis of the cilia in the paired horizontal semicircular canals is directed toward the utricle. When the head rotates to the left, the relative movement of the endolymphatic fluid is toward the right, generating an excitatory response on the left and an inhibitory response on the right. This, in turn, generates compensatory conjugate eye movement to the right so that visual orientation is maintained during head movement. (Adapted from Kelly JP: Vestibular System. In Kandel EK and Schwartz JH (ed): *Principles of Neural Science*. New York: Elsevier, 1981. p 416.)

ity because it not only records nystagmus during eye closure but also documents its intensity under different test conditions. Overall, ENG findings help determine if vestibular function is impaired or if central nervous system (CNS) indicators are present (i.e., vertical nystagmus, disconjugate eye movement). A brief summary of the ENG test battery follows, and its interpretation is presented in Table 28-5.

Eye Movements

To record horizontal and vertical eye movement, electrodes are placed bitemporally, on the forehead, and above and below one eye. As the eyes move, the electrodes detect changes in the polarity of the corneoretinal potential. A two-channel ENG recorder amplifies and records these changes on a strip chart. One channel monitors horizontal eye movement; upward needle deflections reflect movement toward the right and downward deflections represent movement toward the left. Vertical eye movements are recorded on the other channel. The equipment is calibrated so that 1 mm of needle deflection represents 1 degree of eye movement. This allows the examiner to calculate the degrees of eye movement when nystagmus is observed.

Visual Stimulation

The saccade, pursuit, and optokinetic tests evaluate the integrity of the saccadic and pursuit control system. To generate saccadic eye movement, the patient is requested to look alternately at two points spaced 20 degrees apart. The pursuit control system is assessed by having the patient track a slow-moving target. To perform the optokinetic test, a drum with black and white vertical strips is rotated in front of the patient. The patient is requested to watch the strips as they pass by. This should elicit visually induced nystagmus beats. Abnormal findings on any of these tests are indicative of a central lesion (Table 28-5).

Table 28-5. Electronystagmogram interpretation

Test	*Purpose*	*Abnormality*	*Lesion site*
Saccade (calibration)	Evaluates saccadic control system	Ocular dysmetria	CNS
Pursuit (tracking)	Evaluates pursuit control system	Saccadic, disorganized, or disconjugate pursuit	CNS
Optokinetic	Evaluates symmetry of visually produced right & left beating nystagmus	Asymmetry or poorly formed nystagmus	CNS
Gaze test	Records nystagmus, if present, in different eye positions (EO, EC)	Direction-fixed horizontal nystagmus (EC)	Peripheral
Position test	Records nystagmus, if present, in different head positions (EO, EC)	Nystagmus (EO)	CNS
		Direction-fixed nystagmus (EC)	Peripheral or normal
Hallpike maneuver	Records nystagmus, if present, following a rapid change in body and head position	Benign paroxysmal nystagmus	Peripheral
Calorics	Evaluates vestibular function	Symmetric caloric response	Normal
		Unilateral weakness	Peripheral
		Directional preponderance	Peripheral or normal
		Bilateral weakness	Peripheral or CNS
		Lack of fixation suppression	CNS

EO = eyes open; EC = eyes closed.

Gaze Test
Eye movements are recorded as the patient gazes toward the center for 20 seconds, first with the eyes open, then with the eyes closed. The procedure is repeated with the eyes deviated right 20 degrees, then left 20 degrees (Table 28-5).

Positional Test
The patient is placed in different positions: erect, supine, right lateral, left lateral, and supine with the head and neck extended dorsally. In each position, eye movements are recorded for 20 seconds with eyes open, then with eyes closed (Table 28-5).

Dix-Hallpike Maneuver
The patient is moved rapidly from a sitting position to a supine, head-hanging right position. The eyes remain open and are observed for nystagmus. After returning to an erect position, the procedure is repeated with the head hanging left. When the patient experiences vertigo and delayed, rotatory, fatigable nystagmus, the results are consistent with benign paroxysmal nystagmus (peripheral etiology). Nystagmus that is immediate in onset, nonfatigable, and associated with little or no vertigo implicates a central etiology.

Caloric Test
The Fitzgerald-Hallpike binaural bithermal caloric test is used to evaluate vestibular function. The patient is placed in a supine position with the head elevated 30 degrees. In turn, each ear is irrigated for 40 seconds, first with warm (44°C) water, followed later with cool (30°C) water. Eye movements with eyes closed are recorded during and immediately after each irrigation. Warm irrigations induce horizontal nystagmus that beats toward the stimulated side. Nystagmus beating toward the opposite ear occurs with cool irrigations. The response should be suppressed during visual fixation.

Calorics are evaluated for unilateral weakness and directional preponderance. For each irrigation, three beats from the most intense 10-second period are used to calculate the degrees of eye movement (Table 28-6). An ENG report exhibiting left unilateral weakness is displayed in Figure 28-6.

Table 28-6. Electronystagmography: formulas for calculating unilateral weakness and directional preponderance

Unilateral Weakness

Right ear	Left ear
$\frac{RW + RC}{TR} = \quad \%$	$\frac{LW + LC}{TR} = \quad \%$

Note: Unilateral weakness is present when the difference between ears exceeds 25%.

Directional Preponderance

Right beating	Left beating
$\frac{RW + LC}{TR} = \quad \%$	$\frac{LW + RC}{TR} = \quad \%$

Note: Directional preponderance is present when the difference exceeds 29%.

RW = right warm; RC = right cold; LW = left warm; LC = left cold; TR = total response, where TR = RW + RC + LW + LC.

AURAL REHABILITATION

Psychologically, hearing impairment can be devastating. Its impact depends on the degree and type of hearing loss, the involvement of one or both ears, age, and presentation (i.e., sudden or insidious onset), as well as social and vocational considerations. Among head and neck cancer patients, the incidence of hearing loss is relatively low. Generally, afflicted patients exhibit mild to moderate hearing losses. When the loss is irreparable, rehabilitation (counseling, amplification, and therapy) is considered.

During counseling, the audiologic findings are reviewed. The patient also is presented with the advantages and disadvantages of amplification. Included in this discussion are the types of aids available (i.e., body, behind-the-ear, in-the-ear, canal; their adaptability to adverse listening conditions, and the benefit of visual supplementation, that is speech reading). If the patient exhibits a genuine interest in amplification, a hearing aid evaluation is scheduled. This procedure identifies the most suitable hearing aid for each patient. At times, the recommended aid does not meet the patient's approval due to either an undesirable sound quality or an "unflattering" appearance. To ensure consistent use, patient preference is considered, but if possible, it should not supersede optimal performance.

When a patient has limited cochlear reserve, word recognition ability is poor. In this situation, a hearing aid usually enhances sound awareness without significantly improving speech intelligibility. To maximize communication, an appropriate aural rehabilitation program is recommended. Aural rehabilitation includes one or more of the following: patient/family counseling, speech reading, auditory training, speech therapy, and, if needed, an assistive listening device evaluation.

Patient and Family Counseling

Counseling and patient education is an integral part of any rehabilitation program. Hearing loss, its impact on communication, and compensatory measures are reviewed extensively. In addition, the patient is counseled regarding hearing aid use and maintenance. To facilitate the adjustment process, realistic goals are reviewed. Two to four counseling sessions are sufficient for most patients. Some require a structured rehabilitation program involving several other rehabilitation components.

Speech Reading

Because only 40 percent of all English speech sounds are visibly different, speech-reading lessons are more than just lipreading. Instead, patients must be trained to take advantage of many different visual cues such as gestures, facial expressions, and articulatory movements. Patients also are taught to analyze messages by utilizing syntax (word order), phonemic, and contextual cues [10].

Auditory Training

Auditory training attempts to maximize residual hearing by improving the patient's recognition of individual speech sounds in quiet and under adverse listening conditions. However, when word recognition is poor, the primary focus is placed on the extraction of meaningful cues from the prosodic features of speech (i.e., rhythm, voice duration, inflection, stress). Also, if a patient has difficulty adjusting to amplified sound, developing a tolerance for loud sound becomes the initial therapy goal.

Speech Therapy

When a severe to profound hearing loss exists, patients often lose the ability to monitor their own voice. This can result in deviant speech patterns, including loud voice, altered intonation patterns, and articulation errors. To minimize the impact hearing loss has on speech production, patients are trained to monitor their speech with kinesthetic, tactile, and auditory cues.

Assistive Listening Devices

Some patients, although amplified, misinterpret speech under certain conditions (at church, over the telephone, listening to radio or TV). In such cases, a number of assistive listening devices are available such as telephone amplifiers, telephone systems for the deaf, direct audio inputs to televisions and radios, and induction loop or frequency modulated (FM) systems for lecture halls and churches (Figure 28-7). Those devices that suit the patient's need and budget are considered.

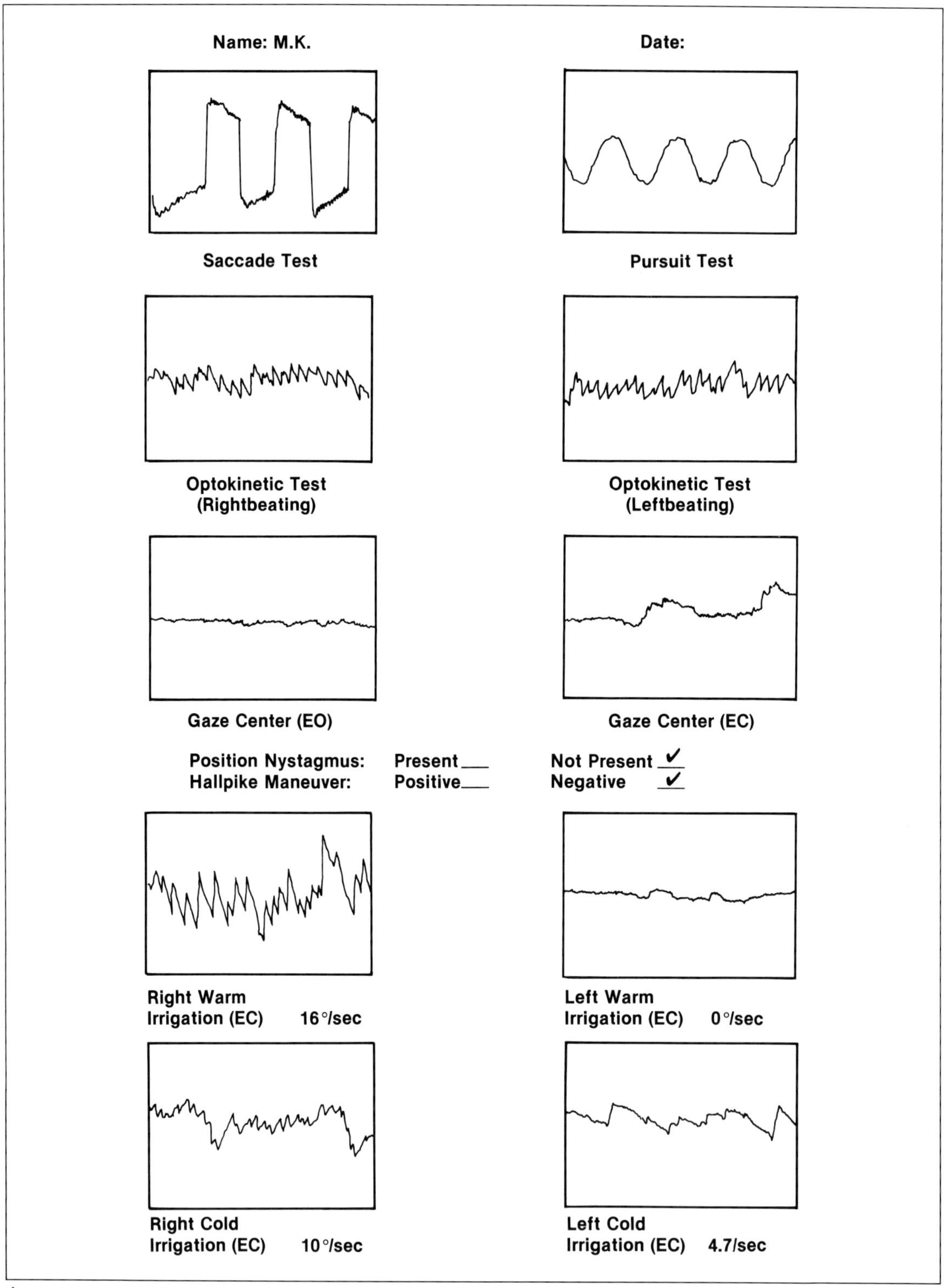
Name: M.K.
Date:
Saccade Test
Pursuit Test
Optokinetic Test (Rightbeating)
Optokinetic Test (Leftbeating)
Gaze Center (EO)
Gaze Center (EC)
Position Nystagmus: Present ___ Not Present ✔
Hallpike Maneuver: Positive ___ Negative ✔
Right Warm Irrigation (EC) 16°/sec
Left Warm Irrigation (EC) 0°/sec
Right Cold Irrigation (EC) 10°/sec
Left Cold Irrigation (EC) 4.7/sec

A

Unilateral Weakness

Right ear	Left ear
$\frac{16°/\text{sec} + 10°/\text{sec}}{30.7} = 85\%$	$\frac{16°/\text{sec} + 4.7°/\text{sec}}{30.7} = 15\%$

Directional Preponderance

Rightbeating	Leftbeating
$\frac{16°/\text{sec} + 4.7°/\text{sec}}{30.7} = 67\%$	$\frac{0°/\text{sec} + 10°/\text{sec}}{30.7} = 33\%$

Comments: Unilateral weakness is present on the left with a directional preponderance to the right.

B

Figure 28-6. ENG report.

Figure 28-7. Telecommunication device for the deaf (TDD). A. Without telephone. B. With telephone.

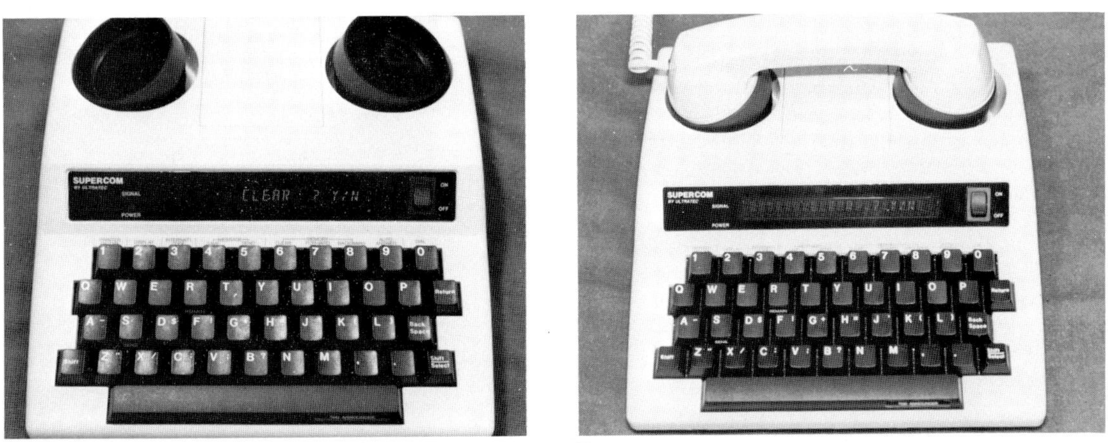

A B

CASE STUDIES

CASE 1

A 27-year-old woman complained of severe episodic vertigo, tinnitus, and decreased unilateral hearing loss (left) spanning several years.

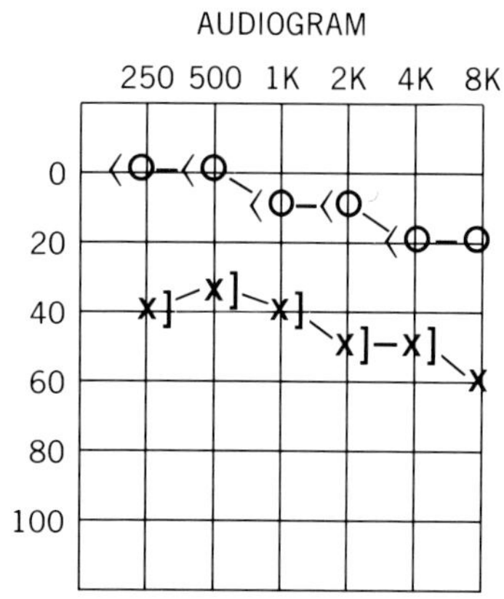

	Right	Left
Tympanogram type	A	A
Stapedial reflexes		
Ipsilateral	Present	Present
Contralateral	Present	Present
Intensity level	90 dBHL	90 dBHL
SRT	15 dBHL	35 dBHL
Word recognition		
@ 40 dBSL	100%	100%
@ 90 dBHL	100%	100%
High-level SISI	100%	100%
Tone decay	Negative	Negative
STAT		

Audiologic Findings

Pure tone and speech audiometry revealed essentially normal hearing on the right. Immittance testing exhibited a normal tympanogram with reflexes present at normal sensation levels. The left ear displayed a mild to moderate sensorineural hearing loss with an excellent word recognition score at 40 dBSL and 90 dBHL. That ear also exhibited a normal tympanogram. However, the stapedial reflex thresholds were obtained at reduced sensation levels, which is indicative of recruitment (a cochlear sign). No tone decay was observed, and the high-level SISI was positive. Overall, the audiologic findings were consistent with cochlear pathology.

Electronystagmography

The following findings were indicative of a peripheral lesion.

Gaze test: Right beating nystagmus
Saccade test: Normal
Pursuit test: Normal
Optokinetic: Well-formed and symmetric nystagmus
Hallpike: Negative
Positional test: Right beating nystagmus
Caloric irrigation:

RW = 16.7 degrees/second
RC = 10.7 degrees/second

LW = 0 degrees/second
LC = 4.7 degrees/second

Unilateral weakness:

$$\frac{RW + RC}{TR} = 85\% \qquad \frac{LW + LC}{TR} = 15\%$$

Difference exceeds 25 percent; indicates left unilateral weakness

Directional preponderance:

Right beating $\frac{RW + LC}{TR} = 66\%$ Left beating $\frac{LW + RC}{TR} = 34\%$

Difference exceeds 29 percent; indicates right directional preponderance

Interpretation

Based on the history, audiologic, and ENG profile, the results possibly are indicative of endolymphatic hydrops. A medical workup was negative for lues, thyroid disease, and diabetes mellitus. Although the findings are consistent with Ménière's disease, this diagnosis is made only after careful sequential observation over months or years. An in-the-ear hearing aid fitted to the left ear was recommended. Because of the excellent word recognition ability, amplification resulted in acceptable rehabilitation.

CASE 2

A 59-year-old man, having a bilateral occupational sensorineural hearing loss, presented with a painless swelling on the palate. Otoscopy was unremarkable. Physical examination of the oral cavity and oropharynx revealed a 4- × 4-cm submucosal lesion at the junction of the hard and soft palate and poor dental hygiene. Biopsy demonstrated a low-grade adenocarcinoma.

Computed Tomography (CT) Scan

Confirmed the previously mentioned lesion; no nasopharyngeal or maxillary sinus invasion was noted. One-third of the posterior hard palate demonstrated frank bony invasion.

Plan

1. Full mouth extractions and alveoloplasty.
2. Subtotal palatectomy and maxillectomy.
3. Palatal prosthesis.

Clinical Course

1. Patient refused surgery for 5 months after the initial evaluation.

2. Reexamination indicated no further progression of tumor.
3. Five months after the initial diagnosis, a left partial maxillectomy and partial palatectomy were performed.
4. Two months after surgery, an intractable left serous otitis media developed (see audiogram). Relief required myringotomy and tube insertion.

Pre- and Postoperative Audiologic Evaluation

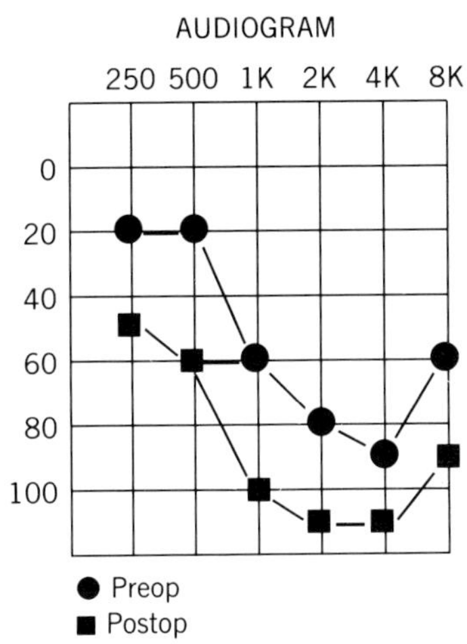

	Preop	Postop
Tympanogram type	A	B
Stapedial reflexes	Absent	Absent
SAT	20 dBHL	50 dBHL
Word recognition	68% @ 90 dBHL	68% @ 100 dBHL

Comments
Preoperatively, the patient had a bilateral, severe, high-frequency sensorineural hearing loss that required a hearing aid. Postoperatively, due to eustachian tube dysfunction secondary to the palatectomy, he developed an intractable serous otitis media. This conductive component superimposed on the sensorineural hearing loss greatly compromised auditory function. During this time, the patient complained of unsatisfactory amplification while aided. Minor surgery, myringotomy, and tube insertion returned hearing function to preoperative levels. A hearing aid was recommended.

CASE 3

A 47-year-old woman had a lifelong history of profound right ear hearing loss. The CT scan revealed a soft-tissue mass in the petrous apex consistent with a primary cholesteatoma (Figure 28-8). The patient was referred for an audiologic evaluation, ENG, and BAER testing.

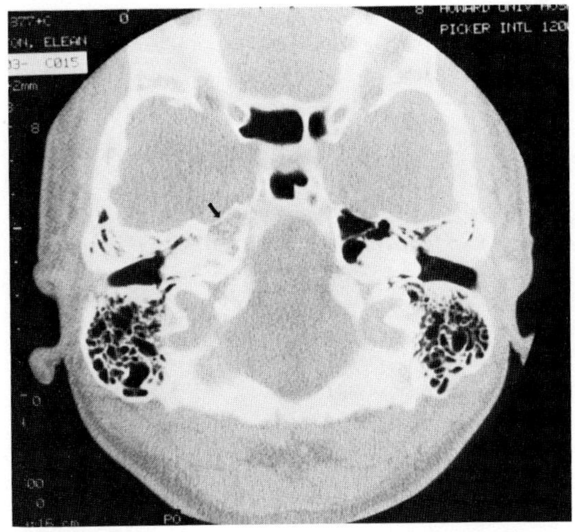

Figure 28-8. Right petrous apex epidermoid cyst (*arrow*).

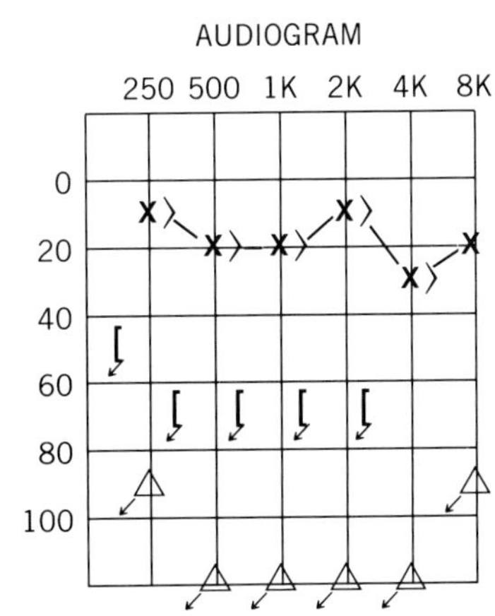

	Right	Left
Tympanogram type	A	A
Stapedial reflexes		
Ipsilateral	Absent	Present
Contralateral	Absent	Present
SRT	No response	5 dBHL
Word recognition		
@ 40 dBSL	Could not establish	100%
@ 90 dBHL	—	100%
BAER	Could not test	Normal
I	—	1.56 msec
III	—	3.84 msec
V	—	5.88 msec
I–V	—	4.32 msec

When a profound hearing loss is present, BAER cannot differentiate between a cochlear and retrocochlear lesion.

Electronystagmography

Gaze test: Right beating nystagmus
Saccade test: Normal
Pursuit test: Normal
Optokinetic: Well-formed and symmetric nystagmus
Hallpike: Negative
Positional test: Right beating nystagmus
Caloric irrigation:

RW = 11.7 degrees/second
RC = 4.7 degrees/second

LW = 19.7 degrees/second
LC = 27.0 degrees/second

Unilateral weakness:

$$\frac{RW + RC}{TR} = 25\% \qquad \frac{LW + LC}{TR} = 75\%$$

Difference exceeds 25 percent; indicates right unilateral weakness

Directional preponderance:

Right beating $\frac{RW + LC}{TR} = 61\%$ Left beating $\frac{LW + RC}{TR} = 39\%$

Difference less than 29 percent; no significant directional preponderance

Interpretation

Pure tone and speech audiometry revealed a slight hearing loss on the left and no measurable hearing on the right. The absent right stapedial reflexes and BAER are nondiagnostic due to the severity of the hearing loss. However, the ENG findings indicate that some degree of vestibular function is present on the affected side.

Clinical Course

Translabyrinthine petrosectomy was proposed. After a discussion of the risks and possible complications, the patient refused surgery. For now, she is being followed closely by her neurologist; sequential ENGs were recommended to assess residual eighth nerve function (vestibular).

CASE 4

A 28-year-old woman's chief complaint was a subtle right-sided hearing loss. The audiologic profile was as follows:

	Right	Left
Tympanogram type	A	A
Stapedial reflexes		
Ipsilateral	Absent	Present
Contralateral	Absent	Present
SRT	15 dBHL	5 dBHL

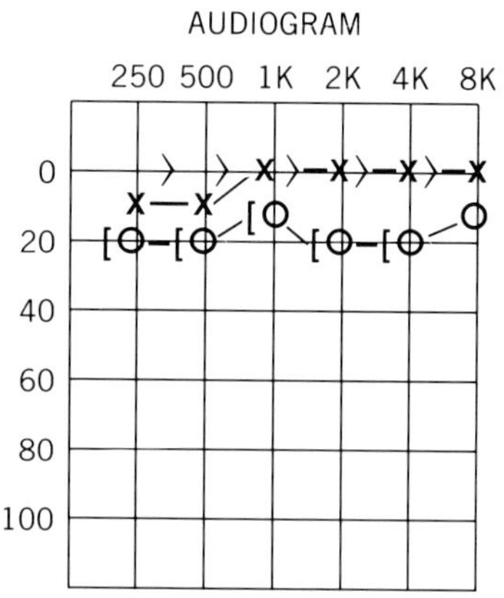

	Right	Left
Word recognition		
@ 40 dBSL	100%	100%
@ 90 dBSL	12%	100%
High-level SISI	0%	100%
Tone decay (STAT)	Positive	Negative
Masking level difference @ 500 Hz $(S_oN_o - S_nN_o)$	0 dB	

Preoperative Audiologic Diagnostics

1. Absent right stapedial reflexes in the presence of normal hearing and middle ear function.
2. Severely reduced right word recognition at high-intensity level.
3. Unable to detect 1-dB increment during high-level SISI test.
4. Positive tone decay.
5. MLD displayed no release from masking at 500 Hz.
6. Interpretation: retrocochlear lesion.

Skull Base Imaging

1. Mastoid series: negative.
2. CT scan of internal auditory canal: cerebellar lesion 3 cm in height and 2 cm in its greatest diameter, extending from cerebellopontine angle into the superior cerebellar cistern (Figure 28-9; see also Chapter 4).

Neurologic Assessment

1. Cranial nerve examination
   a. Moderate sixth nerve palsy with diplopia upon right lateral gaze.
   b. Unable to fully abduct left eye.
   c. Diminished right corneal reflex.
   d. V_1 and V_2 diminished in pinprick and touch on right as compared to the left.
   e. Mild peripheral right facial palsy.
   f. Tongue slightly weak on right versus left.

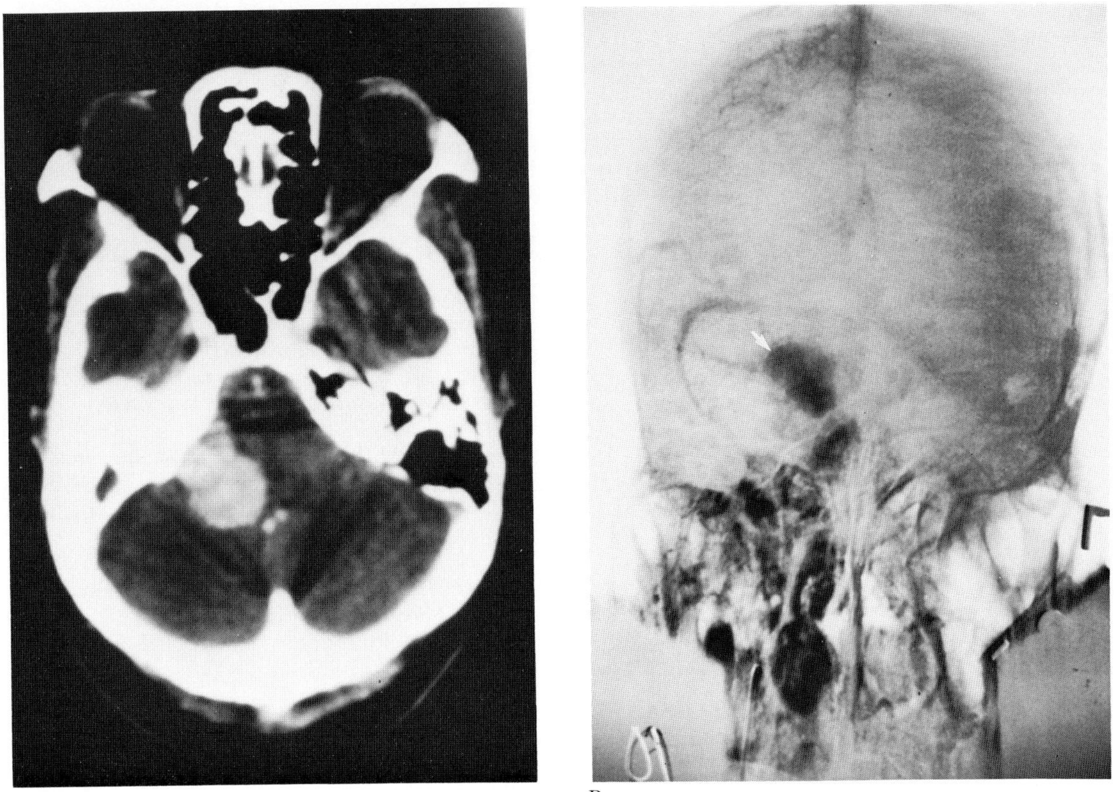

A B

Figure 28-9. Cerebellopontine angle lesion. A. CT scan. B. Anterioposterior angiogram.

g. Interpretation: cranial nerve involvement—V, VI, VII, VIII, and XII.

2. Cerebellar examination
   a. Mild right ocular dysmetria.
   b. Mild dysdiadochokinesia in upper extremities, greater on right.
   c. Minimal right upper extremity dysmetria.
   d. Normal gait and tandem walk.
3. Bilateral vertebral arteriography: vascular displacement of right superior cerebellar artery and right basilar artery.

Surgery

This included a right frontal ventriculostomy and a right suboccipital craniectomy with excision of the cerebellopontine angle epidermoid tumor (see Chapter 13).

Postoperative Audiologic Profile

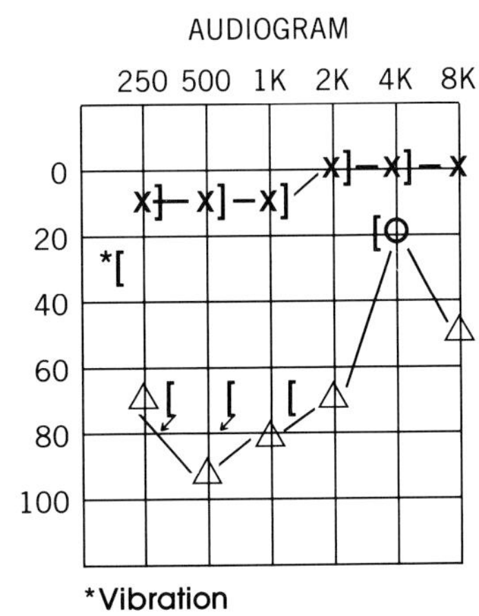

	Right	Left
Tympanogram type	A	A
Stapedial reflexes		
Ipsilateral	No response	Present
Contralateral	No response	Present
SAT	40 dBHL	
SRT	Could not establish	5 dBHL
Word recognition		
@ 40 dBSL	0%	100%
@ 90 dBHL	—	100%

Postoperative Neurologic Diagnosis

1. Slightly decreased blink (right).
2. Seventh motor nerve essentially the same as preoperatively.
3. Normal corneal reflex.
4. Severe sensorineural hearing loss (see audiogram).
5. No weakness of motor nerve V.
6. Normal gait.
7. No dysmetria.

Comments

Although the subjective complaints were subtle, the diagnostic audiologic evaluation strongly suggested a retrocochlear lesion. This was confirmed by CT scan. Because the lesion was greater than 2.5 cm, the eighth nerve was injured during surgery. However, the facial nerve was preserved anatomically, and postoperative function remained normal. Hearing, postoperatively, was severely impaired, but rehabilitative needs were minimal due to normal contralateral hearing.

SUMMARY

Whenever a patient is suspected to have a hearing loss due to the malignant process, chemotherapy, radiation, or surgery, a complete audiologic evaluation is recommended. If irreparable hearing loss exists, rehabilitation begins immediately. For most, day-to-day communication is enhanced with appropriate amplification, counseling, and training.

REFERENCES

1. Borg E: On the neuronal organization of the acoustic middle ear reflex: A physiological and anatomical study. *Brain Res* 49 : 101, 1973.
2. Lynn GE, et al: Binaural masking-level differences in neurological disorders. *Arch Otolaryngol* 107 : 357, 362, 1981.
3. Hannley M, Jerger J, Rivera VM: Relationships among auditory brainstem response, masking level differences and acoustic reflex in multiple sclerosis. *Audiology* 22 : 20, 1983.
4. Olsen WO, Noffsinger D: Masking level differences for cochlear and brainstem lesions. *Ann Otol Rhinol Laryngol* 85 : 820, 1976.
5. Swisher LP: Response to intensity change in cochlear pathology. *Laryngoscope* 76 : 1706, 1966.
6. Schwartz DM, Grant AB: Normative Aspects of the ABR. In Jacobson JT (ed): *The Auditory Brainstem Response*. San Diego: College-Hill, 1985. Pp 65–98.
7. Eggermont J, Don M, Brackman D: Electrocochleography and auditory brainstem electric responses in patients with pontine angle tumors. *Ann Otol Rhinol Laryngol* 89(Suppl 75): 1980, Pp 1–19.
8. Kelly, JP: Vestibular System. In Kandel EK, Schwartz JH (eds): *Principles of Neural Science*. New York: Elsevier, 1981. Pp 406–418.
9. Barber HO, Stockwell CW: *Manual of Electronystagmography*. St. Louis: Mosby, 1976.
10. Sanders DA: *Aural Rehabilitation*. Englewood Cliffs, NJ: Prentice-Hall, 1982.

GLOSSARY

Air-bone gap More than a 10-dB difference between air and bone conduction thresholds for a given ear and frequency; indicates a conductive component to the hearing loss.

Air conduction testing The measurement of pure tone threshold levels with earphones.

Antiphasic Two signals that are 180° out of phase with each other.

Audiogram A graphic representation of air and bone conduction hearing threshold levels between 125 and 8000 Hz.

Audiology The specialty devoted to the assessment and management of hearing-impaired individuals.

Audiometer An electronic device used to evaluate hearing.

Binaural Refers to both ears.

Binaural fusion test A list of two-syllable words where the low and high frequency energy are separated so that high pass energy is presented to one ear and low pass energy is presented to the other. The perception of both is needed for word recognition. Patients with a brainstem lesion may perform poorly on this test. The site of the lesion, however, cannot be determined from this test alone.

Bone conduction testing The measurement of pure tone thresholds using a bone conduction oscillator that typically is placed on the mastoid bone.

dB hearing level (dBHL) The number of decibels above audiometric 0. In 1969 the American National Standards Institute (ANSI) established standard sound pressure levels on a frequency-by-frequency basis for audiometric 0 (0 dBHL on the audiometer's attenuation dial); i.e., 0 dBHL equals 7 dBSPL for 1000 Hz and 25.5 dBSPL for 250 Hz using TDH-39 earphones and MX-AR41 cushions. These standards reflect "normal" hearing sensitivity levels. Therefore, all audiometers are calibrated according to ANSI standards.

dB sensation level (dBSL) The number of decibels above a person's hearing threshold level.

dB sound pressure level (dBSPL) The logarithmic unit of measure that expresses the sound pressure level (SPL) of an acoustic signal in reference to a standard sound pressure such as the least audible sound (0.0002 dyne/cm^2).

Directional preponderance Nystagmus that tends to beat in one direction more than the other during caloric stimulation.

Filtered speech A list of 50 words from which most of the high-frequency energy has been removed using a low pass filter with a cutoff frequency of 500 Hz and an 18 dB/octave rejection rate. The tape-recorded words are presented monaurally at 50 dB above the pure tone average (PTA). A percent correct score is obtained; 70 to 100 percent is considered normal. Patients with temporal lobe lesions frequently exhibit reduced performance in the contralateral ear. Parietal and frontal lobe lesions usually exhibit normal performance.

Frequency The number of cycles per seconds; hertz (Hz).

Homophasic Two stimuli that are in phase with each other; one condition of the MLD requires that both the signal and noise be presented to both ears with the same starting phase.

Monaural Refers to one ear.

Most comfortable level (MCL) The subjective intensity level that speech is comfortably loud.

Pure tone average (PTA) Arithmetic average of the speech frequency thresholds (500 Hz, 1 kHz, and 2 kHz).

Pursuit Also referred to as tracking; an involuntary eye movement that keeps a slowly moving target on the fovea.

Saccades Rapid eye movement; a rapidly moving target (exceeding 90 degrees/second) requires saccadic eye movement to place the target on the fovea; voluntary eye movement generates saccades.

Speech awareness threshold (SAT) The intensity level where speech is detected 50 percent of the time; also referred to as speech detection threshold (SDT); often used when SRT cannot be obtained due to poor word recognition ability.

Speech reception threshold (SRT) The intensity level where phonemically dissimilar words (e.g., ice-cream, baseball) are understood 50 percent of the time; should correlate with a PTA within $\pm 10-12$ dB.

Spondaic words Two-syllable words (e.g., baseball, ice-cream) with equal stress placed on each syllable.

Synthetic sentences identification test (SSI) A group of 10 artificial sentences (e.g., small boat with a picture has become.) that are presented with either an ipsilateral competing message (ICM) or contralateral competing message (CCM). The test is administered at different signal-to-noise ratios. Patients with intra-axial brain stem lesions may show a contralateral ear effect on the SSI/ICM while displaying normal findings on the SSI/CCM. Patients with temporal lobe lesions typically exhibit a bilateral deficit on the SSI/ICM with a contralateral deficit on the SSI/CCM.

29

Prosthodontics

JAMES T. JACKSON

KEY CONCEPTS

Materials; Moulage; Planning Splints; Obturators; Radiation Carrier

MILESTONES

1600 B.C.	Treatise Reconstructive Surgery of Ears and Nose	Elibers Papyrus (Egypt)
1000 A.D.	Dental Restoration with Ivory	Abdulcasis
1470s	Facial Proportions	DeVinci
1570s	Facial Impressions	Tagliacozzi
1800	Prosthetic Appliances and Anesthesia	Fauchard
1850s	Dental Anesthesia	Morton
1868	First Organic Plastic Molding Compound, Acellulose Nitrate	Hyatt
1889	Textbook of Maxillofacial Prosthetics	Martin
1917	Maxillofacial Prosthetics for Ear Injuries	Kazanjian
1939	Liquid Latex Prosthetics	Bulbulian

The head and neck cancer patient, although sharing similar fears with other cancer patients, remains uniquely distinct [1]. The methods and procedures for surgical intervention may result in significant functional disability and facial disfigurement [1,2]. The patient presents to the prosthodontist for rehabilitation services for the restoration of facial integrity and functional losses.

The maxillofacial prosthodontist coordinates and collaborates with the clinicians to provide prostheses for head and neck oncology patients. As a cost-effective alternative to reconstruction, prosthetics can immediately restore function, protect the surrounding tissues, enhance healing, and promote esthetics. Together, these benefits have an immediate psychological effect and provide immeasurable boost to otherwise depressed patients (Table 29-1) [3].

INDICATIONS

Prosthetics are considered when (1) the anticipated defect is too difficult to reconstruct, (2) the malignancy may recur, (3) radiotherapy is being instituted, and (4) surgery is refused (Figure 29-1).

CONTRAINDICATIONS

Poor health, advanced age, very large deformities, and compromised blood supply are con-

Table 29-1. Maxillofacial prosthetic objectives

Maxillofacial prosthetic objectives
Restoration of function
Preservation of esthetics
Tissue protection
Enhancement of healing

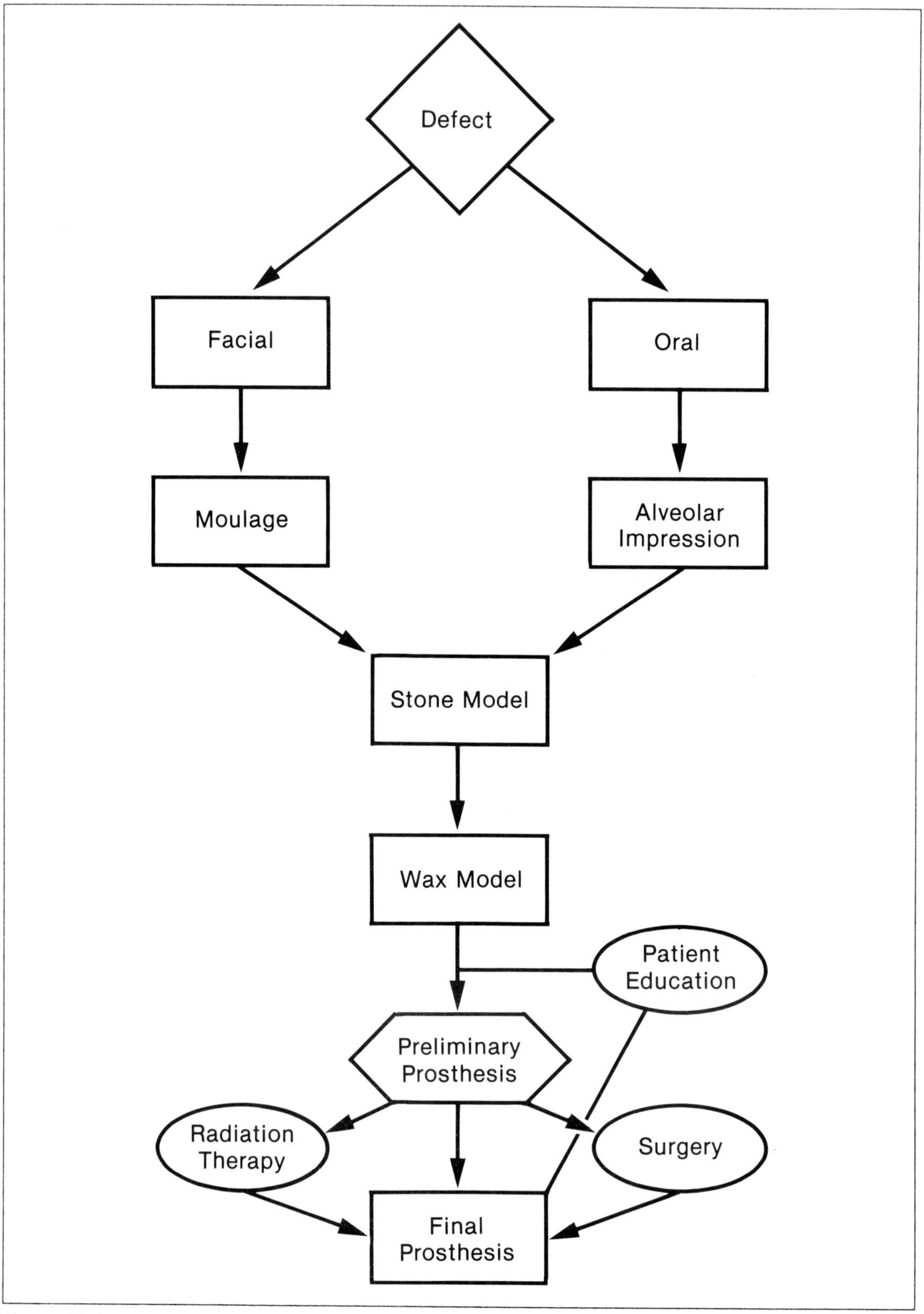

Figure 29-1. Prosthetic dynamics.

traindications to prosthetics for the head and neck oncology patient.

MATERIALS AND METHODS

Although there is no perfect prosthetic material, it should adhere ideally to the following criteria: biocompatibility, esthetic acceptability, durability, and reproducibility (Table 29-2). Some materials such as polyvinylchlorides, polysiloxane, and Silastic 44210 have excellent physical properties. Silicone, easily polymerized and colorized, is popular and has been used with great success. Presently, the most common materials are the resilient synthetic resins, hard acrylic resins, and recent silicone rubbers. All are either self or heat cured [4–6].

Whether the defect is facial or oral, an alginate impression is made and a stone model is fabricated. From this model, a wax or clay pattern simulates the proposed prosthesis. Based on the model and the properties of the material, an initial prosthesis is formulated.

MOULAGE

When necessary, a model or moulage of the face is fabricated to accurately depict the facial relationship of the defect (Figure 29-2) [2].

Technique

With the patient sitting, relaxed and prepared, the alginate is flowed into the defect and onto the face. Plastic breathing tubes are placed in the nostrils or the mouth. Hair, included in the impression, is lubricated with petroleum jelly. The periphery of the area is boxed with wax and modeling clay. The defect is blocked out with petrolatum-impregnated gauze. Strips of gauze impregnated with material is applied to reinforce the moulage. The final thickness is about 1/4 to 3/8 inch thick.

Table 29-2. Characteristics of the ideal prosthetic material

Biocompatible
Pliable
Durable
Lightweight
Translucent
Malleable
Insertable
Inexpensive
Hygienic

Preliminary Prosthesis

After the moulage sets, it is removed, and dental stone is poured into the moulage. A layer of baseplate is adapted to the defect on the stone cast. A wax or trial prosthesis is completed, based on the stone cast. Old photographs aid in the esthetic interpretation of the facial prosthesis. The wax prosthesis is placed on the patient's face and modifications are made until acceptable dimensions and contours are obtained.

PLANNING

Coordination

For the best results, there should be close collaboration between the clinician and the prosthodontist. Preplanning includes a thorough dental evaluation to determine the condition of the remaining teeth and structures after radiotherapy or surgery. The preservation of key teeth—posterior molar and anterior canine—greatly aids rehabilitation. As a general rule, the more hard palate and premaxilla that is conserved, the better the prosthesis. The entire prosthesis is planned prior to resection or therapy to provide support, resist movement, maintain function, and ensure cosmesis.

Patient Education

Comprehensive counseling and patient education precede definitive treatment. The patient is informed, in detail, of the goals and limitations of prosthetic restoration. It includes an honest appraisal of the physical and psychological adjustments necessary for successful prosthetic usage. Continued prosthetic maintenance following definitive treatment is stressed, as well as the future dependence on the prosthesis to attain rehabilitation. Properly informed of the realities of functional and cosmetic restoration, the patient will have a realistic expectation of the quality of life [2].

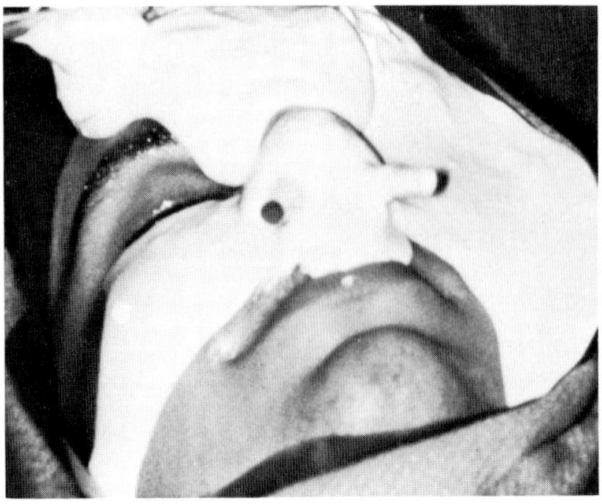

A

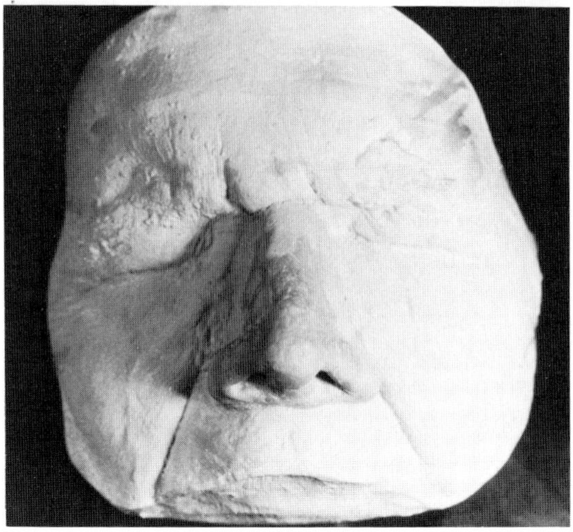

C

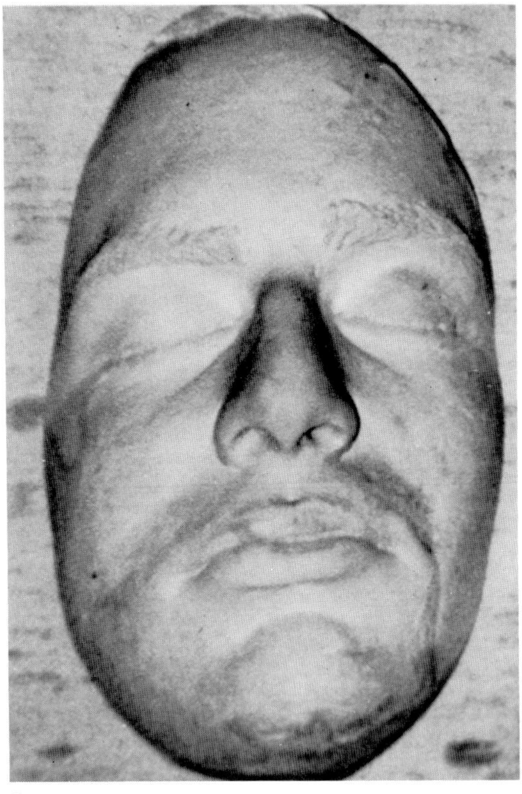

B

Figure 29-2. A. Alginate being poured to create a facial moulage. B. Full-face moulage. C. Three-quarter face moulage.

APPLIANCES

Eye and Orbit

Orbital exenteration including the eyebrow is caused by malignancy, burns, or other severe trauma. The resulting large depression is unsightly (Figure 29-3). However, properly executed, prosthetic restoration is highly satisfactory [2].

Problem

The basic problem is natural reproduction that must match the color, socket contour, and the orbital ridge prominence. A good ocular prosthesis solves two problems: orbital reconstruc-

Figure 29-3. Middle-aged patient with a well-healed orbital socket after orbital exenteration. This defect is ideal for a prosthesis.

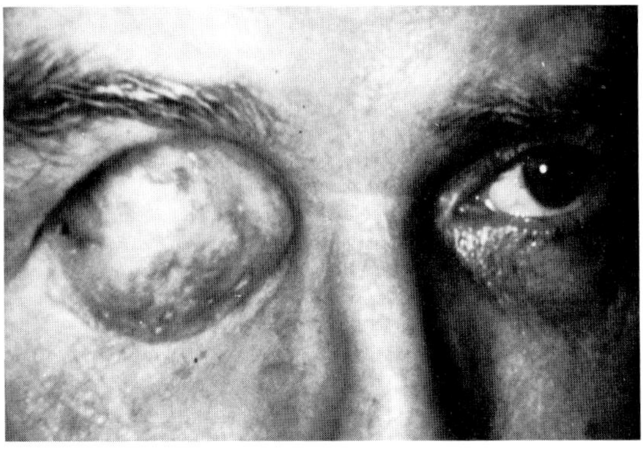

tion and artificial eye retention and removal. The orbital deformity is suited well for a prosthesis that is retained by eyeglass frames [1].

Final Result
A carefully selected artificial eye is affixed permanently, and retention is devised (Figures 29-4 through 29-6). Rather than use natural hair, eyebrows are either modeled or painted on the prosthesis.

Ear
A well-executed prosthetic ear is gratifying for both patient and prosthodontist. Partial or total ear amputation is secondary to dysgenesis, agenesis, surgery, or trauma. Congenital deformities vary from small aural tags, with little resemblance to a normal external ear, to fairly large aural tags, suggestive of an external ear. Prior to prosthodontic fabrication, the tags are removed. Since deformities vary greatly, skill

Figure 29-4. Prosthetic eyes.

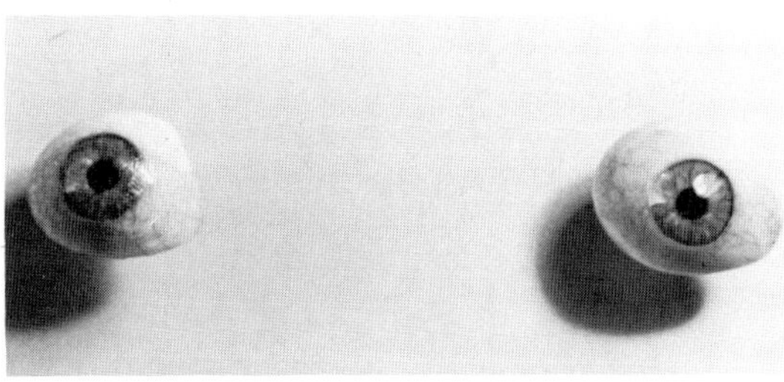

Figure 29-5. Eye prosthesis on a partial midfacial moulage.

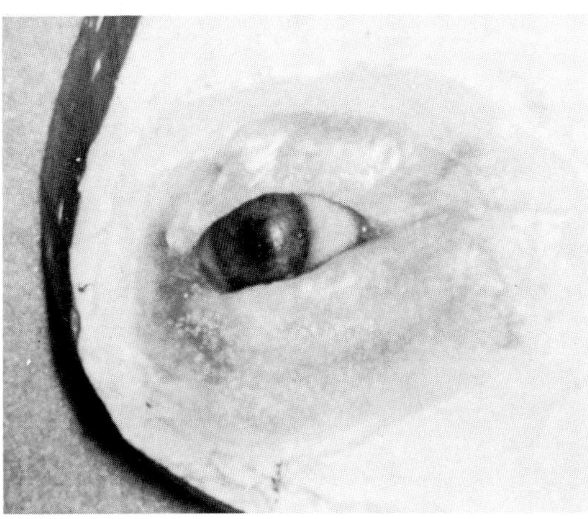

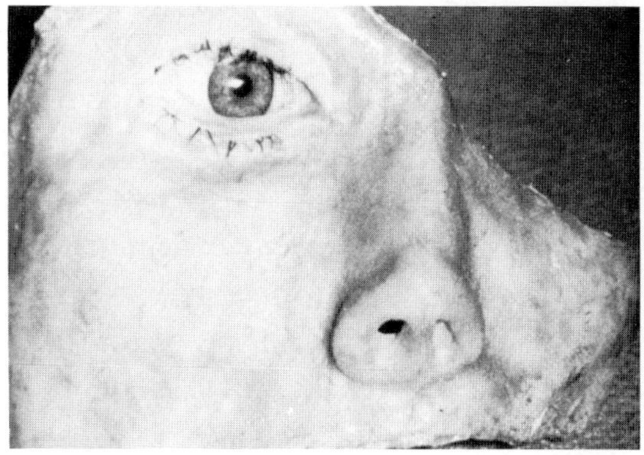

Figure 29-6. Subtotal midfacial prosthesis that includes the eye, nose, and cheek.

and experiences are prerequisites for making a satisfactory prosthesis.

Nose
Due to its central location, total or partial deformities produce serious disfigurement. Many surgeons delay final reconstruction after ablation to monitor recurrent or persistent disease. Some patients, especially when medically unstable, are not surgical candidates. Under these circumstances, a temporary prosthesis is invaluable and more socially acceptable (Figures 29-7 and 29-8) [8,9].

Goals
The degree of success depends on form, color, and adaptation to the defect's margins. Careful selection of an inconspicuous junction line is critical for camouflage.

Technique
Nasal prostheses are fabricated from hollow, elastic materials with thin edges that overlap the margins of the defect. They are retained with a skin adhesive that adapts to the margins of the underlying structures. The sensitive mucous membrane frequently prohibits retentive undercuts.

Maxilla
The most common operation for cancer that creates an intraoral defect is a maxillectomy. This involves removal of the soft palate and/or orbital exenteration [10]. A postmaxillectomy

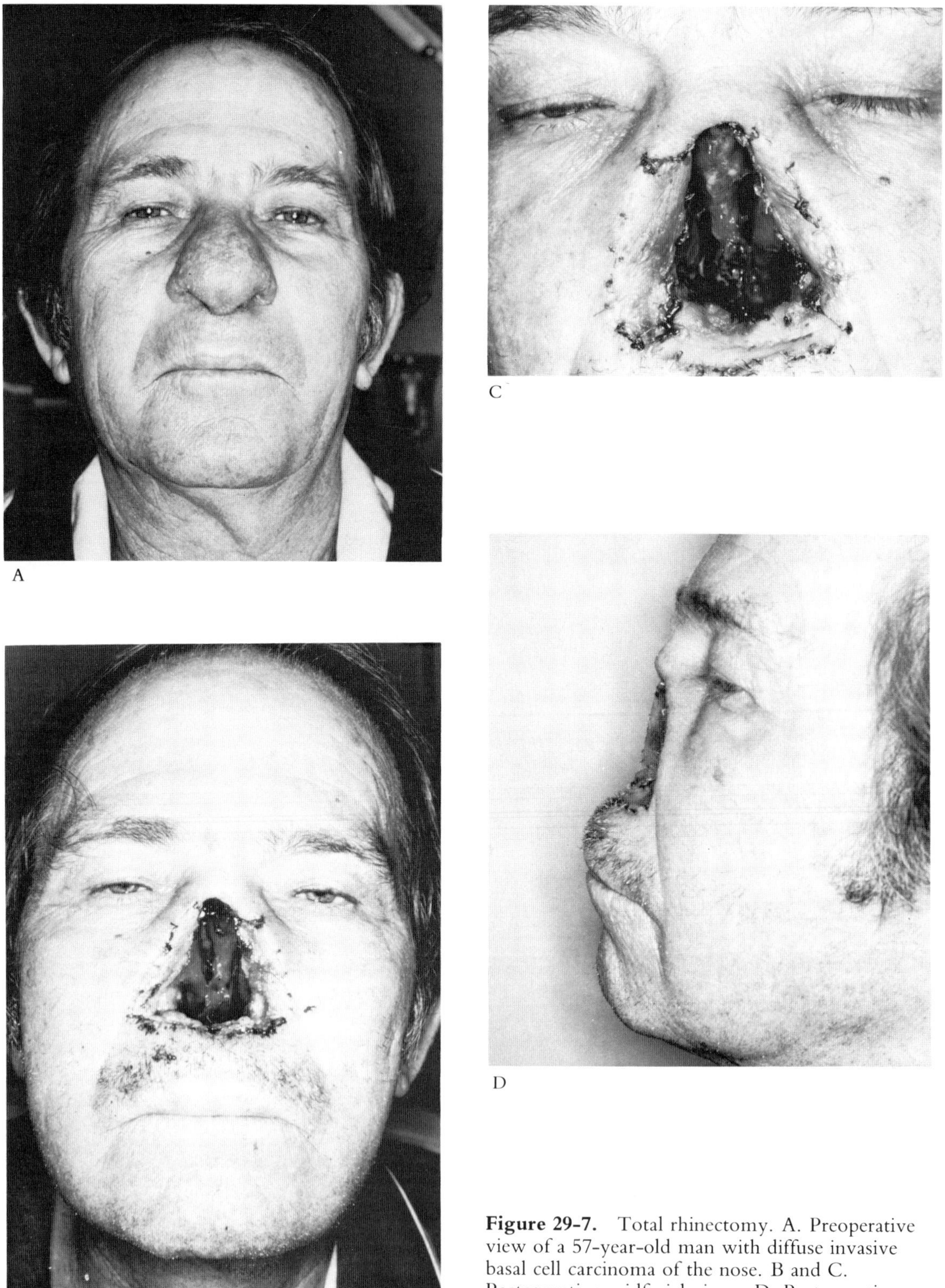

A B C D

Figure 29-7. Total rhinectomy. A. Preoperative view of a 57-year-old man with diffuse invasive basal cell carcinoma of the nose. B and C. Postoperative midfacial views. D. Postoperative lateral view.

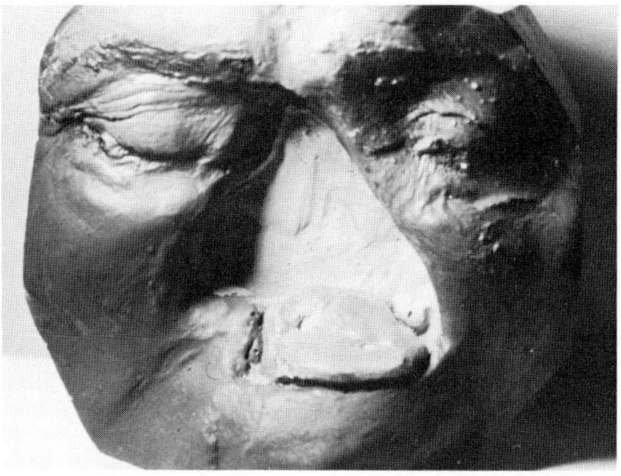

Figure 29-8. Tinted midfacial moulage for a patient with total rhinectomy.

Figure 29-9. Stone model of dental impression.

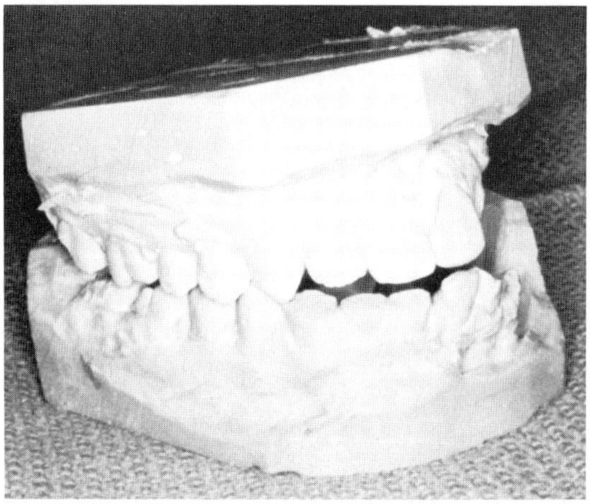

A

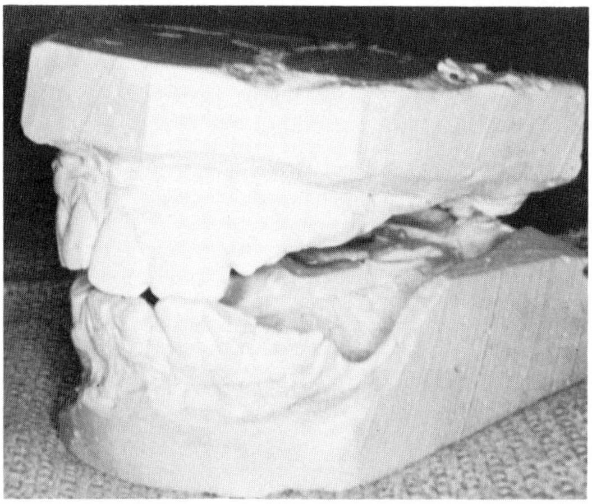

B

defect is a prosthodontic challenge from both a functional and psychological aspect [11]. Satisfactory restorations for rehabilitation require early prosthetic intervention (Figures 29-9 and 29-10).

Obturators

An obturator, for either the dentulous or edentulous patient, eliminates the communication between the oral and orbital cavities. An obturator fits over the defect but not too high into the cavity. An improper fit interferes with healing and causes difficulty with removal and insertion.

Prosthesis

The surgical prosthesis can be converted into a final prosthesis when clasps have been placed preoperatively. As in the edentulous patient, a preliminary prosthesis is inserted within 1 to 2 hours of the time the impression is made. With the surgical prosthesis, the patient immediately resumes swallowing and speech. After 7 to 10 days, an interim prosthesis is created and inserted. The final prosthesis is fabricated months later. With good oral hygiene, a final prosthesis can last 5 to 7 years or longer. When properly fabricated, a maxillary prosthesis produces durable and functional rehabilitation (Figures 29-11 through 29-14).

Figure 29-10. Maxillary obturator with palatal extension.

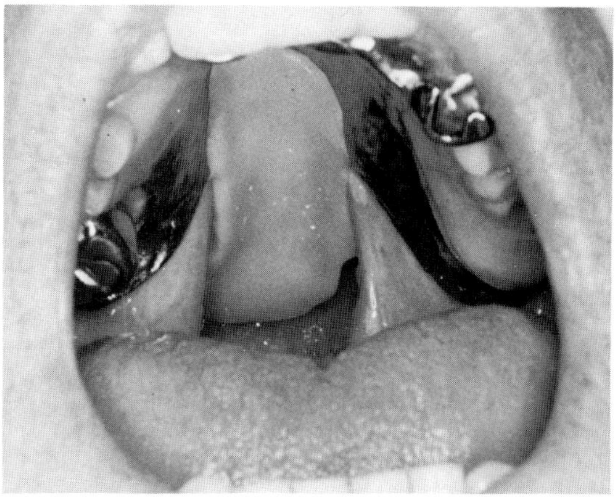

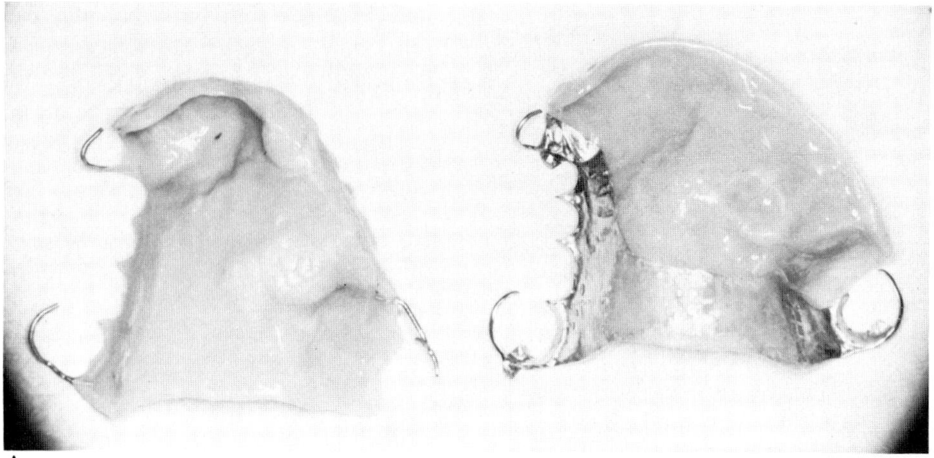

A

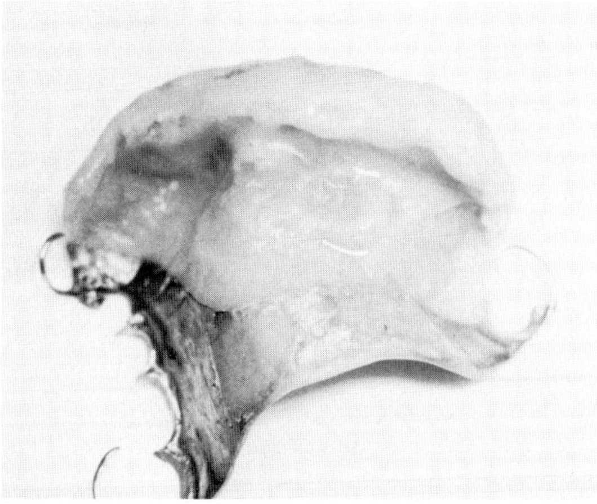

B

Figure 29-11. Palatal-maxillary prosthesis. A. Surgical prosthesis (left); postoperative prosthesis (right). B. Soft Coe-Resilient liner on dorsal surface in preparation for insertion.

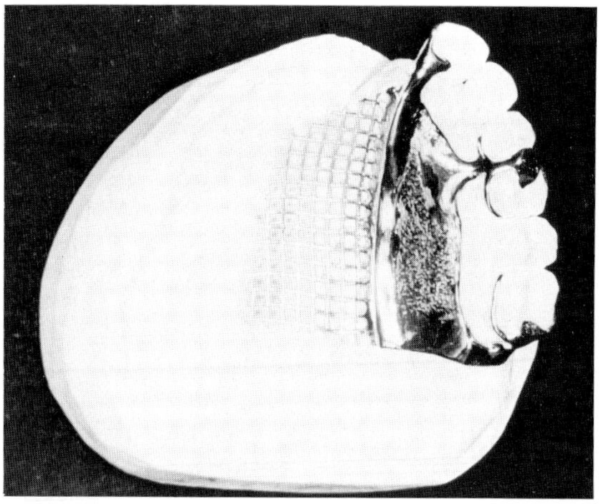

Figure 29-12. Cast chrome cobalt frame for a maxillary obturator (dentulous patient).

Tongue

Tongue prosthetics that reduplicate chewing, swallowing, and speaking are difficult to execute. Static devices achieve limited mobility. Mobile or hinged models are somewhat better. With the assistance of a speech pathologist, a mandibular prosthesis with palatal augmentation can be effective (see Chapter 25).

Goals

1. Reduction in the size of the oral cavity, thereby improving resonance.
2. Direction of food into the esophagus with the aid of a curved prosthetic tongue.
3. Protection of the underlying mucosa.
4. Development of a surface for the residual tongue to contact during speech and swallowing.
5. Improvement in appearance and psychosocial adjustment.

Limitations

Despite these achievements, a tongue and palatal augmentation prosthesis cannot reduplicate

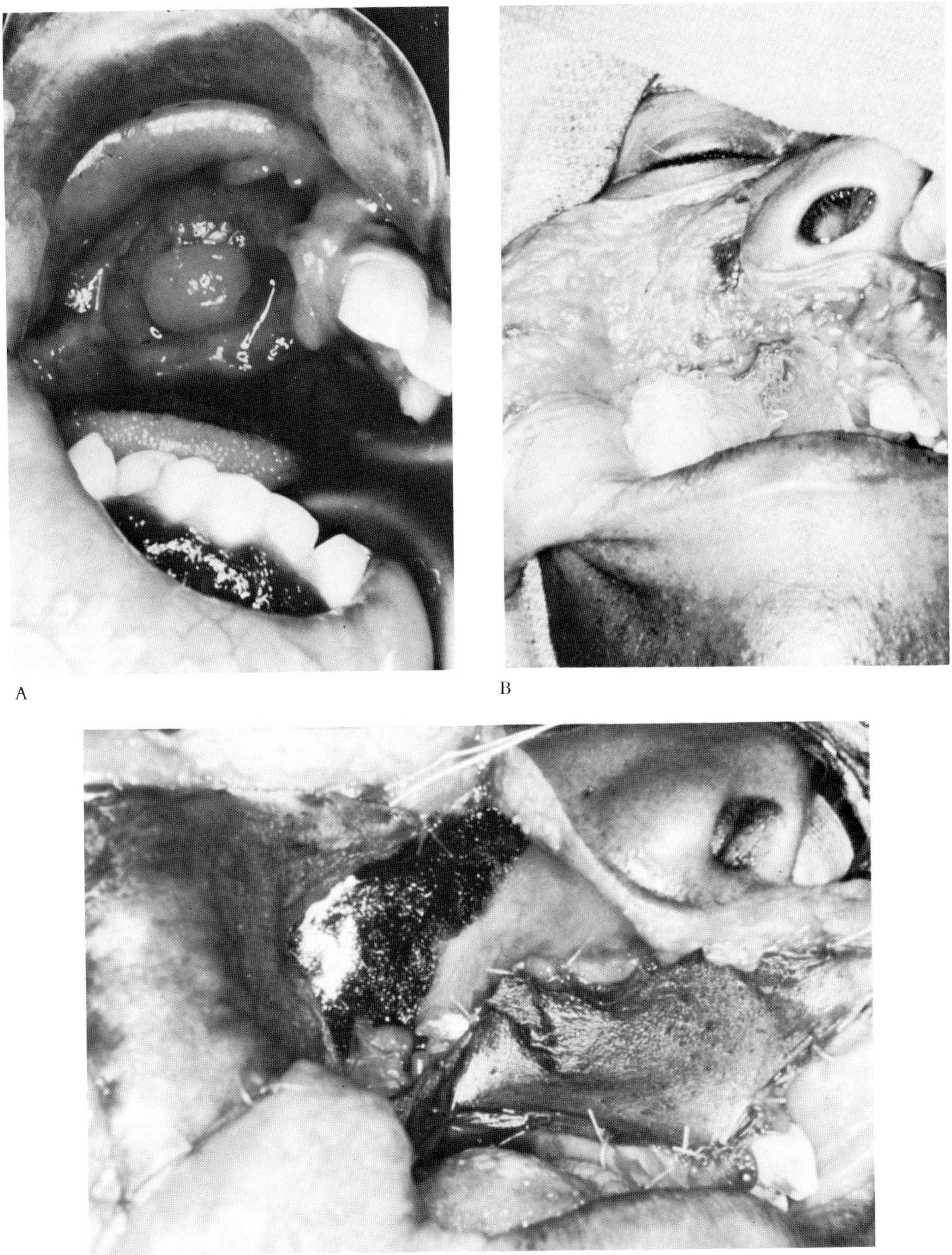

A B C

Figure 29-13. A. View of a 26-year-old man with an ameloblastoma of the right maxilla. B. The surgical approach via a Weber-Ferguson incision. C. Surgical defect after removal of the lesion.

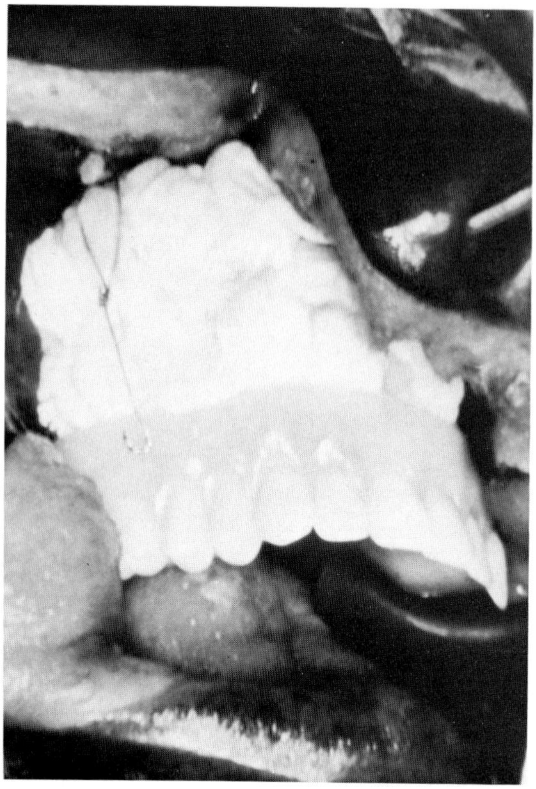

D

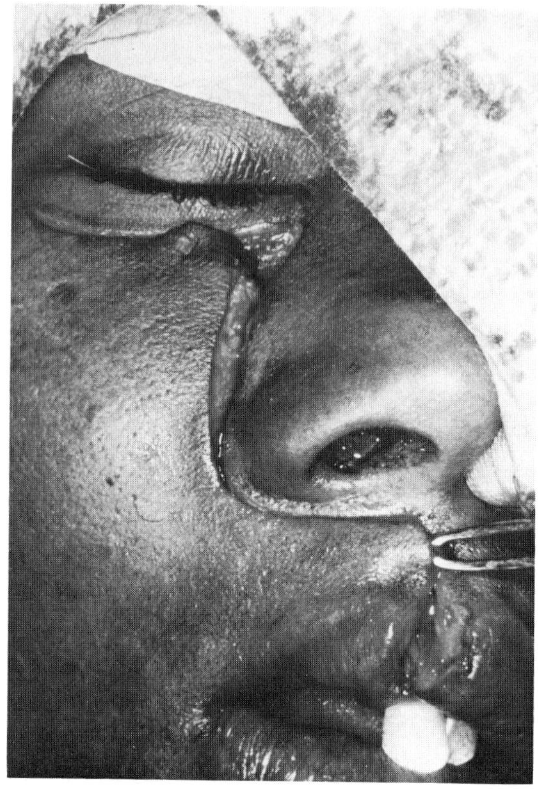

E

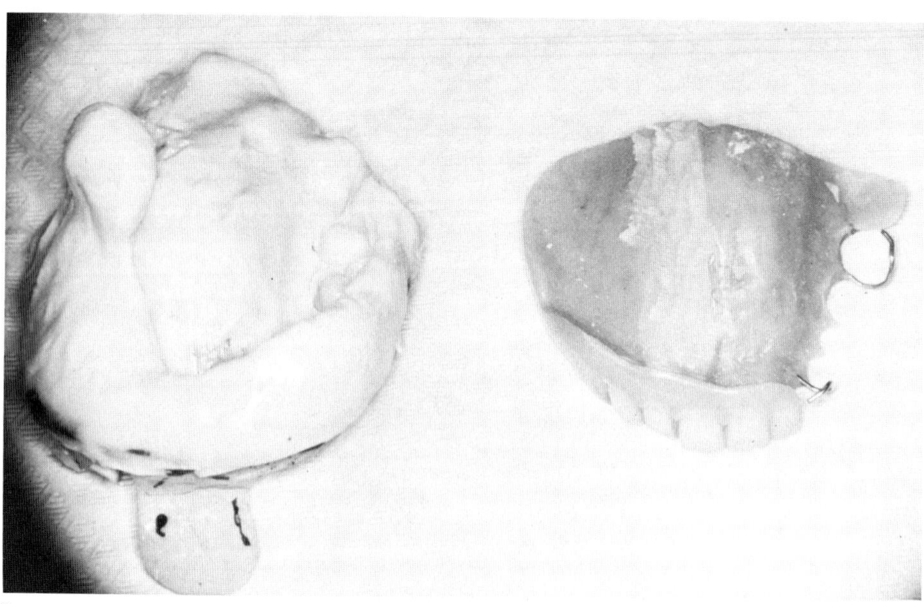

F

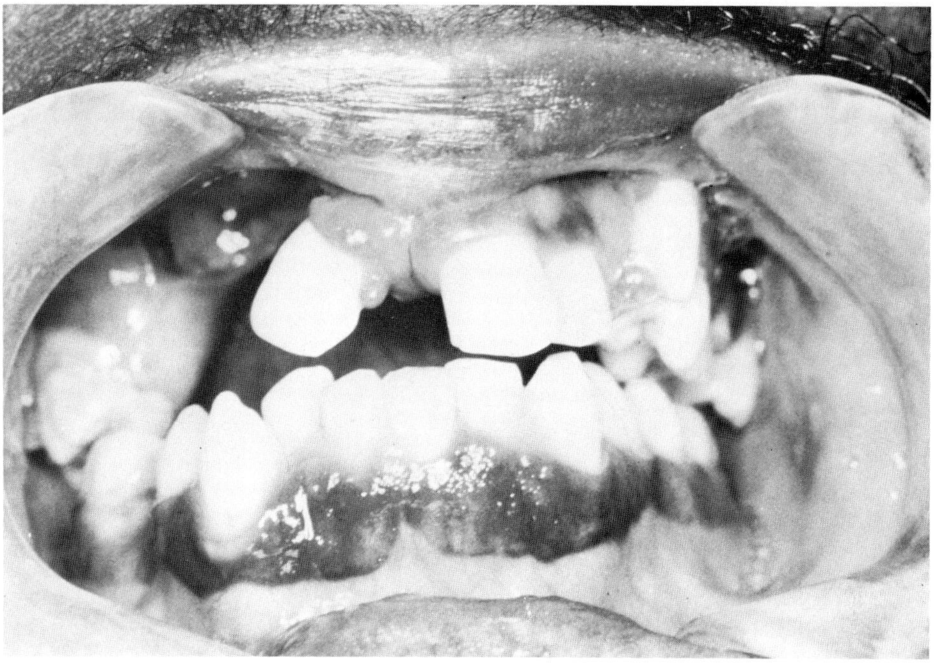

G

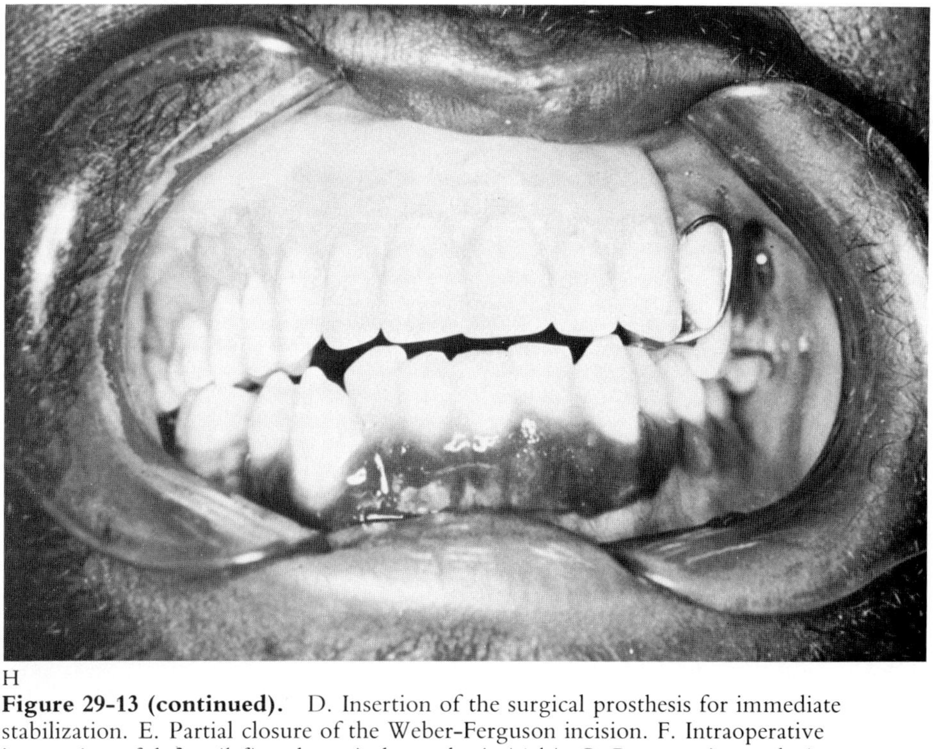

H

Figure 29-13 (continued). D. Insertion of the surgical prosthesis for immediate stabilization. E. Partial closure of the Weber-Ferguson incision. F. Intraoperative impression of defect (*left*) and surgical prosthesis (*right*). G. Preoperative occlusion. H. Postoperative occlusion with final prosthesis.

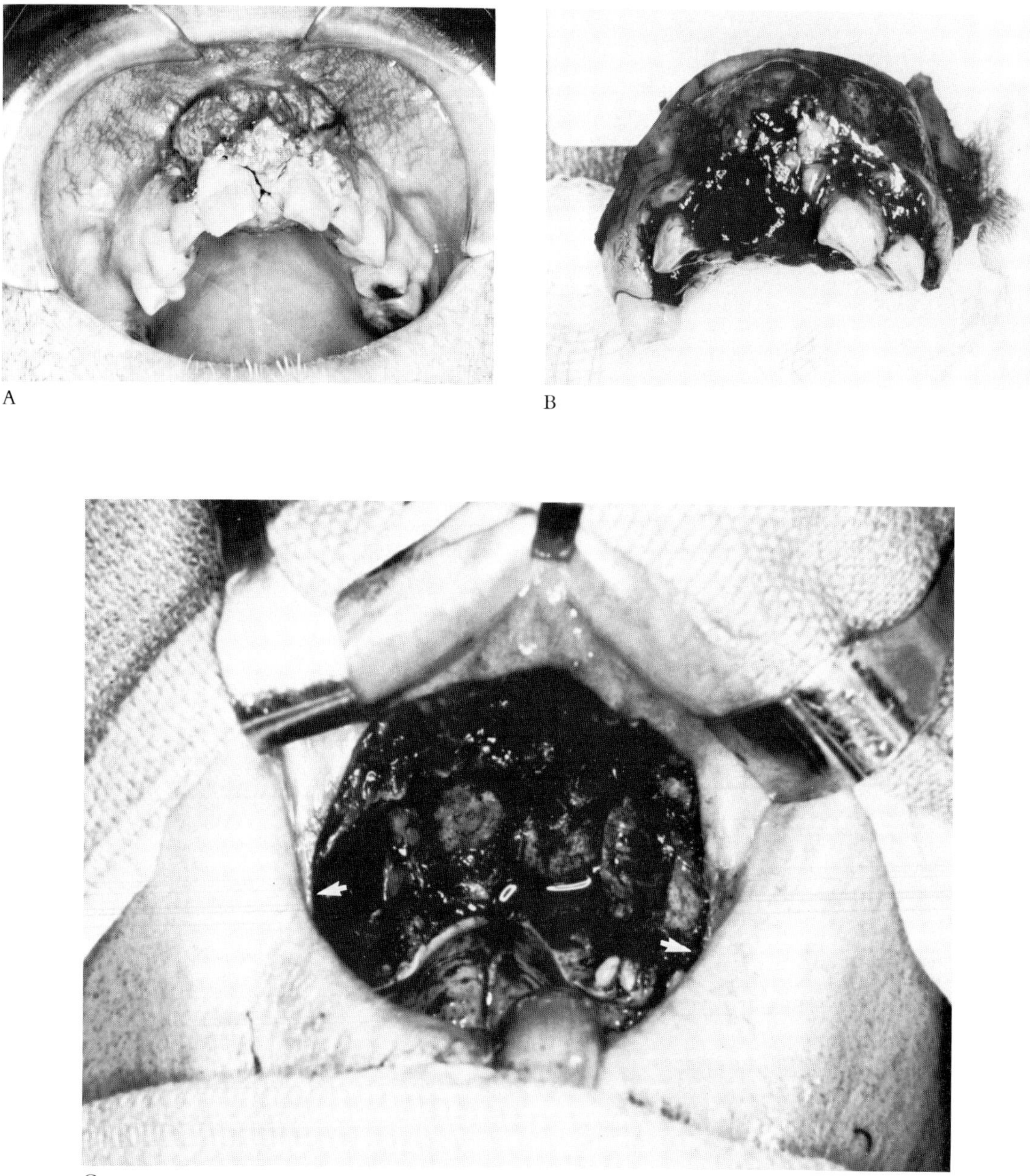

A B C

Figure 29-14. A. Squamous cell carcinoma of the premaxillary gingiva. B. Surgical pathologic specimen. C. Surgical defect, from premolars to premolars. (continued)

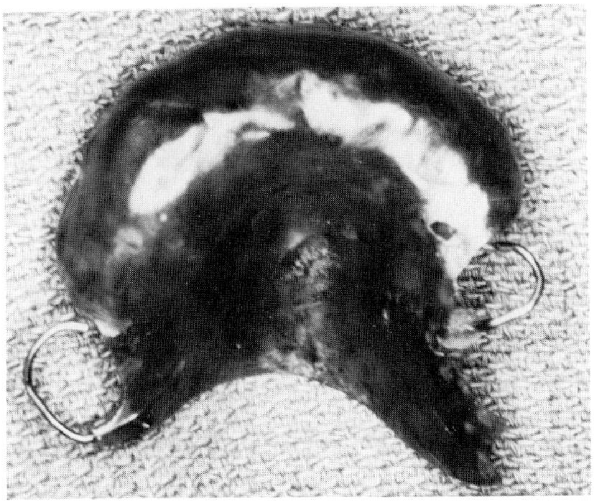

D

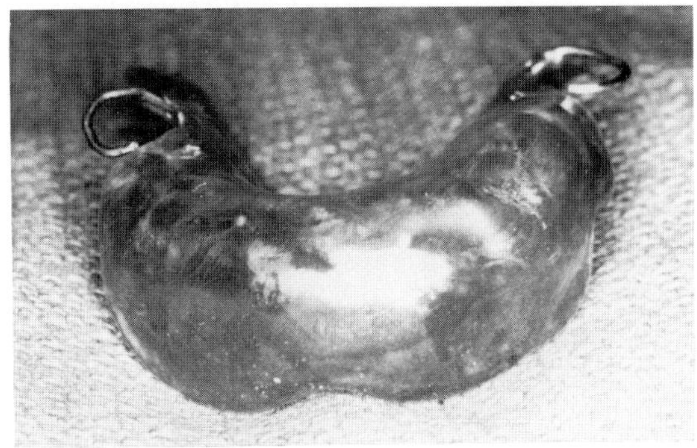

E

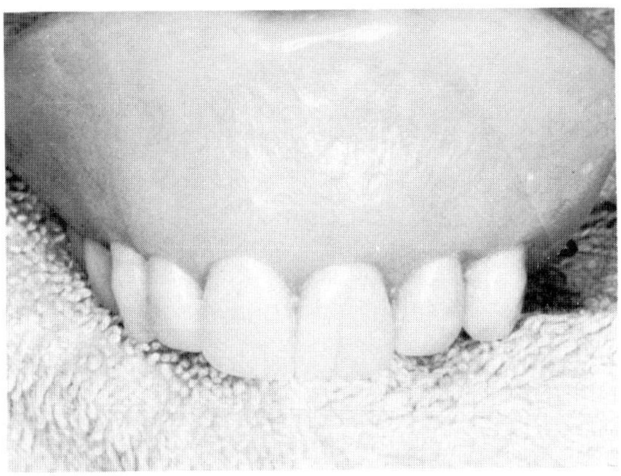

F

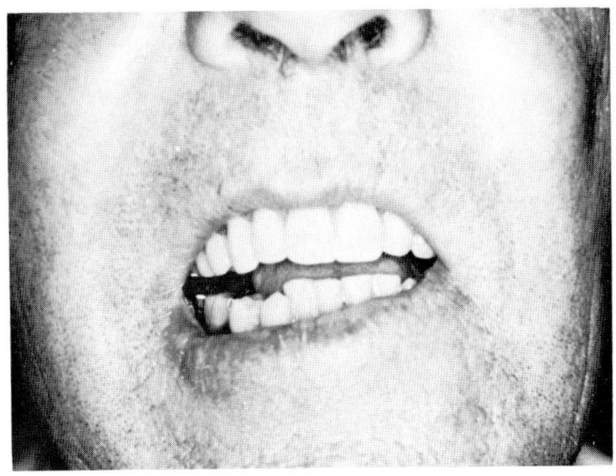

G

Figure 29-14. (continued) D and E. Surgical prosthesis. F and G. Final prosthesis.

normal swallowing and speech. The inflexible, static prosthesis affects articulation and resonance. Xerostomia and fibrosis, secondary to radiotherapy, aggravate these problems.

Palatal Extension

With total glossectomy, the emphasis is on a mandibular prosthesis, whereas with partial glossectomy, a maxillary prosthesis is constructed with palatal extension (see Figure 29-10).

Sometimes the palatal augmentation prosthesis is used as a training prosthesis until the tongue recovers its function. When used as the definitive prosthesis, eating becomes extremely difficult and frustrating. This may be ameliorated with interdental fixation until healing and scarring have occurred.

Mandible

Mandibular reconstruction is preferable to a mandibular prosthesis (see Chapter 23). Surgery restores mandibular continuity and greatly reduces facial distortion. Removal of large portions of tongue precludes restoration of normal speech by either surgery or a prosthesis (see Chapter 25).

Goals

In order of importance, the goals are swallowing, saliva control, speech, mastication, and cosmesis.

Limitations

The prosthetic prognosis deteriorates in proportion to the amount of tissue removed. The other problems associated with mandibulectomy are deviation and soft-tissue loss.

Resection Device

The resection device is used primarily when a patient has teeth remaining in the intact segment after there has been a resection of a portion of the mandible with an accompanying disarticulation of the condyle [1,2]. After mandibulectomy, the mandible deviates ipsilaterally because of tissue scarring and unopposed muscular contraction.

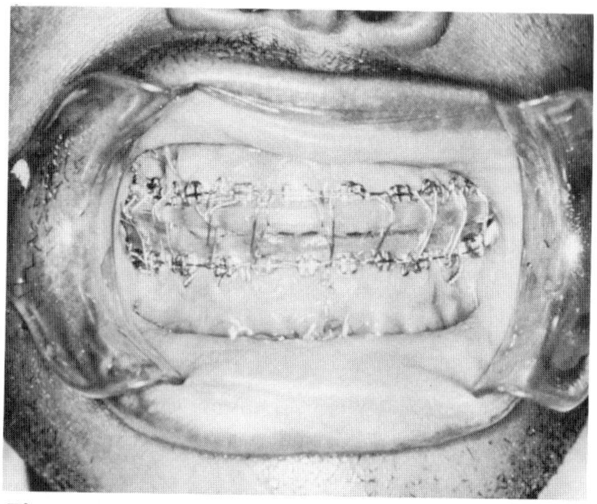

Figure 29-15. Intermaxillary splints and stainless steel wire fixation.

Radiation Carriers

Radiation carriers facilitate irradiation of the oral cavity and oropharynx. These prostheses, classified as locators, stents, or carriers, aid in precise delivery of radiotherapy. Selective oral lesions are treated by positioning a radioactive source such as cesium or radium at a precalculated distance from the tumor. The distance from the radiation source to the lesion is critical and determined by the radiotherapist. The radioactive source is incorporated in the carrier and placed intraorally as long as needed for treatment. The treatment success depends on accurate carrier prosthetic positioning [2].

Figure 29-16. Gunning splints on a dental articulator.

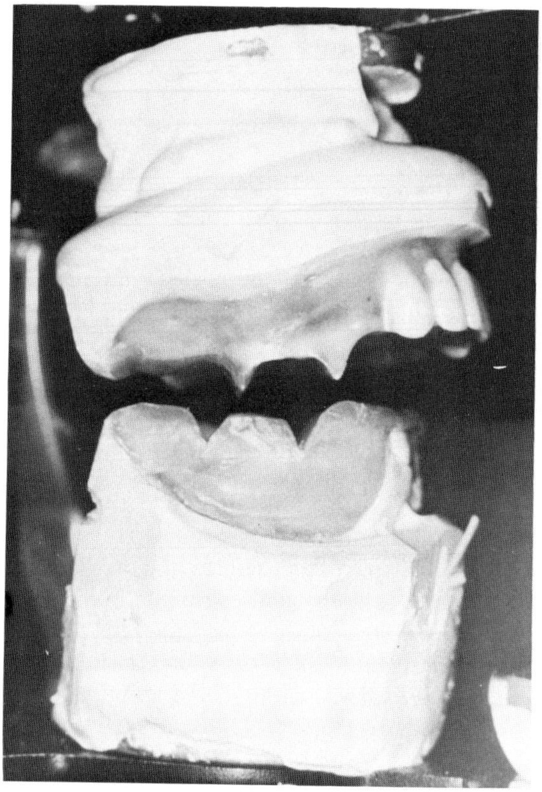

Gunning Splints

Gunning splints are constructed primarily to immobilize fractured segments of the edentulous mouth (Figures 29-15 and 29-16). After the arch bars are added, a hole the size of No. 1/2 round burr is drilled through each side of the lower rim in the first molar area (see Figure 29-14). It is important not to drill into the tissue surface of the splint; this will accommodate circum-mandibular wires that hold the lower segment in place. The surgeon is consulted as to the placement of any wire in the upper splint, since this varies with the type of technique used in maintaining this splint.

FUTURE CHALLENGES

There is a need for more efficient service. Presently, the treatment too often is protracted and incomplete. Often, preoperative consultation between surgeon and the prosthodontist is inadequate or nonexistent. Too little time is provided by surgeons for the construction of temporary or surgical prostheses. There is often an absence of long-range planning and interdisciplinary rehabilitation. In addition, there is minimal or inadequate maintenance of the prostheses. Changes in the defect due to healing or subsequent surgery may require alterations in existing prostheses or construction of new prostheses.

Multiple Prostheses

Frequently, more than one appliance is needed to adequately carry a patient through a rehabilitation program. It is far better to be realistic with a maxillofacial patient than to overstate the benefits of this type of therapy. Close communication between all disciplines concerned with maxillofacial services should be maintained. The introduction of acid etching of enamal to increase the adhesive capacity of resins to tooth structure has improved and simplified many clinical procedures relative to the management of maxillofacial problems [12].

Osseointegration

The introduction of osseointegration by Branemark and his associates [13] led to a renewed interest in the use of dental implants to resolve the problems associated with the fabrication and use of complete dentures and maxillofacial prostheses.

The primary requisite for successful osseointegration is healthy bone. Bone must be of sufficient quantity and quality to permit integration of a stable implant fixture [1].

Osseointegrated dental implants provide a viable alternative to tooth and other oral and maxillofacial replacement structures [13–15]. Success is the culmination of good case selection, thoughtful treatment planning, meticulous clinical and technical attention to detail, and proper maintenance care.

Research

Finally, there is a serious need for research in materials, technical procedures, and instrumentation.

REFERENCES

1. Chalian VA, Drane JB, Standish SM: *Maxillofacial Prosthesis: A Multidisciplinary Practice*. Baltimore: Williams & Wilkins; 1971. Pp 112–120.
2. Beumer III J, Curtis TA, Firtell DN: *Maxillofacial Rehabilitation: Prosthodontic and Surgical Consideration*. St. Louis: Mosby, 1979. Pp 332–350.
3. Parel SM: Advances in rehabilitation for the head and neck cancer patient. *Tex Dent J* 103(6) : 24, 1986.
4. Raptis CN, Knapp JA: Properties of silicone maxillofacial elastamer processed in stone and metal. *J Prosthet Dent* 44(4) : 447, 1980.
5. Munson FT, Heron DF: Facial reconstruction with acrylic resin. *Am J Surg* 53 : 291, 1941.
6. Bulbulian AH: Repair of facial defects with prosthetic using a latex compound. *J Am Dent Assoc* 28 : 559, 1941.
7. Pfinghoeft FA, Shearer HW: Fabrication of plastic facial moulage. *J Prosthet Dent* 25 : 567, 1971.
8. Baird WH: An artificial nose. *Dent Cosmos* 47 : 560, 1905.
9. Baker L: An artificial nose and palate. *Dent Cosmos* 47 : 561, 1905.
10. Strohauer RA: Button obturator for a soft palate defect. *J Prosthet Dent* 43 : 229, 1980.
11. Fattbone L, Edmonds D: A technique for the obturator of anterior maxillary defects with accompanying midfacial tissue loss. *J Prosthet* 58 : 203, 1987.
12. Taylor TD, Gerrow JD, Brudvik JA: Resin bonded components for maxillofacial prosthesis construction: A clinical trial. *J Prosthet Dent* 59 (3) : 334,1988.
13. Branemark PI: Osseointegration and its experimental background. *J Prosthet Dent* 50 : 399, 1983.
14. Jemist T, Salblad PA: The effect of chewing on mandibular complete dentures to osseointegrated over-dentures. *J Prosthet Dent* 55 : 357, 1986.
15. Desjardins RP: Tissue-integrated prosthesis for edentulous patients with normal and abnormal jaw relationship. *J Prosthet Dent* 59 : 180, 1988.

30

Social Services

TOMMYZEE H. SUGGS and THOMASINE LYLES

KEY CONCEPTS

Psychological Reactions; Medical Insurance; Medicare; Medicaid; Hospice; Discharge Planning

MILESTONES

1900	Advocate of Medical Social Work	Cabot
1905	First Department of Medical Social Services (Massachusetts General Hospital)	Cabot and Commons
1920	Public Health Social Work	
1935	Social Security Act	
1939	Rehabilitation and Medical Social Work	
1966	American Society for Hospital Social Work	
1971	Medical Social Services Department as an Accreditation Requirement	Joint Commission Accreditation of Hospitals (JCAH)

Cancer for many patients is a chronic disease, albeit one with significant impact [1]. Whether in remission or while undergoing therapy, cancer patients have special psychological, social, and economic needs (Figure 30-1). Social workers provide casework services and play an important role in helping cancer patients and their families to cope with the illness [2].

EMOTIONAL REHABILITATION

The cancer experience is a sequence of related events proceeding from the first perception of illness, hospitalization, treatment, convalescence, to recurrence and death. Beginning with the diagnosis, the subsequent patient and family reactions establish an adaptation pattern that continues throughout the disease (see Chapter 19).

PSYCHOLOGICAL SUPPORT

Psychological support and guidance are beneficial throughout treatment. The typical psychological responses are anger, denial, alienation, and anxiety. These responses are triggered by fears and misconceptions that are influenced by personal opinions and the experience of others in the patient's life.

Personalized intervention by the social worker greatly eases these concerns about the hospital and treatment. Therapy is distressing for most patients, but early and ongoing social worker intervention reduces fears and anxiety.

PSYCHOLOGICAL REACTIONS

Adaptation

Adaptation in response to illness consists of two general tasks:

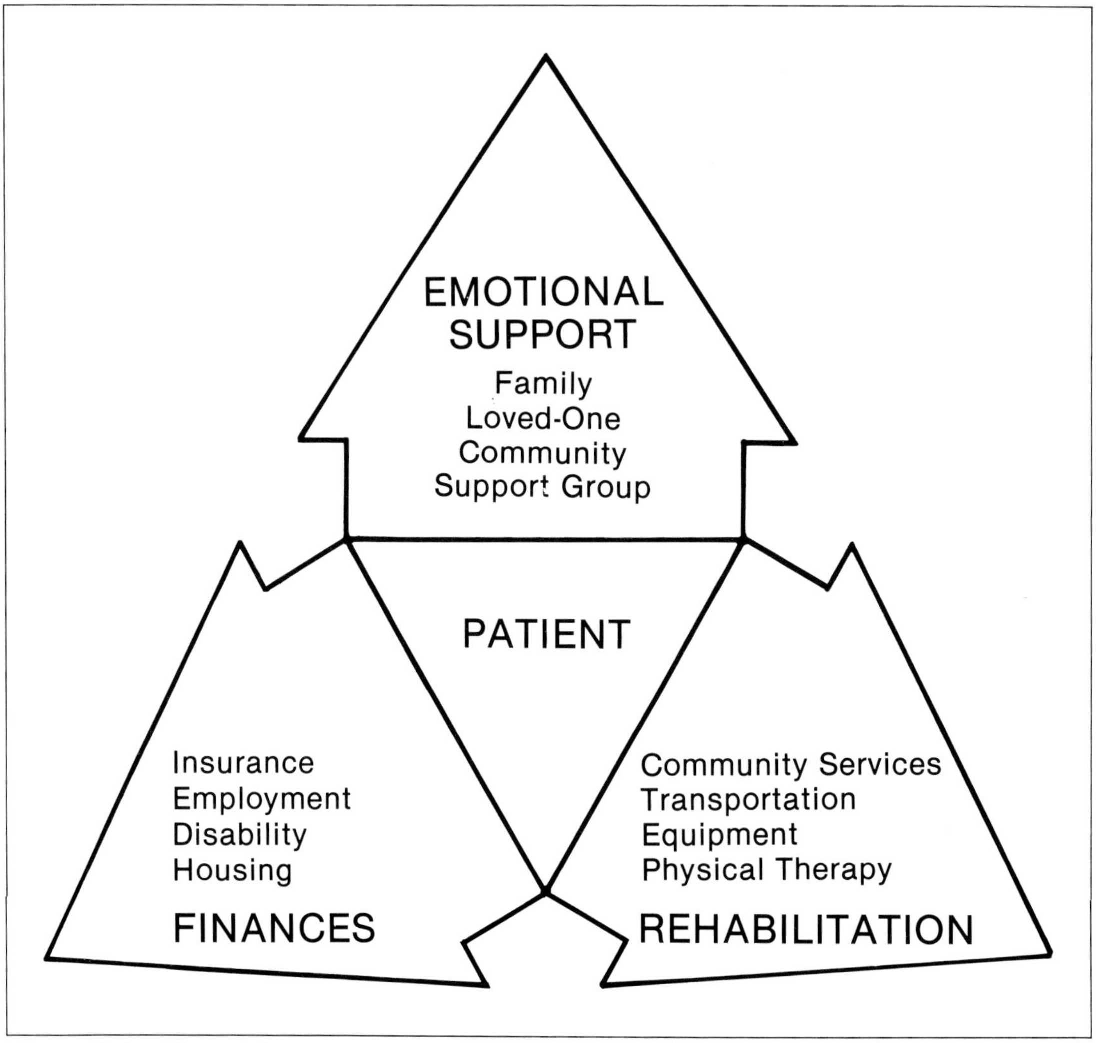

Figure 30-1. The social assessment.

1. Coping with illness and its attendant problems, such as pain or paralysis.
2. Coping with life as it is altered by cancer.

It is very important that health professionals realize the importance of a patient's emotional state following the diagnosis and treatment of head and neck cancer. Many responses such as denial, anxiety, hostility, fear, alienation, and confusion are common throughout the disease course [3].

Denial

The emotional response varies greatly. Some patients easily communicate, while others withdraw and are devastated completely. In most, denial is commonplace, since the emotional impact of the diagnosis clouds and prevents many patients from absorbing important details. Retrospectively, many patients complain of the physician failing to help them cope with the diagnosis. Thus, it is important that physicians repeat and review to allow for the strong emotional reaction to the diagnosis and treatment.

Depression

Once denial passes, depression often follows, but it usually resolves shortly. However, at times following surgery, a more intense form of depression is seen. This depression is most pronounced if accompanied by severe disfigurement. Strong encouragement may be necessary for the patient to continue treatment. Hope overcomes irrational thinking when emotional support is readily available.

Hostility

Some patients are very hostile and angry. It is important that those around the patient understand this hostility and allow for ventilation. Patients should not be made to feel guilty for their anger. They should be assured that the pain and effects of treatment will subside eventually. Family members must also realize that these reactions are normal and that the patient merely requires time and understanding.

MEDICAL INSURANCE

For the cancer patient, effective health insurance is vital. Some patients are covered by private health insurance, others by Medicare and Medicaid. Many are uninsured. Even for those covered by private insurance, significant portions of care must be funded out-of-pocket. Some private insurances do not pay for prescriptions, physical therapy, prostheses, and so on. Most private plans are subsidized by the employer; however, if the patient becomes disabled, loses his or her job, or retires, this coverage is lost. For most patients, the loss of insurance is more devastating than the loss of income. Therefore, one of the social worker's first priorities is to review the patient's medical insurance. Patients lacking health insurance or having inadequate coverage should apply for Medicaid (state funded) or Medicare (federally funded).

Medicare

Medicare is the medical insurance program administered by the Social Security Administration [4]. It is available to persons 65 years old regardless of whether they are retired or still working. It is also available for anyone receiving Social Security benefits for 2 years or who has a chronic kidney disease.

The Medicare Catastrophic Coverage Act of 1988 was repealed at the end of 1989. The Medicare program has two parts. Part A is hospital insurance; Part B is supplementary medical insurance.

Part A: Hospital Insurance

Hospital Insurance (HI), Part A, pays the basic inpatient hospital expenses minus an initial yearly deductible. This deductible changes from year to year, depending on hospital costs. The patient receives a set number of days of inpatient care without additional cost.

Part B: Supplementary Medical Insurance

Most patients, but not all, have both Part A and Part B of Medicare. In Part B, Supplementary Medical Insurance (SMI), there is a deductible for covered medical services and a co-insurance charge. The items covered under Part B are

1. Physician services and supplies (including drugs that cannot be self-administered and also blood-clotting factors for hemophilia cases).
2. Diagnostic x-ray, laboratory, and radiotherapy.
3. Surgical dressings, splints, casts, and other devices.
4. Necessary ambulance service.
5. Rental or purchase of durable medical equipment used in the patient's home, including respirators, oxygen tent, hospital bed, and wheelchair.
6. Home health services.
7. Artificial replacements (not dental) for all or part of an internal body organ, including colostomy bags and supplies.
8. Braces for arm, leg, back, or neck.
9. Artificial legs, arms, and eyes.

Skilled Nursing Facility

If the patient qualifies for skilled care in a nursing home, he or she pays nothing for the first

20 days. For the next 80 days, the patient pays $74.00 per day, and Medicare pays all the remaining recognized charges. No benefits are available after 100 days of care in a benefit period.

Skilled nursing facilities are also covered under Part A. Admission to such a nursing facility must meet strict standards. The only care in nursing homes that Medicare covers is skilled nursing care or skilled rehabilitative care that is provided by a Medicare-certified nursing facility. Most people who enter nursing homes do so to receive custodial care, which is not covered by Medicare.

Home Health Services

Home health services include part-time nursing care, physical therapy, and medical and social services. Medical supplies and some rehabilitation equipment are subject to co-insurance. They are reimbursed at 80 percent of recognized charges.

Special Needs

Patients who have tracheotomies or who require special nutritional support are covered for the equipment. A special form, obtained from the social worker, must be completed (Figure 30-2). In addition, a Certificate of Medical Necessity is completed by the physician (Figure 30-3). Sterile supplies, other than already listed, are purchased by the patient. Medicare numbers are designated by the patient's Social Security number plus a letter suffix.

Medicaid

Medicaid is the state-run medical assistance program, usually under the Department of Human Services. It is for patients whose income or health insurance does not cover the cost of needed health services. Medicaid eligibility is determined by strict regional standards and guidelines. It requires the following verification: name; date of birth; current address/living situation; medical circumstances; income and employment status; monies on hand (savings and/or checking accounts), resources, stocks, bonds, securities, contracts, and personal property (e.g., cars, boats); and other insurance (life and health).

Coverage (District of Columbia)

Medicaid covers all inpatient care, based on fixed charges. It includes transportation to and from a medical facility or physician's office. All but fifty cents on each prescription, most sterile supplies, and durable equipment are covered. A special form is completed for ordering equipment and supplies; this may be obtained from the social worker (see Figure 30-2).

Medical Charities (District of Columbia)

Medical Charities is the "low option" medical assistance program. It covers all the cost of inpatient services (e.g., surgery) but pays only a certain fixed rate for care. It also does not pay for certain medical supplies or equipment and requires the patient to get prescription drugs at designated pharmacies. Not all states have such a plan.

Identification

The Medicaid patient's identification number (District of Columbia) is identified by 11 numbers. The last three numbers denote the coverage. The last three digits for some examples follow:

270 Medical Charities
470 Medical Charities
150 Medicaid
110 Medicaid

There are approximately 90 Medicaid categories. The social worker identifies what services are covered based on the last three digits in each of these categories.

Private Insurance

Insurance coverage for many patients alters treatment plans and dictates follow-up care. Third-party and commercial insurance also have standard rates for procedures performed in and out of the hospital. Insurance coverage determines the length of stay as well as what kinds of outpatient services may be obtained. The insurance designates whether a procedure is "same day admission" or "ambulatory surgery."

GOVERNMENT OF THE DISTRICT OF COLUMBIA
DEPARTMENT OF HUMAN SERVICES
MEDICAL ASSISTANCE PROGRAM

PRIOR AUTHORIZATION REQUEST/APPROVAL

1 PATIENT			2 REQUESTING PROVIDER			
A. RECIPIENT D.C. I.D. NUMBER			A. PROVIDER NUMBER			
B. NAME (LAST, FIRST, M.I.) PRINT			B. NAME (LAST, FIRST, M.I.) PRINT			
C. ADDRESS			C. ADDRESS			
D. TELEPHONE NUMBER	E. DATE OF BIRTH	F. SEX ☐ M ☐ F	D. CITY	STATE	ZIP	E. TELEPHONE NUMBER

3 OTHER HEALTH INSURANCE COVERAGE	4 REQUESTED SERVICE		5 PATIENT LOCATION
ENTER NAME OF POLICYHOLDER AND PLAN NAME AND ADDRESS AND POLICY. IF NONE PLEASE INDICATE.	SURGERY ☐	MEDICAL SUPPLIES OR EQUIPMENT ☐	HOME ☐
	MEDICAL ☐	TRANSPORTATION ☐	NURSING HOME ☐
	DENTAL ☐	EYEWEAR ☐	HOSPITAL INPATIENT ☐
		OTHER ☐	DISCHARGED DATE:

REQUESTED SERVICE DATA

6 DIAG-NOSIS CODE	7 PROCEDURE CODE	8 DESCRIPTION OF SERVICES, DURABLE MEDICAL EQUIPMENT OR SUPPLIES	9 TIME REQUIRED	10 FREQ. OR UNITS	11 ESTIMATED CHARGE ($)	12 APPROVED AMOUNT ($)

13 JUSTIFICATION

____

____

____

____

14 FOR DENTAL USE ONLY

DENOTE TEETH ALREADY MISSING BY "X"; TO BE EXTRACTED BY "/"; X-RAYS TAKEN BY "V"

Q1			FACIAL								FACIAL				Q2
01	02	03	04	05	06	07	08	09	10	11	12	13	14	15	16
RIGHT		PRIMARY TEETH	AA	BB	CC	DD	EE	FF	GG	HH	II	JJ	PRIMARY TEETH		LEFT
			LINGUAL								LINGUAL				
			TT	SS	RR	QQ	PP	OO	NN	MM	LL	KK			
32	31	30	29	28	27	26	25	24	23	22	21	20	19	18	17
Q4			FACIAL								FACIAL				Q3

15 A. SIGNATURE OF REQUESTING PROVIDER — I CERTIFY THAT THE SERVICES REQUESTED ARE MEDICALLY INDICATED AND NECESSARY TO THE HEALTH OF THIS PATIENT AND THAT THE FOREGOING INFORMATION IS TRUE, ACCURATE AND COMPLETE.	B. DATE

DO NOT WRITE BELOW THIS LINE

ACTION

☐ DISAPPROVED	☐ APPROVED AMOUNT $ ________	PRIOR AUTHORIZATION NUMBER	SIGNED	DATE

COMMENTS ______________________________

SUBMIT ORIGINAL AND 1 (ONE) COPY TO D.C. DEPT OF HUMAN SERVICES. IF SERVICE IS APPROVED TRANSCRIBE PRIOR AUTHORIZATION APPROVAL NUMBER TO BILLING FORM. SUBMIT BILLING FORM TO ADDRESS SHOWN IN BILLING MANUAL.

DHS 719A (REVISED 3/81)

Figure 30-2. Prior Authorization Request form required by District of Columbia Medicaid for equipment and supplies.

native. Still others have no fixed address or alternative housing.

Homeless Patients
The patient's living situation is determined during the initial interview. A patient with no fixed address is an obvious discharge problem. There are many concerns for homeless patient. First, most homeless patients have no health insurance or income. An application for Medicaid or Public Assistance may be initiated by the social worker. Meeting basic eligibility requirements and the approval process may take as long as 45 business days in some states.

Shelters
City shelters do not accept nonambulatory or tracheotomy patients or those requiring enteral therapy. In some jurisdictions, small specialized shelters will consider the independent tracheotomized patient. In the District of Columbia, the Community for Creative Nonviolence Infirmary and Christ House are temporary living accommodations that provide food, shelter, medical care, counseling, and assistance for such patients. These facilities have limited capacity and rarely are vacant. Some geographic areas have no such facilities.

Licensed Residences
Hospice care provides invaluable services for the terminal patient. Hospice is a way of dying rather than a place to die. There are both in-home and inpatient programs. The latter accepts patients if the prognosis is 4 weeks or less. A physician to physician contact by telephone is necessary. The social worker provides the social history, financial, and insurance data.

Utilization of Resources
Prior to discharge, a variety of services, equipment, and supplies must be coordinated. Home health agencies such as Visiting Nurse Association, Staff Builders, In-Home Supports, and Upjohn provide nursing care, including dressing changes, tracheotomy care, monitoring of vital signs, and wound care. A health aide can assist with such daily activities as bathing, dressing, meal preparation, and light housekeeping.

Lost Chord Club
The Lost Chord Club is specifically designed for laryngectomy patients (see Chapter 26). Trained members will visit new laryngectomy patients in the hospital. Artificial larynxes are available for demonstration or loan.

I Can Cope/Can Surmount
I Can Cope and Can Surmount are programs designed to help patients and families to understand and cope with the disease. The shared experience is an essential element of the program.

DISCHARGE RESPONSIBILITIES

Social Worker
Discharge planning begins with admission. The coordination and facilitation of services are expedited as the patient's medical condition stabilizes. The social worker's areas of activity and focus are

1. The patient and family's emotional and psychological readiness for discharge.
2. Setting or environment.
3. Medical supplies and equipment.
4. Personal and community resources.
5. Financial resources.
6. Coordination of timely services.
7. Van or ambulance transportation.

Physician
The physician's discharge responsibilities are

1. Communication with the social worker as to the anticipated date of discharge and follow-up care needed.
2. Review of the progress notes of all other health professionals to ensure that discharge is smooth and orderly.
3. Completion of medical supply forms and medical reports.
4. Requests for visiting nurse home visits.
5. Coordination of outpatient radiotherapy or chemotherapy.
6. Prescriptions (generic medications whenever feasible).
7. Patient counseling in regard to analgesics, diet, and medications.

REFERENCES

1. *Coping with Cancer.* Washington, DC: U.S. Department of Health and Human Services, National Institutes of Health, 1980. Pp 1–6, 20–25, 79–82.
2. Disability evaluation under social security. *Fed Reg,* January 6, 1986.
3. *Taking Time.* Washington, DC: U.S. Department of Health and Human Services, National Institutes of Health, 1985. Pp 4, 10–18.
4. *The Medicare Handbook.* Washington, DC: U.S. Dept. of Health and Human Services Health Care Financing Administration, 1989.
5. *What You Need to know About Cancer.* Washington, DC: U.S. Department of Health and Human Services, National Institutes of Health, 1985.
6. *What You Need to Know About Cancer of the Esophagus.* National Institutes of Health, Publication, No. 85–1557. Washington, DC: U.S. Department of Health and Human Services, National Institutes of Health, 1984.

Appendix

HEAD AND NECK CANCER: A PERSONAL ACCOUNT

It was after returning from a business trip to the Virgin Islands in 1977 that I noticed a bloody spot on the soft palate of my mouth. Although I did not like the way it looked, I was convinced it was not cancerous because of the professional medical assurance I had received shortly before leaving. I also had visited my dentist every 6 months and had no indication from him that I had any serious oral problems. The Manhattan ENT Clinic in New York had taken a biopsy from that area before I left for the Islands, and I believed that the area had simply gotten infected. I had failed to return for the results of the analysis as I had promised. The clinic had determined that I had squamous cell carcinoma of the soft palate and that treatment should be started immediately.

Several doctors at Howard University Hospital examined me and determined that the location of the cancer made it inoperable and that radiation was the treatment of choice. The urgency to get started caused my wife and me to fear the worse. I experienced the attitude most people do when confronted with cancer—I asked myself "Why me?" and felt that all was lost.

As I recall, I received the maximum dosage of cobalt 5 times a week for 2 months. With the exception of a loss of weight, burned out salivary glands, and a loss of stamina, I stood up pretty well to the treatment, which was successful in burning out the tumor. I took it all as an outpatient and suffered some occasional vomiting while at the hospital clinic. My doctor advised me that vomiting was an activity common to people suffering from apprehension. I subsequently took the treatments in stride and soon got over what I called the "mortality syndrome" associated with cancer.

In 1982, five years had passed, during which time I was regularly visiting my ENT specialist, oral surgeon, and the hospital's chief surgeon to determine if there had been any recurrence of the wayward cancer cells. In addition to these specialists, I was also seen by a speech pathologist and a psychiatrist in the hospital. There is a school of thought that asserts that most cancers are cured after 5 years of remission. I found it strange that neither my doctors nor I showed any particular relief after the 5-year period had elapsed.

During this 5-year period, I reverted to my favorite pastime activities of drinking and smoking. I strongly believe that these activities, combined with my strong susceptibility to cancer derived from my ancestral linkage, contributed to the recurrence of the tumor in late 1982. It was during this time that a growth was detected on the left side of my neck during a regular visit to my ENT specialist. A CT scan and biopsy quickly exposed it as a malignancy composed of cells similar to those found in my soft palate in 1977. A radical neck dissection was proposed by the ENT specialist, who explained in detail what the procedure entailed. The dissection was performed during the Christmas holidays of 1982.

During that year (1983), another procedure had to be performed due to the presence of another malignancy in the neck area. This oper-

Editor's note: Mr. Marvin Plunkett's long and courageous battle is a graphic case of a head and neck cancer. His personal account, spanning eight years, eloquently illustrates the goals of this textbook.

ation was known as intraoperative radiation, which was also performed at Howard University Hospital. This was a relatively new procedure performed by only a few facilities in the country. It consisted mainly of surgery being performed followed by radiation while the wound was still open. I understand this procedure allowed the radiation to be more effective than shooting it through the outer skin.

The procedure was followed by chemotherapy, which was done on an outpatient basis at a local hospital near my residence. I experienced some of the worst feelings of my life during the time chemotherapy was being administered. I would go into the hospital on a Saturday afternoon and come out the following Sunday afternoon. During that short stay I would break out in sweats, vomit like crazy, had no appetite, and would sleep the remainder of the day after arriving home from the hospital. I would also spend the following Monday asleep. It was discovered, much to the chagrin and surprise of my doctor and me, that another tumor had begun to grow during the time I was receiving the chemotherapy. The chemotherapy was discontinued, and I returned to Howard University Hospital for more surgery.

During the years from 1982 to 1986, I had 11 operations for malignant tumors. My ENT specialist, who performed the operations, made a statement to the effect that treating me was like putting out forest fires.

One other important and relatively unusual operation I received was an insertion of a Infusid pump into my chest. By this time, in late 1986, I had become so consumed with pain that I was taking large doses of morphine at least 4 times a day, along with Percodan and Panadol tablets. The pump would fit into my chest connected to a tube through the top of my brain (directly under the skull) to my spinal cord. The direct route to the spinal cord would reduce the amount of morphine needed to cause it to be more effective. It would totally eradicate the oral ingestion of morphine.

This also was a relatively new procedure that was being practiced in the United States. As one may imagine, it took some time for me to agree to this procedure. I was totally against anything that involved my brain. However, the pain got so bad that I was increasing the oral intake of morphine along with Percodan and Panadol on a daily basis. This resulted in my becoming a zombie-like creature. I could hardly sit without dozing or walk without staggering. Things got so bad that I felt I had no alternative but to submit to the insertion of the pump. Sure enough, the result was fantastic. For a while I had no pain at all.

During the time of my sickness and hospitalization, my family and office staff were very supportive of me and empathized with what I was going through. I believe I am here today because of their support and prayers and my belief in God Almighty. Prior to each operation, my wife would accompany me to the doors of the operating room and meet me in the recovery room after the operation. I believe it was this type of support that helped me endure the operations.

One of the effects of one of the many operations I had was the sacrifice of one of the facial nerves, which caused a paralysis on the left side of my face. By early 1987, that paralysis had spread from my forehead to the left side of my mouth. The crooked mouth, coupled with a lack of saliva, often makes my speech rather difficult to understand. (The lack of saliva, as I mentioned earlier, resulted from the radiation I received during the onset of the first tumor).

Another tumor was detected in early 1987. This tumor was located on the left side of the face around the area of the ear. The method of treatment, as in 1977, was radiation therapy. The difference, as I understand it, is that this was electron beam, a form of low energy radiation, and that in 1977 it was cobalt. The radiation therapy lasted for 6 weeks. Similar to the previous radiation, I lost my hair in the area the radiation was applied. Prior to the radiation, I had developed trouble with the sight in my left eye. I was advised by the attending physician in radiology that I would probably eventually lose the sight in the eye completely, since it was included in the area of the radiation. Prior to the radiation, I had difficulty maintaining my equilibrium unless the eye was covered. Consequently, I began wearing an eye patch. I have noticed the sight in the eye becoming blurred and imagine it will soon be lost.

In spite of what has happened, I thank God regularly for the positive things I have experienced. I am currently up to 195 pounds, which matches my regular weight (190–200). The last time I was discharged from the hospital I weighed 145 pounds.

Currently, my biggest problems are the various side effects of the operations I had. My facial paralysis makes it rather difficult to open my mouth. I am receiving facial and speech exercises from a speech therapist who works with me in an effort to improve my ability to open my mouth, speak, and swallow. I have seen some improvement since working with the speech therapist. I am able to open my mouth a little wider and speak a bit more effectively. In the meanwhile, I am making extensive use of my Waterpik to assist in cleaning the inside of my teeth and rinsing my mouth.

How do I feel about all this? Being raised in the church and a strong believer in God and prayer, I believe that the Lord is keeping me around for some reason. I am especially thankful for his blessings when I see others who are worse off than I; I admit that I often dream of what I would be doing if I were in good health. These dreams enable me to realize the many things we take for granted—that the majority of us never stop to smell the roses. While I realize my condition could still be terminal, I hardly think of it that way. As a matter of fact, I have thought of nothing but living since my first episode of cancer. Who knows, maybe a cure will soon be found and all of this will be behind me and millions of others.

Marvin Lewis Plunkett, Sr.
December 13, 1938–April 17, 1989

INDEX

Index

The abbreviations *f* and *t* stand for figure and table, respectively.